ADVANCES IN
PHARMACOLOGY

VOLUME 39

ADVANCES IN PHARMACOLOGY

VOLUME 39

J. Thomas August
Department of Pharmacology
Johns Hopkins University
Baltimore, Maryland

M. W. Anders
Department of Pharmacology
University of Rochester
Rochester, New York

Ferid Murad
Lake Forest, Illinois

Joseph Coyle
Harvard Medical School
McLean Hospital
Belmont, Massachusetts

ACADEMIC PRESS
San Diego London Boston New York Sydney Tokyo Toronto

This book is printed on acid-free paper. ♾

Academic Press
a division of Harcourt Brace & Company
525 B Street, Suite 1900, San Diego, California 92101-4495, USA
http://www.apnet.com

Academic Press Limited
24-28 Oval Road, London NW1 7DX, UK
http://www.hbuk.co.uk/ap/

International Standard Book Number: 0-12-032940-9

PRINTED IN THE UNITED STATES OF AMERICA
97 98 99 00 01 02 EB 9 8 7 6 5 4 3 2 1

Contents

Sodium Channels and Therapy of Central Nervous System Diseases

Charles P. Taylor and Lakshmi S. Narasimhan

Anti-adhesion Therapy

Carol J. Cornejo, Robert K. Winn, and John M. Harlan

Use of Azoles for Systemic Antifungal Therapy

Carol A. Kauffman and Peggy L. Carver

Pharmacology of Neuronal Nicotinic Acetylcholine Receptor Subtypes

Lorna M. Colquhoun and James W. Patrick

Structure and Function of Leukocyte Chemoattractant

Richard D. Ye and François Boulay

Pharmacologic Approaches to Reperfusion Injury

James T. Willerson

Restenosis: Is There a Pharmacologic Fix in the Pipeline?

Joan A. Keiser and Andrew C. G. Uprichard

Role of Adenosine as a Modulator of Synaptic Activity in the Central Nervous System

James M. Brundege and Thomas V. Dunwiddie

Combination Vaccines

Ronald W. Ellis and Kenneth R. Brown

Pharmacology of Potassium Channels

Maria L. Garcia, Markus Hanner, Hans-Günther Knaus, Robert Koch, William Schmalhofer, Robert S. Slaughter, and Gregory J. Kaczorowski

Contributors

Numbers in parentheses indicate the pages on which the authors' contributions begin.

François Boulay (221) DBMS/Biochimie, CEA/Grenoble, 38054 Grenoble Cedex 9, France

Kenneth R. Brown (393) Regulatory Liaison, Biologics/Vaccines, Merck Research Laboratories, West Point, Pennsylvania 19486

James M. Brundege (353) Department of Pharmacology, University of Colorado Health Sciences Center, Denver, Colorado 80222

Peggy L. Carver (143) College of Pharmacy, University of Michigan, Ann Arbor, Michigan 48109

Lorna M. Colquhoun (191) Division of Neuroscience, Baylor College of Medicine, Houston, Texas 77030

Carol J. Cornejo (99) Department of Surgery, University of Washington, Seattle, Washington 98104

Raymond N. DuBois (1) Departments of Medicine and Cell Biology, Center in Molecular Toxicology, Vanderbilt University Medical Center, Nashville, Tennessee 37232

Thomas V. Dunwiddie (353) Department of Pharmacology and Program in Neuroscience, University of Colorado Health Sciences Center, Denver, Colorado 80222

Ronald W. Ellis (393) Vaccine Research and Development, Astra Research Center Boston, Cambridge, Massachusetts 02139

Maria L. Garcia (425) Department of Membrane Biochemistry & Biophysics, Merck Research Laboratories, Rahway, New Jersey 07065

Markus Hanner (425) Department of Membrane Biochemistry and Biophysics, Merck Research Laboratories, Rahway, New Jersey 07065

John M. Harlan (99) Department of Medicine, Division of Hematology, University of Washington, Seattle, Washington 98195

Gregory J. Kaczorowski (425) Department of Membrane Biochemistry and Biophysics, Merck Research Laboratories, Rahway, New Jersey 07065

Carol A. Kauffman (143) Division of Infectious Diseases, Department of Internal Medicine, Veterans' Affairs Medical Center, University of Michigan Medical School, Ann Arbor, Michigan 48105

Joan A. Keiser (313) Parke-Davis Research Division, Warner Lambert Company, Ann Arbor, Michigan 48105

Hans-Günther Knaus (425) Institute for Biochemical Pharmacology, A-6020 Innsbruck, Austria

Robert Koch (425) Institute for Biochemical Pharmacology, A-6020 Innsbruck, Austria

Lakshmi S. Narasimhan (47) Department of Chemistry, Parke-Davis Pharmaceutical Research Divison, Warner-Lambert Co., Ann Arbor, Michigan 48105

James W. Patrick (191) Division of Neuroscience, Baylor College of Medicine, Houston, Texas 77030

Susan R. Ross (21) Department of Microbiology, University of Pennsylvania, Philadelphia, Pennsylvania 19104-6142

William Schmalhofer (425) Department of Membrane Biochemistry and Biophysics, Merck Research Laboratories, Rahway, New Jersey 07065

Robert S. Slaughter (425) Department of Membrane Biochemistry and Biophysics, Merck Research Laboratories, Rahway, New Jersey 07065

Walter E. Smalley (1) Departments of Medicine and Cell Biology, Veterans' Affairs Medical Center, Vanderbilt University Medical Center, Nashville, Tennessee 37232

Charles P. Taylor (47) Department of Neurological and Neurodegenerative Diseases, Parke-Davis Pharmaceutical Research Divison, Warner-Lambert Co., Ann Arbor, Michigan 48105

Andrew C. G. Uprichard (313) Parke-Davis Research Division, Warner Lambert Company, Ann Arbor, Michigan 48105

James T. Willerson (291) University of Texas–Houston Medical School, Houston, Texas 77030

Robert K. Winn (99) Departments of Surgery, Physiology, and Biophysics, University of Washington, Seattle, Washington 98104

Richard D. Ye (221) Department of Immunology, The Scripps Research Institute, La Jolla, California 92037

Walter E. Smalley
Raymond N. DuBois*

Departments of Medicine and Cell Biology
*Center in Molecular Toxicology
Veterans Affairs Medical Center
Vanderbilt University Medical Center
Nashville, Tennessee 37232

Colorectal Cancer and Nonsteroidal Anti-inflammatory Drugs

I. Introduction

Colorectal cancer is the second leading cause of death from cancer in the United States. Differences in dietary habits and life-styles among populations in different geographic locations have been associated with an altered risk for developing colorectal cancer (Miller *et al.,* 1983; Wynder *et al.,* 1969). Although several studies have shown that persons on a high fat diet with a sedentary life-style have an increased risk for developing cancer of the large intestine, the etiology of colorectal cancer is not clearly understood. Since 1991, several reports indicate an association between an intake of nonsteroidal anti-inflammatory drugs (NSAIDs) and a decreased risk for developing colorectal cancer. Three independent lines of research indicate that a link between NSAID use and colorectal cancer may exist. First, epidemiologic studies indicate a 40–50% reduction in mortality from

Advances in Pharmacology, Volume 39

1054-3589/97/$25.00

colorectal cancer in individuals taking NSAIDs (like aspirin) compared to those not taking these agents. Second, familial adenomatous polyposis (FAP) patients who take sulindac have a significant reduction in adenoma size and number. Third, in animal models of colorectal carcinogenesis, several different NSAIDs exhibit chemoprotective effects, causing a reduction in the frequency and number of premalignant and malignant lesions. The aim of this review is to carefully examine these studies and attempt to offer insight concerning the molecular basis for the chemoprotective effect of NSAIDs. There is hope that more effective chemoprotective agents can be developed in the future, once we have gained a better understanding of the biological basis for the decreased cancer risk caused by NSAIDs.

II. The Adenoma–Carcinoma Sequence

Our current understanding of the development of colon cancer is based on a paradigm developed by Fearon and Vogelstein (1990) utilizing results from epidemiologic, clinical, and genetic studies. More than 95% of colorectal adenocarcinomas arise from adenomatous polyps, and the progression from normal mucosa to adenoma and then to a subsequent carcinoma is thought to typically occur over a 10-year period (Peipins and Sandler, 1994). This progression is the result of a series of mutations affecting multiple genes involved in the regulation of epithelial cell growth, differentiation, and programmed cell death (Bedi *et al.*, 1995; Boland, 1993; Fearon, 1994; Hamilton, 1993; Rustgi, 1993).

This model has important implications for basic and clinical research which involve studies on the temporal relationship among changes in gene expression, mutations of key regulatory genes, and the development of colon cancer. The availability of clinical specimens, such as adenomas and adenocarcinomas, provides the opportunity to determine the sequential points at which genetic changes occur in the progression from normal colonic mucosa to adenoma formation (Eberhart *et al.*, 1994). In autopsy studies, the prevalence of adenomatous polyps in U.S. adults is 30–40% (Peipins and Sandler, 1994), and the detection of many polyps is readily accomplished by endoscopic screening. Most importantly, the incidence of *de novo* polyps is much greater than the incidence of adenocarcinoma, making them a potential "intermediate end point" for trials of colon cancer chemoprevention (Greenberg *et al.*, 1993; Hixson *et al.*, 1994; Landenheim *et al.*, 1995).

III. Prevention of Colon Cancer in Animal Models

In rats, azoxymethane (AOM) treatment reproducibly causes the development of colon cancer. Fifty two weeks following AOM (15 mg/kg) treatment about 80% of the animals develop colon tumors. The precise mechanism by which AOM causes colorectal cancer is unknown; however, several investigators have utilized this model to study the effect of various dietary factors and drugs on preventing the development of colon cancer (Rao *et al.*, 1995; Reddy *et al.*, 1987, 1990, 1992, 1993). Several NSAIDs, including indomethacin, piroxicam, aspirin, ibuprofen, and sulindac, have been shown to suppress AOM-induced colon carcinogenesis in laboratory animals. Rao *et al.* (1995) demonstrated that administration of sulindac in the diet, even as late as 14 weeks after administration of the carcinogen, had a remarkable effect in suppressing colon carcinogenesis in male F344 rats. Additionally, colon tumor volume was reduced by more than 52% in animals fed 160 and 320 ppm sulindac when compared to those fed the control diet. The investigators also demonstrated that prostaglandin levels were much higher in colon tumors than in normal adjacent mucosa and that these levels were markedly suppressed following sulindac treatment. The bulk of these animal studies demonstrate that the effect of NSAIDs to inhibit arachidonic acid conversion to eicosanoid products is linked to their effectiveness in suppressing colon carcinogenesis. It is difficult to assess how well this carcinogen-induced model mimics the events which occur during the development of spontaneous colorectal cancer in humans. However, it is clear that NSAIDs can provide up to a 60% protective effect in some of these animal studies.

IV. Familial Adenomatous Polyposis and NSAIDs

Treatment of familial adenomatous polyposis (FAP) patients with NSAIDs has provided insight into the potential role of eicosanoids in chemoprevention strategies. FAP is an autosomal dominant inherited condition, marked by the development of adenomatous polyps throughout the digestive tract, particularly in the colon. There is wide variability in the severity of the phenotype in humans, and a candidate gene thought to modify the phenotype in mice has been isolated (MacPhee *et al.*, 1995). In 1987, genetic linkage studies identified the chromosome 5q21 locus as the site of the genetic lesion in FAP patients. The adenomatous polyposis coli (APC) gene was subsequently identified at this site, inactivation of which results in FAP (Kinzler *et al.*, 1991; Nishisho *et al.*, 1991; Powell *et al.*, 1992; Su *et al.*, 1993). Over 200 germline mutations of this very large (>100 kb) APC gene have been described and most are predicted to result in a truncated protein that is dysfunctional in its role as a tumor suppressor. Patients with FAP develop hundreds of adenomatous colon polyps in their late teens to early 30s, and adenocarcinoma of the colon will usually develop by the age of 40–50 in those patients who do not undergo prophylactic colectomy. A commonly performed operation for this condition is a subtotal colectomy which leaves a rectal remnant to preserve continence. Periodic sigmoidoscopy is recommended for these patients to remove recurrent polyps. Gardner's syndrome is a particularly aggressive form of familial polyposis that is marked by the formation of adenomatous polyps throughout the gastrointestinal tract and by the presence of desmoid tumors, retinal changes, and osteomas of the skull, mandible, and long bones (Friend, 1990).

The initial observation that sulindac was effective in decreasing the number of adenomatous colon polyps in patients with FAP was made by Waddell and associates in 1983, with an additional follow-up report 6 years later (Waddell *et al.,* 1989; Waddell and Loughry, 1983). Waddell reported a patient with Gardner's syndrome who was being treated with indomethacin for complications of a desmoid tumor (Waddell and Loughry, 1983). Because of a lack of response to indomethacin, treatment was changed to sulindac and the desmoid tumor regressed. Concurrently, the physicians caring for the patient observed a significant decrease in the recurrence of rectal polyps in periodic follow-up screening exams. Based on this finding, several relatives of the index case who also had Gardner's syndrome and other patients with FAP syndrome were offered treatment with sulindac and all patients had a remarkable decrease in the number of polyps noted on serial endoscopic and radiographic exams (Waddell and Loughry, 1983). Since this initial report, there have been several other uncontrolled studies of FAP patients with similar findings (Rigau *et al.,* 1991; Tonelli and Valanzano, 1993; Winde *et al.,* 1993).

Three randomized controlled trials of sulindac treatment for polyps in FAP patients provided additional insights (Giardiello *et al.,* 1993; Labayle *et al.,* 1991; Nugent *et al.,* 1993). Labalye *et al.* (1991) conducted a randomized double-blind, placebo-controlled, crossover trial in patients with FAP who had prior colectomy and ileoanal anastamoses. In this study, patients were given sulindac (100 mg three times daily) or placebo for 4 months, followed by a "wash out" period of 1 month and subsequent crossover to the other treatment arm for an additional 4 months of follow-up. There was a statistically significant decrease in the number of polyps in patients treated with sulindac when compared to those treated with placebo. There was a "temporary" decrease in the number of polyps in the group that was initially treated with placebo; however, subsequent exams by the same blinded endoscopist revealed no decrease in polyp number. Four of the five patients treated with sulindac during the first phase of the trial experienced an increase in the number of polyps during the subsequent placebo phase of the trial.

Giardiello *et al.* (1993) reported the results of a double-blinded, randomized, placebo-controlled study of the effects of sulindac (150 mg twice daily) on polyp regression in patients with FAP. A single observer performed sigmoidoscopy every 3 months. A careful attempt was made to standardize the exam for each patient by tattooing a reference mark in a rectal segment of each patient. Measurements of the first five polyps distal to the reference mark were made using a standard scale passed through the instrument. After

9 months, there was a 44% ($p = 0.014$) decrease in the number of polyps and a 35% ($p < 0.001$) decrease in the mean diameter of polyps in the group of patients treated with sulindac. When the patients were reexamined 3 months after treatment ended, an increase in both the number and the size of polyps was observed in the treated group, although they did not return to the pretreatment baseline. In the placebo group there was an increase in the number and size of polyps. No adverse effects were noted with the therapy, but sulindac did not completely prevent polyp formation in any patient.

Nugent *et al.* (1993) carried out a randomized, placebo-controlled trial of sulindac (200 mg twice daily) in 24 patients with FAP who had duodenal polyposis. Fifteen of these patients who had prior ileoanal anastomoses were examined by serial video sigmoidoscopy before and after 6 months of therapy. In this study, paired videotapes before and after sigmoidoscopy were graded in random order by two reviewers who were blinded to the treatment arm. In the group treated with sulindac the polyp status was improved (decreased) in five, worse in none, and unchanged in two patients. In the placebo-treated group the polyp status was improved in none, worsened in two, and unchanged in five. The overall effect was statistically significant ($p = 0.01$). Studies of cell proliferation in the rectum as measured by 5-bromo-2′-deoxyuridine incorporation revealed a decrease of 11% ($p = 0.01$). There was a trend for decreased duodenal polyposis, but this trend did not reach statistical significance.

In summary, studies evaluating FAP patients have clearly shown that NSAIDs cause polyp regression. This effect is fairly dramatic and occurs within months after therapy has been initiated. The genetic defect and background in FAP patients may account for more significant polyp regression in response to NSAIDs which has not been well documented in patients with sporadic adenomas.

V. NSAIDs and Colorectal Neoplasia

The observation that NSAIDs cause polyp regression in FAP patients encouraged further laboratory investigation and led to a series of human studies examining the relationship between NSAID use and colorectal neoplasia. A randomized clinical trial is the preferred study design because it is informative compared to other study designs. However, there are several problems in designing an NSAID intervention clinical trial. The use of NSAIDs is associated with risks, most notably for gastrointestinal hemorrhage and peptic ulcer disease, and thus, the benefits of cancer prevention must outweigh the risks of adverse effects. A significant percentage of persons in the population at risk for colorectal cancer are already taking aspirin for cardiovascular or other reasons and it would be difficult to restrict its use in a palcebo-controlled trial. The incidence rate for colorectal cancer in the United States among those 65 years and older is relatively low, approximately 300/100,000 persons, and the mortality rate is approximately 150/100,000 (Miller *et al.*, 1983). Therefore, a large-scale clinical trial using colon cancer incidence or mortality as an end point would be time-consuming, expensive, and difficult to manage. In an attempt to overcome some of these problems, adenomatous polyps are being used as surrogate end points in several clinical trials. This is likely to be the most appropriate outcome; however, because of the biological variability of polyps, it is unclear how an effect on polyp formation will relate to the development of colorectal cancer.

Observational studies provide important information that may demonstrate the effectiveness of NSAIDs in preventing cancer and aid in the rational design of randomized clinical trials. Several factors must be considered in the evaluation of these studies, including the source of the study population, the outcome of interest (adenomatous polyp, cancer incidence, cancer mortality), the reliability of the outcome diagnosis, the reliability of the information regarding NSAID exposure, and controls for potential confounding variables.

A. Observational Studies

1. *NSAIDs and the Prevention of Colon Cancer*

There have been several observational studies of the relationship between intake of aspirin or other NSAIDs and the subsequent risk of developing colorectal cancer (Giovannucci *et al.*, 1994; Kune *et al.*, 1988; Muscat *et al.*, 1994; Paganini-Hill *et al.*, 1989; Peleg *et al.*, 1994; Rosenberg *et al.*, 1991; Schreinemachers and Everson, 1994; Suh *et al.*, 1993; Thun *et al.*, 1991). The results of these studies are summarized in Table I.

2. *Retrospective Case Control Studies*

Several retrospective studies of the effect of NSAID use on colorectal cancer incidence have utilized case control methodology. All of these studies demonstrate a protective effect of NSAIDs.

One study was community based (Kune *et al.*, 1988), whereas all others were hospital based. Two studies were based on data designed specifically to assess the effect of NSAIDs on colon cancer (Muscat and Wynder, 1993; Peleg *et al.*, 1994). Most relied on patient and control interviews to determine NSAID exposure history, whereas one study utilized computerized records from a hospital and clinic-based pharmacy (Peleg *et al.*, 1994).

One study controlled for confounding variables by matching (Muscat and Wynder, 1993), whereas others utilized multivariate techniques to control for confounding by sex, age, and race. Two of the studies examined acetaminophen use (an indicator of arthritis which may be a potential con-

TABLE I Summary of Retrospective Case Control Studies of NSAID Use and Colon Cancer Incidence

Setting	*Outcome (N)*	*NSAID/dose*	*Odds ratio (95% CI)*	*Comment*	*Reference*
Population based (Melbourne, Australia	Colon cancer (392)	ASA (weekly use)	0.53 (0.35–0.80)	Adjusted for age, sex, diet, and physical activity (community controls)	Kune *et al.* (1988)
		NANSAID (weekly use)	0.66 (0.47–0.92)		
	Rectal cancer (323)	ASA (weekly use)	0.59 (0.39–0.91)		
		NANSAID (weekly use)	NS		
Hospital based (multiple hospitals)	Colorectal cancer (1326)	Mostly ASA (≥4 days/week)		Adjusted for age, sex, race, religion, physical activity, family history, and educational level (cancer and noncancer controls)	Rosenberg *et al.* (1991)
		<2 years	0.6 (0.4–1.1)		
		2–4 years	0.6 (0.3–1.1)		
		5–9 years	0.5 (0.2–1.0)		
		10+ years	0.3 (0.1–0.7)		
Cancer Center	Colorectal cancer (830)	ASA		Adjusted for age, sex, educational level, and duration of use (cancer controls)	Suh *et al.* (1993)
		<1/day per week	0.83 (1.61–0.43)		
		1–2/day per week	0.49 (0.99–0.24)		
		>2/day per week	0.44 (1.10–0.18)		
County Hospital	Colorectal cancer (97)	ASA		Univariate analysis. Exposure determined by objective review of hospital and clinic pharmacy records (hospital controls)	Peleg *et al.* (1994)
		<1/7 days over 4 years	0.52 (0.30–0.91)		
		>3/7 days over 4 years	0.08 (0.01–0.59)		
		NANSAID			
		<1/4 days over 4 years	0.77 (0.48–1.23)		
		≥1/4 days over 4 years	0.34 (0.15–0.77)		
Hospital based (multiple hospitals)	Colorectal cancer (511)	Mostly ASA (≥3 days/week)	Results for men	Matched-pair odds ratios. Acetaminophen use not associated with a protective effect (hospital cancer and noncancer controls)	Muscat *et al.* (1994)
		1–4 years	0.77 (0.34–1.75)		
		5–9 years	0.93 (0.45–1.97)		
		>9 years	0.47 (0.21–0.94)		
Community based (from trial of fecal occult blood testing for cancer detection)	Colon polyps (147)	Negative controls		Positive controls were those who had tested positive for occult blood. Adjusted for age, sex, and social class	Logan *et al.* (1993)
		Any use of ASA	0.57 (0.3–1.0)		
		Any use of NSAIDs	0.50 (0.3–1.0)		
		Positive controls			
		Any use of ASA	0.72 (0.4–1.3)		
		Any use of NSAIDs	0.69 (0.3–1.4)		

founder) and found no protective effect (Kune *et al.*, 1988; Muscat and Wynder, 1993).

One additional case control study examined the effect of NSAIDs on colorectal adenomas (Logan *et al.*, 1993). The underlying population consisted of participants in a randomized trial of fecal occult blood testing in Nottingham, England. In this study, cases consisted of patients who had adenomas detected on colonoscopy after testing positive for occult blood in their stool. Two control groups were selected from others in the screening trial and were identified on the basis of their screening result: "positive" controls had tested positive for occult blood and "negative" controls had tested negative. Prior exposure to aspirin or nonaspirin NSAIDs was determined by interview. When compared to "negative" controls, the odds ratio for developing polyps was 0.57 (0.3–1.0) for aspirin users and 0.50 (0.3–1.0) for other NSAID users and there was a trend for increased protection with a longer duration (>5 years) of use. A protective effect was also seen when using the "positive" controls; however, this did not reach statistical significance. No protective effect was observed for acetaminophen use.

3. *Prospective Studies*

All but one (Paganini-Hill *et al.*, 1989) of the prospective cohort studies examining the effect of aspirin on the incidence or mortality of colon cancer indicated a protective effect (Giovannucci *et al.*, 1994, 1995; Schreinemachers and Everson, 1994; Thun *et al.*, 1991) (see Table II).

Paganini-Hill *et al.* (1989) reported the results of a cohort study on the relationship between aspirin use and chronic diseases within a California retirement community from 1982 to 1988. Aspirin use was determined by a single questionnaire upon entry into the study and was categorized as daily use, less than daily use, and no use. Incident colon cancers were detected by follow-up of admissions to hospitals and by death certificate reports. The sex- and age-adjusted relative risk of colon cancer among daily users was 1.5 (1.1–2.2). This study was carried out in a retirement community with a predominantly white, well-educated, affluent elderly population. One important limitation of the study is that the exposure to aspirin was only determined at the beginning of the study, thus many of the elderly patients in this population who were initially "nonusers" could have become users during the 9 years of total follow-up.

Thun *et al.* (1991) reported the results of the largest and most frequently cited study of the relationship between aspirin use and colon cancer. The population was a cohort of over a million individuals interviewed by American Cancer Society volunteers with a questionnaire on cancer risks and personal health habits, including medication use. Complete information was available for 662,424 persons for the 6-year study period. Death certificates (indicating the cause of death) were available on 94.1% of the 79,877 persons who died. Exposure to aspirin was determined at the beginning of the survey only and use was categorized as "none," less than once a month, once to 15 times per month, and greater than 16 times a month. The risk of colon cancer mortality was decreased among those who used aspirin, and the protective effect increased with increasing frequency of aspirin use. The relative risk of cancer mortality among men who used aspirin less than once a month was 0.77 (0.61–0.97) and fell to 0.60 (0.40–0.89) among those who used aspirin more than 16 times a month. The relative risk among women was slightly lower. A case-control analysis was done to control for other cancer risk factors: age, body mass index, physical activity, family history, and dietary intake of fiber, vegetables, and fruits. The relative risk among men who used aspirin less than once a month was not changed significantly, 0.84 (0.64–1.12), whereas the decreased risk for those who used aspirin more than 16 times a month was 0.48 (0.30–0.76). The relative risk for women who used aspirin more than 16 times a month was 0.53 (0.32–0.87). The potential limitations of the study, as pointed out by the authors, were the use of cancer mortality instead of cancer incidence as an end point, the lack of any information after the initial interview regarding aspirin use, and the lack of information regarding dosage. Nonetheless, the strong association which persisted after controlling for a variety of other cancer risk factors argued for a protective effect in this population.

The relationship between aspirin use and the development of lung, colon, and breast cancer was examined in a prospective cohort study (Schreinemachers and Everson, 1994). This study utilized data from the National Health and Nutrition Survey (NHANES-I) from 1971 and 1975. Follow-up studies were done on patients in 1982–1984, 1986, and 1987. Exposure to aspirin was defined by those who self-reported aspirin use in the 30 days prior to the initial interview of the study. Cases were determined by interview of the study subjects or surrogates in combination with the review of pertinent hospital, nursing home, and death certificate records. Complete information was available for 12,668 subjects who were followed for an average of 12.4 years. There were 169 colorectal cancers in the study population. There was a decreased risk for developing colon cancer in aspirin users among men younger than 65 years of age, for which the adjusted relative risk of colon cancer was 0.35 (0.17–0.73). This effect was not found across age and gender, however, as there was no statistically significant protective effect demonstrated for older men or for women at any age.

A prospective cohort study in male health professionals reported a decreased risk for both colorectal cancer and adenomatous polyps (Giovannucci *et al.*, 1994). The study was initiated in 1986 among 17,900 male nonphysician health care workers between the ages of 40 and 75. Information was obtained by a mailed questionnaire inquiring about aspirin and other NSAID use, other cancer risks, and clinically diagnosed conditions. Follow-up surveys mailed in 1988, 1990, and 1992 were used to update information on aspirin and NSAID use and to update clinical information,

TABLE II Summary of Prospective Studies of NSAID Use and Colon Cancer

Setting	*NSAID/dose*	*Outcome (N)*	*Relative risk (95% CI)*	*Comment*	*Reference*
Cohort: Residents of California retirement community, 1981–1988 (67,000 person years)	ASA daily use	Colon cancer, incidence (181)	1.5 (1.1–2.2)	Aspirin use determined only on initial interview	Paganini-Hill *et al.* (1989)
Cohort: Participants recruited by American Cancer Society, 1982–1988 (3.9 million person years)	ASA use/month	Colon cancer, mortality (1388)	Results for men	Aspirin use determined only on initial interview. Results for women were similar. Case control analysis adjusted for diet, physical activity, and family history with similar results	Thun *et al.* (1991)
	<1		0.77 (0.61–0.97)		
	1–15		0.69 (0.52–0.93)		
	≥16		0.60 (0.40–0.89)		
Cohort: NHANES-I (study of nutrition and health), 1971–1984 (over 140,000 person years)	ASA use <30 days prior to baseline interview	Colorectal cancer, incidence		High prevalence of aspirin use in the cohort (>50%)	Schreinemachers and Everson (1994)
		Men <65	0.35 (0.17–0.73)		
		Men ≥65	1.21 (0.69–2.10)		
		Women <65	0.78 (0.38–1.59)		
		Women ≥65	1.28 (0.73–2.23)		

Cohort: Male health professionals (nonphysicians), 1986–1990 (41,000 person years)	ASA use two or more times a week reported on three consecutive questionnaires, 1986–90	Colorectal cancer, incidence (50)	0.38 (0.18–0.78)	Adjusted for age, history of polyp, history of endoscopy, family history, diet, smoking, alcohol, and physical activity	Giovannucci *et al.* (1994)
		Colorectal cancer, metastatic disease or death (21)	0.08 (0.01–0.59)		
Cohort: Nurses Health Study, 1980–92 (540,000 person years)	ASA use two or more times a week reported on three consecutive questionnaires, 1986–90	Colorectal cancer, incidence (501)	0.62 (0.44–0.86)	Adjusted for age, family history, diet, smoking, alcohol, and physical activity	Giovannucci *et al.* (1995)
		Duration of use			
		1–4 years	1.06 (0.78–1.45)		
		5–9 years	0.84 (0.55–1.28)		
		10–19 years	0.70 (0.41–1.20)		
		≥20 years	0.56 (0.36–0.90)		
Randomized controlled trial of male physicians (54,188 person years in aspirin group)	ASA 325 mg every other day	Colorectal cancer (228)	1.15 (0.80–1.65)	The only available randomized trial. This study was terminated after 4 years	Gann *et al.* (1993); Physician's Health Study Group (1995)
		Colorectal polyps (263)	0.86 (0.68–1.10)		

including any diagnosis of cancer or adenomatous polyps as well as information pertaining to any endoscopic procedure that had been performed on the participants. Multivariate analysis controlled for age, history of polyps, history of lower endoscopy, family history of cancer, smoking, body mass index, physical activity, intake of red meat, vitamin E, and alcohol. There was a marked decrease in the risk for colorectal cancer among the aspirin users of 0.68 (0.52 to 0.92) who had reported aspirin use on the initial questionnaire only. Among those who consistently noted aspirin use on three consecutive questionnaires (1986, 1988, 1990), the relative risk of colorectal cancer was 0.35 (0.16 to 0.75). The effect on the relative risk of advanced cancers (those presenting with metastasis or mortality) was more marked with a relative risk of 0.51 (0.32 to 0.84) among those who noted aspirin use on the first interview only and a relative risk of 0.08 (0.01 to 0.59) among those who noted use on all three questionnaires. Excluding those patients who had diagnostic tests for overt and occult rectal bleeding, there was also a decreased risk for the development of incident adenomatous polyps of 0.65 (0.42 to 1.02). There was not enough information on the use of nonaspirin NSAIDs to determine an anticancer effect. This study was unique because it evaluated the prior use of endoscopic tests and the ability to control for several other potentially confounding factors in the multivariate analysis. The effect of aspirin on adenomas detected by endoscopy is subject to detection bias, but by excluding cases that were done because of bleeding, this bias was minimized.

An even more recent study reported the results of a cohort study of 89,446 women as a part of the Nurses Health Study (Giovannucci *et al.*, 1995). This was a longitudinal study of nurses that was designed to assess risk factors for cancer and heart disease. Information on risk factors and medical outcomes was obtained by questionnaire every 2 years. The duration of use was estimated from the questionnaires and by the length of prior use noted on the initial questionnaire. The prevalence of aspirin use in this population was high. For any given interview, approximately 40–60% of respondents reported the use of aspirin two or more times a week. Information from three consecutive interviews indicated that 15% of the subjects reported regular aspirin use on all three interviews. There were 501 colorectal cancers identified from follow-up questionnaires and confirmed by review of the medical record. The relative risk for colorectal cancer among those who consistently reported aspirin use over consecutive interviews was 0.62 (0.44–0.86). When the effect was examined by the duration of use, there was a statistically significant trend for an increasing effect over time of continuous use. In fact, the protective effect for colorectal cancer did not become statistically significant until there were 10 or more years of continuous use. During the study period, women who took aspirin were slightly more likely (21.5 to 17.6%) to have lower gastrointestinal endoscopy for diagnostic or screening reasons than those who were not taking aspirin.

However, the diagnosis of a large (>1 cm) adenoma on endoscopy for fecal blood was less likely among those on aspirin (3.2 to 4.0%), suggesting that any decrease in the colorectal cancer rate was not due to the removal of polyps in the aspirin group.

An additional prospective study of polyp recurrence demonstrated a protective effect of aspirin (Greenberg *et al.,* 1993). This study was done as part of a randomized polyp prevention trial and was designed to assess the effects of other chemopreventive agents (β-carotene, combination of vitamin C, vitamin E, or placebo) in patients who had undergone a prior polypectomy. Aspirin use was determined by interviews that took place on entry and every 6 months while enrolled in the study. The 793 patients were classified as nonusers (75%), intermittent users (12%), or consistent users (13%) based on whether they noted aspirin use on none, one, or both of the interviews. Polyps were detected by colonoscopy at 1 year. The relative risk for polyps at 1 year was 0.52 (0.31–0.89) for the consistent aspirin users and there was no effect noted for other nonsteroidal drugs.

B. Clinical Trials

1. Sulindac and Sporadic Polyps

Two clinical trials have examined the effect of sulindac on "sporadic" adenomatous polyps (i.e., those occurring outside of the setting of FAP) (Hixson *et al.,* 1993; Landenheim *et al.,* 1995). One randomized clinical trial in patients with previously identified polyps determined that there was no dramatic effect of sulindac therapy in reducing the number of size of polyps (Landenheim *et al.,* 1995). In this study, patients who had polyps identified by flexible sigmoidoscopy were randomized to receive either sulindac (150 mg twice daily) or placebo for 4 months. Follow-up colonoscopy with polypectomy was performed at 4 months, and the number and size of any residual polyps were noted. The difference in the rates of disappearance of polyps in the treated (5/22) and placebo (3/22) groups was not statistically different. Closer analysis of the data in this report indicates that the actual study population of interest was much smaller than 44 patients. Out of the initial 22 patients in the treatment group, 4 did not complete the study. Closely examining the histology from the remaining 18 patients in the treatment group revealed that 3 had "no" histology, 5 had hyperplastic polyps, and 1 had a lymphoid follicle. Furthermore, assuming that all 3 of the patients with "no" histology had hyperplastic polyps leaves only 9 patients in the treated group with documented adenomas. In the placebo group, 3 patients had "no" histology and 7 had hyperplastic polyps which leaves 12 patients with documented adenomas. Only 1 adenoma disappeared in the 9 patients with adenomas on sulindac treatment and none of the 12 patients in the placebo group had a documented adenoma disappear. This study confirmed the results of a smaller (7–9 patients), uncontrolled study (Hixson *et al.,* 1993) which failed to demonstrate a clear therapeutic benefit of NSAIDs on sporadic colon polyps.

The effect of NSAIDs on left-sided polyps was the outcome measured in both of these studies. It is important to point out that these studies examined a very small number of patients and would not be capable of detecting less than a 50% response. Also, NSAIDs may have a regional effect, as reported in an animal study (Liu *et al.,* 1995). Investigators have demonstrated that NSAIDs prevent the development of AOM-induced colon cancers predominately in the right colon with much less of an effect on left-sided colonic lesions (DuBois, 1995; Liu *et al.,* 1995).

2. Aspirin and Colorectal Cancer Incidence

The results of a randomized clinical trial among male physicians did not demonstrate a protective effect of aspirin in reducing the risk of colorectal cancer at a dose of 325 mg every other day. The intention of this study was to evaluate the effects of aspirin in preventing myocardial infarction and β-carotene in preventing cancer (Physician's Health Study Group, 1995). In this study, 22,071 U.S. physicians were randomly assigned to receive placebo, aspirin and placebo, β-carotene and placebo, or β-carotene and aspirin. Among the exclusion criteria were prior histories of peptic ulcer disease or cancer, or current NSAID use. Subjects completed a questionnaire every 6 months, and potential cases of cancer were reviewed by an end points committee that was blinded to the treatment. Information regarding gastrointestinal bleeding and diagnosis of colon polyps were also obtained via questionnaire, and the source of the bleeding (as reported by the patient) was recorded. Because of the marked effect of aspirin on decreasing the incidence of myocardial infarction, the study was terminated after only 4 years of follow-up (Physicians' Health Study Group, 1989). The mean age of the study subjects was 53 years and no protective effect of aspirin was observed. There was no statistically significant trend for a decrease in the self-reported diagnosis of polyps among those who were treated with aspirin (RR 0.86, 95% CI 0.68–1.10).

Thus, this randomized trial, which evaluates the relationship between aspirin use and colorectal cancer, does not show a positive effect. This is not consistent with almost all of the observational studies. The strength of the randomized design is that many of the biases associated with observational studies can be avoided. However, this study was not originally designed to evaluate the effect of aspirin on colorectal cancer. It is possible that the aspirin dose (325 mg every other day) or duration (4 years) was insufficient to provide a protective effect. The patients with cancer taking aspirin did not exhibit the expected increased risk for gastrointestinal bleeding when compared to those on placebo. Others (Giovannucci *et al.,* 1995) have indicated that it may take up to a decade of continuous aspirin use before a significant protective effect occurs in a cohort of women.

VI. Molecular Targets of NSAIDs

NSAIDs were designed by pharmaceutical companies primarily to inhibit prostaglandin production by inhibiting the enzyme, prostaglandin endoperoxide synthase (cyclooxygenase). There are at least two prostaglandin endoperoxide synthase isoforms present in humans, which are referred to as cyclooxygenase-1 (COX-1) (Yokoyama and Tanabe, 1989) and cyclooxygenase-2 (COX-2) (Hla and Neilson, 1992). Both of these enzymes possess cyclooxygenase and peroxidase activities which convert arachidonate to PGG_2 by inserting two oxygen molecules and then reducing this intermediate to PGH_2 (Marnett, 1992; Smith and Marnett, 1991).

In most circumstances, COX-1 is a constitutively expressed gene, and therefore levels of this protein do not fluctuate in response to stimuli such as cytokines or growth factors (Vane, 1994). Expression of COX-2 can be induced by a variety of agents, including growth factors and cytokines, which accounts for its alternative designation (mitogen-inducible prostaglandin G/H synthase) (DuBois *et al.*, 1994; Jones *et al.*, 1993; Kujubu *et al.*, 1991). These enzymes are of particular clinical relevance because they are the target of NSAIDs. Aspirin acetylates a serine in the substrate-binding site in these two related hemoproteins and, in the case of COX-1, completely blocks substrate utilization (Shimokawa and Smith, 1992). In COX-2, aspirin blocks PGH_2 formation, but oxygenase activity persists with the subsequent conversion of arachidonate to 15(R)HETE (Capdevila *et al.*, 1995; Holtzman *et al.*, 1992; Meade *et al.*, 1993). Furthermore, the recombinant COX-2 enzyme has a different sensitivity to NSAID inhibition than COX-1 (Meade *et al.*, 1993).

Studies were carried out to determine if cyclooxygenase expression was upregulated in colonic carcinomas obtained by endoscopic biopsy or surgical resection. Eberhart *et al.* (1994) reported that of 14 human colonic carcinomas screened, 12 had increased COX-2 mRNA, and of 14 unpaired adenomas screened, 43% had increased levels of COX-2 mRNA. The decrease in incidence of elevated COX-2 expression in benign adenomas is not surprising, considering that adenomas are precursors to carcinomas and are expected to express a different array of gene products. Indeed, the fact that there is a marked elevation of COX-2 mRNA in the adenomas, when compared to normal adjacent mucosa, may indicate that increased expression of COX-2 is involved in the progression to a transformed state. Therefore, the increased COX-2 levels in adenomas may be useful as a prognostic marker for tumorigenesis in the intestinal epithelium. Studies from other laboratories have confirmed these findings and show that COX-2 protein levels are increased in a significant number of colorectal carcinomas as well (Kargman *et al.*, 1995). Using immunohistological evaluation of colorectal cancer tissue sections, another group has shown that COX-2 protein is predominantly expressed in transformed epithelial cells and in some endothelial cells in the tumor (Sano *et al.,* 1995). However, COX-1 expression was low in both normal mucosa and tumor samples. More extensive patient studies will have to be performed before any definite conclusions can be drawn about the feasibility of utilizing COX-2 levels as a prognostic marker.

The authors' laboratory has demonstrated that expression of COX-2 in a nontransformed intestinal epithelial cell line results in an altered phenotype. The cells become more adherent to extracellular matrix components (like laminin), have markedly delayed transit through the G_1 phase of the cell cycle, and are resistant to undergo apoptosis (DuBois *et al.,* 1996; Tsujii and DuBois, 1995). These phenotypic changes are reversed by treatment with the NSAID sulindac sulfide. Other groups have reported that NSAIDs at high concentrations can directly induce programmed cell death in cultured cells (Lu *et al.,* 1995; Piazza *et al.,* 1995), which may not be related to their ability to inhibit cyclooxygenase. Additional research is underway to delineate the precise mechanism for the effect of NSAIDs on programmed cell death.

VII. Summary

The authors have presented a concise review of the studies which evaluate the risk of colorectal cancer among NSAID users. Animals studies have clearly documented a protective effect of NSAIDs in preventing colon cancers in a carcinogen-induced (AOM) model. NSAIDs are protective in the animal model, even if given 14 weeks after administration of the carcinogen, indicating that they must be playing a role very early in the adenoma-to-carcinoma sequence of events. Several studies have indicated that treatment of FAP patients with NSAIDs causes a regression of adenomas that were already present prior to initiation of NSAID therapy. Many epidemiological studies have examined the relationship between aspirin use and colorectal cancer. Most of these studies have shown a marked decrease in the relative risk (40–50%) of colorectal cancer among continuous aspirin users. The appropriate dose and duration of aspirin treatment for optimal effects are still unknown. Future work, directed at the molecular basis for the chemoprotective effects of NSAIDs in humans, may reveal strategies for the development of better chemopreventive agents.

One effect shared by all NSAIDs is their ability to inhibit cyclooxygenase. Presently, it is not clear whether inhibition of cyclooxygenase-1 or -2 effects on other signaling pathways are required for the protective effect of aspirin and other NSAIDs. The authors and others have demonstrated that COX-2 is upregulated from 2- to 50-fold in 85–90% of colorectal adenocarcinomas, which makes the COX-2 enzyme a possible target. Drugs are currently under development at several pharmaceutical companies that preferentially inhibit either COX-1 or COX-2. If COX-2 is found to be a relevant target in the prevention of colorectal cancer, then these newly developed, more selective NSAIDs may play a role in future chemoprevention strategies.

Acknowledgments

The authors thank Georgia and Louise Hanson, Mark Peeler, Chris Williams, and Dan Beauchamp for providing helpful editorial assistance. R.N.D. acknowledges support from the A. B. Hancock, Jr. Memorial Laboratory, Lucille P. Markey Charitable Trust, U.S. Public Health Services Grants DK 47297-01A1 (R.N.D.), P30 ES00267 (R.N.D.), and the Veterans Administration Merit Grant (R.N.D.). R.N.D. is a recipient of a VA Research Associate career development award, Boehringer Ingelheim New Investigator Award, and is an AGA Industry Research Scholar. W. S. is an AGA Industry Research Scholar.

References

Bedi, A., Pasricha, P. J., Akhtar, A. J., Barber, J. P., Bedi, G. C., Giardiello, F. M., Zehnbauer, B. A., Hamilton, S. R., and Jones, R. J. (1995). Inhibition of apoptosis during development of colorectal cancer. *Cancer Res* **55,** 1811–1816.

Boland, C. R. (1993). The biology of colorectal cancer. Implications for pretreatment and follow-up management. *Cancer (Philadelphia)* **71,** 4180–4186.

Capdevila, J. H., Morrow, J. D., Belosludtsev, Y. Y., Beauchamp, D. R., DeBois, R. N., and Falck, J. R. (1995). The catalytic outcomes of the constitutive and the mitogen inducible isoforms of prostaglandin H2 synthase are markedly affected by glutathione and glutathione peroxidase(s). *Biochemistry* **34,** 3325–3337.

DuBois, R. N. (1995). Nonsteroidal anti-inflammatory drug use and sporadic colorectal adenomas. *Gastroenterology* **108,** 1310–1314.

DuBois, R. N., Tsujii, M., Bishop, P., Awad, J. A., Makita, K., and Lanahan, A. (1994). Cloning and characterization of a growth factor-inducible cyclooxygenase gene from rat intestinal epithelial cells. *Am. J. Phys.* **266,** G822–G827.

DuBois, R. N., Shao, J., Sheng, H., Tsujii, M., and Beauchamp, R. D. (1996). G_1 delay in intestinal epithelial cells overexpressing prostaglandin endoperoxide synthase-2. *Cancer Res.* **56,** 733–737.

Eberhart, C. E., Coffey, R. J., Radhika, A., Giardiello, F. M., Ferrenbach, S., and DuBois, R. N. (1994). Up-regulation of cyclooxygenase 2 gene expression in human colorectal adenomas and adenocarcinomas. *Gastroenterology* **107,** 1183–1188.

Fearon, E. R. (1994). Molecular genetic studies of the adenoma-carcinoma sequence. *Adv. Intern. Med.* **39,** 123–147.

Fearon, E. R., and Vogelstein, B. (1990). A genetic model for colorectal tumorigenesis. *Cell (Cambridge, Mass.)* **61,** 759–767.

Friend, W. G. (1990). Sulindac suppression of colorectal polyps in Gardner's syndrome. *Am. Fam. Physician* **41,** 891–894.

Gann, P. H., Manson, J. E., Glynn, R. J., Buring, J. E., and Hennekens, C. H. (1993). Low-dose aspirin and incidence of colorectal tumors in a randomized trial [see comments]. *J. Natl. Cancer Inst.* **85,** 1220–1224.

Giardiello, F. M., Hamilton, S. R., Krush, A. J., Piantadosi, S., Hylind, L. M., Celano, P., Booker, S. V., Robinson, C. R., and Offerhaus, G. J. (1993). Treatment of colonic and rectal adenomas with sulindac in familial adenomatous polyposis. *N. Engl. J. Med.* **328,** 1313–1316.

Giovannucci, E., Rimm, E. B., Stampfer, M. J., Colditz, G. A., Ascherio, A., and Willett, W. C. (1994). Aspirin use and the risk for colorectal cancer and adenoma in male health professionals. *Ann. Intern. Med.* **121,** 241–246.

Giovannucci, E., Egan, K. M., Hunter, D. J., Stampfer, M. J., Colditz, G. A., Willett, W. C., and Speizer, F. E. (1995). Aspirin and the risk of colorectal cancer in women. *N. Engl. J. Med.* **333,** 609–614.

Greenberg, E. R., Baron, J. A., Freeman, D. H. J., Mandel, J. S., and Haile, R. (1993). Reduced risk of large-bowel adenomas among aspirin users. *J. Natl. Cancer Inst.* **85,** 912–916.

Hamilton, S. R. (1993). The molecular genetics of colorectal neoplasia. *Gastroenterology* **105,** 3–7.

Hixson, L. J., Earnest, D. L., Fennerty, M. B., and Sampliner, R. E. (1993). NSAID effect on sporadic colon polyps. *Am. J. Gastroenterol.* **88,** 1652–1656.

Hixson, L. J., Alberts, D. S., Krutzsch, M., Einsphar, J., Brendel, K., Gross, P. H., Paranka, N. S., Baier, M., Emerson, S., and Pamukcu, R. (1994). Antiproliferative effect of nonsteroidal antiinflammatory drugs against human colon cancer cells. *Cancer Epidemiol. Biomarkers Prev.* **3,** 433–438.

Hla, T., and Neilson, K. (1992). Human cyclooxygenase-2 cDNA. *Proc. Natl. Acad. Sci. U.S.A.* **89,** 7384–7388.

Holtzman, M. J., Turk, J., and Shornick, L. P. (1992). Identification of a pharmacologically distinct prostaglandin H synthase in cultured epithelial cells. *J. Biol. Chem.* **267,** 21438–21445.

Jones, D. A., Carlton, D. P., McIntyre, T. M., Zimmerman, G. A., and Prescott, S. M. (1993). Molecular cloning of human prostaglandin endoperoxide synthase type II and demonstration of expression in response to cytokines. *J. Biol. Chem.* **268,** 9049–9054.

Kargman, S., O'Neill, G., Vickers, P., Evans, J., Mancini, J., and Jothy, S. (1995). Expression of prostaglandin G/H synthase-1 and -2 protein in human colon cancer. *Cancer Res.* **55,** 2556–2559.

Kinzler, K. W., Nilbert, M. C., Su, L. K., Vogelstein, B., Bryan, T. M., Levy, D. B., Smith, K. J., Preisinger, A. C., Hedge, P., McKechnie, D., *et al.* (1991). Identification of FAP locus genes from chromosome 5q21. *Science* **253,** 661–665.

Kujubu, D. A., Fletcher, B. S., Varnum, B. C., Lim, R. W., and Herschman, H. R. (1991). TIS10, a phorbol ester tumor promoter-inducible mRNA from Swiss 3T3 cells, encodes a novel prostaglandin synthase/cyclooxygenase homologue. *J. Biol. Chem.* **266,** 12866–12872.

Kune, K. A., Kune, S., and Watson, L. F. (1988). Colorectal cancer risk, chronic illnesses, operations, and medications: Case control results from the Melbourne Colorectal Cancer Study. *Cancer Res.* **48,** 4399–4404.

Labayle, D., Fischer, D., Vielh, P., Drouhin, F., Pariente, A., Bories, C., Duhamel, O., Trousset, M., and Attali, P. (1991). Sulindac causes regression of rectal polyps in familial adenomatous polyposis. *Gastroenterology* **101,** 635–639.

Landenheim, J., Garcia, G., Titzer, D., Herzenberg, H., Lavori, P., Edson, R., and Omary, M. B. (1995). Effect of sulindac on sporadic colonic polyps. *Gastroenterology* **108,** 1083–1087.

Liu, T., Mokuolu, A. O., Rao, C. V., Reddy, B. S., and Holt, P. R. (1995). Regional chemoprevention of carcinogen-induced tumors in rat colon. *Gastroenterology* **109,** 1167–1172.

Logan, R. F., Little, J., Hawtin, P. G., and Hardcastle, J. D. (1993). Effect of aspirin and nonsteroidal anti-inflammatory drugs on colorectal adenomas: Case-control study of subjects participating in the Nottingham faecal occult blood screening programme. *B.M.J.* **307,** 285–289.

Lu, X., Xie, W., Reed, D., Bradshaw, W. S., and Simmons, D. L. (1995). Nonsteroidal antiinflammatory drugs cause apoptosis and induce cyclooxygenase in chicken embryo fibroblasts. *Proc. Natl. Acad. Sci. U.S.A.* **92,** 7961–7965.

MacPhee, M., Chepenik, K., Liddell, R., Nelson, K., Siracusa, L., and Buchberg, A. (1995). The secretory phospholipase A2 gene is a candidate for the *Mom1* locus, a major modifier of Apc^{min}-induced intestinal neoplasia. *Cell (Cambridge, Mass.)* **81,** 957–966.

Marnett, L. (1992). Aspirin and the potential role of prostaglandins in colon cancer. *Cancer Res.* **52,** 5575–5589.

Meade, E. A., Smith, W. L., and DeWitt, D. L. (1993). Differential inhibition of prostaglandin endoperoxide synthase (cyclooxygenase) isozymes by aspirin and other non-steroidal anti-inflammatory drugs. *J. Biol. Chem.* **268,** 6610–6614.

Miller, A. B., Howe, G. R., and Jain, M. (1983). Food items and food groups as risk factors in a case-control study of diet and colon cancer. *Int. J. Cancer* **32,** 155–162.

Muscat, J. E., and Wynder, E. L. (1993). Anti-inflammatory drugs and rheumatoid arthritis. *J. Natl. Cancer Inst.* **85,** 921–922.

Muscat, J. E., Stellman, S. D., and Wynder, E. L. (1994). Nonsteroidal antiinflammatory drugs and colorectal cancer. *Cancer (Philadelphia)* **74,** 1847–1854.

Nishisho, I., Nakamura, Y., Miyoshi, Y., Miki, Y., Ando, H., Horii, A., Koyama, K., Utsunomiya, J., Baba, S., and Hedge, P. (1991). Mutations of chromosome 5q21 genes in FAP and colorectal cancer patients. *Science* **253,** 665–669.

Nugent, K. P., Farmer, K. C., Spigelman, A. D., Williams, C. B., and Phillips, R. K. (1993). Randomized controlled trial of the effect of sulindac on duodenal and rectal polyposis and cell proliferation in patients with familial adenomatous polyposis. *Br. J. Surg.* **80,** 1618–1619.

Paganini-Hill, A., Chao, A., Ross, R. K., and Henderson, B. E. (1989). Aspirin use and chronic diseases: A cohort study of the elderly. *B.M.J.* **299,** 1247–1250.

Peipins, L. A., and Sandler, R. S. (1994). Epidemiology of colorectal adenomas. *Epidemiol. Rev.* **16,** 273–297.

Peleg, II, Maibach, H. T., Brown, S. H., and Wilcox, C. M. (1994). Aspirin and nonsteroidal anti-inflammatory drug use and the risk of subsequent colorectal cancer. *Arch. Intern. Med.* **154,** 394–399.

Physicians' Health Study Group. (1989). Final report on the aspirin component of the ongoing Physicians' Health Study. *N. Engl. J. Med.* **321,** 129–135.

Physicians' Health Study Group (1995). Preliminary report: Findings from the aspirin component of the ongoing Physicians' Health Study. *N. Engl. J. Med.* **318,** 262–264.

Piazza, G. A., Rahm, A. L., Krutzsch, M., Sperl, G., Paranka, N. S., Gross, P. H., Brendel, K., Burt, R. W., Alberts, D. S., Pamukcu, R., and Ahnen, D. J. (1995). Antineoplastic drugs sulindac sulfide and sulfone inhibit cell growth by inducing apoptosis. *Cancer Res.* **55,** 3110–3116.

Powell, S. M., Zilz, N., Beazer-Barclay, Y., Bryan, T. M., Hamilton, S. R., Thibodeau, S. N., Vogelstein, B., and Kinzler, K. W. (1992). APC mutations occur early during colorectal tumorigenesis. *Nature (London)* **359,** 235–237.

Rao, C. V., Rivenson, A., Simi, B., Zang, E., Kelloff, G., Steele, V., and Reddy, B. S. (1995). Chemoprevention of colon carcinogenesis by sulindac, a nonsteroidal anti-inflammatory agent. *Cancer Res.* **55,** 1464–1472.

Reddy, B. S., Maruyama, H., and Kelloff, G. (1987). Dose-related inhibition of colon carcinogenesis by dietary piroxicam, a nonsteroidal antiinflammatory drug, during different stages of rat colon tumor development. *Cancer Res.* **47,** 5340–5346.

Reddy, B. S., Nayini, J., Tokumo, K., Rigotty, J., Zang, E., and Kelloff, G. (1990). Chemoprevention of colon carcinogenesis by concurrent administration of piroxicam, a nonsteroidal antiinflammatory drug with D,L-alpha-difluoromethylornithine, an ornithine decarboxylase inhibitor, in diet. *Cancer Res.* **50,** 2562–2568.

Reddy, B. S., Tokumo, K., Kulkarni, N., Aligia, C., and Kelloff, G. (1992). Inhibition of colon carcinogenesis by prostaglandin synthesis inhibitors and related compounds. *Carcinogenesis (London)* **13,** 1019–1023.

Reddy, B. S., Rao, C. V., Rivenson, A., and Kelloff, G. (1993). Inhibitory effect of aspirin on azoxymethane-induced colon carcinogenesis in F344 rats. *Carcinogenesis* (*London*) **14,** 1493–1497.

Rigau, J., Pique, J. M., Rubio, E., Planas, R., Tarrech, J. M., and Bordas, J. M. (1991). Effects of long-term sulindac therapy on colonic polyposis. *Ann. Intern. Med.* **115,** 952–954.

Rosenberg, L., Palmer, J. R., Zauber, A. G., Washauer, M. E., Stolley, P. D., and Shapiro, S. (1991). A hypothesis: Nonsteroidal anti-inflammatory drugs reduce the incidence of large-bowel cancer. *J. Natl. Cancer Inst.* **83,** 355–358.

Rustgi, A. K. (1993). Molecular genetics and colorectal cancer. *Gastroenterology* **104,** 1223–1225.

Sano, H., Kawahito, Y., Wilder, R. L., Hashiramoto, A., Mukai, S., Asai, K., Kimura, S., Kato, H., Kondo, M., and Hla, T. (1995). Expression of cyclooxygenase-1 and -2 in human colorectal cancer. *Cancer Res.* **55,** 3785–3789.

Schreinemachers, D. M., and Everson, R. B. (1994). Aspirin use and lung, colon, and breast cancer incidence in a prospective study. *Epidemiology* **5,** 138–146.

Shimokawa, T., and Smith, W. L. (1992). Prostaglandin endoperoxide synthase. The aspirin acetylation region. *J. Biol. Chem.* **267,** 12387–12392.

Smith, W. L., and Marnett, L. J. (1991). Prostaglandin endoperoxide synthase: Structure and catalysis. *Biochim. Biophys. Acta* **1083,** 1–17.

Su, L. K., Vogelstein, B., and Kinzler, K. W. (1993). Association of the APC tumor suppressor protein with catenins. *Science* **262,** 1734–1737.

Suh, O., Mettlin, C., and Petrelli, N. J. (1993). Aspirin use, cancer, and polyps of the large bowel. *Cancer* (*Philadelphia*) **72,** 1171–1177.

Thun, M. J., Namboodiri, M. M., and Heath, C. W. J. (1991). Aspirin use and reduced risk of fatal colon cancer. *N. Engl. J. Med.* **325,** 1593–1596.

Tonelli, F., and Valanzano, R. (1993). Sulindac in familial adenomatous polyposis. *Lancet* **342,** 1120–1120.

Tsujii, M., and DuBois, R. N. (1995). Alterations in cellular adhesion and apoptosis in epithelial cells overexpressing prostaglandin endoperoxide synthase-2. *Cell* (*Cambridge, Mass.*) **83,** 493–501.

Vane, J. (1994). Towards a better aspirin. *Nature* (*London*) **367,** 215–216.

Waddell, W. R., and Loughry, R. W. (1983). Sulindac for polyposis of the colon. *J. Surg. Oncol.* **24,** 83–87.

Waddell, W. R., Gasner, G. F., Cerise, E. J., and Loughry, R. W. (1989). Sulindac for polyposis of the colon. *Am. J. Surg.* **157,** 175–178.

Williams, C. W., Luongo, C., Radhika, A., Zhang, T., Lamps, L. W., Nanney, L. B., Beauchamp, R. D., and DuBois, R. N. (1996). Elevated cyclooxygenase-2 levels in *Min* mouse adenomas. *Gastroenterology* **111,** 1134–1140.

Winde, G., Gumbinger, H. G., Osswald, H., Kemper, F., and Bunte, H. (1993). The NSAID sulindac reverses rectal adenomas in colectomized patients with familial adenomatous polyposis: Clinical results of a dose-finding study on rectal sulindac administration. *Int. J. Colorectal Dis.* **8,** 13–17.

Wynder, E. L., Kajitani, T., Ishikawa, S., Dodo, H., and Takano, A. (1969). Environmental factors of cancer of colon and rectum. II. Japanese epidemiological data. *Cancer* (*Philadelphia*) **23,** 1210–1220.

Yokoyama, C., and Tanabe, T. (1989). Cloning of human gene encoding prostaglandin endoperoxide synthase and primary structure of the enzyme. *Biochem. Biophys. Res. Commun.* **165,** 888–894.

Susan R. Ross

Department of Microbiology
University of Pennsylvania
Philadelphia, Pennsylvania 19104-6142

Mouse Mammary Tumor Virus and the Immune System

I. Introduction

Mammary cancer in mice has been studied for almost a century, when it was recognized in the 1890s that certain inbred strains developed tumors in this tissue (Nandi and McGrath, 1973). Subsequently, it was shown that some mammary tumors were caused by a milk-borne transmissible agent (Bittner, 1936; Heston *et al.*, 1945). This agent, which was found to be a retrovirus, is called mouse mammary tumor virus (MMTV) (Duesberg and Cardiff, 1968). Genetic studies also showed that there was an inherited form of breast cancer in mice and that foster-nursing, high tumor incidence pups on low tumor incidence mothers did not always free the offspring of mammary tumors (Bentvelzen and Daams, 1969). The inherited form of the disease in mice was caused by the germ line transmission of an ac-

Advances in Pharmacology, Volume 39

1054-3589/97/$25.00

tive, endogenous MMTV provirus (Varmus *et al.*, 1972; Bentvelzen and Daams, 1969).

The study of MMTV has proven to be important to a number of different areas in addition to providing an animal model of mammary tumorigenesis. MMTV was the first mammalian "gene" shown to encode DNA sequences that caused increased transcription in response to glucocorticoid hormones (Yamamoto, 1985). As a result, much of the evidence that mammalian transcription factors interacted with specific DNA sequences came about from studies of how glucocorticoid receptors induced MMTV expression. MMTV DNA sequences have also been used to direct the expression of transforming genes to mammary cells in transgenic mice, and a number of mouse models of breast cancer caused by different oncogenes have been created (Cardiff and Muller, 1993). Developmental biologists are currently studying the role that the cellular oncogenes activated by MMTV play in prenatal development (Nusse, 1988); many of these novel oncogenes were identified solely by their association with MMTV-induced mammary tumors.

More recently, endogenous and exogenous MMTVs have generated interest because one of the virus-encoded proteins possesses superantigen activity. The existence of superantigens expressed from endogenous MMTVs has profound effects on the immune repertoire of mice, as discussed later. Moreover, this protein plays a critical role in the ability of MMTV to infect mice because it allows the virus to amplify within cells of the immune system. The discovery of the MMTV superantigen protein has provided new insights into how viruses can subvert the biology of their host.

II. Endogenous and Exogenous Mouse Mammary Tumor Viruses

MMTV is a B-type retrovirus and can be transmitted exogenously as viral particles through milk or endogenously via the germ line as stably integrated proviruses (Nandi and McGrath, 1973; Moore *et al.*, 1979) (Fig. 1). The milk-borne infectious particles are produced by mammary gland cells. The exogenous forms of the virus are referred to as MMTV, with the virus substrain given in parentheses, i.e., MMTV(C3H) is an exogenous form of the virus found in the milk of C3H/He inbred mice. The endogenous copies of MMTV are called *Mtv* loci and are numbered in order of their discovery. Most commonly used inbred strains of mice have from two to eight *Mtv* loci (Kozak *et al.*, 1987). As with all endogenous retroviruses, *Mtv* loci represent the infection of germ cells or early embryos with exogenous viruses that are then maintained in the germ line. Approximately 50 different *Mtv* loci located at different chromosomal sites have been identified.

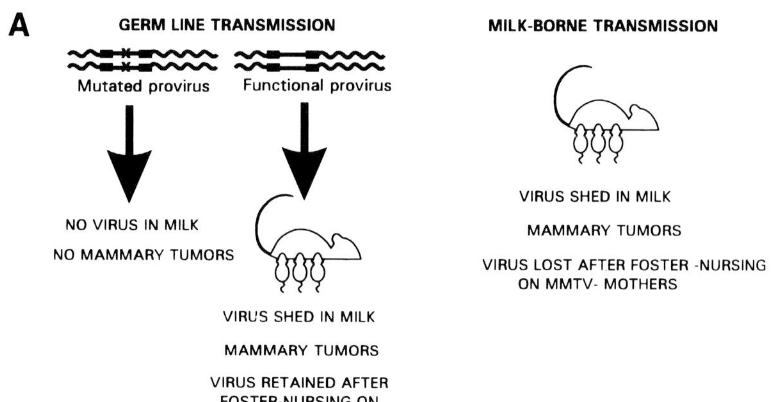

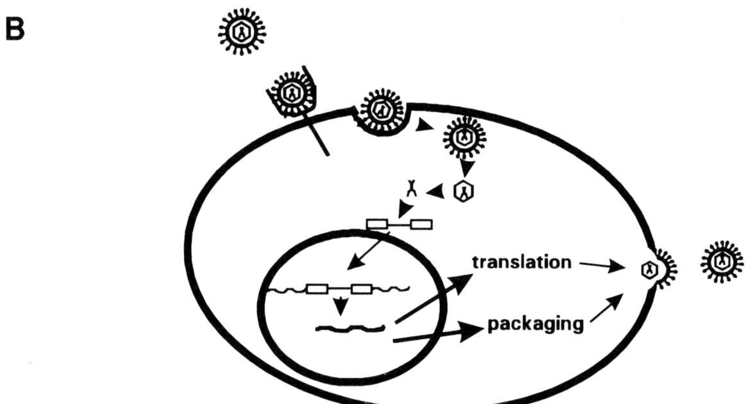

FIGURE 1 MMTV transmission pathways. (A) Endogenous MMTVs that are transmitted through the germ line can either produce functional virions or sustain mutations, usually in the protein-coding regions, that prevent their transmission. Mice with active, unmutated endogenous MMTVs cannot be freed of virus by nursing on nonviremic mothers. MMTV infection of mice that have exogenous and not functional endogenous proviruses can lose the milk-borne virus after nursing on virus-free mothers. (B) The retroviral infection of cells. Retroviruses usually infect somatic cells; in the rare case where infection of a germ cell occurs, the provirus is passed to subsequent generations.

These loci can be distinguished from each other by restriction fragment length polymorphisms (Kozak *et al.*, 1987; Tomonari *et al.*, 1993).

Most endogenous MMTV proviruses do not produce infectious particles. Some *Mtv* loci have mutations or deletions in protein coding regions (Kozak *et al.*, 1987) (Fig. 1A), whereas others are not expressed in the mammary gland. Some inbred strains of mice, such as GR, have infectious endogenous proviruses that can be transmitted to other strains of mice as exogenous MMTVs [i.e., MMTV(GR)] (Michalides *et al.*, 1978) (Fig. 1A). Female GR mice develop mammary tumors after their first pregnancy and do not survive past 1 year of age, most likely because of *in situ* infection of the mammary gland (Muhlbock, 1965).

A. Genome and Encoded Proteins

MMTV has a typical retrovirus genome, with the coding regions for the viral capsid, envelope, and polymerase proteins flanked by 5′ and 3′ long terminal repeats (LTR) (Fig. 2A). Two major RNAs are transcribed, both of which initiate in the 5′ LTR, a full-length genomic transcript of 8.5 kb and a spliced RNA of 3.8 kb (Coffin, 1990). The genomic transcript, which is packaged in the virion (Fig. 1B), encodes the group-specific antigen (Gag) capsid and reverse transcriptase proteins (Pol). The virion envelope proteins (Env) are translated from the spliced mRNA. Two Env polypeptides are produced by protease cleavage of a polyprotein precursor. The cell surface (SU) and transmembrane (TM) polypeptides associate to form the

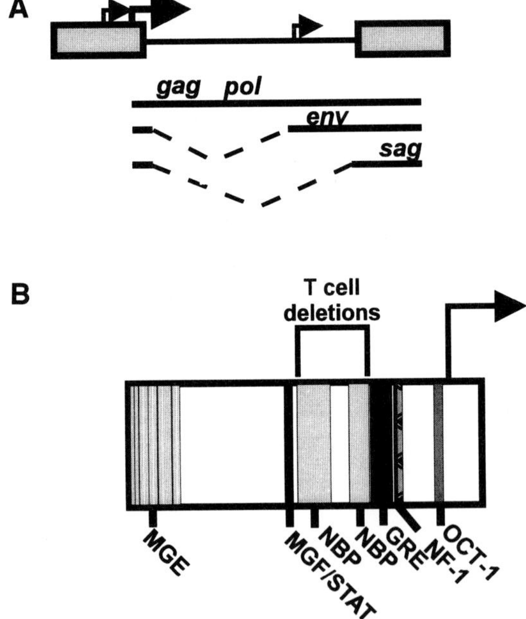

FIGURE 2 Map of integrated MMTV. (A) The three major transcripts described in the text are shown. The large arrow denotes the major transcription initiation site; small arrows denote other reported sites, as described in the text. (B) Relative position of the major transcriptional regulatory sequences. MGE, mammary gland enhancer; MGF/STAT, STAT consensus sequence; NBP, negative binding protein; GRE, glucocorticoid response element; NF-1, nuclear factor 1; Oct-1, octamer binding factor 1.

two domains of the viral protein responsible for MMTV binding to its cellular receptor (Hilkens *et al.*, 1983).

When sequencing of the virus began in the late 1980s, it was discovered that the MMTV LTR contained an open reading frame (ORF) (Donehower *et al.*, 1981). This ORF peptide was the first retroviral protein shown to be encoded in an LTR and for many years its function was unknown. It is now known to encode a protein with superantigen activity (see later). The ORF or superantigen (Sag) protein may be made from an alternatively spliced transcript, which has been described in some cell types (van Ooyen *et al.*, 1983; Wheeler *et al.*, 1983) (Fig. 2A). This 1.7-kb RNA initiates in the 5′ LTR, using the same splice donor site as the *env* mRNA and a splice acceptor site just upstream of the 3′ LTR.

B. Regulation of MMTV Transcription

For most retroviruses, including MMTV, the LTRs contain the major transcription start site and the regulatory regions necessary for determining the level of RNA produced by cells containing integrated proviruses. One of the earliest observations made about MMTV was that pregnancy or glucocorticoids and progesterone dramatically increased viral transcription and, as a consequence, virus production, as much as 50-fold (Bittner, 1958). The progestin/glucocorticoid receptor antagonist RU486 inhibits this induction. The DNA sequences controlling the hormone responsiveness, termed the glucocorticoid response elements (GRE), are responsible for the upregulation of virus production that occurs during lactation, when glucocorticoid and progesterone levels are elevated (Yamamoto, 1985) (Fig. 2B). The GREs also confer responsiveness to a number of other steroid hormones, including androgens and mineralcorticoids, because of cross-recognition of the receptors with the consensus DNA-binding site (Yamamoto, 1985; Beato *et al.*, 1995). Steroid hormones other than progesterone or glucocorticoids are probably not biologically important for the regulation of MMTV transcription during lactation, however.

A number of additional regulatory elements located near the start of transcription have been found to contribute to the regulation of MMTV transcription in various cultured cell lines. These include binding sites for the NF-1, Oct-1, and TFIID transcription factors (Toohey *et al.*, 1990; Mink *et al.*, 1992; Cordingley *et al.*, 1987). As expected for a virus transmitted through milk, there are sequences within the LTR that confer mammary gland-specific expression (Choi *et al.*, 1987; Ross *et al.*, 1990; Mok *et al.*, 1992) (Fig. 2B). Viral transcripts can also be found in lymphoid tissues (Henrard and Ross, 1988); the sequences controlling MMTV expression in B and T cells have not yet been defined. However, a number of variant MMTVs have been described, all with deletions or substitution mutations of the same region of the LTR (Fig. 2B); these viruses with altered LTRs are associated with T-cell lymphomas (Dekaban *et al.*, 1984; Michalides, 1983; Yanagawa *et al.*, 1993). Evidence shows that the deletions or alterations affect the binding of factors that negatively regulate transcription in lymphoid and other cells (Hsu *et al.*, 1988; Ross *et al.*, 1990; Mink *et al.*, 1990).

Although the major transcription start site is found in the LTR, there have been several reports of additional initiation sites within MMTV. Phorbol ester-inducible transcripts that initiate in the *env* gene have been found in some T-cell lymphomas (Elliott *et al.*, 1988; Miller *et al.*, 1992) (Fig. 2A). Reuss and Coffin (1995) have proposed that the sag RNA could initiate within env because they observed transcription initiation in a cultured early B-cell line transfected with a construct lacking the 5′ LTR; transcription from this promoter was dependent on regulatory sequences in the 3′ LTR. Finally, an additional promoter located upstream of the major transcription initiation site in the LTR has been described (Gunzburg *et al.*, 1993) (Fig. 2A). Whether any of these novel promoters play a role in the transcription of viral genes, thereby affecting virus life cycle *in vivo*, awaits experiments in which mutations are introduced into the novel promoter sequences within the context of the virus.

Many of the *Mtv* loci are also transcribed; however, they often show a different tissue-specific pattern and timing of expression. For example, *Mtv*-7 and -9 are only expressed at high levels in lymphoid tissue, whereas *Mtv*-17 RNA is found at significant levels only in mammary gland (Ross and Golovkina, 1995; Golovkina *et al.*, 1996). The LTRs of the different endogenous MMTVs are remarkably homologous to each other outside the superantigen hypervariable coding region (Brandt-Carlson *et al.*, 1993; see later). Indeed, the promoters and hormone regulatory elements among the different MMTVs are almost identical (Brandt-Carlson *et al.*, 1993). Interestingly, there is a consensus sequence for the STAT family of transcription factors upstream from the transcription start site (position 519 to 528 bp) that may determine whether the different MMTVs are expressed in the lymphoid or mammary gland (Golovkina *et al.*, 1997). Members of the STAT family of transcription factors have been shown to be important for the increased transcription of milk protein genes in response to prolactin in mammary gland cells and for the response of a number of genes to cytokines such as interleukin-2 (IL-2) in lymphoid cells (Schindler and Darnell, 1995). The MMTVs expressed in mammary gland have a different STAT consensus sequence in their LTR (CTCAA(T/G)T(G/C)AA) compared to those expressed in lymphoid tissue (CGC AAGT CAA), and functional evidence shows that this sequence affects the tissue-specific transcription of the virus (Qin *et al.*, 1997). Whether these STAT sequences confer increased MMTV transcription in response to prolactin in mammary gland or to cytokines such as IL-2 in lymphoid cells is not yet known.

C. Mechanism of Tumorigenesis

MMTV is a nonacute-transforming retrovirus, i.e., it does not encode its own oncogene. Instead, MMTV causes mammary tumors by integrating next to cellular oncogenes and activating their transcription (Nusse, 1988; Peters, 1991). MMTV works through a unique set of oncogenes that were not previously identified prior to their association with MMTV-induced tumors. These *int* (for integration site) oncogenes are, for the most part, not normally expressed in mammary or any other adult tissue. Instead, several *int* genes have been shown to be important in prenatal development (Rijsewijk *et al.,* 1987; Thomas and Capecchi, 1990; Nusse, 1988).

Both virgin and multiparous females, but not males, develop MMTV-induced mammary gland tumors (Nandi and McGrath, 1973). However, pregnancy reduces the latency and increases the incidence of mammary tumor induction. The effect of pregnancy is twofold. First, as described in the preceding section, the induction of MMTV transcription by glucocorticoid and progesterone hormones and perhaps prolactin increases virus production, leading to higher infection levels. Second, the mammary gland epithelial cells undergo cell division in response to lactogenic hormones, which may allow for more efficient infection.

Because MMTV integrates relatively randomly in the genome, as do all retroviruses, the activation of cellular oncogenes is a stochastic event. Thus, the more MMTV particles produced, the more cells become infected, increasing the likelihood that oncogene activation and hence mammary tumors will be induced. An early effective measurement of virus load in a mouse was the incidence and latency of tumor formation in nursed offspring (Nandi and McGrath, 1973). The offspring of an animal that shed high titer virus in its milk would show a high tumor incidence, with a latency of less than 6 to 7 months. In contrast, fewer offspring of a mouse that produced little virus would develop tumors and the latency of this tumor formation was increased. This delay in tumor incidence is probably significant for the reproductive life span of the mouse, as described later.

Because MMTV is expressed at high levels in mammary gland and the sequences controlling this tissue-specific expression are well defined, the LTR has been used to direct the expression of a number of linked oncogenes to this tissue (Cardiff and Muller, 1993). Indeed, the first patented transgenic mouse was one in which the c-*myc* oncogene was expressed under the control of the MMTV LTR (Stewart *et al.,* 1984); this mouse developed lymphomas and mammary gland tumors. Usually only one or a few clonal tumors develop in the various MMTV–oncogene transgenic mice that have been generated, indicating that expression of a single oncogene is not sufficient for transformation. These models of mammary tumorigenesis are being used to study the role of specific oncogenes in the transformation process. In addition, because the transgenic mice are genetically predisposed to mammary gland cancer, they can be used for carcinogen testing and for the development of pharmacological strategies for treating this type of cancer.

III. Superantigens and Their Interaction with T Cells

A large proportion of T cells in mammals have heterodimeric receptors made up of α and β chains (Fig. 3). Both the α and β chains have a variable and a constant region. The constant region contains the transmembrane and dimerization domains, whereas the α and β variable region forms the binding site for the recognition of antigen. Most antigens are recognized as peptide fragments presented in the groove of one of two proteins encoded in the major histocompatibility complex (MHC), called Class I and Class II, that are expressed on the surface of antigen-presenting cells (APCs) (Fig. 3). These peptides are generated by the intracellular processing of proteins. Peptide fragments can be generated from proteins expressed in the APCs themselves. Alternatively, foreign peptides can be generated after infection with viruses and other organisms or by endocytosis of proteins. The T-cell receptor (TCR) binds to both the antigenic peptide and the MHC.

In contrast to traditional peptide antigens, which are presented in the groove of the MHC Class I and II proteins, superantigens for the most part bind outside this groove. Moreover, unlike peptide antigens, which must interact with both the α and the β chains of the TCR, superantigens apparently only bind to the β chain (Fig. 3). Mice and humans have only about 20 and 60 different variable region β chain genes, respectively, and over 100 α variable regions in their genomes (Janeway and Travers, 1994). Like immunoglobulin molecules, the α and β proteins are assembled from several domains joined together during splicing of the mRNA. It has been estimated that a mouse may make as many as 10^{16} different T cells, each bearing a different combination of the $\alpha\beta$ chains (Janeway and Travers, 1994). As a result, about 1 in 10^5 or 10^6 T cells can respond to a peptide antigen. Because

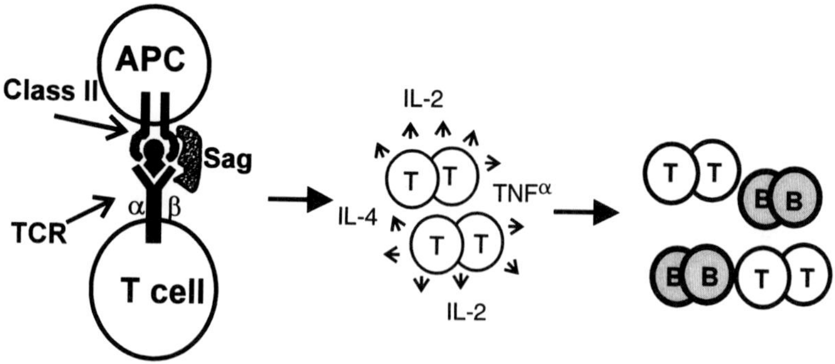

FIGURE 3 Diagram of superantigen interaction with APCs and T cells.

superantigens interact with the β chain and not with the groove formed by α and β together, these proteins are successfully presented to a much higher percentage of T lymphocytes, usually on the order of 5 to 20%, depending on the frequency with which that Vβ chain appears in the T-cell population (Marrack and Kappler, 1990).

A. Bacterial Superantigens

A number of pathogenic bacteria produce superantigens that bind to the Vβ chain of the TCR. For example, Staphyloccus A and B produce enterotoxins SEA and SEB, respectively, that have superantigen activity and interact with specific Vβ-bearing T cells in humans and mice (Marrack and Kappler, 1990). Two other properties of bacterial superantigens make them unique from peptide antigens. First, there is no evidence that bacterial superantigens go through an intracellular processing pathway and are presented by APCs as intact proteins after they bind to the MHC Class II proteins on the cell surface (Marrack and Kappler, 1990). Second, all known superantigens are presented only by the MHC Class II and not Class I proteins. Unlike the MHC Class I protein, which is found on virtually all cell types. Class II molecules are expressed on professional APCs, such as B cells, dendritic cells, and macrophages. Only the T-helper subsets, which express the coreceptor CD4, and not cytolytic T cells, which express CD8, interact with Class II$^+$ APCs; thus, superantigens stimulate predominantly those T cells that activate other cells of the immune system. In some cases, however, the affinity of the Vβ chain for the superantigen is so strong that CD8$^+$ T cells can also bind superantigen presented by Class II molecules.

B. Superantigen Presentation Results in Immune Cell Stimulation

In addition to the α and β chains, the TCR contains a complex of four proteins, termed CD3, that are responsible for transducing signals to the cell upon binding to antigen. Of these four proteins, the ξ chain is thought to be responsible for signaling (Janeway and Travers, 1994). When traditional antigens or superantigens are presented by APCs and bind to the TCR, activation of a number of tyrosine kinases occurs in the responding T cell. These include the fyn and lck tyrosine kinases. As a result of the signal transduction cascade, transcription of lymphokines, such as IL-2 and IL-4, is activated. The production of these cytokines leads to the proliferation of T cells and bystander cells, such as B cells and macrophages (Fig. 3).

Because superantigens are recognized by a large percentage of T cells, stimulation results in a measurable increase in the percentage of Vβ-specific T cells. For example, the staphylococcal toxin SEB interacts with Vβ8$^+$ T cells, which normally represent about 25% of the total T-cell population in mice. After injection of SEB into mice, however, the percentage of Vβ8$^+$-bearing cells increases to >60% (White *et al.*, 1989; Janeway *et al.*, 1989). Moreover, there are measurable increases in the numbers of B cells in these animals. This ability of superantigens to cause massive cellular proliferation can be lethal to the host. It is thought that the production of lymphokines and tumor necrosis factor α in response to the toxin produced by *Staphylococcus aureus*, TSST-1, is what causes toxic shock in humans (Bohach *et al.*, 1990).

After superantigen stimulation, the activated T cells undergo apoptosis. In adults that are infected with a superantigen-producing bacteria, T-cell numbers decline to their preinfection levels. In contrast, in newborn animals injected with bacterial superantigens, there are fewer cognate T cells than are found in untreated animals (White *et al.*, 1989). This is thought to be due to shaping of the immune repertoire during neonatal life. If a bacterial superantigen is introduced into a mouse during this period, it is mistaken for a self-antigen, and the T cells capable of recognizing it are deleted from the population by the same mechanism that occurs with other self-reactive T cells.

C. Endogenous MMTVs and Their Relationship to *Mls* Loci

As described earlier, endogenous MMTV proviruses are present in the germ line of all inbred mice, and different strains contain distinct proviruses at various genomic locations. Endogenous MMTVs have been shown to genetically cosegregate with a set of genes called the minor lymphocyte stimulating (*Mls*) loci (Dyson *et al.*, 1991; Frankel *et al.*, 1991; Woodland *et al.*, 1992). The *Mls* genes were originally identified by their ability to stimulate T-cell proliferation in mixed cultures of spleen cells from mice of different genetic backgrounds that were matched at the major histocompatibility complex locus (Festenstein, 1973). It was later shown that this stimulation was of specific Vβ-bearing T cells, i.e., that the *Mls* genes encoded self-superantigens (Kappler *et al.*, 1988; MacDonald *et al.*, 1988). In addition to causing the proliferation of specific classes of Vβ^+ T cells *in vitro*, the *Mls* genes cause the deletion of these same T cells during shaping of the immune repertoire because they are recognized as self-antigens. Similar to bacterial superantigens, neonatal infection of mice by MMTV results in the slow deletion of Sag-cognate T cells (Marrack *et al.*, 1991; Ignatowicz *et al.*, 1992).

Shortly after the discovery that the *Mtv* and *Mls* loci were identical, it was shown that the ORF protein had superantigen activity (Acha-Orbea *et al.*, 1991; Choi *et al.*, 1991). The MMTV Sag protein is a type II membrane glycoprotein (extracellular C terminus and cytoplasmic N terminus) of approximately 45 kDa apparent molecular mass (Choi *et al.*, 1992; Brandt-

Carlson and Butel, 1991; Korman *et al.*, 1992) (Fig. 4A). There are a number of potential protease (i.e., Arg-Lys-Arg-Arg) cleavage sites in the protein. Unlike bacterial superantigens, evidence suggests that cleavage is required for presentation of the MMTV Sag by APCs (Park *et al.*, 1995) and that it is found as an 18.5-kDa peptide on the surface of cells (Winslow *et al.*, 1994). Detailed biochemical analysis of the MMTV Sag has been hampered by its low abundance in cells.

The *sag* genes of the various *Mtv* loci are very homologous at both the nucleotide and the amino acid level except for their 30 C-terminal amino acids (Fig. 4B), which have been called the hypervariable domain. The C-terminal extracellular domain contacts the Vβ chain of the T-cell receptor and determines the specificity of this interaction (Yazdanbakhsh *et al.*, 1993). Indeed, the different *Mtv* and MMTV Sag proteins can be grouped together by the sequences of their hypervariable domain; Sag proteins that fall into the same group generally interact with the same Vβ-bearing T cells (Fig. 4B).

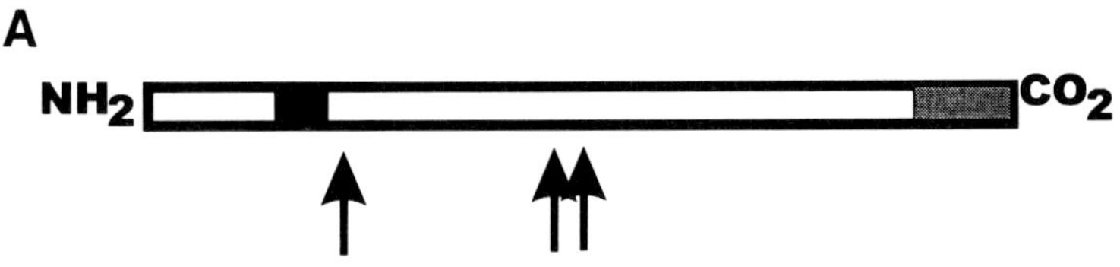

B

```
MMTV                                                                   Vβ
               280
MMTV(C3H)      YIYLGTGM-H FWGKIFH-TK EGTVAGLIEH YS-AKTYGMS YYE-     14,15
MMTV (GR)      ........-. ....V..-.. ..A....... ..-....... ..D-     14
II-TES         ........-S I......-.. .....A.... ..-....... ..D-     14
BALB14         ........MS L......Y.. G..MTA.... ..-....... ..D-     14

MMTV (C4)      YVYRGTGM-R DLNLFFKSRE EVQKH-LIDS ID-ALPL--S Y---     2
BALBcV,BALB2   ........-. ...V...... .....-.... .K ....--. .---     2
Mtv-DDO        ...L...L-I H.KV..N... ..K..-..E. .K-.....-A .---     2

MMTV (SW)      YIYLGTGM-N FWGKIFDYTE EGAIAKIIYN IKYTHGGRIG FDPF     6
Mtv-7          .......... .......... .......L.. M.......V. ....     6
Mtv-43         .......... .......... .......L.. M......... ....     6
```

FIGURE 4 Diagram of the MMTV Sag protein. (A) Structure of the protein. The black box denotes the transmembrane domain whereas the stippled box denotes the hypervariable domain. The three arrows show the relative position of the protease cleavage sites. (B) Sequence of the C-terminal hypervariable domains of several MMTVs. Dots denote identical sequence; dashes denote no amino acid. Data taken from Brandt-Carlson *et al.*, 1993 [MMTV(C3H), MMTV(GR), MMTV(SW), *Mtv*-7, *Mtv*-43; Golovkina *et al.*, 1997 (BALB14, BALB2); Wajjwalku *et al.*, 1995 (II-TES); Jouvin-Marche *et al.*, 1993 (MMTV-DDO); Hodes *et al.*, 1993 (BALBcV); and Shakhov *et al.*, 1993 [MMTV(C4)].

IV. Infection of the Mammary Gland via the Immune System

The discovery that the *Mtv* and *Mls* loci were one and the same was a major breakthrough in the fields of both virology and immunology. The role of the *Mls* loci in shaping the immune repertoire had long been a subject of investigation for immunologists and these results explained their genetic segregation. For virologists, the identification of a viral protein that affected cells of the immune system helped explain how lymphoid cells were involved in virus transmission. The remainder of this review describes how the Sag protein works to facilitate the MMTV infection of cells of the immune system, leading to mammary gland infection.

A. Genetic Studies

After the discovery that there was an infectious agent that could be transmitted through milk to nursing pups, it was found that not all strains of mice were equally able to be infected with MMTV. Notably, the C57BL mouse strain and its derivatives were shown to have very low mammary tumor incidence when foster nursed on C3H/He mice known to transmit virus either to their own pups or to other mouse strains, such as BALB/c (Muhlbock and Dux, 1972). Genetic studies mapped one major resistance gene to the MHC locus in C57BL mice (Muhlbock and Dux, 1972).

C57BL mice may contain an additional virus resistance gene. Classical backcrossing studies demonstrated that there was an additional resistance locus in C57 mice that could be genetically segregated from the MHC locus (Dux, 1972). These genetic studies have been confirmed using B10.BR mice, which have the same MHC allele as susceptible strains on a C57BL/10 background. However, B10.BR mice are less infected by MMTV(C3H) in comparison with the MMTV-susceptible strain, C3H/HeN, when nursed on the same C3H/HeN MMTV$^+$ mothers (Golovkina and Ross, unpublished). Backcrosses between C3H/HeN and B10.BR mice indicate that there is a single, recessive resistance gene in the C57BL/10 background that controls resistance to infection. It has also been reported that a gene in the B10.BR background decreases the effectiveness of endogenous Sag presentation (Pullen *et al.*, 1989).

An additional gene thought to contribute to resistance to MMTV infection is the lipopolysaccharide sensitivity allele (*lps*). A substrain of C3H mice maintained at the Jackson Laboratory (C3H/HeJ) had a spontaneous mutation of this allele in the 1960s; C3H/HeJ mice are 60 times less sensitive to killing by *lps* than are other substrains of C3H mice, such as C3H/HeN. This resistance allele (*lps*^{r}) also results in decreased B-cell proliferation and other immune system effects in response to this endotoxin (Coutinho, 1976). Interestingly, C3H/HeJ mice show a much lower level of infection by

MMTV(C3H) than do C3H/HeN mice and they develop fewer mammary tumors with a much longer latency (Outzen *et al.*, 1985). This indicates that there is overlap between the *lps* response and MMTV infection pathways.

One possible mechanism by which this occurs is at the level of transcription. *lps* can upregulate transcription from the endogenous *Mtv*-9 locus in B cells (Carr *et al.*, 1985; King and Corley, 1990). Stimulation of T cells by Sag or B cells by T-cell cytokines may also increase viral RNA synthesis through the same pathways as *lps*. For example, if virus transcription in C3H/HeJ mice is lower than in C3H/HeN mice, decreased virion production would result. As a result, C3H/HeJ would be less infected than C3H/HeN mice and develop fewer mammary tumors. It is not known, however, whether all MMTVs, including the exogenous viruses such as MMTV(C3H), are transcriptionally regulated by *lps* or what DNA sequences within *Mtv*-9 confer *lps* responsiveness.

B. Other Studies Implicating the Immune System

In addition to genetic studies, a number of investigators reported that MMTV antigens could be detected in cells of the immune system, such as B and T cells (Moore *et al.*, 1979). Similarly, transplantation experiments in which thymic or splenic lymphocytes from infected mice were injected into naive animals showed that virus transfer could occur (Tsubura *et al.*, 1988; Held *et al.*, 1993a). However, these studies did not show that cells of the immune system were required for MMTV infection.

The first direct evidence that the immune system was involved in MMTV infection was obtained when Squartini and colleagues (1970) showed that neonatal thymectomy of newborn mice infected through milk had a much lower incidence of mammary tumors than sham-operated mice. Similarly, nude mice were also shown to be relatively resistant to MMTV-induced tumors (Tsubura *et al.*, 1988). Transplantation experiments into nude mice indicated that T cells were the most efficient at transmitting virus (Tsubura *et al.*, 1988); however, other investigators have found that injecting MMTV-infected B cells into naive mice results in infection of both lymphoid and mammary gland cells (Waanders *et al.*, 1993).

C. How the MMTV Sag Protein Functions in the Infection Pathway

1. Role of T Cells

Mls loci were originally identified because of their ability to stimulate the cellular division of a large percentage of T cells in mixed lymphocyte cultures (Festenstein, 1973). In addition to stimulating cell division, viral and bacterial Sags cause T cells to secrete cytokines that cause B-cell expansion (Fig. 3). Thus, a major effect of Sag presentation is the creation of dividing T and B cells.

It is well known that most retroviruses, with the exception of the human immunodeficiency virus (HIV), can only infect actively dividing cells (Fritsch and Temin, 1977; Roe *et al.*, 1983; Lewis and Emerman, 1994). Evidence indicates that retroviral replication complexes are not able to cross the nuclear membrane; as a result, the double-stranded DNA copy of genomic RNA that will integrate into chromosomes can only enter the nucleus during nuclear membrane breakdown (Roe *et al.*, 1993; Lewis and Emerman, 1994). It was hypothesized that a major role for the MMTV Sag protein during the acquisition of the milk-borne virus by uninfected pups might be to cause T-cell stimulation (Fig. 5). This would result in the creation of actively dividing populations of T, B, and other bystander cells that could be easily infected by virus. In the absence of Sag-responsive T cells, viral infection would be inefficient because there would be few, if any, actively dividing, infection-competent cells.

The hypothesis that Sag cognate T cells were required for virus infection was tested using mice transgenic for the MMTV(C3H) Sag (Golovkina *et al.*, 1992). The presence of endogenous MMTVs in the genome causes the deletion of all Vβ-bearing T cells that recognize the Sags encoded by these loci during the shaping of the immune repertoire, as described earlier. Transgenic mice that expressed the MMTV(C3H) Sag protein under the control of the MMTV LTR deleted cognate Vβ14-bearing T cells (Fig. 5). When these mice were nursed on C3H/HeN mothers that produced milk-borne MMTV(C3H), they were resistant to infection relative to their nontransgenic littermates that retained cognate T cells (Fig. 5).

These results were later confirmed for a different exogenous MMTV, called SW virus (Held *et al.*, 1993b). Unlike MMTV(C3H), this virus interacts with $V\beta 6^+$ T cells because of sequence differences in its Sag hypervariable region (Fig. 4B). The Sag protein encoded by *Mtv*-7, which is highly homologous to that of the SW virus, also causes the deletion of $V\beta 6^+$ T cells. Held and colleagues (1993b) showed that inbred mouse strains containing *Mtv*-7 were resistant to the SW but not the MMTV(C3H) virus.

That Sag presentation was critical to the milk-borne infection pathway also explained why C57BL mice were resistant to milk-borne MMTV(C3H). Most strains of mice have germ line copies of two different MHC Class II genes, I-E and I-A. However, C57BL mice and related strains have a genomic deletion of their I-E gene. Most of the MMTV-encoded Sags are only efficiently presented by I-E and not I-A (Simpson *et al.*, 1993). Because they lack the Class II I-E molecule, there is no Sag presentation in C57BL mice and, as a result, little or no stimulation of cognate T cells can occur. Hence, MMTV infection is inefficient. Indeed, it has been shown that C57BL/6

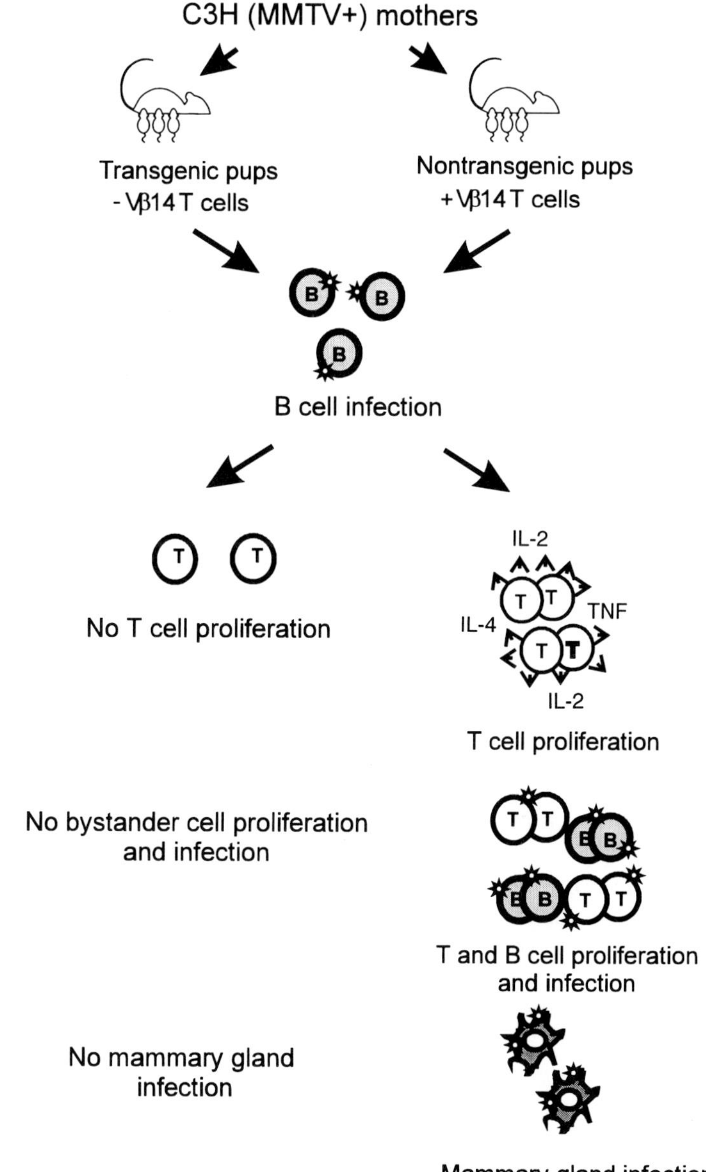

FIGURE 5 MMTV infection pathway in nontransgenic and superantigen-transgenic mice.

mice transgenic for I-E are easily infected by milk-borne MMTV(C3H) (Pucillo *et al.*, 1993).

T cells become infected with MMTV (Michalides *et al.*, 1982; Dudley and Risser, 1984; Ball *et al.*, 1985). Studies have shown that MMTV infection occurs after the transfer of T cells from infected animals to naive mice (Tsubura *et al.*, 1988). It is also known that T lymphoma cell lines are capable of producing virus particles (Meyers *et al.*, 1989), and it has been shown that primary T cells shed virus (Dzuris *et al.*, 1997). Moreover, variant MMTVs that have deletions in their LTRs are known to cause T-cell lymphomas (Yanagawa *et al.*, 1993), presumably through integration next to cellular oncogenes. These deletions may remove negative transcription regulatory regions and cause increased lymphoid cell expression of the virus and the adjacent oncogene (Hsu *et al.*, 1988; Theunissen *et al.*, 1989). The deletions also encompass the Sag hypervariable coding region; it remains to be determined whether the lack of a functional Sag protein plays a role in lymphomagenesis. It is also not known if MMTV infection of T cells is required for virus transmission to the mammary gland.

Because MMTV infection occurs during the shaping of the immune repertoire in neonatal life and because infection is persistent, there is a gradual deletion of Sag cognate T cells (Ignatowicz *et al.*, 1992). Mice infected with MMTV(C3H), for example, have less than 10% the normal Vβ14-bearing T cells by about 10 weeks of age and the remaining cognate T cells are anergic (Ignatowicz *et al.*, 1992). It is possible that this loss of functional cognate T cells results in an immune system that is tolerant to MMTV-infected cells later in life and prevents recognition, for example, of mammary tumors. There is some precedent for this effect of MMTV in viral immunity. The deletion of V$\beta 6^+$ T cells in mice that have the *Mtv*-7 locus results in lack of an immune response to polyoma virus-induced tumors. In contrast, inbred strains of mice that lack the *Mtv*-7 locus have V$\beta 6^+$ T cells, can mount a cellular immune response, and are resistant to tumors induced by this virus (Lukacher *et al.*, 1995). Whether a similar loss of immune response occurs during MMTV infection is not known.

Therefore, at minimum, the role of the MMTV-encoded Sag protein is to stimulate cognate T cells and this stimulation is a requisite step in the infection pathway. Whether T cells are important for other steps is yet to be determined. B-cell infection is also critical, as described in the next section.

2. *Role of B Cells*

Superantigens can be presented by a number of different Class II$^+$ APCs to cognate T cells, including B cells, macrophages, and dendritic cells. B cells present in the Peyer's patches of the gut were shown to be the first cells infected when newborn mice acquire MMTV through suckling on viremic mothers (Karapetian *et al.*, 1994). A similar infection of B cells is seen in the draining lymph node when MMTV virions are injected in the footpad of adult mice (Waanders *et al.*, 1993). Indeed, B-cell infection is necessary to milk-borne MMTV transmission, since mice that lacked B cells because of targeted mutagenesis of the immunoglobulin heavy chain gene (Igμ) were unable to be infected with MMTV; no deletion of cognate T cells occurred in these animals and their mammary glands did not acquire virus (Beutner *et al.,* 1994). Interestingly, there is a deletion of cognate T cells by endogenous *Mtv*-encoded Sags in the Igμ knockout mice, indicating that there are other APCs, such as dendritic cells, epithelial cells, and macrophages, that function to present endogenous superantigens during the shaping of the immune repertoire. That these other APCs only present endogenous Sags indicates that they do not become infected during the course of an exogenous MMTV infection, perhaps because they lack the receptor for the virus or do not actively undergo cell division during this process.

Therefore, the infection of B cells in the Peyer's patches of the gut is the first step in the MMTV infection pathway and these cells serve as APCs for cognate T cells (Fig. 5). After Sag presentation by B cells, both $CD4^+$ and $CD8^+$ T cells become infected (Waanders *et al.,* 1993) and presumably cytokine production occurs. This in turn leads to the proliferation of B cells. It has been shown that B cells of the IgG class are amplified in the draining lymph node of mice injected with the SW virus and that these cells are MMTV infected (Held *et al.,* 1994a). This amplification is not dependent on the retroviral infection of additional cells because it occurs in the presence of 3′azido-3′-deoxythymidine (AZT), an inhibitor of retrovirus replication. However, as is the case with T cells, it is still not known whether B-cell infection is required for transmission of the virus to the mammary gland.

No evidence exists for a Sag-independent pathway of MMTV transmission and only MMTVs with functional *sag* genes can be transmitted through milk (Golovkina *et al.,* 1995). The acquisition of a *sag* gene in the MMTV genome probably allows this virus to take maximum advantage of its host's biology. The main target tissue for MMTV is the mammary gland. The epithelial cells of the mammary gland undergo proliferation at about 3–4 weeks of age (during puberty) and in response to the hormonal stimulus provided by pregnancy. Because of the requirement for cell division, MMTV most likely only efficiently infects cells during these two periods. Thus, MMTV can reside and amplify in the cells of the immune system during the neonatal period until efficient infection of the mammary gland can occur.

3. *Role of Endogenous Viruses*

Some endogenous retroviruses in mice and other species have been shown to confer resistance to exogenous viruses, primarily through the expression of envelope proteins that interfere with virus binding to the cell surface receptor. In contrast, it is thought that expression of the MMTV envelope protein does not prevent reinfection of a cell. MMTV-induced mammary tumors often have multiple independent proviral integrations characteristic of a cell that has been reinfected (Nusse and Varmus, 1982; Nusse *et al.,* 1985). Thus, if endogenous MMTVs conferred resistance to exogenous virus infection, this protection would likely involve a different mechanism. MMTV is thus far unique among the murine and perhaps other retroviruses in encoding a Sag whose activity it uses as part of its infection pathway. Because this protein causes profound deletion of cognate T cells when expressed from the *Mtv* loci, any mouse that is infected with an exogenous virus encoding a Sag with the same specificity as its endogenous loci cannot be infected with this virus. As a result, these mice do not acquire exogenous MMTV in the mammary gland nor do they develop mammary tumors (Fig. 5) (Golovkina *et al.*, 1992; Held *et al.*, 1993b).

A number of new endogenous and exogenous MMTVs with different Vβ specificities have been described. These viruses have been found in previously existing stocks of mice (Yoshimoto *et al.*, 1994; Ando *et al.*, 1995; Shakhov *et al.*, 1993). Interestingly, most of the infectious viruses encode Sags that interact with different Vβ-bearing T cells than those encoded by the endogenous loci. One exception is SW virus, which is only weakly tumorigenic (Held *et al.*, 1992). This predicts that there is a natural selection for tumorigenic or highly infectious MMTVs that produce Sag proteins capable of stimulating cognate T cells and against viruses that do not have this ability.

This prediction has been borne out in the laboratory. In the case of MMTV(C3H) Sag transgenic mice, the MMTV(C3H) virus was totally lost from a pedigree after three generations (Golovkina *et al.*, 1993). Similarly, the SW virus was eliminated from *Mtv*-7-containing mice after two generations (Held *et al.*, 1993b).

This elimination of infectious virus is beneficial to mice. Inheritance of an endogenous *sag* with the same Vβ specificity as an exogenous virus should increase the reproductive life span of the mouse. MMTV(C3H) very efficiently causes tumors in both BALB/c and C3H/HeN mice, about 95% incidence and an average latency of 6 to 7 months in breeding females (Nandi and McGrath, 1973). In MMTV(C3H) Sag transgenic mice, the virus load is reduced several orders of magnitude and the average latency of tumor formation more than doubles (Golovkina *et al.*, 1993). As a result, breeding females develop mammary tumors after their peak reproductive period. Although this increase in latency has little effect on litter number and size in the laboratory setting, it is probably significant in the wild, where the average life span is less than 1 year (Sage, 1981). Moreover, tumor-bearing animals are less able to nurse their young and are more susceptible to opportunistic infection.

Balanced against the selective pressure to retain endogenous copies of MMTV to protect against exogenous infection is the pressure to retain only those copies of the virus that are not infectious. Inbred strains of mice that retain an infectious endogenous provirus, such as GR, very rapidly succumb to mammary tumors. This would imply that the GR *Mtv*-2 locus has recently integrated into the mouse genome and that with time it would accumulate a mutation(s) that would inactivate its tumorigenic activity. This inactivation can be the result of mutations that prevent functional virus capsid protein synthesis or the modulation of the tissue-specific expression of the virus.

Interestingly, all of the known defective Mtv proviruses have mutations in their protein-coding regions or in the transcriptional regulatory regions, but not in their *sag* genes, further confirming that it is advantageous for mice to retain these genes.

V. Conclusions and Perspectives

MMTV represents a unique virus in that its sole route of natural infection is through milk. Because the mammary gland cell is the ultimate target for this virus, it is not surprising that MMTV acquired the ability to replicate and amplify in cells of the lymphoid system of newborn, nursing pups. A number of other viruses have been shown to encode superantigen proteins. The actual viral protein that has superantigen activity has only been identified for one of these viruses, rabies, a neurotropic rhabdovirus (Lafon *et al.*, 1994). It is not clear why a virus that infects cells of the nervous system would encode such a protein, although it has been suggested that the N protein superantigen could cause immunosuppression, resulting in increased virus spread.

A superantigen activity has also been associated with cytomegalovirus (CMV), a member of the herpes virus family (Dobrescu *et al.*, 1995). The gene product that encodes this activity has not yet been identified and it is also not known what role such a protein might play in the virus life cycle. However, because CMV is an opportunistic pathogen associated with HIV infection, it has been suggested that some of the T-cell loss that occurs in AIDS could be the result of the CMV-encoded superantigen. It seems likely that there will be other viruses and pathogens that also use superantigen-like proteins to either infect or disable cells of the immune system.

Additional questions remain to be answered with regard to endogenous superantigens. It has been suggested that the deletion of cognate T cells might be beneficial to the mouse in addition to conferring protection against MMTV infection (Marrack and Kappler, 1990). For example, a mouse that has endogenous *Mtv* loci and deletes those $V\beta^+$ T cells that are stimulated by a Staph superantigen would not develop the severe pathologies associated with infection by that bacteria. It is not known whether any other species besides mice contain such germ line genes, although it has been reported that MMTV *sag* homologous sequences can be found in humans (Indraccolo *et al.*, 1995). Even if humans and other species do not have endogenous superantigen genes, understanding how shaping the immune repertoire affects the response to microorganisms and other pathogens will lead to the development of therapies for the treatment of infections. For example, for viruses that rely on superantigen activity to invade their host or cause pathogenic effects, one could envision an antiviral therapy that involves deletion of the T-cell targets of the superantigen or prevents the activation of these cells. Finally, since it is thought that retroviral genes were originally derived from their host, it may be that the MMTV acquired the coding region for a host protein that is involved in immunoregulation. An understanding of where the superantigen proteins arose may result in new insights about the immune system.

Acknowledgments

I acknowledge the helpful discussions with the members of my laboratory, especially Tatyana Golovkina and John Dzuris, and my collaborator, Jaquelin Dudley. This work was supported by NIH Grants R01 CA45954 and CA52646.

References

Acha-Orbea, H., Shakhov, A. N., Scarpellino, L., Kolb, E., Muller, V., Vessaz-Shaw, A., Fuchs, R., Blochlinger, K., Rollini, P., Billotte, J., Sarafidou, M., MacDonald, H. R., and Diggelman, H. (1991). Clonal deletion of Vβ14-bearing T cells in mice transgenic for mammary tumor virus. *Nature (London)* **350,** 207–210.

Ando, Y., Wajjwalku, W., Niimi, N., Hiromatsu, K., Morishima, T., and Yoshikai, Y. (1995). Concomitant infection with exogenous mouse mammary tumor virus encoding I-E-dependent superantigen in I-E-negative mouse strain. *J. Immunol.* **154,** 6219–6226.

Ball, J., Arthur, L., and Dekaban, G. (1985). The involvement of type-B retrovirus in the induction of thymic lymphomas. *Virology* **140,** 159–182.

Beato, M., Herrlich, P., and Schutz, G. (1995). Steroid hormone receptors: Many actors in search of a plot. *Cell (Cambridge, Mass.)* **83,** 851–857.

Bentvelzen, P., and Daams, J. H. (1969). Hereditary infections with mammary tumor viruses in mice. *J. Natl. Cancer Inst. (U.S.)* **43,** 1025–1035.

Beutner, U., Draus, E., Kitamura, D., Rajewsky, K., and Huber, B. T. (1994). B cells are essential for murine mammary tumor virus transmission, but not for presentation of endogenous superantigens. *J. Exp. Med.* **179,** 1457–1466.

Bittner, J. J. (1936). Some possible effects of nursing on the mammary gland tumor incidence in mice. *Science* **84,** 162.

Bittner, J. J. (1958). Genetic concepts in mammary cancer in mice. *Ann. N.Y. Acad. Sci.* **71,** 943–975.

Bohach, G. A., Fast, D. J., Nelson, R. D., and Schlievert, P. M. (1990). Staphylococcal and streptococcal pyrogenic toxins involved in toxic shock syndrome and related illnesses. *CRC Crit. Rev. Microbiol.* **17,** 251–272.

Brandt-Carlson, C., and Butel, J. S. (1991). Detection and characterization of a glycoprotein encoded by the mouse mammary tumor virus long terminal repeat gene. *J. Virol.* **65,** 6051–6060.

Brandt-Carlson, C., Butel, J. S., and Wheeler, D. (1993). Phylogenetic and structural analysis of MMTV LTR ORF sequences of exogenous and endogenous origins. *Virology* **185,** 171–185.

Cardiff, R. D., and Muller, W. J. (1993). Transgenic mouse models of mammary tumorigenesis. *Cancer Surv.* **16,** 97–113.

Carr, J., Traina-George, V. L., and Cohen, J. (1985). Mouse mammary tumor virus gene expression regulated in trans by *Lps* locus. *Virology* **147,** 210–213.

Choi, Y., Kappler, J. W., and Marrack, P. (1991). A superantigen encoded in the open reading frame of the 3′ long terminal repeat of the mouse mammary tumor virus. *Nature* (*London*) **350**, 203–207.

Choi, Y., Marrack, P., and Kappler, J. W. (1992). Structural analysis of a mouse mammary tumor virus superantigen. *J. Exp. Med.* **175**, 847–862.

Choi, Y. C., Henrard, D. H., Lee, I., and Ross, S. R. (1987). The mouse mammary tumor virus long terminal repeat directs expression in epithelial and lymphoid cells of different tissues in transgenic mice. *J. Virol.* **61**, 3013–3019.

Coffin, J. M. (1990). Retroviridae and their replication. *In* "Virology" (B. N. Fields and D. M. Knipe, eds.), pp. 1437–1500. Raven Press, New York.

Cordingley, M. G., Riegel, A. T., and Hager, G. L. (1987). Steroid-dependent interaction of transcription factors with the inducible promoter of mouse mammary tumor virus in vivo. *Cell* (*Cambridge, Mass.*) **48**, 261–270.

Coutinho, A. (1976). Identification of the spleen B-cell defect in C3H/HeJ mice. *Scand. J. Immunol.* **5**, 129–140.

Dekaban, G., Ball, J., Robey, W., Arthur, L., and McCarter, J. (1984). Molecular biological characterization of a highly leukaemogenic virus isolated from the mouse. IV. Viral proteins. *J. Gen. Virol.* **65**, 1791–1802.

Dobrescu, D., Ursea, B., Pope, M., Asch, A. S., and Posnett, D. N. (1995). Enhanced HIV-1 replication in Vβ12 T cells due to human cytomegalovirus in monocytes: Evidence for a putative herpesvirus superantigen. *Cell* (*Cambridge, Mass.*) **82**, 753–763.

Donehower, L. A., Huang, A. L., and Hager, G. L. (1981). Regulatory and coding potential of the mouse mammary tumor virus long terminal redundancy. *J. Virol.* **37**, 226–238.

Dudley, J., and Risser, R. (1984). Amplification and novel locations of endogenous mouse mammary tumor virus genomes in mouse T-cell lymphomas. *J. Virol.* **49**, 92–101.

Duesberg, P. H., and Cardiff, R. D. (1968). Structural relationships between the RNA of mammary tumor virus and those of other RNA tumor viruses. *Virology* **49**, 92–101.

Dux, A. (1972). Genetic aspects in the genesis of mammary cancer. *In* "RNA Viruses and Host Genome in Oncogenesis" (P. Emmelot and P. Bentvelzen, eds.), pp. 301–308. North-Holland Publ., Amsterdam.

Dyson, P. J., Knight, A. M., Fairchild, S., Simpson, E., and Tomonari, K. (1991). Genes encoding ligands for deletion of Vβ11 T cells cosegregate with mammary tumour virus genomes. *Nature* (*London*) **349**, 531–532.

Dzuris, J. L., Golovkina, T. V., and Ross, S. R. (1997). Both T and B cells shed infectious moose mammary tumor virus. Submitted for publication.

Elliott, J., Pohajdak, B., Talbot, D., Shaw, J., and Paetkau, V. (1988). Phorbol diester-inducible, cyclosporine-suppressible transcription from a novel promoter within the mouse mammary tumor virus env gene. *J. Virol.* **62**, 1373–1380.

Festenstein, H. (1973). Immunogenetic and biological aspects of *in vitro* lymphocyte allotransformation (MLR) in the mouse. *Transplant. Rev.* **15**, 62–88.

Frankel, W. N., Rudy, C., Coffin, J. M., and Huber, B. T. (1991). Linkage of *Mls* genes to endogenous mammary tumour viruses of inbred mice. *Nature* (*London*) **349**, 526–528.

Fritsch, E. F., and Temin, H. M. (1977). Inhibition of viral DNA synthesis in stationary chicken embryo fibroblasts infected with avian retroviruses. *J. Virol.* **24**, 461–469.

Golovkina, T. V., Piazzon, I., Nepomnaschy, I., Buggiano, de Olano Viela, M., and Ross, S. R. Generation of a tumorigenic milk-borne mouse mammary tumor virus by recombination between endogenous and exogenous viruses. (Submitted for publication.) (1997).

Golovkina, T. V., Chervonsky, A., Dudley, J. P., and Ross, S. R. (1992). Transgenic mouse mammary tumor virus superantigen expression prevents viral infection. *Cell* (*Cambridge, Mass.*) **69**, 637–645.

Golovkina, T. V., Prescott, J. A., and Ross, S. R. (1993). Mouse mammary tumor virus-induced tumorigenesis in sag transgenic mice; a laboratory model of natural selection. *J. Virol.* **67**, 7690–7694.

Golovkina, T. V., Dudley, J. P., Jaffe, A., and Ross, S. R. (1995). Mouse mammary tumor viruses with functional superantigen genes are selected during in vivo infection. *Proc. Natl. Acad. Sci. U.S.A.* **92**, 4848–4832.

Golovkina, T. V., Prakash, O., and Ross, S. R. (1996). Endogenous mouse mammary tumor virus *Mtv*-17 is involved in *Mtv*-2-induced tumorigenesis in GR mice. *Virology* **218**:14–22.

Gunzburg, W. H., Heinemann, F., Wintersperger, S., Miethke, T., Wagner, H., Erfle, V., and Salmons, B. (1993). Endogenous superantigen expression controlled by a novel promoter in the MMTV long terminal repeat. *Nature* (*London*) **364**, 154–158.

Held, W., Shakhov, A. N., Waanders, G., Scarpellino, L., Luethy, R., Kraehenbuhl, J.-P., MacDonald, H. R., and Acha-Orbea, H. (1992). An exogenous mouse mammary tumor virus with properties of *Mls*-1a (*MTv*-7). *J. Exp. Med.* **175**, 1623–1633.

Held, W., Shaknow, A. N., Izui, S., Waanders, G. A., Scarpellino, L., MacDonald, H. R., and Acha-Orbea, H. (1993a). Superantigen-reactive $CD4^+$ T cells are required to stimulate B cells after infection with mouse mammary tumor virus. *J. Exp. Med.* **177**, 359–366.

Held, W., Waanders, G., Shakhov, A. N., Scarpellino, L., Acha-Orbea, H., and Robson-MacDonald, H. (1993b). Superantigen-induced immune stimulation amplifies mouse mammary tumor virus infection and allows virus transmision. *Cell* (*Cambridge, Mass.*) **74**, 529–540.

Held, W., Waanders, G. A., Achta-Orbea, H., and MacDonald, H. R. (1994a). Reverse transcriptase-dependent and -independent phases of infection with mouse mammary tumor virus: Implications for superantigen function. *J. Exp. Med.* **180**, 2347–2351.

Held, W., Waanders, G. A., MacDonald, H. R., and Acha-Orbea, H. (1994b). MHC class II hierarchy of superantigen presentation predicts efficiency of infection with mouse mammary tumor virus. *Int. Immunol.* **6**, 1403–1407.

Henrard, D., and Ross, S. R. (1988). Endogenous mouse mammary tumor virus is expressed in several organs in addition to the lactating mammary gland. *J. Virol.* **62**, 3046–3049.

Heston, W. E., Deringer, M. K., and Andervont, H. B. (1945). Gene-milk agent relationship in mammary tumor development. *J. Natl. Cancer Inst.* (*U.S.*) **5**, 289–307.

Hilkens, J., van der Zeust, B., Buijs, F., Kroezen, V., Bluemink, N., and Hilgers, J. (1983). Identification of a cellular receptor for mouse mammary tumor virus and mapping of its gene to chromosome 16. *J. Virol.* **45**, 140–147.

Hodes, R. J., Novick, M. B., Palmer, L. D., and Knepper, J. E. (1993). Association of a V beta 2-specific superantigen with a tumorigenic milk-borne mouse mammary tumor virus. *J. Immunol.* **150**, 1422–1428.

Hus, C.-L. L., Fabritius, C., and Dudley, J. (1988). Mouse mammary tumor virus proviruses in T-cell lymphomas lack a negative regulatory element in the long terminal repeat. *J. Virol.* **62**, 4644–4652.

Ignatowicz, L., Kappler, J., and Marrack, P. (1992). The effects of chronic infection with a superantigen-producing virus. *J. Exp. Med.* **175**, 917–923.

Indraccolo, S., Günzburg, W. H., Leib-Mosch, C., Erfle, V. and Salmons, B. (1995). Identification of three human sequences with viral superantigen-specific primers. *Mamm. Genome* **6**, 339–344.

Janeway, C. A., Jr., and Travers, P. (1994). "Immunobiology." Garland Publishing, New York.

Janeway, C. A., Jr., Yagi, J., Katz, M. E., Jones, B., Vroegop, S., and Buxser, S. (1989). T cell responses to *Mls* and to bacterial proteins that mimic its behavior. *Immunol. Rev.* **107**, 61–68.

Jouvin-Marche, E., Marche, P. N., Six, A., Liebe-Gris, C., Voegtle, D., and Cazenave, P.-A. (1993). Identification of an endogenous mouse mammary tumor virus involved in the clonal deletion of Vβ2 T cells. *Eur. J Immunol.* **23**, 2758–2764.

Kappler, J. W., Staerz, U., White, J., and Marrack, P. C. (1988). Self-tolerance eliminates T cells specific for *Mls*-modified products of the major histocompatibility complex. *Nature* (*London*) **332**, 35–40.

Karapetian, O., Shakhov, A. N., Kraehenbuhl, J.-P., and Acha-Orbea, H. (1994). Retroviral infection of neonatal Peyer's patch lymphocytes: The mouse mammary tumor virus model. *J. Exp. Med.* **180,** 1511–1516.

King, L. B., and Corley, R. B. (1990). Lipopolysaccharide and dexamethasone induce mouse mammary tumor proviral gene expression and differentiation in B lymphocytes through distinct regulatory pathways. *Mol. Cell. Biol.* **10,** 4211–4220.

Korman, A. J., Bourgarel, P., Meo, T., and Rieckhof, G. E. (1992). The mouse mammary tumor virus long terminal repeat encodes a type II transmember glycoprotein. *EMBO J.* **11,** 1901–1905.

Kozak, C., Peters, G., Pauley, R., Morris, V., Michalides, R., Dudley, J., Green, M., Davisson, M., Proksh, O., Vaidya, A., Hilgers, J., Verstraeten, A., Hynes, N., Diggelmann, H., Peterson, D., Cohen, J. C., Dickson, C., Sarkar, N., Nusse, R., Varmus, H., and Callahan, R. (1987). A standardized nomenclature for endogenous mouse mammary tumor viruses. *J. Virol.* **61,** 1651–1654.

Lafon, M., Scott-Algara, D., Marche, P. N., Cazenave, P., and Jouvin-Marche, E. (1994). Neonatal deletion and selective expansion of mouse T cells by exposure to rabies virus nucleocapsid superantigen. *J. Exp. Med.* **180,** 1207–1215.

Lewis, P. F., and Emerman, M. (1994). Passage through mitosis is required for oncoretroviruses but not for the human immunodeficiency virus. *J. Virol.* **68,** 510–516.

Lukacher, A. E., Ma, Y., Carroll, J. P., Abromson-Leeman, S. R., Laning, J. C., Dorf, M. E., and Benjamin, T. L. (1995). Susceptibility to tumors induced by polyoma virus is conferred by an endogenous mouse mammary tumor virus superantigen. *J. Exp. Med.* **181,** 1683–1692.

MacDonald, H. R., Schneider, R., Lees, R. K., Howe, R. C., Acha-Orbea, H., Festenstein, H., Zinkernagel, R. M., and Hengartner, H. (1988). T-cell receptor Vβ use predicts reactivity and tolerance to *Mls*a-encoded antigens. *Nature (London)* **332,** 40–45.

Marrack, P., and Kappler, J. (1990). The staphylococcal enterotoxins and their relatives. *Science* **248,** 705–711.

Marrack, P., Kushnir, E., and Kappler, J. (1991). A maternally inherited superantigen encoded by mammary tumor virus. *Nature (London)* **349,** 524–526.

Meyers, S., Gottlieb, P. D., and Dudley, J. P. (1989). Lymphomas with acquired mouse mammary tumor virus proviruses resemble distinct prethymic and intrathymic phenotypes defined in vivo. *J. Immunol.* **142,** 3342–3350.

Michalides, R. (1983). Lymphomagenesis by endogenous mouse mammary tumor virus in the GR mouse strain. *In* "Mechanisms of B-Cell Neoplasia" (J. Western-Schnurr, ed.), pp. 196–198. Editiones Roche, Hoffman LaRoche, Basel.

Michalides, R., van Deemter, L., Nusse, R., and van Nie, R. (1978). Identification of the *Mtv*-2 gene responsible for early appearance of mammary tumors in the GR mouse by nucleic acid hybridization. *Proc. Natl. Acad. Sci. U.S.A.* **75,** 2368–2372.

Michalides, R., Wagenaar, E., Hilkens, J., Hilgers, J., Groner, B., and Hynes, NE. (1982). Acquisition of proviral DNA of mouse mammary tumor virus in thymic leukemia cells from GR mice. *J. Virol.* **43,** 819–829.

Miller, C. L., Garner, R., and Paetkau, V. (1992). An activation-dependent, T-lymphocyte-specific transcriptional activator in the mouse mammary tumor virus env gene. *Mol. Cell. Biol.* **12,** 3262–3272.

Mink, S., Ponta, H., and Cato, A. C. B. (1990). The long terminal repeat region of the mouse mammary tumour virus contains multiple regulatory elements. *Nucleic Acids Res.* **18,** 2017–2023.

Mink, S., Hartig, E., Jennewein, P., Doppler, W., and Cato, A. C. B. (1992). A mammary cell-specific enhancer in mouse mammary tumor virus DNA is composed of multiple regulatory elements including binding sites for CTF/NF1 and novel transcription factor, mammary cell-activating factor. *Mol. Cell. Biol.* **11,** 4906–4918.

Mok, E., Golovkina, T. V., and Ross, S. R. (1992). A mouse mammary tumor virus (MMTV) mammary gland enhancer confers tissue-specific, but not lactation-dependent expression in transgenic mice. *J. Virol.* **66,** 7529–7532.

Moore, D. H., Long, C. A., Vaidya, A. B., Sheffield, J. B., Dion, A. S., and Lasfargues, E. Y. (1979). Mammary tumor viruses. *Adv. Cancer Res.* **29,** 347–418.

Muhlbock, O. (1965). Note on a new inbred mouse strain GR/A. *Eur. J. Cancer* **1,** 123–124.

Muhlbock, O., and Dux, A. (1972). MTV-variants and histocompatibility. *In* "Fundamental Research on Mammary Tumours" (J. Mouriquand, ed.), pp. 11–20. INSERM, Paris.

Nandi, S., and McGrath, C. M. (1973). Mammary neoplasia in mice. *Adv. Cancer Res.* **17,** 353–414.

Nusse, R. (1988). The *int* genes in mammary tumorigenesis and in normal development. *Trends Genet.* **4,** 291–295.

Nusse, R., and Varmus, H. E. (1982). Many tumors induced by the mouse mammary tumor virus contain a provirus integrated in the same region of the host genome. *Cell (Cambridge, Mass.)* **31,** 99–109.

Nusse, R., van Ooyen, A., Rijsewijk, F., van Lohuizen, M., Schuuring, E., and Van'T Veer, L. (1985). Retroviral insertional mutagenesis in murine mammary cancer. *Proc. R. Soc. London, Ser. B* **226,** 3–13

Outzen, H. C., Corrow, D., and Shultz, L. D. (1985). Attenuation of exogenous murine mammary tumor virus virulence in the C3H/HeJ mouse substrain bearing the *Lps* mutation. *JNCI, J. Natl. Cancer Inst.* **75,** 917–923.

Park, C. G., Jung, M., Choi, Y., and Winslow, G. M. (1995). Proteolytic processing is required for viral superantigen activity. *J. Exp. Med.* **181,** 1899–1904.

Peters, G. (1991). Inappropriate expression of growth factor genes in tumors induced by mouse mammary tumor virus. *Semin. Virol.* **2,** 319–328.

Pucillo, C., Cepeda, R., and Hodes, R. J. (1993). Expression of a MHC Class II transgene determines superantigenicity and susceptibility to mouse mammary tumor virus infection. *J. Exp. Med.* **178,** 1441–1445.

Pullen, A. M., Marrack, P., and Kappler, J. W. (1989). Evidence that *Mls*-2 antigens with delete Vβ3+ T cells are controlled by multiple genes. *J. Immunol.* **142,** 3033–3037.

Qin, W., Golovkina, T. V., Nepomnaschy, V., Buggiano, V., Piazzon, I., and Ross, S. R. (1977). A STAT site in the mouse mammary tumor virus long terminal repeat determines mammary gland expression *in vivo* (in preparation).

Reuss, F. U., and Coffin, J. M. (1995). Stimulation of mouse mammary tumor virus superantigen expression by an intragenic enhancer. *Proc. Natl. Acad. Sci. U. S. A.* **92,** 9293–9297.

Rijsewijk, F., Schuermann, M., Wagenaar, E., Parren, P., Weigel, D., and Nusse, R. (1987). The Drosophila homolog of the mouse mammary oncogene *int*-1 is identical to the segment polarity gene wingless. *Cell (Cambridge, Mass.)* **50,** 649–657.

Roe, T., Reynolds, T. C., Yu, G., and Brown, P. O. (1983). Integration of murine leukemia virus DNA depends on mitosis. *EMBO J.* **12,** 2099–2108.

Ross, S. R., and Golovkina, T. V. (1995). The role of endogenous *Mtvs* in resistance to MMTV-induced mammary tumors. *In* "Viral Superantigens" (K. Tomonari, ed.). CRC Press, Boca Raton, FL (in press).

Ross, S. R., Hsu, C.-L., Choi, Y., Mok, E., and Dudley, J. P. (1990). Negative regulation in correct tissue-specific expression of mouse mammary tumor virus in transgenic mice. *Mol. Cell. Biol.* **10,** 5822–5829.

Sage, R. D. (1981). Wild mice. *In* "The Mouse" (H. L. Foster, J. D. Small, and J. G. Fox, eds.), Vol. 1, pp. 40–90. Academic Press, New York.

Schindler, C., and Darnell, J. E., Jr. (1995). Transcriptional responses to polypeptide ligands: The JAK-STAT pathway. *Annu. Rev. Biochem.* **64,** 621–651.

Shakhov, A. N., Wang, H., Acha-Orbea, H., Pauley, R. J., and Wei, W.-Z. (1993). A new infectious mammary tumor virus in the milk of mice implanted with C4 hyperplastic alveolar nodules. *Eur. J. Immunol.* **23,** 2765–2769.

Simpson, E., Dyson, P. J., Knight, A. M., Robinson, P. J., Elliott, J. I., and Altmann, D. M. (1993). T-cell receptor repertoire selection by mouse mammary tumor viruses and MHC molecules. *Immunol. Rev.* **131,** 93–115.

Squartini, F., Olivi, M., and Bolis, G. B. (1970). Mouse strain and breeding stimulation as factors influencing the effect of thymectomy on mammary tumorigenesis. *Cancer Res.* **30,** 2069–2072.

Stewart, T. A., Pattengale, P. K., and Leder, P. (1984). Spontaneous mammary adenocarcinomas in transgenic mice that carry and express MTV/myc fusion genes. *Cell (Cambridge, Mass.)* **38,** 627–637.

Theunissen, H. J. M., Paardekooper, M., Maduro, L. J., Michalides, R. J. A. M., and Nusse, R. (1989). Phorbol ester-inducible T-cell-specific expression of variant mouse mammary tumor virus long terminal repeats. *J. Virol.* **63,** 3466–3471.

Thomas, K. R., and Capecchi, M. R. (1990). Targeted disruption of the murine *int*-1 proto-oncogene resulting in severe abnormalities in midbrain and cerebellar development. *Nature (London)* **346,** 847–850.

Tomonari, K., Fairchild, S., and Rosenwasser, O. A. (1993). Influence of viral superantigens on Vβ- and Vα-specific positive and negative selection. *Immunol. Rev.* **131,** 131–168.

Toohey, M. G., Lee, J. W., Huang, M., and Peterson, D. O. (1990). Functional elements of the steroid hormone-responsive promoter of mouse mammary tumor virus. *J. Virol.* **64,** 4477–4488.

Tsubura, A., Inaba, M., Imai, S., Murakami, A., Oyaizu, N., Yasumizu, R., Ohnishi, Y., Tanaka, H., Moril, S., and Ikehara, S. (1988). Intervention of T-cells in transportation of mouse mammary tumor virus (milk factor) to mammary gland cells in vivo. *Cancer Res.* **48,** 6555–6559.

van Ooyen, A. J., Michalides, R. J., and Nusse, R. (1983). Structural analysis of a 1.7kb mouse mammary tumor virus-specific RNA. *J. Virol.* **46,** 362–370.

Varmus, H. E., Bishop, J. M., Nowinski, R. C., and Sarker, N. H. (1972). Mammary tumour virus specific nucleotide sequences in mouse DNA. *Nature (London)* **238,** 189–191.

Waanders, G. A., Shakhov, A. N., Held, W., Karapetian, P., Acha-Orbea, H., and MacDonald, H. R. (1993). Peripheral T cell activation and deletion induced by transfer of lymphocyte subsets expressing endogenous or exogenous mouse mammary tumor virus. *J. Exp. Med.* **177,** 1359–1366.

Wajjwalku, W., Ando, Y., Niimi, N., and Yoshikai, Y. (1995). A novel exogenous mouse mammary tumor virus encoding MHC class II H2E-independent superantigen specific for Tcr-Vβ14. *Immunogenetics* **41,** 156–158.

Wheeler, D. A., Butel, J. S., Medina, D., Cardiff, R. D., and Hager, G. L. (1983). Transcription of mouse mammary tumor virus: identification of a candidate mRNA for the long terminal repeat gene product. *J. Virol.* **46,** 42–52.

White, J., Herman, A., Pullen, A. M., Kubo, R., Kappler, J. W., and Marrack, P. (1989). The Vβ-specific superantigen staphylococcal enterotoxin B: Stimulation of mature T cells and clonal deletion in neonatal mice. *Cell (Cambridge, Mass.)* **56,** 27–35.

Winslow, G. M., Marrack, P., and Kappler, J. W. (1994). Processing and major histocompatibility complex binding of the MTV7 superantigen. *Immunity* **1,** 23–33.

Woodland, D. L., Lund, F. E., Happ, M. P., Blackman, M. A., Palmer, E., and Corley, R. B. (1992). Endogenous super-antigen expression is controlled by mouse mammary tumor proviral loci. *J. Exp. Med.* **174,** 1255–1258.

Yamamoto, K. (1985). Steroid receptor regulated transcription of specific genes and gene networks. *Annu. Rev. Genet.* **19,** 209–252.

Yanagawa, S.-I., Kakimi, K., Tanaka, H., Murakami, A., Nakagawa, Y., Kubo, Y., Yamada, Y., Hiai, H., Kuribayashi, K., Amsuda, T., and Ishimoto, A. (1993). Mouse mammary tumor virus with rearranged long terminal repeats causes murine lymphomas. *J. Virol.* **67,** 112–118.

Yazdanbakhsh, K., Park, C. G., Winslow, G. M., and Choi, Y. (1993). Direct evidence for the role of COOH terminus of mouse mammary tumor virus superantigen in determining T cell receptor Vβ specificity. *J. Exp. Med.* **178**, 737–741.

Yoshimoto, T., Nagase, H., Nakano, H., Matsuzawa, A., and Nariuchi, H. (1994). A Vβ8.2-specific superantigen from exogenous mouse mammary tumor virus carried by FM mice. *Eur. J. Immunol.* **24**, 1612–1619.

Charles P. Taylor*
Lakshmi S. Narasimhan†

*Department of Neurological and Neurodegenerative Diseases
and †Department of Chemistry
Parke-Davis Pharmaceutical Research Division
Warner-Lambert Co.
Ann Arbor, Michigan 48105

Sodium Channels and Therapy of Central Nervous System Diseases

Voltage-dependent Na^+ channels have long been recognized targets for anti-arrhythmic and local anesthetic drugs. Since the mid-1980s, Na^+ channels have become widely accepted as the primary target of anticonvulsants with pharmacological profiles similar to phenytoin, carbamazepine, and lamotrigine. Results from animal models and a few preliminary clinical trials suggest that this class of drugs may also offer significant potential for reducing the neuronal damage caused by ischemic stroke, head trauma, and perhaps certain neurodegenerative diseases. Studies using site-directed mutations of Na^+ channels with electrophysiology have provided extensive insight into both the physiology and the interaction of drug molecules with ion channels. This review includes an introduction to Na^+ channel structure, molecular biology, and physiology as they relate to pharmacology. A review of several *in vitro* actions of Na^+ channel blockers is provided. Neuroprotective actions with a variety of Na^+ channel blockers in models of central nervous system disease in animals and *in vitro* models are reviewed. Although

Advances in Pharmacology, Volume 39

1054-3589/97/$25.00

many voltage-dependent Na^+ channel blockers have additional pharmacological targets, the hypothesis that anticonvulsant and neuroprotective actions result from the blockade of Na^+ channels is explored.

I. Introduction

It has been appreciated since the landmark studies of Hodgkin and Huxley (1952) that voltage-gated Na^+ channels are responsible for the action potential of axonal nerve fibers. Since that time, a wealth of information has accumulated on the localization, structure, molecular biology, and function of Na^+ channels and on the drugs that modify them. Functional Na^+ channels are located not only in axonal membranes, but also in cell bodies and dendrites of neurons of the mammalian brain (Westenbroek *et al.*, 1989). Most Na^+ channels are sensitive to the specific blocker tetrodotoxin (TTX), which has been used to pharmacologically define Na^+ channels. TTX-sensitive channels cause action potential propagation in dendrites (Colling and Wheal, 1994; Stuart and Sakmann, 1994; Callaway and Ross, 1995) and amplify synaptic potentials and other subthreshold potentials, facilitating their propagation along dendritic structures (Schwindt and Crill, 1995; Stuart and Sakmann, 1995; Hu and Hvalby, 1992). The hallmark of Na^+ channels is their short open time, which leads to action potentials in nerve fibers that last about 1 msec. The blockade of Na^+ channels by TTX is independent of membrane voltage [except in some cases, hyperpolarization increases block, see Patton and Goldin (1991)]. In contrast, a class of voltage-dependent Na^+ channel blockers represented by lidocaine, phenytoin, carbamazepine, and lamotrigine block channels significantly only if cells are depolarized, with little drug action at hyperpolarized membrane potentials. Such voltage-dependent Na^+ channel blockers are a major subject of this review.

In many or even all neuronal preparations, very small persistent Na^+ currents arise from sustained or repeated Na^+ channel openings. These persistent currents last much longer than the 1 to 5 msec of action potentials (Llinas and Sugimori, 1980; Stafström *et al.*, 1985; French *et al.*, 1990; Stys *et al.*, 1993; reviewed by Taylor, 1993). Persistent Na^+ current is only 2 to 5% as large as the maximal Na^+ current activated during action potentials, but it may be important for several physiological and pathophysiological functions. Persistent currents are sensitive to TTX and have single-channel properties suggesting that they arise from the same class of Na^+ channels responsible for action potentials (Alzheimer *et al.*, 1993b; Brown *et al.*, 1994b; Moorman *et al.*, 1990). Persistent Na^+ currents probably result from a mode shift in Na^+ channel gating to a state with a reduced likelihood of inactivation, allowing multiple channel openings (Brown *et al.*, 1994a; Alzheimer *et al.*, 1993a; Keynes, 1994). The voltage dependence of activation for persistent Na^+ currents is somewhat different than for peak Na^+ current, with persistent current activating at significantly less depolarized voltage than rapid current (Brown *et al.,* 1994a). Persistent Na^+ currents can cause long-lasting depolarizing plateau potentials that result in bistable membrane voltage (Llinas and Sugimori, 1980; Steinberg, 1990; French *et al.,* 1990; Cerne and Spain, 1995). Bistability means that membrane voltage is stable near rest potential, but if neurons become depolarized momentarily, they tend to depolarize almost completely and to remain depolarized for a long time. Although Na^+-dependent plateaus have been observed mostly in preparations when repolarizing K^+ currents are blocked, the persistent Na^+ current underlying plateau potentials may still influence the behavior of neurons in a variety of circumstances, particularly during situations of abnormal excitability or deprivation of energy substrate. Similar bistable membrane potentials are also associated with inward current from the voltage dependence of NMDA-type glutamate receptors (Flatman *et al.,* 1983).

It is likely that the bistability of membrane voltage conferred by persistent Na^+ conductance (French *et al.,* 1990) is involved with the repeated depolarizing waves associated with seizures, spreading depression and the sustained depolarizations of ischemic brain tissues (Nedergaard and Hansen, 1993; Nedergaard and Astrup, 1986; Hansen, 1985). Persistent inward Na^+ currents may cause or trigger the pronounced increase of intracellular Na^+ concentration observed during hypoxia (Hansen, 1985; Kass *et al.,* 1992; LoPachin and Stys, 1995). It is remarkable and perhaps not coincidental that the blockade of either NMDA conductance or Na^+ conductance results in anticonvulsant (Rogawski and Porter, 1990) and neuroprotective actions (Taylor and Meldrum, 1995), as either type of conductance can lead to prolonged neuronal depolarization.

Therefore, drugs that selectively block voltage-sensistive Na^+ channels and particularly persistent Na^+ currents are a reasonable choice for treating epilepsy, stroke, cerebral ischemia, and head trauma. The local anesthetic and anti-arrythmic action of voltage-dependent Na^+ channel blockers has been reviewed previously, (e.g., Catterall, 1987). This review focuses on recent advances in the structure and function of Na^+ channels and on the molecular and neurological disease targets of novel Na^+ channel blockers.

II. Structure and Function of Voltage-Dependent Na^+ Channels

A single Na^+ channel α subunit protein molecule spans the plasma membrane (see Fig. 1) and is thought to comprise an independent Na^+ selective channel. Studies with molecular biological approaches, particularly site-directed mutagenesis of Na^+ channel proteins and functional expression of mutant channels have pinpointed regions that are involved in different functions of the channel; these studies were reviewed previously by Catterall

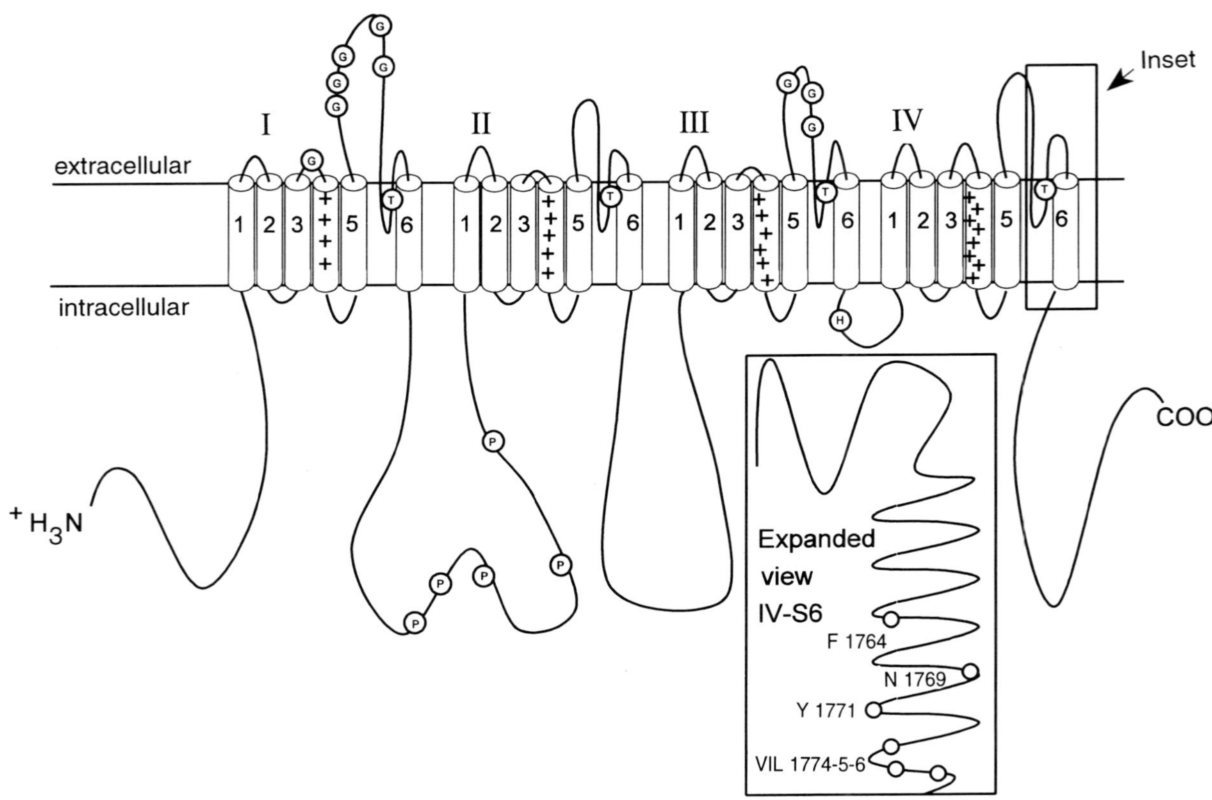
Inset
I
II
III
IV
extracellular
intracellular
+H3N
COO-
Expanded
view
IV-S6
F 1764
N 1769
Y 1771
VIL 1774-5-6

(1992). Each α subunit molecule consists of four homologous domains (I–IV) and each domain consists of six transmembrane segments (S1–S6). Each membrane-spanning segment is an amphipathic α helix of about 22 amino acids. Between each of the six transmembrane segments and particularly between each of the four larger domains are extensive regions that fold out from the membrane. Highly charged S4 segments of each domain (marked with "+" charges in Fig. 1) transduce transmembrane electrical voltage by moving across the transmembrane electrical field. This movement causes conformational changes that result in opening or "gating" of the ion-conducting pathway. Opening of the channel, also called "activation," allows sodium ions to passively enter the cell down the Na^+ concentration gradient, depolarizing the membrane.

The regions between the S5 and the S6 segments in all four domains fold so as to form part of the extracellular mouth of the channel, and the S6 segments line the ion-conducting pore. Mutations or chimeras formed from specific regions of Na^+ channels alter channel properties such as Ca^{2+} and Na^+ ion selectivity (Heinemann *et al.*, 1992). Although the three-dimensional structure of Na^+ channels is not known, most researchers (Kallen *et al.*, 1993; Guy and Durell, 1994; Noda *et al.*, 1986) assume that the transmembrane segments of each of the four domains fold similarly to models of voltage-sensitive potassium channel proteins. K^+ channels exist as a tetramer of identical subunits (Guy and Conti, 1990; Durell and Guy, 1992) rather than a single protein with four domains. Each of the four subunits of a K^+ channel is thought to exist as a closely packed group of transmembrane helices arranged in a "rosette" around the central ion-conducting pore (Durell and Guy, 1992). Presumably, the four homologous domains of Na^+ channels act much as the four identical subunits of a K^+ channel.

In addition to the main (260 kDa) α subunit of Na^+ channels, there are two auxilliary subunits that copurify with the α protein, the β-1 subunit (36 kDa) and the β-2 subunit (33 kDa). The functions of β subunits are subsidiary to the α subunit of Na^+ channels because the basic physiology and the action of several toxins and drugs with isolated α subunits are

FIGURE 1 Na^+ channel structure, including regions of the protein that have been associated with various functions. Modified from Catterall (1992) with kind permission from the American Physiological Society. T, the TTX-binding site; H, the crucial portion of the inactivation gate; +, the charged portion that senses membrane voltage and is necessary for activation gating; P, phosphorylation sites along an extensive cytosolic loop that is absent in skeletal muscle and eel electroplax (Trimmer and Agnew, 1989). G, sites of extracellular glycosylation (Trimmer and Agnew, 1989). (Inset) An expanded view of the domain IV-S6 region, crucial for the binding of local anesthetics (Ragsdale *et al.*, 1994) and phenytoin. Numbering of amino acid residues begins at the amino (NH_2) terminus and continues sequentially through approximately 1800 amino acids toward the carboxyl (COOH) terminus. See text for details.

similar to those of native Na^+ channels (West *et al.*, 1992b; Ragsdale *et al.*, 1994; Joho *et al.*, 1990b). Na^+ channel β-1 subunits are found in association with brain, cardiac, and skeletal muscle Na^+ channels, whereas β-2 subunits are found only with brain Na^+ channels. β-2 subunits of brain channels bind to the α subunit via covalent disulfide bonds. The rate and voltage dependence of inactivation of Na^+ currents from cloned α subunits expressed in *Xenopus* oocytes (Isom *et al.*, 1992) or mammmalian cells (Isom *et al.*, 1995b) are altered by the coexpression of β-1 subunits. Furthermore, the number of toxin-binding sites and density of Na^+ currents in mammalian cells is greatly increased by the coexpression of β-1 subunits, suggesting that β-1 subunits are involved in the folding or membrane incorporation of α subunits (Catterall, 1992). In addition, β-2 subunits increase the functional expression of Na^+ current, alter the voltage dependence and kinetics of channel gating, and cause a surprising increase in the membrane infolding of *Xenopus* oocytes (Isom *et al.*, 1995a). These findings indicate that β-1 and β-2 subunits modulate the expression and function of α subunits and possibly alter other cell functions. No drugs are known to interact directly with β subunits; therefore the α subunit is the primary target of drug discovery to date.

A. Genetic Subtypes and Mutations of Na^+ Channels

Rat Na^+ channel α subunits are coded by several distinct genes or paralogs, each of which has an ortholog (corresponding gene) in other mammalian species. The gene products in rats have been divided into several categories (Table I) and mapped to defined gene loci (Table II). In several cases, the human genes have been identified and cloned (Tables I and II) (Burgess *et al.*, 1995; Kallen *et al.*, 1993). The main ion-conducting α subunit of each of these subtypes is a single gene product of about 1800 amino acids. The remainder of this section discusses the molecular biology and structural analysis of mammalian brain Na^+ channel α subunits.

1. Clones, Amino Acid Sequences, Homology, and Spontaneous Mutations

The cloned and functionally expressed Na^+ channel α subunit proteins from rat brain are called type I, type II, type III, and type VI (Kallen *et al.*, 1993; Trimmer *et al.*, 1989; Catterall, 1992; Noda *et al.*, 1986; Schaller *et al.*, 1995). To avoid confusion, the gene locus names will be used in addition to the protein names because the locus designations are consistent in different species. For example, Scn1a is used for the rat gene and SCN1A for the human gene. The use of gene locus names to describe gene products is useful because protein designations tend to differ depending on when they were first described, whereas the gene locus names are consistent and based on sequence relationships. The known rat brain Na^+ channels are listed in Table I. It is likely that additional mammalian brain Na^+ channels remain

TABLE I Cloned Na^+ Channel α-Subunit cDNAs

Gene locus (see table II) (species)	*AA identify*[a] *w/rat type II*	*Alpha subunit names*	*Sites of expression (TTX sensitivity)*	*Number of AA residues*	*Predicted m_r (kDa)*	*GenBank or PIR accession number for sequence*	*Molecular biology reference*
Not identified (electric eel)	62.6%	—	Electroplax (TTX sensitive)	1820	208	X01119	Noda *et al.* (1984)
Scn1a (rat)	88.0%	Type I, NaCh1	Brain (TTX sensitive)	2009	229	X03638	Noda *et al.* (1986)
Scn2a (rat)	—	Type II, NaCh2	Brain (TTX sensitive)	2005	228	X03639 human: M94055 (Ahmed *et al.*, 1992)	Schmidt and Catterall (1986); Noda *et al.* (1986) splice var. IIA: Auld *et al.* (1988)
Scn3a (rat)	87.3%	Type III, NaCh3	Brain (neonate) (TTX sensitive)	1951	221	Y00766	Kayano *et al.* (1988)
Scn4a (mouse)	73.0%	SkM 1	Skeletal muscle (TTX sensitive)	1840	209	PIR: JN0007 human:PIR: JS0648 (George *et al.*, 1992b)	Trimmer *et al.* (1989); Kallen *et al.* (1990)
Scn5a (mouse)	66.1%	h1, SkM2	Heart, immature skeletal muscle (TTX resistant)	2018	227	PIR: A33996 human: M77235 (Gellens *et al.*, 1992)	Rogart *et al.* (1989); White *et al.* (1991)
SCN6A (human)		HUMNACH	Heart, uterus			human: M91556 (George *et al.*, 1992a)	
Snc7a (mouse)		Na-G	Glial cells			(partial sequence)	Gautron *et al.* (1992)
Scn8a (mouse, rat)	75.5%	NaCh6	Neuron and glial cells	1976	225	rat: L39018; mouse: U26707	Schaller *et al.* (1995) Burgess *et al.* (1995)
Not identified (rat)	60.0%	TTXi	Sensory neurons (TTX resistant)	1957	220	X92184	Akopian *et al.* (1996) Sangameswaran *et al.*, (1996)
Scn9a (rabbit)		Nas	Schwann cells (glia)	1984			Belcher *et al.* (1995)

[a] Identities were calculated with the Bestfit program of the Wisconsin Package (Genetics Computer Group, Madison, WI) using default parameters.

TABLE II Chromosome Locations of Na^+ Channel α-Subunit Genes[a]

Gene locus (human chromosome location)	*α-subunit name or ortholog protein name*	*Human mapping reference (if human sequence available)*	*Map location of orthologous genes*	*Ortholog mapping reference*
SCN1A (2q24)	Type I brain	Malo *et al.* (1994a)	Mouse: chr 2 Rat: chr 3	Malo *et al.* (1991)
SCN2A (2q23–24.1)	Type II brain	Litt *et al.* (1989)	Mouse: chr 2 Rat: chr 3	Malo *et al.* (1991); Ahmed *et al.* (1992) Zha *et al.* (1994)
SCN3A (2q24–31)	Type III brain	Malo *et al.* (1994b)	Mouse: chr 2 Rat: chr 3	Malo *et al.* (1991)
SCN4A (17q23.1–25.3)	SkM1 Skeletal muscle	George *et al.* (1991) George *et al.* (1992b)	Mouse: chr 11	Ambrose *et al.* (1992)
SCN5A (3p21)	HHIA (heart TTX resistant)	George *et al.* (1995) Gellens *et al.* (1992)	Mouse: chr 9	Schleef *et al.* (1993)
SCN6A (2q21–23)	Heart, uterus HUMNACH	George *et al.* (1994)		
SCN7A (2q36–37)	Glia	Potts *et al.* (1993)	Mouse: chr 2	Potts *et al.* (1993)
SCN8A (12q13)	Brain, spinal cord	Burgess *et al.* (1995)	Mouse: chr 15	Burgess *et al.* (1995)
Scn9a (unidentified)	Schwann cells	—	Mouse: chr 2	Belcher *et al.* (1995)

[a] Adapted from Burgess *et al.* (1995) with permission.

to be discovered and described. Furthermore, it is clear that splice variants of each Na^+ channel gene occur with important functional consequences. For example, type II channels are expressed in adult cells as an alternatively spliced variant called type IIA (Auld *et al.,* 1988, 1990) that has similar functional properties to type II and differs by seven amino acids out of approximately 1800. Because these splice varients are identical except in one small region, type IIA channels would not be distinguished from type II by techniques such as the RNase protection assay unless the assay is sensitive enough to detect the alternatively spliced exon.

Each α subunit protein contains approximately 1800 amino acids. The different gene products from brain (Scn1a, Scn2a, Scn3a, Scn8a) are assumed to produce similar structures, as they have 75 to 88% overall amino acid identity. However, the amino acid sequence identity is only about 60% between brain channels and Na^+ channels from peripheral sensory neurons, skeletal muscle, or cardiac tissue (Table I). Conservative amino acids (similar in chemical properties, but not necessarily identical) account for 90 to 94% of the differences between the sequences of Scn1a, Scn2a, and Scn3a Na^+ channels. Therefore, it is postulated that these three channels are recently diverged by gene duplication. The relatedness between various Na^+ channel genes is shown by a "dendrogram" in Fig. 2. A dendrogram depicts sequence similarity between amino acids in aligned sequences determined by an automated sequence alignment and comparison procedure (BESTFIT program). In the dendrogram, percentage similarity is shown by the distance between branch points. Although dendrogram analysis does not directly determine the genetic similarity between channel sequences, distances on the dendrogram give an approximation of both the genetic and the structural relatedness between channel types.

The genes encoding brain Na^+ channels (SCN1A, SCN2A, SCN3A, and SCN8A), as well as genes expressed in other tissues, have been mapped to specific human, mouse, and rat chromosomes (Table II). For each Na^+ channel gene, the human chromosome locus has been mapped, often by *in situ* hybridization of fluorescently labeled cloned DNA sequences to specific chromosome bands (Burgess *et al.,* 1995). Four human cDNAs have been cloned (see Table I column 7 for references to cDNA databases).

Comparison of amino acid sequences of the rat Na^+ channel genes reveals high homology in several specific regions of the channel. For example, several transmembrane regions are almost completely conserved across all the known Na^+ channel genes, and when substitutions occur, the substituted amino acids are mostly chemically similar (Trimmer and Agnew, 1989). Other highly conserved regions comprise voltage sensors, Na^+ selectivity filters, and the inactivation gate (Fig. 3A). In contrast, relatively little homology occurs between Na^+ channel sequences within cytosolic loops such as between domains I and II (Fig. 3B). The I–II loop is shortened in skeletal muscle Na^+ channels (Scn4a and Scn5a) and also has deletions in the TTX-resistant sensory neuronal channel and the type III channel (Scn3a). The

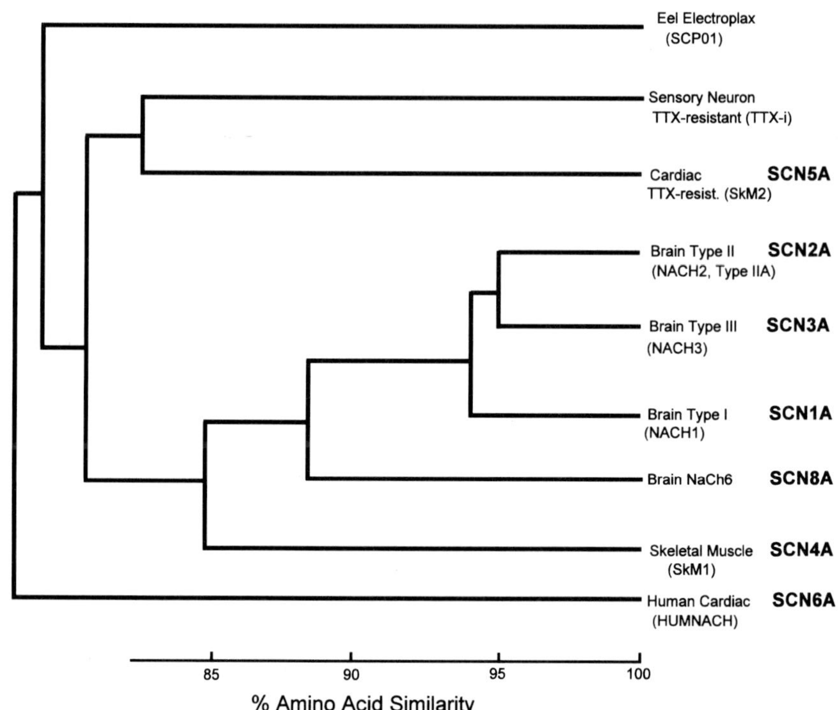

FIGURE 2 Dendrogram showning genetic similarity between sequences of cloned rat Na^+ channels. Analysis was based on published amino acid sequences, and distance was determined by the Bestfit program of the Wisconsin Package using default parameters (Version 8, Sep. 1994, Genetics Computer Group, Madison, WI). The percentage sequence similarity (identical or chemically similar amino acid residues at each position), using the full amino acid sequence, is indicated on the abscissa and was determined from a comparison table (Staden, 1982) based on the relatedness odds matrix analysis of Dayhoff (1996). Note that the genetic distance between brain channels (type I, II, III, and VI) is less than the distance from these channels to other Na^+ channel types expressed in heart, skeletal muscle, glia, or sensory neurons. However, the recently cloned type VI channel of brain (Scn8a) appears to be significantly distant from other brain channels, and the TTX-insensitive channel of the peripheral nerve is even more distant. As might be expected, the eel electroplax channel (SCP01) is relatively distantly related to mammalian channels. In cases that human clones are available (see Table II), the similarity between the human clone and the corresponding (orthologous) rat clone is usually within 1 to 3%.

I–II cytosolic loop is the major region of both Na^+ channels and Ca^{2+} channels that is modulated by phosphorylation or GTP-dependent proteins. Because of sequence variations in this region, the I–II loop was chosen for the production of subtype-specific antibodies (see later).

Extracellular loops within domains I and III contain sites that are highly glycosylated (Trimmer and Agnew, 1989a); post-translational glycosylation is required for normal membrane incorporation and function of Na^+ channels (Schmidt and Catterall, 1986).

A

Domain III-IV cytosolic loop of rat channels (inactivation gate w/ critical sequence [**IFM**]):

```
Gene    1474 (Amino acid sequence number)                       1525
Scn2a   DNFNQQKKKF GGQDIFMTEE QKKYYNAMKK LGSKKPQKPI PRPANKFQGM VF
Scn1a   ---------- ---------- ---------- ---------- ---G------ --
Scn3a   ---------- ---------- ---------- ---------- ---------- --
Scn4a   ---------- --K------- ---------- ---------- ---Q--I--- -Y
Scn5a   ---------L ---------- ---------- ---------- ---L--Y--F I-
Scn8a   ---------- ---------- ---------- ---------- ---L--I--I --
Scn9a   ---------L ---------- ---------- ---------- ---L--Y--F --
```

Domain IV, segment 6 (local anesthetic [**FNY**] and inactivation gate [**VIL**] binding sites):

```
        1755                  1776
Scn2a   FFVSYIIISF LVVVNMYIAV IL
Scn1a   ---------- ---------- -
Scn3a   ---------- ---------- -
Scn4a   --C------- -I-------I -
Scn5a   --TT------ -I-------I -
Scn8a   ---------- -I----C--I -
Scn9a   --TT------ -I-------- -
```

Single-letter amino acid codes:

A Alanine	I Isoleucine	R Arginine
C Cysteine	K Lysine	S Serine
D Aspartic acid	L Leucine	T Threonine
E Glutamic acid	M Methionine	V Valine
F Phenylalanine	N Asparagine	W Tryptophan
G Glycine	P Proline	Y Tyrosine
H Histidine	Q Glutamine	

FIGURE 3 (A) Alignment of amino acid sequences for seven cloned rat Na^+ channels in regions of interest (single-letter amino acid designations are shown at bottom). Amino acid sequence numbers (top line) correspond to the type II channel (Scn2a) and are shown for comparison. The multiple alignments were generated using the Pileup program with default parameters (Program Manual for the Wisconsin Package, Version 8, Sept., 1994, Genetics Computer Group, Madison, WI). The type II sequence is shown at the top because it is the most common in brain; other clones are shown in order of their gene locus names rather than the order from the analysis (Scn5a, 9a, 4a, 2a, 3a, 1a, 8a), which corresponds to the branch sequence in the dendrogram (Fig.2). Identical amino acids from other channel subtypes are shown with a hyphen (-) and deletions by dots (·). Nonhomologous amino acids are shown in bold print if they are chemically dissimilar from the type II seqence. The alignment of amino acids in III–IV intracellular loop and in the IV–S6 (see Fig. 1 for orientation) shows that sequences comprising the inactivation gate and the putative binding site for local anesthetics are almost completely conserved and that substitutions are mostly chemically similar. Transmembrane segments were identified by comparison to the reported sequence of Scn5a in the Swissprot database (Wisconsin Package). The multiple alignments shown here and in B were extracted from the multiple alignment of the complete α-subunit channel proteins. (B) As in A except showing alignment of amino acids in the cytosolic I–II loop. There are large variations in sequence between different channel α proteins, including deletions in skeletal muscle channels (Scn4a and Scn5a), in type III channels (Scn3a), and in a sequence expressed in glial cells (Scn9a). Consensus sequences for protein phosphorylation of the Scn2a channel by cytosolic kinases are shown by symbols [cyclic A kinase (*), protein kinase C ($), casein kinase (#), both cAMP and PKC in same region (&)]. Consensus sites were identified using the Motifs program of the Wisconsin Package.

B

Domain I-II cytosolic loop (phosphorylation sites of Scn2a shown above sequence):

```
     459                                              & &                  513
Scn2a    EAQAAA.... AA.ASAESRD FSGAGGIGVF SESSSVASKL SSKSEKELKN RRKKKKQKEQ
Scn1a    A--Q--.... --T--EH--E P-A-...-RL -D---E---- ----A--RR- ----R-----
Scn3a    ---.-V.... --.---A--- ---I--L-EL L----E---- ----A--WR- ----RR-R-H
Scn4a    -LE....... .......... .......... .......... .......... ...-A-AAQA
Scn5a    ALT....... .......... ...IR-VDTV -R--LEM-P- APVTNH-R-S K-R-R....L
Scn8a    ------MATS -GTV-EDAIE EE-ED-V-S. PR---EL--- ----A--RR- ----R----L
Scn9a    VLE....... .......... ...AL--DTT -LQ-HSG-P- A-KNAN-RRP -V--R....V

     514               #     $                        *       $       $    571
Scn2a    AGEEEK..ED AVRKSASEDS IRKKGFQFSL EGSRLTYEKR FSSPHQSLLS IRGSLFSPRR
Scn1a    S-G---.DD- EFH--E---- --R---R--I --N------- Y--------- ----------
Scn3a    LEGNHRADG- RFP--E---- VKRRS-LL-- D-NP--GDKK LC-------- ----------
Scn4a    LESG-EADG- PTHNKDCNG- L......... .......... .......... ..........
Scn5a    SSGT-DGGD- RLP--D---G P-........ .......... .ALNQL--TH GLSRTSMRP-
Scn8a    SEG---GDPE K-F--E--YG M-R-A-RLP. .DN-I..GRK --IMN----- -P--P-LS-H
Scn9a    SEGSTD..DN RSPQ-DPYNQ R-........ .......... .....M-F.. .LGLSSGR--

     572  *                 #          ##      &   *                       625
Scn2a    NSRASLFNFK GR.VKDIGSE NDFADDEHST FEDNDSRRDS LFVPHRHGER RP.....SNV
Scn1a    ---T---S-R --.A--V--- ---------- ----E----- ----R----- -N.....--L
Scn3a    --KT-I-S-R --.A--V--- ---------- ---SE----- ------P--- -N.....--.
Scn4a    .......... .......... ......DA-. G-KGPP-PSC .......... ..........
Scn5a    S--G-I-T-R ..R.R-Q--- A------N-- AGESE-H-T- -L--WPLRHP SAQGQPGPGA
Scn8a    --KS-I-S-G DPSVR-P--- -E-------- V-ESEG---- --I-I-AR-- -SSYSGY-GY
Scn9a    A-HG-V-H-R APS.Q--SFP DGITP-DGVF HG-QE---G- ILLGR....G AGQTGPLPRS

     626                       #                                           674
Scn2a    SQASRASRGI PTLPMNGKMH SAVDCNGVVS LVGGPSALTS PVGQLLPE.. .........G
Scn1a    --T--S--ML AG--A----- -T-------- ------VP-- --------VI IDKPATDDN-
Scn3a    .......... .......... .......... .......... .......... .........-
Scn4a    .......... .......... .......... .......... .......... ..........
Scn5a    -........A -GYVL---RN -T-------- -L-AGD-EAT SPGSY-LRPM VLDRPPDTTT
Scn8a    --C--S--IS -A.CAQREAN -T-------- -I-PGS.... HIGR--LRQR LRW.......
Scn9a    P........L -QS-NP-RR. .....H-EEG QL-VPTGELT AGA....... ..........

     675 # #          *                                         721
Scn2a    TTTETEIRKR RSS..SYHVS MDLLEDP.SR QRAMSMASIL TNTMEELEES
Scn1a    ------M--- ---------- --F----SQ- ---------- ---V------
Scn3a    ------V--- -L-..--QI- -EM---SSG- --S--I---- ----------
Scn4a    .......... .......... .......... ....-AD-AI SDA------A
Scn5a    PSE-PGGPQM LTPQAP...C A-GF-E-GA- ---L-AV-V- -SAL------
Scn8a    ...KLRRKAL D-F..-FYGP TR--RTEGQN -QHNERG..H KHAS------
Scn9a    ....P-GPAL HTTGQKSFL- AGY-NE-FRA -----VV--M -SVI------
```

FIGURE 3 *(continued)*

Several spontaneous mutations of skeletal muscle Na^+ channels have been characterized in humans, and the location of mutations has been mapped to individual amino acids of the Na^+ channel sequence (Cannon, 1996). These mutations underlie several inherited forms of muscular paralysis and myotonia. Myotonia occurs if inactivation is slow, with paralysis if inactivation is absent or enhanced. A single mutant amino acid in cardiac Na^+ channels causes an inherited form of long Q-T syndrome cardiac arrhythmias

(Bennett *et al.*, 1995b). Long Q-T is caused by the incomplete inactivation of cardiac Na^+ current. To date, no genetic diseases in humans are known to result from mutations to Na^+ channels of brain. However, in mice, genetic inactivation of Scn8a results in a loss of evoked transmission at the neuromuscular juction, with paralysis and early lethalitity (Kohrman *et al.*, 1996; Burgess *et al.*, 1995). A single amino acid substitutuion in the mouse Scn8a results in ataxia and reduced cerebellar Purkinje cell spiking (Kohrman *et al.*, 1996).

2. Distribution of Channel Subtypes in Brain

The anatomical distribution of Na^+ channel subtypes has been studied with site-directed antibodies generated to the hypervariable cytosolic loop between domains I and II of Na^+ channel proteins (Westenbroek *et al.*, 1989). Type IIA channels predominate in mammalian forebrain tissues, but type I channels are present in greater abundance than type IIA in spinal cord. Type IIA channels of forebrain are found in greater densities in axons and proximal dendritic regions than in cell bodies. Type I channels are found in greater density in cell bodies and dendrites than in axons, but are present everywhere at lower density than type IIA channels. Type III channels are found in significant amounts only in immature brain. Type VI channels have been described, but distribution in brain tissues has not been studied using site-directed antibodies.

In situ mRNA hybridization studies indicate the localization of cell bodies manufacturing the various Na^+ channel types. These studies generally agree with those using site-directed antibodies (Beckh *et al.*, 1989). In addition, they provide evidence that type VI channels are widely expressed in neurons and glia of brain and peripheral nerves (Schaller *et al.*, 1995).

3. Percentage of Total Purified Na^+ Channels by Immunoprecipitation or RNase Protection Assays

Using site-directed antibodies and immunoprecipitation, the proportion of various Na^+ channel types has been estimated in solubilized homogenates of various rat brain areas (Gordon *et al.*, 1987). Approximately 80% of ^{32}P-labeled Na^+ channels of neocortex are type IIA, with about 14% being type I. The quantitative contribution of type VI channels has not been studied with site-directed antibodies, but results from an RNase protection assay indicate that type VI mRNA is at least as common as type I, II, III, IIIA, or IIIB mRNA (Schaller *et al.*, 1995). The reason for the apparent discrepancy between immunoprecipitation and hybridization results is not known. Additional studies measuring the amount of protein products with types I, II, IIA, III, and VI are needed, as protein expression does not correlate exactly with mRNA expression.

B. Two-Dimensional Structure and Site-Directed Mutagenesis of Function

1. TTX Blockade

Several studies show that amino acid residues at the extracellular mouth of the channel are crucial for the specific high-affinity binding and blockade of Na^+ channels by tetrodotoxin. It is thought that the guanidine moiety of TTX and the arginine residues of polypeptide toxins such as μ-conotoxins bind to negatively charged carboxyl residues at the channel mouth. If these residues are modified by acidification of the extracellular medium or by site-directed mutations, TTX blockade is lost. For example, neutralizing the single glutamic acid residue at position 387 causes a severe loss of tetrodotoxin sensitivity in cloned Na^+ channels (Noda *et al.*, 1989). Mutagenesis of glutamate residues in homologous extracellular areas of the three other domains also greatly attenuates TTXs action (Terlau *et al.*, 1991). Other mutations in the same region cause cardiac channels to become more sensitive to TTX (Satin *et al.*, 1992). Mutations to amino acids located very near to the TTX-sensitive residues, at locations 1422 and 1714, from lysine and alanine to negatively charged glutamate residues, cause type II sodium channels expressed in *Xenopus* oocytes to lose their selectivity for Na^+ ions and to become permeable and selective for Ca^{2+} ions (Heinemann *et al.*, 1992). Therefore, the TTX-binding site (Fig. 1) is on the external mouth of the channel, very close to the ion selectivity filter. These and other studies with site-directed mutations of K^+ channels (Miller, 1991) suggest that the S5 and S6 segments line the ion-conducting pathway (Fig. 1).

2. Voltage Sensor and Channel Activation

Several investigators independently proposed that positively charged arginine residues in the S4 transmembrane portion of Na^+ channels are moved by the electrostatic force of membrane depolarization, sensing cellular depolarization and causing channel opening. Most models propose that positively charged arginine residues move toward the extracellular side of the membrane in response to depolarization, causing a "gating current" and a conformational change that very rapidly allows Na^+ ions to permeate the sodium channel. This hypothesis has been confirmed by site-directed mutagenesis (Flieg *et al.*, 1994; Auld *et al.*, 1990; Stuhmer *et al.*, 1989). The crucial residues are shown by (+) notations in Fig. 1. Individual mutations of charged S4 arginine residues to cysteine by Yang *et al.* (1996) have shown that the accessibility of mutated residues to the extracellular medium is dependent on membrane voltage. These experiments show that physical movement of the S4 transmembrane region is surprisingly extensive, with several amino acids moving from a location accessible from the cytosol when hyperpolarized to an externally accessible location when depolarized. Furthermore, only one of five charged residue is buried within the channel protein at any particular membrane voltage; the other charged residues are exposed either to the internal or to the external medium. These results account nicely for the postulated movement of 2.5 elementary charges in each S4 completely across the membrane potential field during gating (Hirschberg *et al.*, 1996).

Studies with cysteine mutations (Yang *et al.*, 1996) also show that immobilizing the S4 region in domain IV with methanethiosulfonate reagents prevents inactivation. Thus, movement of the IV–S4 region may directly couple inactivation to the same voltage sensors required for activation. Note that the IV–S4 region is located between the III–IV cytosolic loop and the IV–S6 regions comprising the inactivation gate (see Section II,B,3). Immobilization of mutated IV–S4 regions by methanethiosulfonate reagents may also alter the voltage-dependent drug block of Na^+ channels (see Section II,D), but this idea as yet has not been tested.

Previously, a helical twisting motion of the transmembrane helices located in the areas marked with (+) was proposed to account for transducing conformational changes into an ion channel opening (Catterall, 1986, 1992; Durell and Guy, 1992). However, twisting movement is not required to explain the data of Yang *et al.* (1996). These data may be explained by the sliding movement of the tethered but highly charged S4 segments within an "ion channel" that is permeable only to the charged S4 segment itself (Yang *et al.*, 1996). The sliding S4 model also accounts for the movement of two charged arginine residues in the S4 segment of domain IV from one side to the other of the cell membrane during voltage changes.

3. Inactivation Gate

The "inactivation gate" that closes about 1 msec after channel opening has been studied with molecular biological techniques. It has been known for some time that cytosolic treatment with proteolytic enzymes can abolish inactivation, leading to large, prolonged sodium currents (e.g., Gonoi and Hille, 1987). This is thought to occur because proteolysis cleaves away part of the channel protein, preventing closure of the inactivation gate. Studies of the inactivation process are of interest with respect to voltage-dependent Na^+ channel blockers because these drugs mimick inactivation in several ways (see Section II,D). Antibodies directed toward the cytosolic loop of amino acids between motifs III and IV reduce inactivation when applied from the cytosol (Vassilev *et al.*, 1989), and mutant channels with deletions of amino acids in this region lack normal inactivation (Patton *et al.*, 1992). Mutagenesis of single amino acids in the cytosolic loop between motifs III and IV shows that three amino acids in particular (Ile-Phe-Met at positions 1488–1490, labeled "H" in Fig. 1) are necessary for normal inactivation to occur (West *et al.*, 1992a). If all of these three amino acids are changed or if only the Phe residue at position 1489 is changed to a Gln residue, inactivation is greatly decreased. In this case, voltage clamp commands to

0 mV cause sodium currents that last for many hundreds of milliseconds rather than only 1–2 msec in wild-type channels. In addition, single channel recordings from mutant channels show long-lasting bursts of openings rather than the very short duration openings of wild-type channels. Furthermore, mutations to the cytosolic mouth of the channel in motif IV, domain 6, diminish inactivation, suggesting that these residues (at locations 1774–1776) define the binding site for the inactivation gate on the channel mouth (McPhee *et al.*, 1994, 1995). These various results suggest that several amino acid residues, particularly Phe1489, are involved in a rapid and high-affinity conformational change with folding of the III–IV loop across the cytosolic mouth of the ion channel, blocking the ion-conducting pathway and causing inactivation (West *et al.*, 1992a).

C. Modulation of Na^+ Channels by Cytosolic Factors

Na^+ channel function can be modulated by cytosolic phosphorylation of the α subunit protein by protein kinase C, or by cAMP-dependent protein kinase (Numann *et al.*, 1994; Li *et al.*, 1993). Channel function is also modulated by a G-protein coupled mechanism on the α subunit (Ma *et al.*, 1994). Phosphorylation by either kinase can reduce peak current and slow the time course of inactivation. These interactions are thought to occur within the large cytoplasmic loop between domains I and II. Amino acids of the I–II loop thought to be targets of cytosolic kinases are shown in Fig. 3B. To date, modulation by G-proteins or phosphorylation have not been the target of therapeutic drugs, possibly because such drug interactions would also modify many other proteins in addition to Na^+ channels.

D. Site-Directed Mutations and Voltage-Dependent Block

Site-directed mutations have been used to study Na^+ channel block by local anesthetics (Ragsdale *et al.*, 1994). Local anesthetics also block nicotinic acetylcholine-gated channels, where blockade is abolished by mutations in the extracellular side of the channel pore (Charnet *et al.*, 1990). In contrast to K^+ channels, blockade of Na^+ channels by etidocaine is sharply reduced by mutations to the cytosolic side of motif IV, segment 6, including residues 1764 and 1771 (see inset to Fig. 1) (Ragsdale *et al.*, 1994). Other mutations in this region enhance etidocaine block or alter the permeability selectivity of the channel. These amino acids are adjacent to others necessary for the normal inactivation of native channels (1774 to 1776). Therefore, the local anesthetic-binding site is physically close to the selectivity filter of the channel and to the binding site of the inactivation gate. Furthermore, the local anesthetic-binding site is homologous to the site where verapamil binds onto voltage-gated Ca^{2+} channels (Striessnig *et al.*, 1990). As elegant as these studies are, they do not rule out the possibility of additional sites on Na^+ channels that might contribute to the binding of local anesthetics. For example, site-directed mutations of amino acids on the other three S6 segments (in domains I, II, and III) were not studied.

Additional studies with mutations of type IIA rat brain Na^+ channels (Ragsdale *et al.*, 1996) indicate that substitutions at positions 1764 or 1771 decrease the blocking action of phenytoin and lidocaine and, to a lesser extent, decrease the action of other anti-arrhythmics (quinidine and flecainide). These subtitutions are the same as those that decrease block by etidocaine (Ragsdale *et al.*, 1994). Therefore, all of the voltage-dependent Na^+ blocking agents studied so far appear to have overlapping binding sites on sodium channels at the cytosolic part of the IV–S6 region (see inset to Fig. 1). It is likely that many other voltage-dependent Na^+ channel blockers bind to related, if not identical, sites on mammalian Na^+ channels (see Section III,B,2).

Phenytoin, lidocaine, and other anticonvulsant and local anesthetic compounds that are functionally related, including carbamazepine, lamotrigine, riluzole, and a number of others (Table II), block Na^+ channels in a voltage-dependent manner. Block is minimal when membranes are hyperpolarized prior to a test pulse, but block is pronounced if membranes are slightly depolarized prior to testing (Hondeghem and Katzung, 1977; Hille, 1977; Willow *et al.*, 1985; Ragsdale *et al.*, 1991). This has been called the modulated receptor hypothesis for local anesthetic action (Hondeghem and Katzung, 1977; Hille, 1977), which also accounts for the enhanced blocking action of these compounds in response to rapid trains of action potentials (McLean and MacDonald, 1983, 1986; Adler *et al.*, 1986). The blocking action of phenytoin does not depend on the completion of inactivation, as phenytoin still blocks single-channel Na^+ currents when rapid inactivation is removed by cytosolic treatment with proteolytic enzymes (Quandt, 1988). This was interpreted as an interaction of phenytoin molecules with the "slow" inactivated state (Quandt, 1988). However, block of enzyme-modified channels could also result from an interaction of drugs with another conformational state of the channel, such as the movement of gating charge leading to channel opening (Kuo and Bean, 1994b).

Recent results indicate that neither phenytoin nor lidocaine require channel opening or slow inactivation to produce use-dependent blockade. Repetitive depolarizing pulses that do not open Na^+ channels or cause slow inactivation (depolarizations to −40 mV) cause increased blockade with phenytoin or lidocaine (Ragsdale *et al.*, 1996). In contrast, the anti-arrhythmic drug quinidine, requires repetitive channel opening for potent blockade (depolarizations to 0 mV) (Ragsdale *et al.*, 1996). Thus, inactivation (either slow or fast) may not be necessary for voltage-dependent blockers to act, even though these compounds are often described as "stabilizing the inactivated state" (see discussion below). Blockade by phenytoin does not require channel opening (Kuo and Bean, 1994b), and so is different than the simple open channel block described with other kinds of agents.

A separate analysis of cardiac Na^+ channels (Bennett *et al.*, 1995a) shows that elimination of rapid inactivation by either intracellular enzyme treatment or site-directed mutagenesis decreases high-affinity, use-dependent blockade by lidocaine. These investigators conclude that lidocaine binds with high affinity to the rapid inactivated state because of the site-directed mutagenesis result and also because the kinetics of lidocaine block are more rapid than the onset of slow inactivation. In any case, it is clear that the binding of local anesthetic and anticonvulsant drugs is increased by conformational changes of the channel protein induced by depolarization; conversely, drug unbinding is enhanced by conformational changes induced by hyperpolarization.

E. Biophysical Studies of Voltage-Dependent Na^+ Channel Blockade

The electrophysiological analysis by Kuo and Bean (1994b) suggests that inactivation of the Na^+ channels behaves like the binding of a ligand (the inactivation gate, see "H" in Fig. 1) to the channel pore, with binding affinity a function of channel conformation. In the Kuo model, the affinity for closing the inactivation gate increases 27-fold with each of four sequential states of increasing channel activation (channels open only after reaching the fifth activational state). Thus, inactivation proceeds many thousands of times faster when channels are fully activated than when they are at rest. Nevertheless, inactivation proceeds measurably whenever any of the four activational steps are reached by membrane depolarization, even without channel opening. This model is shown schematically by a "state diagram" in Fig. 4. In the original publication (Kuo and Bean 1994b), each transition between states was represented by a fitted rate constant, several of which depend on membrane voltage.

Kuo and Bean (1994b) used the same kinetic model to describe binding (and blockade of Na^+ channels) by phenytoin molecules. The only difference was much slower kinetics with phenytoin binding than with inactivation gate "binding." Therefore, in the presence of phenytoin, Na^+ channels appear to "inactivate" more readily than without drug, but drug-induced "inactivation" takes several orders of magnitude longer to develop or to be relieved than physiological inactivation. In the Kuo and Bean model, drugs like phenytoin appear to enhance inactivation only because inactivation and drug-induced block both prevent channels from opening and because both phenomena have similar voltage dependencies. These authors speculate that inactivation and drug binding may be completely independent processes that depend on similar conformational changes associated with channel activation. Others have proposed that phenytoin and lamotrigine bind to

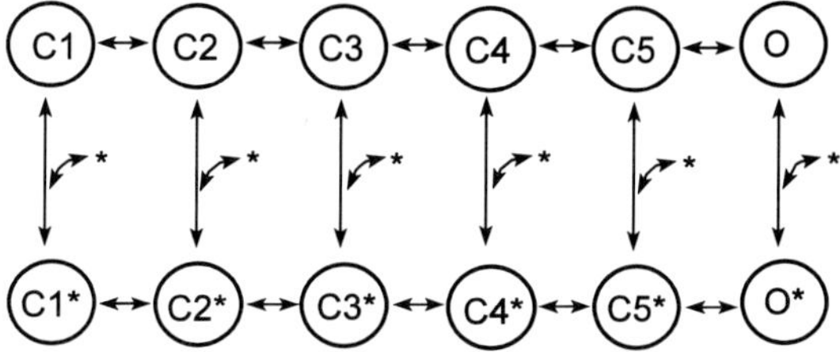

FIGURE 4 State diagram corresponding to numerical model of rapid inactivation and for phenytoin binding. Modified from Kuo and Bean, (1994b) with kind permission from Cell Press. (Note: this figure is simplified from the original publication.) This model is compatible with several previous models of Na^+ channel activation (e.g., Vandenberg and Bezanilla, 1991). C1 to C5 denote sequential closed states prior to channel opening, and O denotes the open or ion-conducting state. Inactivation can occur in the completely inactive state (C1) but is much more likely with increasing activation of the channel (C2 to O). With computational numerical analysis, the voltage dependences for rates of inactivation and rates of recovery from inactivation were fit closely to experimental data. The same model (with different rate constants) was used to fit the voltage dependence of channel block (or recovery from block) with phenytoin; in this case, the rates for drug binding are approximately 4000 times slower than for inactivation, but are otherwise similar. Either inactivation or drug binding in the diagram corresponds to the binding of a particle that blocks the channel and is represented by the C(*) and O(*) states. Rate constants were estimated and modeled numerically for each of the forward and reverse transitions in the diagram (Kuo and Bean, 1994b). The rates of transistion between each of the different closed states are voltage dependent (depolarization favors transition to higher-numbered states). Therefore, the affinities for drug binding are also voltage dependent (see text).

the "slow inactivated state" of Na^+ channels because block develops slowly and still occurs when the inactivation gate is modified by proteolytic enzymes (Xie *et al.,* 1995a; Quandt, 1988). However, the Kuo model appears to account for a greater amount of biophysical data, including the voltage-dependent time course of recovery from drug blockade (Kuo and Bean, 1994b).

A second analysis by Kuo and Bean (1994a) shows that the on-binding rate for phenytoin blockade is concentration dependent but that the off-binding rate is independent of concentration (τ approximately 10 sec with cells held at −70 mV). The relatively slow off-binding rate accounts for accumulated block with repetitive depolarizations (use-dependent block). The combination of on- and off-binding rates and several other independent analyses define blocking affinity for phenytoin (K_m) at about 6 μM in depolarized cells. An important implication is that therapeutically relevant concentrations of phenytoin (approximately 8 μM) block about half of the Na^+ channels, but only if cells remain depolarized for 5–10 sec or more. This may explain why therapeutic dosages of phenytoin do not alter "interictal spikes" in the EEG or action potentials from synaptic excitation; each of these depolarizing events last less than 200 msec. However, sustained depolarizations (as in seizures or ischemia) greatly enhance the blocking action of phenytoin and similar drugs. Furthermore, Kuo and Bean (1994a) conclude that phenytoin binding occurs to the state associated with "fast inactivation" rather than slow inactivation because the range of voltages affecting the kinetics of drug block extends beyond the range of voltages causing detectible slow inactivation.

III. Chemical Structures of Na^+ Channel Blockers

A. Tetrodotoxin and Saxitoxin

Tetrodotoxin and saxitoxin are derived from the poisonous puffer fish and from marine microorganisms, respectively. They are structurally similar toxins that bind with high affinity to Na^+ channels, preventing ion conduction by plugging the external opening of the ion channel (Fig. 5). They are voltage-insensistive blockers, meaning that they bind with the same high affinity regardless of the voltage across the cell membrane. The binding of these toxins is presumed to originate from chemical interactions between the charged nitrogen atoms of the guanidine moiety of TTX and the electronegative oxygen atoms of glutamate residues at the mouth of the channel (Hille, 1975). This model, proposed in the mid-1970s, still appears to be valid today, based on a number of recent studies. Because the toxins bind regardless of the state of the Na^+ channel, they potently block the axonal conduction of action potentials and have little therapeutic potential because they interfere with basic brain functions such as the control of skeletal muscles necessary for breathing. However, they are useful tools because of their specificity for Na^+ channels. For example, anticonvulsant-like or neuroprotective actions of TTX *in vitro* are unlikely to arise from any mechanism other than the blockade of Na^+ channels.

B. Phenytoin and Anticonvulsants (Voltage-Dependent Blockers)

Figure 5 shows the chemical structures of a variety of synthetic compounds that block Na^+ channels. Except for TTX and saxitoxin, all compounds are voltage-dependent blockers. Additional pharmacological actions unrelated to Na^+ channels are caused by some of these compounds; the best known of these are listed parenthetically in Table III. Table IV summarizes the *in vivo* neuroprotective actions of these various compounds; anticonvulsant pharmacology is summarized elsewhere (Rogawski and Porter, 1990). Most of these compounds share several pharmacological properties, including anticonvulsant and neuroprotective action (see later).

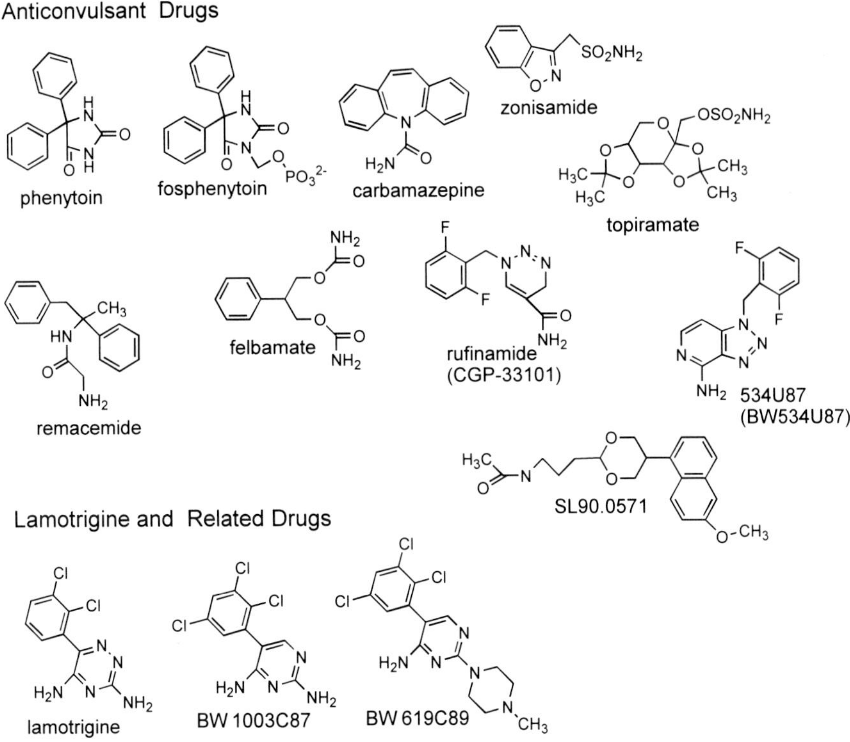

Lidocaine and structurally-related compounds

lidocaine

mexiletine

ralitoline

CI-953

PD 85639

FIGURE 5 Chemical structures of anticonvulsants and neuroprotective drugs active at Na^+ channels. All of these compounds are discussed in the text or in Table III, except for 534U87 (Glaxo-Wellcome) and SL90.0571 (Synthelabs); which are potential anticonvulsant drugs in early stages of development.

Mixed Ca^{2+} and Na^+ Channel Blockers

verapamil

flunarizine

lifarizine (RS 87567)

lomerizine (KB-2796)

CNS 1237

Other Na^+ Channel Modulators

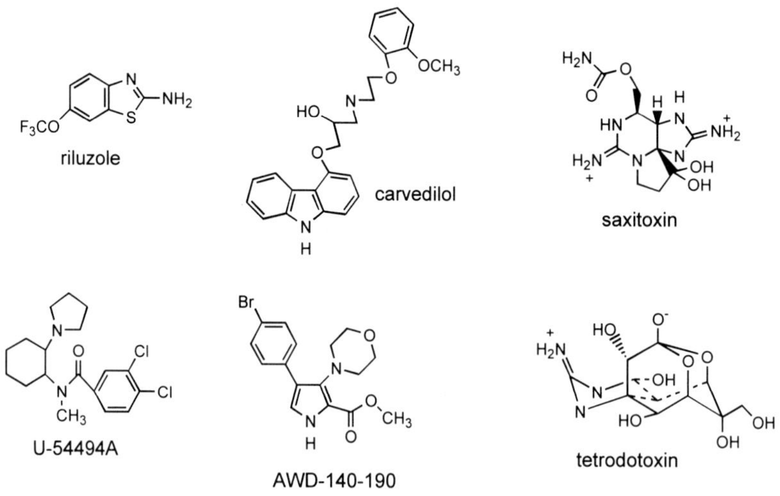

FIGURE 5 *(continued)*

1. Discovery by Maximal Electroshock

Several Na^+ modulators have been discovered by screening from a large pharmaceutical bank of compounds. Empirically, some compounds prevent seizures in mice or other laboratory animals caused by maximal electroshock delivered to the forebrain (Krall *et al.*, 1978). Although the maximal electroshock test is sensitive to drugs with other anticonvulsant mechanisms, Na^+ channel modulators discovered in this manner include phenytoin, carbamazepine, lamotrigine, zonisamide, felbamate, topiramate, CI953, ralitoline, and several others (see Fig. 5). Only since the early 1980s have biochemical and electrophysiological tools become available that enable the convenient characterization of voltage-dependent Na^+ channel blockers *in vitro* (see next section). Results with these compounds *in vitro* are summarized in Table III and in the following section.

2. Use of Toxin Probes (Veratridine), BTX Binding, and V-Clamp Methods

A number of specific toxins in addition to TTX alter the function of Na^+ channels. In particular, veratridine and batrachotoxinin are lipid-soluble alkaloids that alter channel activation and inactivation such that a large percentage of channels remain open at resting membrane potentials (i.e., the conducting state of the channel is stabilized by toxin binding, probably by an allosteric interaction). Veratridine and batrachotoxinin also prevent rapid inactivation. These toxins have been used as selective high-affinity probes of sodium channel function and they compete with the action of several drugs that are voltage-dependent blockers (see later). Studies of these and several other distinct types of Na^+ channel toxins and their associated binding sites have been previously reviewed (Catterall, 1980, 1992; Catterall *et al.*, 1992).

The interaction of various blockers with Na^+ channels has been investigated using electrophysiology or, alternatively, by competition of drug molecules with veratridine *in vitro* or with batrachotoxinin receptor binding *in vitro* (see Table III). Preapplication of voltage-dependent blockers prevents the depolarizing action of veratridine in a competitive-like manner (Rando *et al.*, 1986), suggesting that veratridine may require channel opening to bind. This may underlie the action of anticonvulsants (Willow and Catterall, 1982), anti-arrhythmics (Sheldon *et al.*, 1994), and local anesthetics (McNeil *et al.*, 1985; Postma and Catterall, 1984) to inhibit the binding of radiolabeled batrachotoxin. Furthermore, evidence with batrachotoxin binding suggests that lidocaine, phenytoin, and carbamazepine each interact with a common site or closely related sites on Na^+ channels (Zimanyi *et al.*, 1989).

Lamotrigine and the structurally related compounds BW1003C87 and BW619C89 each inhibit the veratridine-induced release of neurotransmitters, but not K^+-induced release (Leach *et al.*, 1991). This is also strong evidence of a direct interaction of drugs with Na^+ channels (see Table III).

Recently, tritiated lifarizine has been studied as a high-affinity probe of Na^+ channels (MacKinnon *et al.*, 1995) and previously, tritiated PD85639 was shown to bind to purified or native Na^+ channels (Thomsen *et al.*, 1993).

TABLE III Actions of Various Compounds at Voltage-Dependent Na^+ Channels

Compound name (additional targets)	*Na^+ channel electrophysiology*	*BTX binding (K_i or IC_{50})*	*Veratrine block (IC_{50})*
Tetrodotoxin (none)	V-independent block (voltage clamp IC_{50} = approximately 10 n*M*)	Assay conventionally done in TTX	22 n*M* (vs cell death); 60 n*M* (vs Asp release) (Lysko *et al.*, 1995); 15 n*M* (vs ion flux) (Hays *et al.*, 1991)
Lidocaine (K^+ channels)	Use and V-dependent block (voltage clamp) (Ragsdale *et al.*, 1991) and cardiac cells (Bean *et al.*, 1983)	113 μ*M* (Zimanyi *et al.*, 1989) 265 μ*M* (Hays *et al.*, 1991)	97 μ*M* (vs ion flux) (Hays *et al.*, 1991)
Mexiletine (Ca^{2+} channels)	Use and V-dependent block (cardiac cells) (Herring *et al.*, 1983)	18 μ*M* (Sheldon *et al.*, 1994)	
Phenytoin (Ca^{2+} channels)	Use and V-dependent block 6–10 μ*M* (voltage clamp) (Willow *et al.*, 1985; Ragsdale *et al.*, 1991; Kuo and Bean 1994a)	40 μ*M* (Willow and Catterall, 1982) 69 μ*M* (Zimanyi *et al.*, 1989)	21 μ*M* (vs Glu release) (Leach *et al.*, 1986); 23 μ*M* (vs ion flux) (Hays *et al.*, 1994)
Carbamazepine	V-dependent block (voltage clamp) (Ragsdale *et al.*, 1991; Willow *et al.*, 1985)	131 μ*M* (Willow and Catterall, 1982) 286 μ*M* (Zimanyi *et al.*, 1989)	30 μ*M* (vs Glu release) (Waldmeier *et al.*, 1995)
Lamotrigine	Use and V-dependent block (voltage clamp) (Xie *et al.*, 1995a) repetitive firing (Cheung *et al.*, 1992)	114 μ*M* (Cheung *et al.*, 1992)	21 μ*M* (vs Glu release) (Leach *et al.*, 1986)
BW1003C87			1.6 μ*M* (vs Glu release) (Okiyama *et al.*, 1995)
BW619C89			5.3 μ*M* (vs Glu release) (Leach *et al.*, 1993)
Zonisamide	V-dependent block (voltage clamp) (Schauf, 1987)		
Riluzole	Use and V-dependent block 0.2 μ*M* (voltage clamp) (Hebert *et al.*, 1994; Benoit and Escande, (1991)		4 μ*M* (vs ion flux) (Hays *et al.*, 1994)
Topiramate	Repetitive firing (Coulter *et al.*, 1993)		
Rufinamide	Repetitive firing (Karolchyk, 1996)		

Felbamate (NMDA block)	V-dependent block 30 μM (voltage clamp) (Pisani *et al.*, 1995)		
Flunarizine (Ca^{2+} channels)	V-dependent block (Kiskin *et al.*, 1993)	0.35 μM (Pauwels *et al.*, 1990)	0.12 μM (vs cell death) (Pauwels *et al.*, 1990)
Lifarizine (RS-87476) (Ca^{2+} channels)	V-dependent block (voltage clamp) (Kiskin *et al.*, 1993; N. A. Brown *et al.*, 1994b; McGivern *et al.*, 1995)	0.119 μM (Pauwels *et al.*, 1990)	1.6 μM (myocytes) (Pauwels *et al.*, 1990) 0.3 μM (vs cell death) (May *et al.*, 1995)
Lomerizine (KB-2796) (Ca^{2+} channels)	V-dependent block (voltage clamp) (McGivern *et al.*, 1994)	0.026 μM (McGivern *et al.*, 1994)	
U54494A	V-dependent block (voltage clamp) (Zhu and Im, 1992)		
PD 85639	V-dependent block (voltage clamp) (Ragsdale *et al.*, 1993)	0.046 μM (Thomsen *et al.*, 1993)	5 μM (vs cell death) (Hays *et al.*, 1991)
Ralitoline	Repetitive firing block (current clamp) (Rock *et al.*, 1991) V-dependent block (voltage clamp) (Fischer *et al.*, 1992)	25 μM (Rock *et al.*, 1991)	
CI953	Repetitive firing block (current clamp) (Rock *et al.*, 1991)	29 μM (Rock *et al.*, 1991)	
Verapamil (Ca^{2+} channels)	Use and rapid V-dependent block (voltage clamp) (Ragsdale *et al.*, 1991)	2.5 μM (Pauwels *et al.*, 1990)	2.5 μM (vs cell death) (Pauwels *et al.*, 1990)
Carvedilol (β-adrenergic)			0.306 μM (vs cell death) 1.7 μM (vs Asp release) (Lysko *et al.*, 1994)
CNS1237 (Ca^{2+} channels)	Use-dependent block (voltage clamp) (Goldin, 1995; Margolin *et al.*, 1994)		
AWD 140–190 (anticonvulsant)	Use and V-dependent block (voltage clamp) (Rostock *et al.*, 1995)		
Remacemide (NMDA antagonist) (anticonvulsant)	Use and V-dependent block (voltage clamp) (Sanchez and Harris, 1995) repetitive firing block (current clamp) (Wami *et al.*, 1996)		
Enadoline (κ opiate agonist)			Glu release via microdialysis probe (Millan *et al.*, 1995)
Besipirdine (cholinergic agonist, alpha-2 adrenergic)		5.5μm (Tang *et al.*, 1995)	30 μM (vs. NA release) (Tang *et al.*, 1995)

TABLE IV Neuroprotective Actions in Hypoxia/Ischemia of Drugs Blocking Na^+ Channels

Drug	In vitro *model*	In vivo *model*
Tetrodotoxin	Hippocampal slice[a] (Weber and Taylor, 1994; Boening *et al.*, 1989; Kass *et al.*, 1992) optic nerve[c] (Stys *et al.*, 1992b) neuronal culture (Lynch *et al.*, 1995; Tasker *et al.*, 1992 Strijbos *et al.*, 1996) spinal explant culture[e] (Rothstein and Kuncl, 1995)	Gerbil or rat forebrain[b] ischemia (Lysko *et al.*, 1995; Yamasaki *et al.*, 1991) isolated rat head[d] (Xie *et al.*, 1994) rat cardiac arrest (Prenen *et al.*, 1988)
Lidocaine (anticonvulsant)	Hippocampal slice (Weber and Taylor, 1994; Lucas *et al.*, 1989; Fried *et al.*, 1995); optic nerve (Stys, 1995; Stys *et al.*, 1992a)	Rabbit forebrain ischemia (Rasool *et al.*, 1990)
Mexiletine	Optic nerve (Stys and Lesiuk, 1996)	
Phenytoin (anticonvulsant)	Hippocampal slice (Weber and Taylor, 1994; Stanton and Moskal, 1991) optic nerve (Fern *et al.*, 1993)	MCAO[f] (Murakami and Furui, 1994; Rataud *et al.*, 1994; Boxer *et al.*, 1990) gerbil forebrain ischemia (Taft *et al.*, 1989) Levine rat pup[g] (Hayakawa *et al.*, 1994a)
Carbamazepine (anticonvulsant)		MCAO (Murakami and Furui, 1994; Rataud *et al.*, 1994)
Lamotrigine (anticonvulsant)		MCAO (Smith and Meldrum, Murakami and Furui, 1994) gerbil forebrain ischemia (Wiard *et al.*, 1995)
BW1003C87		MCAO (Torp *et al.*, 1993; Meldrum *et al.*, 1992) MCAO w/reperfusion (Gaspary *et al.*, 1994) rat forebrain ischemia (Lekieffre and Meldrum, 1993) Levine rat pup (Gilland *et al.*, 1994) rat head trauma[h] (Okiyama *et al.*, 1995)
BW619C89		MCAO (Chen *et al.*, 1995; Smith *et al.*, 1993; Leach *et al.*, 1993) rat forebrain ischemia (Smith *et al.*, 1993) rat head trauma (Sun and Faden, 1995; Tsuchida *et al.*, 1996)
Zonisamide (anticonvulsant)		Levine rat pup (Hayakawa *et al.*, 1994b)

Riluzole (anticonvulsant)	Spinal explant culture[e] (Rothstein and Kuncl, 1995) cerebellar granule cells in culture (Dessi *et al.*, 1993) hippocampal slice (Malgouris *et al.*, 1994)	Gerbil forebrain ischemia (Pratt *et al.*, 1992) MCAO (Wahl *et al.*, 1993; Pratt *et al.*, 1992) ALS mice[i] (Gurney *et al.*, 1996) MPTP monkeys[j] (Benazzouz *et al.*, 1995)
Felbamate (anticonvulsant)	Hippocampal slice (Wallis and Panizzon, 1995; Wallis *et al.*, 1992) neocortical cell culture (Kanthasamy *et al.*, 1995)	Levine rap pup (Wasterlain *et al.*, 1992)
Flunarizine (anticonvulsant)	Hippocampal slice (Hara *et al.*, 1990) hippocampal cell culture (Hara *et al.*, 1993b)	Rat forebrain ischemia (Van Reempts *et al.*, 1986) rat cardiac arrest (Xie *et al.*, 1995b; Lu *et al.*, 1990; Wauquier *et al.*, 1989) Levine rat pup (Silverstein *et al.*, 1986)
Lifarizine		Cat MCAO (Kucharczyk *et al.*, 1993) mouse MCAO (C. M. Brown *et al.*, 1995a) rat cardiac arrest (Xie *et al.*, 1995b)
Lomerizine	Hippocampal slice (Hara *et al.*, 1990) hippocampal cell culture (Hara *et al.*, 1993b)	Herbil forebrain (Yoshidomi *et al.*, 1989) MCAO (Hara *et al.*, 1993a)
CNS1237		MCAO (Goldin, 1995)
Remacemide		rat forebrain ischemia (Ordy *et al.*, 1992)
Enadoline (anticonvulsant)		MCAO (cats) (Fujisawa *et al.*, 1993) rat forebrain (Hayward *et al.*, 1993)

[a] Rat hippocampal slices deprived of oxygen and glucose.
[b] Global forebrain temporary ischemia.
[c] Rat optic nerve *in vitro* deprived of oxygen.
[d] Arrested perfusion.
[e] Rat spinal organotypic cultures in glutamate uptake inhibitor.
[f] Rat unilateral middle cerebral artery occlusion.
[g] Neonatal rat unilateral carotid occlusion with hypoxia.
[h] Brain damage from trauma.
[i] Transgenic mice with mutant superoxide dismutase gene (symptoms similar to ALS).
[j] Monkeys treated with MPTP, producing symptoms similar to Parkinson's disease.

IV. Undesirable Side Effects Related to Ion Channel Blockade

A. Cardiovascular Effects

Anticonvulsant drugs such as phenytoin and anti-arrhythmic agents such as lidocaine typically cause arrhythmias or decrease heart rate at high dosages. These actions may be attributed to the blockade of Na^+, K^+, or Ca^{2+} channels in heart muscle. Anticonvulsant Na^+ channel blockers also reduce systemic blood pressure at high dosages. Hypotension probably results from the blockade of L-type Ca^{2+} channels in vascular smooth muscle, leading to arterial relaxation. These nonspecific effects of Na^+ blockers on other cation channels illustrate the pharmacological similarity among Na^+, K^+, and Ca^{2+} channel types that will continue to challenge the discovery of novel and specific ion channel modulators.

B. Central Nervous System

Several Na^+ channel blockers have been associated with tremors, myoclonus, and seizures, and occasionally status epilepticus in clinical use (Nelson and Hoffman, 1994), particularly at high dosages relative to those needed for anticonvulsant or anti-arrhythmic actions. It is likely that these effects are caused by some interaction of drug with ion channels, although this has not been clearly demonstrated. It is not clear whether Na^+ channels or other ion channels such as K^+ channels are involved. It is well known that the blockade of cerebral K^+ channels causes seizures (Yamaguchi and Rogawski, 1992). With phenytoin treatment, precipitation of seizures in humans is relatively uncommon even with high dosages (Osorio *et al.,* 1989). However, seizures precipitated with anti-arrhythmic drugs such as lidocaine and mexiletine are more of a problem clinically (Brown *et al.,* 1995b; Brown *et al.,* 1995; Denaro and Benowitz, 1989). These have been studied in animals (e.g., Stone and Javid, 1988; Alexander *et al.,* 1986).

V. Therapeutic Use of Voltage-Dependent Na^+ Blockers

A. Epilepsy

In animal seizure models, phenytoin-like anticonvulsants prevent tonic extensor seizures in rodents from maximal electroshock, reduce the severity of seizures and raise the threshold for afterdischarges in the kindling model (Rogawski and Porter, 1990). However, these compounds generally lack activity against clonic seizures from the GABA antagonists pentylenetetrazole or bicuculline and fail to prevent clonic seizures from other chemical convulsants such as strychnine or excitatory amino acids. Furthemore, phenytoin-like drugs have little or no activity against spontaneous absence seizures in rats (Michelitti *et al.*, 1985). Phenytoin and carbamazepine prevent long-duration, seizure-like events in rat brain slices *in vitro* caused by the removal of extracellular Ca^{2+} ions (Leschinger *et al.*, 1993). This profile of activity is shared by several novel anticonvulsants, including carbamazepine, lamotrigine, topiramate, zonisamide, ralitoline, CI953, U49524E, and the local anesthetic lidocaine (Krall *et al.*, 1978; Rogawski and Porter, 1990), suggesting that their mechanisms are related. As might be expected, the strength of experimental evidence that each compound interacts with Na^+ channels varies; many relevant references are included in Table II. A detailed review of anticonvulsant pharmacology and clinical use of these agents for treatment of epilepsy (phenytoin, carbamazepine, lamotrigine, zonisamide, topiramate) is included in Levy *et al.* (1995) and will not be repeated here.

The primary anticonvulsant mechanism of these compounds seems to be the voltage-dependent blockade of Na^+ channels. However, there is relatively little direct evidence to support this hypothesis other than similar pharmacological profiles in a panel of animal seizure models and evidence for blockade of Na^+ channels. It is still possible that anticonvulant action arises by some other pharmacological property. Direct support for a Na^+ channel hypothesis for anticonvulsant action derives from experiments with rat hippocampal slices *in vitro* (Taylor *et al.*, 1996; Burack *et al.*, 1995). Low concentrations of TTX cause anticonvulsant-like effects *in vitro* similar to those of phenytoin or carbamazepine. The anticonvulsant action of TTX in this model is not likely to arise from any mechanism other than blockade of Na^+ channels. TTX blocked long-duration, seizure-like activity at low concentrations that did not reduce unitary evoked potentials significantly. Therefore, only a small percentage of the total Na^+ channels need to be blocked in order for significant anticonvulsant actions to occur.

Although it is postulated that the anticonvulsant action of the agents shown in Table IV results from the inhibition of voltage-gated Na^+ channels, it is not known whether action potentials or other events related to Na^+

TABLE V Action of PD 85639 and TTX on Na^+ Channels without Anticonvulsant Effects (Drugs Given by IP Injection)[a]

Drug	*BTX binding (IC_{50})*	*MES (ED_{50})*	*Ataxia (ED_{50})*	*Comment*
Phenytoin	181 μM	7.5 mg/kg	46 mg/kg	
Lidocaine	265 μM	8.7 mg/k	41 mg/kg	
TTX	—	Not active (0.015 mg/kg)	Not active (0.015 mg/kg)	Lethal at 0.025 mg/kg
PD 85639	0.145 μM	Not active (30 mg/kg)	Approximate 20 mg/kg	Lethal at 100 mg/kg

[a] Data from Hays *et al.* (1991).

channel opening are inhibited to prevent seizure activity. Studies indicate that persistent Na^+ currents (see Section I) are blocked not only by TTX, but also by relevant concentrations of phenytoin (Segal, 1994; Chao and Alzheimer, 1995). Furthermore, persistent bursts of single Na^+ channel openings that have been described in several preparations (Brown *et al.*, 1994a; Keynes, 1994; Alzheimer *et al.*, 1993a,b) are blocked by phenytoin to a greater extent than are brief openings (Segal *et al.*, 1995). Phenytoin has anticonvulsant-like actions in single neurons of hippocampal cell cultures made "epileptogenic" by sustained treatment with kynurenic acid that is subsequently withdrawn (Segal, 1994). In this model, persistent TTX-sensitive plateau potentials are blocked by 8 μM phenytoin, whereas bursts of action potentials are unaltered. This finding also suggests that phenytoin reduces persistent Na^+ currents without blocking action potentials. Additional studies are needed to determine whether a particular profile of drug kinetics of Na^+ channel block and unblock might provide significant advantages for anticonvulsant therapy (see next section).

A recent report describes changes in the ratio of Na^+ channel expression between types I and II in epileptic human brain tissue (Lombardo, *et al.*, 1996). This finding raises the possibility that subtype-specific Na^+ channel blockers (see Section VI,A.) might eventually be of special benefit to patients with refractory epilepsy. However, this concept remains to be tested.

I. Time Dependence of Block and Lack of Anticonvulsant Action with TTX and PD 85639

Many voltage-dependent Na^+ blockers produce anticonvulsant effects in animals (Rogawski and Porter, 1990). However, certain compounds (PD 85639, possibly lomerizine, also TTX, see Table III) have no significant anticonvulsant activity *in vivo*. Tetrodotoxin is of course lethal when given in moderately high dosages, but a careful study with the maximal electroshock test in mice did not reveal anticonvulsant actions at doses just below those causing respiratory depression and death (Table V). Likewise, no anticonvulsant effects were seen with PD 85639, which binds with high affinity to Na^+ channels (Thomsen *et al.*, 1993) and prevents veratridine-induced ion flux and batrachotoxinin binding in rat brain tissues (Hays *et al.*, 1991). The lack of anticonvulsant action with TTX *in vivo* may arise from its lack of voltage dependence. However, TTX causes anticonvulsant-like actions *in vitro*, where respiratory depression is not a problem (see previous paragraphs). With PD 85639, the absence of anticonvulsant action may result from extremely slow binding kinetics (Ragsdale *et al.*, 1993). Therefore, it appears that specific types of voltage and time dependence of Na^+ blocking actions are necessary for anticonvulsant effects in animal models.

B. Neuropathic Pain

Some voltage-dependent Na^+ channel blockers [carbamazepine (Tanelian and Brose, 1991), low-dose systemic lidocaine (Rowbotham *et al.*, 1991; Bach *et al.*, 1990), phenytoin (Yajnik *et al.*, 1992), mexiletine (Dejgard *et al.*, 1988), tocainide (Lindström and Lindblom, 1987)] are used to treat neuropathic pain (Tanelian and Brose, 1991; Galer, 1995), such as from trigeminal neuralgia (Green and Selman, 1991), diabetic neuropathy, postherpetic neuralgia (Thompson and Bones, 1985), cancer (Kloke *et al.*, 1991), and other forms of sensory nerve damage or infection. Such neuropathic pain may originate from increased numbers of Na^+ channels in sensory nerve fibers and hence increased spontaneous action potentials in peripheral nerves (Devor *et al.*, 1992). There is extensive plasticity in the expression of Na^+ channels following axotomy (Waxman *et al.*, 1994; England *et al.*, 1996), suggesting that it might be possible to selectively block neuropathic pain by selectively blocking up-regulated channels. The same compounds listed above are also active in various animal models of neuropathic pain (Foong and Satoh, 1983; Kamei *et al.*, 1992; Chaplan *et al.*, 1995; lamotrigine: Nakamura-Craig and Follenfant, 1995). Analgesia with Na^+ channel blockers has been attributed to the reduction of abnormal tonic firing of nociceptor neurons (Yaari and Devor, 1985; Woolf and Wiesenfeld-Hallin, 1985).

C. Neuroprotection

1. Stroke and Global Ischemia

Activation of Na^+ channels may contribute significantly to depolarization and loss of ion homeostasis from brain ischemia. It has been noted that the down-regulation of voltage-dependent Na^+ channels during hypoxia may be a survival strategy for diving turtles, whose brains are deprived of oxygen for extended periods (Perez-Pinzon *et al.*, 1992). There is substantial evidence from animal models that Na^+ channel blockers are neuroprotective in global and focal ischemia. Data relating to TTX, phenytoin, riluzole, lamotrigine, BW619C89, lifarizine, and several other drugs are summarized in Table IV. Although the neuroprotective actions of glutamate antagonists and other treatments that directly limit the entry of Ca^{2+} into cellular cytosol have been appreciated for several years (Choi, 1988, 1990; Siesjö, 1988), only recently have blockers of Na^+ entry received serious attention as potential neuroprotective agents.

Several voltage-dependent Na^+ channel blockers reduce brain damage from ischemia at doses that are relatively free from side effects, in marked contrast to excitatory amino acid antagonists or L-type Ca^{2+} channel blockers. For example, lamotrigine, BW619C89, riluzole, and phenytoin reduce brain damage in the rat middle cerebral artery occlusion model of focal stroke at dosages that do not cause ataxia or significant cardiovascular effects. The extent of neuroprotection in focal ischemia models with phenytoin, lamotrigine, or BW619C89 is comparable to that seen with noncompetitive NMDA antagonists (Boxer *et al.*, 1990; and B. S. Meldrum, D. Lekieffre, S. E. Smith and R. Torp, unpublished results).

Unlike neuroprotective excitatory amino acid antagonists, Na^+ channel blockers prevent hypoxic damage to mammalian white matter *in vitro* in a model with isolated rat optic nerve segments (Stys and Lesiuk, 1996; Stys 1995; Stys *et al.*, 1992a, 1992b). Therefore, Na^+ channel modulators may offer advantages for treating certain types of strokes or neuronal trauma where damage to white matter tracts is prominent. It has been proposed that these drugs block sustained Na^+ currents in hypoxic white matter *in vitro* (Stys *et al.*, 1993), thereby reducing hypoxic Na^+ loading and subsequent Ca^{2+} influx via the Na/Ca exchanger of the plasma membrane (Lehning *et al.*, 1996; LoPachin and Stys, 1995; Stys et al., 1992b).

Many of the drugs listed in Table III have actions in addition to Na^+ channel blockade, and it might be argued that neuroprotection is caused by other mechanisms. However, TTX is significantly neuroprotective in several models both *in vitro* and *in vivo*, suggesting that sodium channel blockade alone may account for neuroprotection with some of these agents. Furthermore, phenytoin, riluzole, and lamotrigine and its derivatives have been studied extensively and generally act at other pharmacological sites only with greater concentrations than those modulating Na^+ channels. Several other drugs (Table III) reported to be neuroprotective in rodent models of ischemia with different putative mechanisms such as Ca^{2+} entry block (verapamil), κ opiate agonism (enadoline), NMDA receptor antagonism (felbamate, remacemide), or β-adrenergic blockade (carvedilol) also produce Na^+ channel blockade. Thus, Na^+ channel blockade may account, at least in part, for neuroprotection with a rather broad range of pharmacological agents.

Results from an initial multicenter placebo-controlled clinical trial of lifarizine for acute therapy in stroke have been reported (Squire *et al.*, 1995). Although lifarizine (like flunarizine and lomerizine) blocks several types of cation channels, some of its actions have been attributed to Na^+ channel blockade. In this preliminary study, drug-treated patients did not have a significantly better outcome than placebo-treated patients. However, there was a decided trend toward better outcome with drug treatment (Squire *et al.*, 1995).

Clinical trials in stroke or head injury have been or will soon be initiated for several of the Na^+ channel blockers discussed earlier. These include fosphenytoin, a water-soluble prodrug of phenytoin (Warner-Lambert), BW619C89 (Glaxo-Wellcome), riluzole (Rhône-Poulenc Rorer), and remacemide (Astra-Arcus).

2. *Head Trauma*

To date, the only relevant data are from animal models with the compounds BW619C89, BW1003C87, and riluzole (Table IV). Administration of BW1003C87 15 min after traumatic injury reduced regional brain edema in a rat fluid percussion model. BW619C89 given before injury attenuated CA1 and CA3 cell damage and behavioral deficits from fluid percussion in rats. Other voltage-dependent Na^+ channel blockers have not been studied extensively in brain trauma. However, it is likely that other voltage-dependent Na^+ channel blockers will also reduce neuronal necrosis from head trauma, as several other protective mechanisms relevant for ischemic stroke are also relevant for head trauma in animal models. Necrosis following head trauma is thought to result mostly from ischemia caused by disruption of normal blood flow (Yamakami and McIntosh, 1989) secondary to cerebral edema (Soares *et al.*, 1992).

3. Amyotrophic Lateral Sclerosis and Neurodegenerative Diseases

The neurological disease known as amyotrophic lateral sclerosis (ALS) in the United States or motor neuron disease in the United Kingdom is characterized by the progressive degeneration of spinal and neocortical motoneurones, leading to the paralysis of skeletal muscles. Afflicted patients usually die from respiratory failure within 3 to 5 years of diagnosis. Drug treatment of this disorder is in its infancy, but somewhat promising results have been obtained in controlled clinical studies with the voltage-dependent Na^+ channel blocker riluzole. Chronic treatment significantly prolonged survival in a subset of patients with bulbar onset of the disease (Bensimon *et al.*, 1994; Lacomblez *et al.*, 1996). Clinical results with riluzole for ALS have been confirmed in a second placebo-controlled study; the combined results led to the approval of riluzole (Rilutek) by the U.S. Food and Drug administration for the treatment of ALS. It is notable that riluzole is also active in several models of ischemia, including middle cerebral artery occlusion in rats and global forebrain ischemia in gerbils and rats (Table III). Riluzole blocks glutamate release in several models *in vitro* and partially reduces damage *in vivo* from application of the glutamate agonist quinolinic acid to brain tissue (Mary *et al.*, 1995). However, it is not yet clear whether riluzole reduces only nonvesicular (Ca-independent) transmitter release, as is the case with several other Na^+ channel blockers. Riluzole also blocks K^+ channels (Benoit and Escande, 1993), inhibits certain NMDA-dependent responses (Hubert *et al.*, 1994; Malgouris *et al.*, 1994; Debono *et al.*, 1993; Doble, 1996), and, in at least one model, reduces neurotransmitter release in a pertussis toxin-sensitive manner (Doble *et al.*, 1992). Clearly, not all of these actions arise from Na^+ channel blockade. Although the molecular target of the neuroprotective actions of riluzole has not been definitely established, it is a reasonable to postulate that neuroprotection arises primarily from its actions as a use- and voltage-dependent Na^+ channel blocker (Hebert *et al.*, 1994; Benoit and Escande, 1991) in much the same manner as phenytoin or lidocaine.

It is worth noting that both riluzole and TTX (Rothstein and Kuncl, 1995) have neuroprotective actions in an *in vitro* model designed to mimic ALS

(Rothstein *et al.,* 1993). Anticonvulsant drugs such as phenytoin, lamotrigine, and others may also offer promise for delaying the symptoms of ALS if this hypothesis is correct. However, carefully controlled clinical studies will be needed to test this idea. Riluzole may also be useful in treating Parkinson's disease, based on preliminary results in a model with monkeys (Benazzouz *et al.,* 1995).

4. Biochemical Scheme for Neuroprotective Action of Na^+ Channel Blockers

Electrophysiological results (see Section II,E.) indicate that phenytoin, lidocaine, lamotrigine, and functionally related Na^+ channel blockers are more effective during conditions of cellular depolarization sustained for seconds than under resting conditions. Therefore, these drugs have little effect on normal neuronal signaling but block Na^+ channels under pathological conditions such as seizures or ischemia.

Several ideas about the neuroprotective mechanism are incorporated in a schematic diagram (Fig. 6) that shows the contribution of Na^+ influx from voltage-dependent Na^+ channels during seizures or ischemia. Na^+ influx from the opening of Na^+ channels causes cellular depolarization that contributes to undesirable functions (opening of Ca^{2+} channels and Ca^{2+}-dependent glutamate release, opening of K^+ channels, relief from magnesium-dependent block of NMDA-type glutamate receptors). Because Na^+ channel opening occurs at a fairly early stage in the biochemical cascade from ischemia and generally accelerates other changes, selective Na^+ channel blockers may moderate a wide variety of detrimental actions that occur

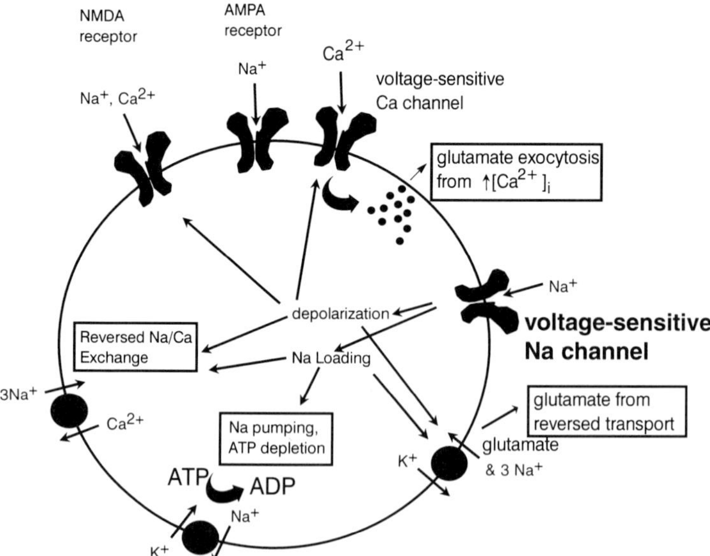

FIGURE 6 The biochemical steps between blockade of Na^+ channels and neuroprotection. See text for details.

later in the cascade. The relative lack of behavioral side effects of voltage-dependent Na^+ channel blockers may offer advantages over other anti-ischemic mechanisms that disrupt normal brain function or blood flow at neuroprotective dosages.

TTX significantly reduces Na^+ influx in rat hippocampal slices depolarized by hypoxia (Kass *et al.,* 1992). In addition, low concentrations of lidocaine reduce Na^+ loading of neurons during anoxia (Fried *et al.,* 1995). Cellular Na^+ loading causes several detrimental changes (inflow of Cl^- to balance net charge and consequent cellular swelling, reversal of Na^+/Ca^{2+} transport, reversal of carrier-mediated glutamate, GABA, hydrogen ion and monoamine transport, etc.). Reduced cellular Na^+ loading would be particularly beneficial during energy deprivation because it would spare cellular ATP. In neurons, ATP is mostly used to fuel the Na^+/K^+ membrane pump. ATP is depleted early in the cascade of event, in brain ischemia (Hansen, 1985), and ATP depletion presumably causes many subsequent detrimental effects. In support of this idea, ATP depletion is reduced by phenytoin pretreatment in rats subjected to forebrain ischemia (Kinouchi *et al.,* 1990) and with lidocaine in hippocampal slices exposed to anoxia (Fried *et al.,* 1995). Maintaining cellular ATP at higher levels would delay or prevent many of the subsequent negative effects in the cascade of biochemical events caused by ischemia.

Transport of Ca^{2+} out of neurons is significantly dependent on the Na^+/Ca^{2+} exchanger of plasma membranes that is driven by the resting transmembrane gradient for Na^+. It is now generally accepted that the exchanger can act in reverse to cause net Ca^{2+} influx when neurons are depolarized or loaded with Na^+ (Kiedrowski *et al.,* 1994; Koch and Barish, 1994). Reversed Na^+/Ca^{2+} exchange may be a major path for Ca^{2+} influx during hypoxia in mammalian white matter *in vitro* (Stys *et al.,* 1992b), as previously demonstrated in ischemic cardiac tissues during reperfusion (Grinwald and Brosnahan, 1987). Studies with hypoxic hippocampal slices *in vitro* (Zhang and Lipton, 1995) show that cellular Na^+ loading from the activation of Na^+ channels releases Ca^{2+} from neuronal mitochondria into the cytosol, as previously observed in vascular smooth muscle (Borin *et al.,* 1994). In hippocampal slices, blockade of Na^+ channels by lidocaine reduces the sustained cytosolic elevation of free Ca^{2+} (Zhang and Lipton, 1995). Most investigators agree that sustained increases in cytosolic-free Ca^{2+} lead to ischemic necrosis (Choi, 1987, 1990; Siesjo, 1988).

Na^+ channel blockade with TTX (Xie *et al.,* 1994) or with other voltage-dependent Na^+ channel blockers (Tagaki *et al.,* 1994; Xie *et al.,* 1995b) delays the onset of hypoxic depolarization [spreading depression-like loss of ion homeostasis (Nedergaard and Hansen, 1993; Hansen 1985)], which is a serious load on brain energy stores (Nedergaard and Astrup, 1986) and which may contribute to cellular damage during ischemia (Alexis *et al.,* 1996; Iijima *et al.,* 1992; Gill *et al.,* 1992; Chen *et al.,* 1993; Hossman, 1996). *In vitro,* phenytoin inhibits spreading depression in retinal tissue, supporting this idea (Chebabo and DoCarmo, 1991). The anti-ischemic actions of several Na^+ channel modulators [including lamotrigine derivatives BW1003C87 (Gaspary *et al.*, 1994) and BW619C89; CNS1237; riluzole] and the mixed cation channel blockers flunarizine and lifarizine, as well as other compounds [e.g., the κ opiate antagonist enadoline (Millan *et al.*, 1995)], have been ascribed to reduced ischemic glutamate release. Glutamate release during ischemia can result from mechanisms fundamentally different from physiological vesicular glutamate release. Several studies, reviewed in Szatkowski and Attwell, (1994), indicate that ischemic glutamate release in several models has little or no Ca^{2+} dependence and is mediated by reversed Na^+-dependent glutamate transport. In hippocampal slices deprived of oxygen and glucose, application of TTX markedly reduces glutamate overflow (Taylor *et al.*, 1995). Reducing ischemic glutamate release may be a major mode of neuroprotective action of voltage-dependent Na^+ channel blockers.

VI. Future Developments

A. Drugs with Na^+ Channel Subtype Specificity

Presently, there are no voltage-dependent Na^+ blocking drugs known to have pronounced selectivity for one subtype of Na^+ channel over another. (Tetrodotoxin is relatively selective for certain neuronal Na^+ channels, being relatively less potent for blockade of Na^+ channels in cardiac muscle, glia, and certain peripheral sensory neurons.) However, the idea of a novel therapeutic compound with very selective properties for blockade of one subtype of neuronal Na^+ channels with little action on other Na^+ or Ca^{2+} channels is attractive. The recent cloning and functional expression of various Na^+ channels subtypes provides a number of useful systems for the potential discovery of subtype-selective blocking drugs. However, the high degree of homology between Na^+ channel sequences in the putative local anesthetic binding region (IV–S6 region, Fig. 3A) suggests that blockers selective for one channel subtype may be difficult to find unless an alternate drug-binding region is discovered.

Lidocaine is more potent for blocking TTX-sensitive channels of sensory neurons than for TTX-resistant channels if neuronal membrane voltage is held the same for both channel types (Roy and Narahashi, 1992). However, because block by lidocaine is dependent on the degree of inactivation, this may result from a larger degree of resting inactivation with TTX-sensitive channels than from a true difference in drug sensitivity between channel subtypes. A similar situation was reported for the blockade of voltage-sensitive Ca^{2+} channels, in which four Ca^{2+} channel subtypes have varying sensitivity to the voltage-sensitive blocking drug mibefradil (Bezprozvanny and Tsien, 1995). In this case, the subtype "selectivity" of mibefradil arose from differences in the voltage dependence of inactivation of the various channel subtypes. The channels showing inactivation at more negative voltages were the most sensitive to blockade. K_i values for mebefradil calculated for inactivated channels (which occur with different voltage dependences in different Ca^{2+} channel subtypes) were similar for the four channel subtypes (Bezprozvanny and Tsien, 1995).

B. Selective Kinetics of Block (Neuroprotection vs. Epilepsy)

Various local anesthetics, anti-arrhythmics, and anticonvulsants prevent hypoxic neuronal damage in isolated rat optic nerve. Within this group of compounds, there appears to be an increased potency of neuroprotection (relative to potency of action potential block) with voltage-dependent Na^+ blockers that increases the conduction delay of action potentials under nonhypoxic conditions (Stys and Lesiuk, 1996; Stys, 1995). Delayed conduction may correlate with rapid open channel block, which has been reported with the quaternary amine derivatives of local anesthetics in voltage clamp experiments (Khodorov, 1991). Neuroprotection in the isolated optic nerve preparation has been reported with relatively little decrement in action potential amplitude with lidocaine and mexiletine (Stys and Lesiuk, 1996; Stys *et al.,* 1992a; Stys, 1995), which share some characteristics of open channel block. The trend of increased action with rapid open channel blockade is not evident for anticonvulsant action in animals, and there may be significant differences between the optimal kinetics or voltage dependence of neuroprotection and other actions such as prevention of seizures. However, additional studies are needed to test this idea thoroughly.

VII. Closing Comments

Since the mid-1930s, voltage-dependent Na^+ channel blockers have provided invaluable therapy for the medical treatment of epilepsies and for certain types of neuropathic pain. More recently, their potential use for the treatment of acute ischemic stroke, traumatic brain injury, and neurodegenerative diseases is becoming appreciated. Molecular and electrophysiological studies have provided considerable insight into their molecular mode of action. It is hoped that modern techniques of drug discovery will allow the discovery of even more effective and more selective agents in the future. However, additional basic studies continue to be needed to better define the essential elements of anticonvulsant, analgesic, and neuroprotive actions and to distinguish among these so that more effective agents with fewer undesirable actions can be discovered.

Acknowledgments

Special thanks to many colleagues, especially Miriam Meisler (University of Michigan) for discussions of Na^+ channel genes and sequences and for help with an earlier version of the manuscript. Thanks are also due to William Catterall (University of Washington), Bruce Bean (Vollum Institute), and David Rock (Parke-Davis Research) for sharing insights and to Brian Meldrum (Institute of Psychiatry, London) for useful discussions. Unpublished data with several new AEDs was obtained from Pharmaprojects (PJB Publications, Ltd., Richmond, U.K.), a proprietary pharmaceutical industry database. Support provided by Parke-Davis Research, Division of Warner-Lambert Co.

References

Adler, E. M., Yarri, Y., David, G., and Selzer, M. E. (1986). Frequency-dependent action of phenytoin on lamprey spinal axons. *Brain Res.* **362,** 271–280.

Ahmed, C. M., Ware, D. H., Lee, S. C., Patten, C. D., Ferrer-Montiel, A. V., Schinder, A. F., McPherson, J. D., Wagner-McPherson, C. B., Wasmuth, J. J., Evans, G. A., and Montal, M. (1992). Primary structure, chromosomal localization and functional expression of a voltage-gated sodium channel from human brain. *Proc. Natl. Acad. Sci. U. S. A.* **89,** 8220–8224.

Akopian, A. N., Sivilotti, L., and Wood, J. N. (1996). A tetrodotoxin-resistant voltage-gated sodium channel expressed by sensory neurons. *Nature (London)* **379,** 257–262.

Alexander, G. J., Kopeloff, L. M., Alexander, R. B., and Chatterjie, N. (1986). Mexiletine: Biphasic action on convulsive seizures in rodents. *Neurobehav. Toxicol. Teratol.* **8,** 231–235.

Alexis, N. E., Back, T., Zhao, W., Dietrich, W. D., Watson, B. D., and Ginsberg, M. D. (1996). Neurobehavioral consequences of induced spreading depression following photothrombic middle cerebral artery occlusion. *Brain Res.* **706,** 273–282.

Alzheimer, C., Schwindt, P. C., and Crill, W. E. (1993a). Postnatal development of a persistent Na+ current in pyramidal neurons from rat sensorimotor cortex. *J. Neurophysiol.* **69,** 290–292.

Alzheimer, C., Schwindt, P. C., and Crill, W. E. (1993b). Modal gating of Na+ channels as a mechanism of persistent Na+ current in pyramidal neurons from rat and cat sensorimotor cortex. *J. Neurosci.* **13,** 660–673.

Ambrose, C., Cheng, S., Fontaine, B., Nadeau, J. H., MacDonald, M., and Gusella, J. F. (1992). The alpha-subunit of the skeletal muscle sodium channel is encoded proximal to Tk-1 on mouse chromosome 11. *Mamm. Genome* **3,** 151–155.

Auld, V. J., Goldin, A. L., Krafte, D. S., Marshall, J., Dunn, J. M., Catterall, W. A., Lester, H. A., Davidson, N., and Dunn, R. J. (1988). A rat brain Na^+ channel alpha subunit with novel gating properties. *Neuron* **1,** 449–461.

Auld, V. J., Goldin, A. L., Krafte, D. S., Catterall, W. A., Lester, H. A., Davidson, N., and Dunn, R. J. (1990). A neutral amino acid change in segment IIS4 dramatically alters the gating properties of the voltage-dependent sodium channel. *Proc. Natl. Acad. Sci. U. S. A.* **87,** 323-327.

Bach, F. W., Jensen, T. S., Kastrup, J., Stigsby, B., and Dejgard, A. (1990). The effect of intravenous lidocaine on nociceptive processing in diabetic neuropathy. *Pain* **40,** 29–34.

Bean, B. P., Cohen, C. J., and Tsien, R. W. (1983). Lidocaine block of cardiac sodium channels. *J. Gen. Physiol.* **81,** 613–642.

Beckh, S., Noda, M., Lübbert, H., and Numa, S. (1989). Differential regulation of three sodium channel messenger RNAs in the rat central nervous system during development. *Nature (London)* **8,** 3611–3616.

Belcher, S. M., Zerillo, C. A., Levenson, R., Ritchie, J. M., and Howe, J. R. (1995). Cloning of a sodium channel alpha subunit from rabbit Schwann cells. *Proc. Natl. Acad. Sci. U. S. A.* **92,** 11034–11038.

Benazzouz, A., Borad, T., Dubedat, P., Boireau, A., Stutzmann, J., and Gross, C. (1995). Riluzole prevents MPTP-induced parkinsonism i the rhesus monkey: A pilot study. *Eur. J. Pharmacol.* **284**, 299–307.

Bennett, P. B., Valenzuela, C., Chen, L.-Q., and Kallen, R. G. (1995a). On the molecular nature of the lidocaine receptor of cardiac Na+ channels—Modification of block by alterations in the alpha-subunit II-IV interdomain. *Circ. Res.* **77**, 584–592.

Bennett, P. B., Yazawa, K., Makita, N., and George, A. L. J. (1995b). Molecular mechanism of an inherited cardiac arrhythmia. *Nature (London)* **376**, 683–685.

Benoit, E., and Escande, D. (1991). Riluzole specifically blocks inactivatied Na channels in myelinated nerve fibre. *Pfluegers Arch.* **419**, 603–609.

Benoit, E., and Escande, D. (1993). Fast K channels are more sensitive to riluzole than slow K channels in myelinated nerve fibre. *Pfluegers Arch.* **422**, 536–538.

Bensimon, G., Lacomblez, L., and Meininger, V. A. (1994). Controlled trial of riluzole in amyotrophic lateral sclerosis. *N. Engl. J. Med.* **330**, 585–591.

Bezprozvanny, I., and Tsien, R. W. (1995). Voltage-dependent blockade of diverse types of voltage-gated Ca^{2+} channels expressed in Xenopus oocytes by the Ca^{2+} channel antagonist mebefradil (RO 40-5967). *Mol. Pharmacol.* **48**, 540–549.

Boening, J. A., Kass, I. S., Cottrell, J. E., and Chambers, G. (1989). The effect of blocking sodium influx on anoxic damage in the rat hippocampal slice. *Neuroscience* **33**, 263–268.

Borin, M. L., Tribe, R. M., and Blaustein, M. P. (1994). Increased intracellular Na+ augments mobilization of Ca2+ from SR in vascular smooth muscle cells. *Am. J. Physiol.* **266**, C311–C317.

Boxer, P. A., Cordon, J. J., Mann, M. E., Rodolosi, L. C., Vartanian, M. G., Rock, D. M., Taylor, C. P., and Marcoux, F. W. (1990). Comparison of phenytoin with noncompetitive N-methyl-D-aspartate antagonists in a model of focal brain ischemia in rat. *Stroke* **21**, 47–51.

Brown, A. M., Schwindt, P. C., and Crill, W. E. (1994a). Different voltage dependence of transient and persistent Na+ currents is compatible with modal-gating hypothesis for sodium channels. *J. Neurophysiol.* **71**, 2562–2565.

Brown, C. M., Calder, C., Linton, C., Small, C., Kenny, B. A., Spedding, M., and Patmore, L. (1995a). Neuroprotective properties of lifarizine compared with those of other agents in a mouse model of focal ischemia. *Br. J. Pharmacol.* **115**, 1425–1432.

Brown, D. L., Ransom, D. M., Hall, J. A., Leicht, C. H., Schroeder, D. R., and Offord, K. P. (1995b). Regional anesthesia and local anesthetic-induced systemic toxicity: Seizure frequency and accompanying cardiovascular changes. *Anesth. Analg. (Cleveland)* **81**, 321–328.

Brown, N. A., Kemp, J. A., and Seabrook, G. R. (1994b). Block of human voltage-sensitive Na+ currents in differentiated SH-SY5Y cells by lifarizine. *Br. J. Pharmacol.* **113**, 600–606.

Burack, M. A., Stasheff, S. F., and Wilson, W. A. (1995). Selective suppression of in vitro electrographic seizures by low-dose tetrodotoxin: A novel anticonvulsant effect. *Epilepsy Res.* **22**, 115–126.

Burgess, D. L., Kohrman, D. C., Galt, J., Plummer, N. W., Jones, J. M., Spear, B., and Meisler, M. H. (1995). Mutation of a new sodium channel gene, SCN8A, in the mouse mutant 'motor endplate disease.' *Nat. Genet.* **10**, 461–465.

Callaway, J. C., and Ross, W. N. (1995). Frequency-dependent propagation of sodium action potentials in dendrites of hippocampal CA1 pyramidal neurons. *J. Neurophysiol.* **74**, 1395–1403.

Cannon, S. C. (1996). Ion-channel defects and aberrant excitability in myotonia and periodic paralysis. *Trends Neurosci.* **19**, 3–10.

Catterall, W. A. (1980). Neurotoxins that act on voltage-sensititve sodium channels in excitable cells. *Annu. Rev. Pharmacol. Toxicol.* **20**, 15–43.

Catterall, W. A. (1986). Voltage-dependent gating of sodium channels: Correlating structure and function. *Trends Neurosci.* **9**, 7–10.

Catterall, W. A. (1987). Common modes of drug action on Na+ channels: Local anesthetics, antiarrhythmics, and anticonvulsants. *Trends Neurosci.* **8,** 57–65.
Catterall, W. A. (1992). Cellular and molecular biology of voltage-gated sodium channels. *Physiol. Rev.* **72,** S15–S48.
Catterall, W. A., Trainer, V., and Baden, D. G. (1992). Molecular properties of the sodium channel: A receptor for multiple neurotoxins. *Bull. Soc. Pathol. Exot.* **85,** 481–485.
Cerne, R., and Spain, W. J. (1995). Bistability in the dendrites of rat neocortical pyramidal cells is mediated by persisitent sodium current. *Soc. Neurosci. Abstr.* **21,** 585.
Chao, T. I., and Alzheimer, C. (1995). Effects of phenytoin on the persistent Na+ current of mammalian CNS neurones. *NeuroReport* **6,** 1778–1780.
Chaplan, S. R., Bach, F. W., Shafer, S. L., and Yaksh, T. L. (1995). Prolonged alleviation of tactile allodynia by intravenous lidocaine in neuopathic rats. *Anesthesiology* **83,** 775–785.
Charnet, P., Labarca, C., Leonard, R. J., Vogelaar, N. J., Czyzyk, L., Gouin, A., Davidson, N., and Lester, H. A. (1990). An open-channel blocker interacts with adjacent turns of alpha-helices in the nicotinic acetylcholine receptor. *Neuron* **4,** 87–95.
Chebabo, S. R., and DoCarmo, R. J. (1991). Phenytoin and retinal spreading depression. *Brain Res.* **551,** 16–19.
Chen, J., Graham, S. H., and Simon, R. P. (1995). A comparison of the effects of a sodium channel blocker and an NMDA antagonist upon extracellular glutamate in rat focal cerebral ischemia. *Brain Res.* **699,** 121–124.
Chen, Q., Chopp, M., Bodzin, G., and Chen, H. (1993). Temperature modulation of cerbral depolarization during focal cerebral ischemia in rats: Correlation with ischemic injury. *J. Cereb. Blood Flow Metab.* **13,** 389–394.
Cheung, H., Kamp, D., and Harris, E. (1992). An in vitro investigation of the action of lamotrigine on neuronal voltage-activated sodium channels. *Epilepsy Res.* **13,** 107–112.
Choi, D. W. (1987). Ionic dependence of glutamate neurotoxicity. *J. Neurosci.* **7,** 369–379.
Choi, D. W. (1988). Glutamate neurotoxicity and diseases of the nervous system. *Neuron* **1,** 623–634.
Choi, D. W. (1990). Methods for antagonizing glutamate neurotoxicity. *Cerebrovasc. Brain Metab. Rev.* **2,** 105–147.
Colling, S. B., and Wheal, H. V. (1994). Fast sodium action potentials are generated in the distal apical dendrites of rat. *Neurosci. Lett.* **172,** 73–96.
Coulter, D. A., Sombati, S., and DeLorenzo, R. J. (1993). Selective effects of topiramate on sustained repetitive firing and spontaneous bursting in cultured hippocampal neurons. *Epilepsia* **34**(Suppl. 2):123 (Abstract).
Dayhoff, M. O. ed. (1996). "Atlas of Protein Structure," Natl. Biomed. Res. Found., Washington, DC.
Debono, M. W., Le Guern, J., Canton, T., Doble, A., and Pradier, L. (1993). Inhibition by riluzole of electrophysiological responses mediated by rat kainate and NMDA receptors expressed in Xenopus oocytes. *Eur. J. Pharmacol.* **235,** 283–289.
Dejgard, A., Petersen, P., and Kastrup, J. (1988). Mexiletine for treatment of chronic painful diabetic neuropathy. *Lancet* **1,** 9–11.
Denaro, C. P., and Benowitz, N. L. (1989). Poisoning due to class 1B antiarrhythmic drugs. Lignocaine, mexiletine and tocainide. *Med. Toxicol. Adverse Drug Exper.* **4,** 412–428.
Dessi, F., Ben Ari, Y., and Charriaut Marlangue, C. (1993). Riluzole prevents anoxic injury in cultured cerebellar granule neurons. *Eur. J. Pharmacol.* **250,** 325–328.
Devor, M. (1994). The pathophysiology of damaged peripheral nerves. *In "Textbook of Pain"* (P. D. Wall and R. Melzack, eds.) Edinburgh: Churchill Livingstone, p. 79–100.
Doble, A., Hubert, J. P., and Blanchard, J. C. (1992). Pertussis toxin pretreatment abolishes the inhibitory effect of riluzole and carbachol on D-[3H]aspartate release from cultured cerebellar granule cells. *Neurosci. Lett.* **140,** 251–254.
Doble, A. (1996). The pharmacology and mechanism of action of riluzole. *Neurol.* **47**(Suppl. 4), S233–S241.

Durell, S. R., and Guy, H. R. (1992). Atomic scale structure and functional models of voltage-gated potassium channels. *Biophys. J.* **62,** 238–247.

England, J. D., Happel, L. T., Kline, D. G., Gamboni, F., Thouron, C. L., Liu, Z. P., and Levinson, S. R. (1996). Sodium channel accumulation in humans with painful neuromas. *Neurol.* **47,** 272–276.

Fern, R., Ransom, B. R., Stys, P., and Waxman, S.G. (1993). Pharmacological protection of CNS white matter during anoxia: Actions of phenytoin, carbamazepine and diazepam. *J. Pharmacol. Exp. Ther.* **266,** 1549–1555.

Fischer, W., Bodewei, R., and Satzinger, G. (1992). Anticonvulsant and sodium channel blocking effects of ralitoline in different screening models. *Naunyn-Schmiedeberg's Arch. Pharmacol.* **346,** 442–452.

Flatman, J. A., Schwindt, P. C., Crill, W. E., and Stafström, C. E. (1983). Multiple actions of N-methyl-D-aspartate on cat neocortical neurons in vitro. *Brain Res.* **266,** 169–173.

Flieg, A., Fitch, J. M., Goldin, A. L., Rayner, M. D., Starkus, J. G., and Ruben, P. C. (1994). Point mutations in IIS4 alter activation and inactivation of rat brain IIA Na channels in Xenopus oocyte macropatches. *Pfluegers Arch.* **427,** 406–412.

Foong, F. W., and Satoh, M. (1983). Analgesic potencies of non-narcotic, narcotic and anesthetic drugs as determined by the bradykinin-induced biting-like responses in rats. *Jpn. J. Pharmacol.* **33,** 933–938.

French, C. R., Sah, P., Buckett, K. J., and Gage, P. W. (1990). A voltage-dependent persistent sodium current in mammalian hippocampal neurons. *J. Gen. Physiol.* **95,** 1139–1157.

Fried, E., Amorim, P., Chambers, G., Cottrell, J. E., and Kass, I. S. (1995). The importance of sodium for anoxic transmission damage in rat hippocampal slices: mechanisms of protection by lidocaine. *J. Physiol. Lond.* **489,** 557–565.

Fujisawa, H., Dawson, D., Browne, S. E., MacKay, K. B., Bullock, R., and McCulloch, J. (1993). Pharmacological modification of glutamate neurotoxicity in vivo. *Brain Res.* **629,** 73–78.

Galer, B. S. (1995). Neuropathic pain of peripheral origin: Advances in pharmacological treatment. *Neurology* **45,** Suppl. 9, S17–S25.

Gaspary, H. L., Simon, R. P., and Graham, S. H. (1994). BW1003C87 and NBQX but not CGS19755 reduce glutamate release and cerebral ischemic necrosis. *Eur. J. Pharmacol.* **262,** 197–203.

Gautron, S., Dossantos, G., Pintohenrique, D., Koulakoff, A., Gros, F., and Berwaldnetter, Y. (1992). The glial voltage-gated sodium channel: Cell-specific and tissue-specific messenger RNA expression. *Proc. Natl. Acad. Sci. U. S. A.* **89,** 7272–7276.

Gellens, M. E., George, A. L., Jr., Chen, L., Chahine, M., Horn, R., Brachi, R. L., and Kallen, R. G. (1992). Primary stucture and functional expression of the human cardiac tetrodotoxin-insensitive voltage-dependent sodium channel. *Proc. Natl. Acad. Sci. U. S. A.* **89,** 554–558.

George, A. L., Jr., Ledbetter, D. H., Kallen, R. G., and Barchi, R. L. (1991). Assignment of a human skeletal muscle sodium channel alpha-subunit gene (SCN4A) to 17q23.1-25.3. *Genomics* **9,** 555–556.

George, A. L., Jr., Knittle, T. J., and Tamkun, M. M. (1992a). Molecular cloning of an atypical voltage-gated sodium channel expressed in human heart and uterus: Evidence for a distinct gene family. *Proc. Natl. Acad. Sci. U. S. A.* **89,** 4893–4897.

George, A. L., Jr., Komisarof, J., Kallen, R. G., and Barchi, R. L. (1992b). Primary structure of the adult human skeletal muscle voltage-dependent sodium channel. *Ann. Neurol.* **32,** 131–137.

George, A. L., Jr., Knops, J. F., Han, J., Finley, W. H., Knittle, T. J., Tamkun, M. M., and Brown, G. B. (1994). Assignment of a human voltage-dependent sodium channel alpha-subunit gene (SCN6A) to 2q21-q23. *Genomics* **19,** 395–397.

George, A. L., Jr., Varkony, T. A., Drabkin, H. A., Han, J., Knops, J. F., Finley, W. H., Brown, G. B., Ward, D. C., and Haas, M. (1995). Assignment of the human heart tetrodotoxin-resistant voltage-gated Na+ channel alpha-subunit gene (SCN5A) to band 3p21. *Cytogenet. Cell Genet.* **68**, 67–70.

Gill, R., Andinè, O., Hillered, L., Persson, l., and Hagberg, H. (1992). The effect of MK-801 on cortical spreading depression in the penumbra zone following focal ischemia in the rat. *J. Cereb. Blood Flow Metab.* **12**, 371–379.

Gilland, E., Puka Sundvall, M., Andine, P., Bona, E., and Hagberg, H. (1994). Hypoxic-ischemic injury in the neonatal rat brain: Effects of pre- and post-treatment with the glutamate release inhibitor BW1003C87. *Brain Res.: Dev. Brain Res.* **83**, 79–84.

Goldin, S.M. (1995). Neuroprotective use-dependent blockers of Na+ and Ca2+ channels controlling presynaptic release of glutamate. *Ann. N. Y. Acad. Sci.* **765**, 210–229.

Gonoi, T., and Hille, B. (1987). Gating of Na channels: Inactivation modifiers dicriminate among models. *J. Gen. Physiol.* **89**, 253–274.

Gordon, D., Merrick, D., Auld, V. J., Dunn, R., Goldin, A. L., Davidson, N., and Catterall, W. A. (1987). Tissue-specific expression of the R_I and R_{II} sodium channel subtypes. *Proc. Natl. Acad. Sci. U. S. A.* **84**, 8682–8686.

Green, M. W., and Selman, J. E. (1991). Review article: The medical management of trigeminal neuralgia. *Headache* **31**, 588–592.

Grinwald, P. M., and Brosnahan, C. (1987). Sodium imbalance as a cause of calcium overload in post-hypoxic reoxygenation injury. *J. Mol. Cell. Cardiol.* **19**, 487–495.

Gurney, M. E., Cutting, F. B., Zhai, P., Doble, A., Taylor, C. P., Andrus, P. K., and Hall, E. D. (1996). Benefit of vitamin E, riluzole and gabapentin in a transgenic model of familial ALS. *Ann. Neurol.* **39**, 147–157.

Guy, H. R., and Conti, F. (1990). Pursuing the structure and function of voltage-gated channels. *Trends Neurosci.* **13**, 201–206.

Guy, H. R., and Durell, S. R. (1994). Using sequence homology to analyze the structure and function of voltage-gated ion channel proteins. *Soc. Gen. Physiol. Ser.* **49**, 197–212.

Hansen, A. J. (1985). Effect of anoxia on ion distribution in the brain. *Physiol. Rev.* **65**, 101–148.

Hara, H., Ozaki, A., Yoshidomi, M., and Sukamoto, T. (1990). Protective effect of KB-2796, a new calcium antagonist, in cerebral hypoxia and ischemia. *Arch. Int. Pharmacodyn. Ther.* **304**, 206–218.

Hara, H., Harada, K., and Sukamoto, T. (1993a). Chronological atrophy after transient middle cerebral artery occlusion in rats. *Brain Res.* **618**, 251–260.

Hara, H., Yokota, K., Shimazawa, M., and Sukamoto, T. (1993b). Effect of KB-2796, a new diphenylpiperizine Ca2+ antagonist, on glutamate-induced neurotoxicity in rat hippocampal primary cell cultures. *Jpn. J. Pharmacol.* **61**, 361–365.

Hayakawa, T., Hamada, Y., Maihara, T., Hattori, H., and Mikawa, H. (1994a). Phenytoin reduces neonatal hypoxic-ischemic brain damage in rats. *Life Sci.* **54**, 387–392.

Hayakawa, T., Higuchi, Y., Nigami, H., and Hattori, H. (1994b). Zonisamide reduces hypoxic-ischemic brain damage in neonatal rats irrespective of its anticonvulsive effect. *Eur. J. Pharmacol.* **257**, 131–136.

Hays, S. J., Schwarz, R. D., Boyd, D. K., Coughenour, L. L., Dooley, D. J., Rock, D. M., and Taylor, C. P. (1991). PD 85639: A potent inhibitor of Na+ influx into rat neocortical slices. *Soc. Neurosci. Abstr.* **17**, 956.

Hays, S. J., Rice, M. J., Ortwine, D. F., Johnson, G., Schwarz, R. D., Boyd, D. K., Copeland, L. F., Vartanian, M. G., and Boxer, P. A. (1994). Substituted 2-benzothiazoles as sodium flux inhibitors: Quantitative structure-activity relationships and anticonvulsant activity. *J. Pharma. Sci.* **83**, 1425–1432.

Hayward, N. J., McKnight, A. T., and Woodruff, G. N. (1993). Neuroprotective effect of the kappa-agonist enadoline (CI-977) in rat models of focal cerbral ischaemia. *Eur. J. Pharmacol.* **5**, 961–967.

Hebert, T., Drapeau, P., Pradier, L., and Dunn, R. J. (1994). Block of rat brain IIA sodium channel α subunit by the neuroprotective drug riluzole. *Mol. Pharmacol.* **45**, 1055–1060.

Heinemann, S. H., Terlau, H., Stuhmer, W., Imoto, K., and Numa, S. (1992). Calcium channel characteristics confered on the sodium channel by single mutations. *Nature* (*London*) **356,** 441–443.

Herring, S., Bodewei, R., and Wollenberger, A. (1983). Sodium current in freshly isolated and in cultured single rat myocardial cells: Frequency and voltage-dependent block by mexiletine. *J. Mol. Cell. Cardiol.* **15,** 431–444.

Hille, B. (1975). The receptor for tetrodotoxin and saxitoxin: A structural hypothesis. *Biophys. J.* **15,** 615–619.

Hille, B. (1977). Local anesthetics: Hydrophilic and hydrophobic pathways for the drug-receptor reaction. *J. Gen. Physiol.* **69,** 497–515.

Hirschberg, B., Rovner, A., Lieberman, M., and Patlack, J. (1995). Transfer of twelve charges is needed to open skeletal muscle Na channels. *J. Gen. Physiol.* **106,** 1053–1068.

Hodgkin, A. L., and Huxley, A. F. (1952). A quantitative description of membrane current and its application to conduction and excitation in nerve. *J. Physiol.* (*London*) **117,** 500–544.

Hondeghem, L. M., and Katzung, B. G. (1977). Time- and voltage-dependent interaction of antiarrhythmic drugs with cardiac sodium channels. *Biochim. Biophys. Acta* **472,** 373–398.

Hossmann, K. A. (1996). Periinfarct depolarizations. *Cerebrovasc. Brain Metab. Rev.* **8,** 195–208.

Hu, G. Y., and Hvalby, O. (1992). Glutamate-induced action potentials are preceded by regenerative prepotentials in rat hippocampal pyramidal cells in vitro. *Exp. Brain Res.* **88,** 485–494.

Hubert, J. P., Delumeau, J. C., Glowinski, J., Premont, J., and Doble, A. (1994). Antagonism by riluzole of entry of calcium evoked by NMDA and veratridine in rat cultured granule cells: evidence for a dual mechanism of action. *Br. J. Pharmacol.* **113,** 261–267.

Iijima, T., Mies, G., and Hossmann, K. A. (1992). Repeated negative DC deflections in rat cortex following middle cerebral artery occlusion are abolished by MK-801: Effect on volume of ischemic injury. *J. Cereb. Blood Flow Metab.* **12,** 727–733.

Isom, L. L., DeJongh, K. S., Patton, D. E., Reber, B. F. X., Offord, J., and Charbonneau, H. (1992). Primary structure and functional expression of the beta 1 subunit of the rat brain sodium channel. *Science* **256,** 839–842.

Isom, L. L., Ragsdale, D. S., DeJongh, K. S., Westenbroek, R., Reber, B. F. X., Scheuer, T., and Catterall, W. A. (1995a). Structure and function of the beta-2 subunit of sodium channels, a transmembrane glycoprotein with a CAM motif. *Cell* (*Cambridge, Mass.*) **83,** 433–442.

Isom, L. L., Scheuer, T., Brownstein, A. B., Ragsdale, D. S., Murphy, B. J., and Catterall, W. A. (1995b). Functional co-expression of the beta 1 and type IIA alpha subunits of sodium channels in a mammalian cell line. *J. Biol. Chem.* **270,** 3306–3312.

Joho, R. H., Moorman, J. R., VanDongen, M. J., Kirsch, G. E., Silberg, H., Schuster, G., and Brown, A. M. (1990). Toxin and kinetic profile of rat brain type III sodium channels expressed in *Xenopus* oocytes. *Mol. Brain Res.* **7,** 105–113.

Kallen, R. G., Sheng, Z., Yang, J., Chen, L., Rogart, R. B., and Barchi, R. L. (1990). Primary structure and expression of a sodium channel characteristic of denervated and immature rat skeletal muscle. *Neuron* **4,** 233–242.

Kallen, R. G., Cohen, S. A., and Barchi, R. L. (1993). Structure, function and expression of voltage-dependent sodium channels. *Mol. Neurobiol.* **7,** 383–428.

Kamei, J., Hitosugi, H., Kawahima, N., Aoki, T., Ohhashi, Y., and Kasuya, Y. (1992). Antinociceptive effect of mexiletine in diabetic mice. *Res. Commun. Chem. Pathol. Pharmacol.* **77,** 245–248.

Kanthasamy, A. G., Matsumoto, R. R., Gunasekar, P. G., and Truong, D. D. (1995). Excitoprotective effect of felbamate in cultured cortical neurons. *Brain Res.* **705,** 97–104.

Karolchyk, M. A. (1996). Rufinamide (CGP-33101): A triazole derivative anticonvulsant. Southborough, MA: International Business Communications (oral conference presentation).

Kass, I. S., Abramowicz, A. E., Cottrell, J. E., and Chambers, G. (1992). The barbiturate thiopental reduces ATP levels during anoxia but improves electrophysiological recovery and ionic homeostasis in the rat hippocampal slice. *Neuroscience* **49**, 537–543.

Kayano, T., Noda, M., Flockerzi, H., Takahashi, H., and Numa, S. (1988). Primary structure of rat brain sodium channel III deduced from the cDNA sequence. *FEBS Lett.* **228**, 187–194.

Keynes, R. D. (1994). Bimodal gating of the Na+ channel. *Trends Neurosci.* **17**, 58–61.

Khodorov, B. I. (1991). Role of inactivation in local anesthetic action. *Ann. N. Y. Acad. Sci.* **625**, 225–248.

Kiedrowski, L., Brooker, G., Costa, E., and Wroblewski, J. T. (1994). Glutamate impairs neuronal calcium extrusion while reducing sodium gradient. *Neuron* **12**, 295–300.

Kinouchi, H., Imaizumi, S., Yoshimoto, T., and Motomiya, M. (1990). Phenytoin affects metabolism of free fatty acids and nucleotides in rat cerebral ischemia. *Stroke* **21**, 1326–1332.

Kiskin, N. I., Chizhmakov, I. V., Tsyndrenko, A. Y., Krishtal, O. A., and Tegtmeier, F. (1993). R56865 and flunarizine as Na(+)-channel blockers in isolated Purkinje neurons of rat cerebellum. *Neuroscience* **54**, 575–585.

Kloke, M., Hoffken, K., Olbrich, H., and Schmidt, C. G. (1991). Anti-depressants and anticonvulsants for the treatment of neuropathic pain syndromes in cancer patients. *Onkologie* **14**, 40–43.

Koch, R. A., and Barish, M. E. (1994). Perturbation of intracellular calcium and hydrogen ion regulation in cultured mouse hippocampal neurons by reduction of the sodium ion concentration gradient. *J. Neurosci.* **14**, 2585–2593.

Kohrman, D. C., Harris, J. B., and Meisler, M. H. (1996). Mutation detection in the *med* and *med*^{J} alleles of the sodium channel *Scn8a*: Unusual splicing due to a minor class AT-AC intron. *J. Biol. Chem.* 271, 17576–17581.

Kohrman, D. C., Smith, M. R., Goldin, A. L., Harris, J., and Meisler, M. H. (1996). A missense mutation in the sodium channel Scn8a is responsible for cerebellar ataxia in the mouse mutant *jolting*. *J. Neurosci.* **16**, 5993–5999.

Krall, R. L., Penry, J. K., White, B. G., Kupferberg, H. J., and Swinyard, E. A. (1978). Antiepileptic drug development: II. Anticonvulsant drug screening. *Epilepsia* **19**, 409–428.

Kucharczyk, J., Mintorovitch, J., Moseley, M. E., Asgari, H. S., Sevick, R. J., Derugin, N., Norman, D., Leach, M. J., Swan, J. H., Eisenthal, D., Dopson, M., and Nobbs, M. (1993). Ischemic brain damage: Reduction by sodium-calcium ion channel modulator RS- 87476. *Stroke* **24**, 1063–1067.

Kuo, C. C., and Bean, B. P. (1994a). Slow binding of phenytoin to inactivated sodium channels in rat hippocampal neurons. *J. Pharmacol. Exp. Ther.* **46**, 716–725.

Kuo, C. C., and Bean, B. P. (1994b). Na+ channels must deactivate to recover from inactivation. *Neuron* **12**, 819–829.

Lacomblez, L., Bensimon, G., Leigh, P. N., Guillet, P., and Meininger, V. (1996). Dose-ranging study of riluzole in amyotrophic lateral sclerosis. *Lancet* **347**, 1425–1428.

Leach, M. J., Marden, C. M., and Miller, A. A. (1986). Pharmacological studies on lamotrigine, a novel potential antiepileptic drug: II. neurochemical studies on the mechanism of action. *Epilepsia* **27**, 490–497.

Leach, M. J., Baxter, M. G., and Critchley, M. A. (1991). Neurochemical and behavioral aspects of lamotrigine. *Epilepsia* **32**, S4–S8.

Leach, M. J., Swan, J. H., Eisenthal, D., Dopson, M., and Nobbs, M. (1993). BW619C89, a glutamate release inhibitor, protects against focal cerbral ischemic damage. *Stroke* **24**, 1063–1067.

Lehning, E. J., Doshi, R., Isaksson, N., Stys, P. K., and LoPachin, R. M., Jr. (1996). Mechanisms of injury-induced calcium entry into peripheral nerve myelinated axons: Role of reverse sodium-calcium exchange. *J. Neurochem.* **66**, 493–500.

Lekieffre, D., and Meldrum, B.S. (1993). The pyrimidine derivative, BW 1003C87, protects CA1 and striatal neurons following transient severe forebrain ischaemia in rats. A microdialysis and histological study. *Neurosci.* **56**, 93–99.

Leschinger, A., Stabel, J., Igelmund, P., and Heinemann, U. (1993). Pharmacological and electrographic properties of epileptiform activity induced by elevated K+ and lowered Ca2+ and Mg2+ concentration in rat hippocampal slices. *Exp. Brain Res.* **96,** 230–240.

Levy, R. H., Mattson, R. H., and Meldrum, B.S., eds. (1995). "Antiepileptic Drugs," 4th ed. Raven Press, New York.

Li, M., West, J. W., Numann, R., Murphy, B. J., Scheuer, T., and Catterall, W. A. (1993). Convergent regulation of sodium channels by protein kinase C and cAMP-dependent protein kinase. *Science* **261,** 1439–1442.

Lindström, P., and Lindblom, U. (1987). The analgesic effect of tocainide in trigeminal neuralgia. *Pain* **28,** 45–50.

Litt, M., Luty, J., Kwak, M., Allen, L., Magenis, R. E., and Mandel, G. (1989). Localization of a human brain sodium channel gene (SCN2A) to chromosome 2. *Genomics* **5,** 204–208.

Llinas, R., and Sugimori, M. (1980). Electrophysiological properties of *in vitro* Purkinje cell somata in mammalian cerebellar slices. *J. Physiol.* (*London*) **305,** 171–195.

Lombardo, A. J., Kuzniecky, R., Powers, R. E., and Brown, G. B. (1996). Altered brain sodium channel transcript levels in human epilepsy. *Brain Res. Mol. Brain Res.* **35,** 84–90.

LoPachin, R. M., and Stys, P. (1995). Elemental composition and water content of rat optic nerve myelinated axons and glial cells: Effects of *in vitro* anoxia and reoxygenation. *J. Neurosci.* **15,** 6735–6746.

Lu, H. R., Van Reempts, J., Haseldonckx, M., Borgers, M., and Janssen, P. A. J. (1990). Cerebroprotective effects of flunarizine in an experimental rat model of cardiac arrest. *Am. J. Emerg. Med.* **8,** 1–6.

Lucas, L. F., West, C. A., Rigor, B. M., and Schurr, A. (1989). Protection against cerebral hypoxia by local anesthetics: a study using brain slices. *J. Neurosci. Methods* **28,** 47–50.

Lynch, J. J., 3rd, Yu, S. P., Canzoniero, L. M., Sensi, S. L., and Choi, D. W. (1995). Sodium channel blockers reduce oxygen-glucose deprivation-induced cortical neuronal injury when combined with glutamate receptor antagonists. *J. Pharmacol. Exp. Ther.* **273,** 554–560.

Lysko, P. G., Webb, C. L., and Feuerstein, G. (1994). Neuroprotective effects of carvedilol, a new antihypertensive, as a Na+ channel modulator and glutamate transport inhibitor. *Neurosci. Lett.* **171,** 77–80.

Lysko, P. G., Webb, C. L., Yue, T., Gu, J. G., and Feuerstein, M.D. (1995). Neuroprotective effects of tetrodotoxin as a Na+ channel modulator and glutamate release inhibitor in cultured rat cerebellar neurons and in gerbil global brain ischemia. *Stroke* **25,** 2476–2482.

Ma, J. Y., Li, M., Catterall, W. A., and Scheuer, T. (1994). Modulation of brain Na+ channels by a G-protein-coupled pathway. *Proc. Natl. Acad. Sci. U. S. A.* **91,** 12351–12355.

MacKinnon, A. C., Wyatt, K. M., McGivern, J. G., Sheridan, R. D., and Brown, C. M. (1995). [^{3}H]-Lifarizine, a high affinity probe for inactivated sodium channels. *Br. J. Pharmacol.* **115,** 1103–1109.

Malgouris, C., Daniel, M., and Doble, A. (1994). Neuroprotective effects of riluzole on N-methyl-D-aspartate- or veratridine-induced neurotoxicity in rat hippocampal slices. *Neurosci. Lett.* **177,** 95–99.

Malo, D., Schurr, E., Dorfman, J., Canfield, V., Levenson, R., and Gros, P. (1991). Three brain sodium channel alpha-subunit genes are clustered on the proximal segment of mouse chromosome 2. *Genomics* **10,** 666–672.

Malo, M. S., Blanchard, B. J., Andresen, J. M., Srivastava, K., Chen, X. N., Li, X., Jabs, E. W., Korenberg, J. R., and Ingram, V. M. (1994a). Localization of a putative human brain sodium channel gene (SCN1A) to chromosome band 2q24. *Cytogenet. Cell Genet.* **67,** 178–186.

Malo, M. S., Srivastava, K., Andresen, J. M., Chen, X. N., Korenberg, J. R., and Ingram, V. M. (1994b). Targeted gene walking by low stringency polymerase chain reaction: Assignment of a putative human brain sodium channel gene (SCN3A) to chromosome 2q24-31. *Proc. Natl. Acad. Sci. U. S. A.* **91,** 2975–2979.

Margolin, L. D., Knapp, A. G., and Sharma, R. (1994). Block of voltage-gated sodium currents by the novel acenapthyl guanidine, CNS 11237. *Soc. Neurosci. Abstr.* **20,** 718.

Mary, V., Wahl, F., and Stutzmann, J. M. (1995). Effect of riluzole on quinolinate-induced neuronal damage in rats: Comparison with blockers of glutamatergic neurotransmission. *Neurosci. Lett.* **201,** 92–96.

May, G. R., Rowand, W. S., McCormack, J. G., and Sheridan, R. D. (1995). Neuroprotective profile of lifarizine (RS-87476) in rat cerebrocortical neurones in culture. *Br. J. Pharmacol.* **114,** 1365–1370.

McGivern, J. G., Patmore, L., and Sheridan, R. D. (1995). Effects of the neuroprotective agent, KB-2796, on the voltage-dependent sodium current in mouse neuroblastoma, N1E-115. *Br. J. Pharmacol.* (Proc. Suppl.), 137P.

McGivern, J. G., Patmore, L., and Sheridan, R. D. (1995). Actions of the novel neuroprotective agent, lifarizine (RS-87476), on voltage-dependent sodium currents in the neuroblastoma cell line, N1E-115. *Br. J. Pharmacol.* **114,** 1738–1744.

McLean, M. J., and Macdonald, R. L. (1983). Multiple actions of phenytoin on mouse spinal cord neurons in cell culture. *J. Pharmacol. Exp. Ther.* **227,** 779–789.

McLean, M. J., and Macdonald, R. L. (1986). Carbamazepine and 10,11-epoxycarbabamazepine produce use- and voltage-depndent limitation of rapidly firing action potentials of mouse central neurons in cell culture. *J. Pharmacol. Exp. Ther.* **238,** 727–738.

McNeil, E. T., Lewandowski, G. A., Daly, J. W., and Crevling, C. R. (1985). [3H]Batrachotoxinin A 20-α-bezoate binding to voltage-sensitive sodium channels: A rapid and quantitative assay for local anesthetic activity in a variety of drugs. *J. Med. Chem.* **28,** 381–388.

McPhee, J. C., Ragsdale, D. S., Scheuer, T., and Catterall, W. A. (1994). A mutation in segment IV S6 disrupts fast inactivation of sodium channels. *Proc. Natl. Acad. Sci. U. S. A.* **91,** 12346–12350.

McPhee, J. C., Ragsdale, D. S., Scheuer, T., and Catterall, W. A. (1995). A critical role for transmembrane segment IVS6 of the sodium channel alpha subunit in fast inactivation. *J. Biol. Chem.* **270,** 12025–12034.

Meldrum, B. S., Swan, J. H., Leach, M. J., Millan, M. H., Gwinn, R., Kadota, K., Graham, S. H., Chen, J., and Simon, R. P. (1992). Reduction of glutatmate release and protection against ischemic brain damage by BW1003C87. *Brain Res.* **593,** 1–6.

Michelitti, G., Vergnes, M., Marescaux, C., Reis, J., Depaulis, A., Rumbach, L., and Warter, J. M. (1985). Antiepileptic drug evaluation in a new animal model: Spontaneous petit mal epilepsy in the rat. *Arzneim.-Forsch.* **35,** 483–485.

Millan, M. H., Chapman, A. G., and Meldrum, B. S. (1995). Dual inhibitory action of enadoline (CI977) on release of amino acids in the rat hippocampus. *Eur. J. Pharmacol.* **279,** 75–81.

Miller, C. (1991). Annus mirabilis for potassium channels. *Science* **252,** 1092–1096.

Moorman, J. R., Kirsch, G. E., VanDongen, M. J., Joho, R. H., and Brown, A. M. (1990). Fast and slow gating of sodium channels encoded by a single mRNA. *Neuron* **4,** 243–252.

Murakami, A., and Furui, T. (1994). Effects of the conventional anticonvulsants, phenytoin, carbamazepine and valproic acid on sodium-potassium-adenosine triphosphatase in acute ischemic brain. *Neurosurgery* **34,** 1047–1051.

Nakamura-Craig, M. and Follenfant, R. L. (1995). Effect of lamotrigine in the acute and chronic hyperalgesia induced by PGE_2 and in the chronic hyperalgesia in rats with streptozotocin-induced diabetes. *Pain* **63,** 33–37.

Nedergaard, M., and Astrup, J. (1986). Infarct rim: Effect of hyperglycemia on direct current potential and [14C]2- deoxyglucose phosphorylation. *J. Cereb. Blood Flow Metab.* **6,** 607–615.

Nedergaard, M., and Hansen, A. J. (1993). Characterization of cortical depolarizations evoked in focal cerebral ischemia. *J. Cereb. Blood Flow Metab.* **13,** 568–574.

Nelson, L. S., and Hoffman, R. S. (1994). Mexiletine overdose producing status epilepticus without cardiovascular abnormalities. *J. Toxicol., Clin. Toxicol.* **32,** 731–736.

Noda, M., Shimizu, S., Tanabe, T., Takai, T., Kayano, T., Ikeda, T., Takahashi, H., Nakayama, H., Kanaoka, Y., Minamino, N., Kangawa, K., Matsuo, H., Raftery, M., Hirose, T., Inayama, S., Hayashida, H., Miyata, T., and Numa, S. (1984). Primary structure of *Electrophorus-electricus* sodium channel deduced from complimentary DNA sequence. *Nature (London)* **312,** 121–127.

Noda, M., Ikeda, M., Kayano, T., Suzuki, H., Takeshima, H., Kurasaki, M., Takahashi, H., and Numa, S. (1986). Existence of distinct sodium channel messenger RNAs in rat brain. *Nature (London)* **320,** 188–192.

Noda, M., Suziki, S., Numa, S., and Stuhmer, W. (1989). A single point mutation confers tetrodotoxin and saxitoxin insensitivity on the sodium channel II. *FEBS Lett.* **259,** 213–216.

Numann, R., Hauschka, S. D., Catterall, W. A., and Scheuer, T. (1994). Modulation of skeletal muscle sodium channels in a satellite cell line by protein kinase C. *J. Neurosci.* **14,** 4226–4236.

Okiyama, K., Smith, D. H., Gennarelli, T. A., Simon, R. P., Leach, M., and McIntosh, T. K. (1995). The sodium channel blocker and glutamate release inhibitor BW1003C87 and magnesium attenuate regional cerebral edema following experimental brain injury in the rat. *J. Neurochem.* **64,** 802–809.

Ordy, J. M., Volpe, B., Murray, R., Thomas, G., Bialobok, P., Wengenack, T. M., and Dunlap, W. (1992). Pharmacological effects of remacemide and MK-801 on memory and hippocampal CA1 damage in the rat four-vessel occlusion (4-VO) model of global ischemia. *In "The Role of Neurotransmitters in Brain Injury."* (M. Globus and W. D. Dietrich, eds.), New York: Plenum Press, p 83–92.

Osorio, I., Burnstine, T. H., Remler, B., Manon Espaillat, R., and Reed, R. C. (1989). Phenytoin-induced seizures: A paradoxical effect at toxic concentrations in epileptic patients. *Epilepsia* **30,** 230–234.

Palmer, G. C., Cregan, E. F., Borrelli, A. R., and Willett, F. (1995). Neuroprotective properties of the uncompetitive NMDA receptor antagonist remacemide hydrochloride. *Ann. N. Y. Acad. Sci.* **765,** 236–247.

Patton, D. E., and Goldin, A. L. (1991). A voltage-dependent gating transition induces use-dependent block by tetrodotoxin of rat IIA sodium channels expressed in Xenopus oocytes. *Neuron* **7,** 637–647.

Patton, D. E., West, J. W., Catterall, W. A., and Goldin, A. L. (1992). Amino acid residues required for fast Na+-channel inactivation: Charge neutralizations and deletions in the III-IV linker. *Proc. Natl. Acad. Sci. U. S. A.* **89,** 10905–10909.

Pauwels, P. J., VanAssouw, H. P., Peeters, L., and Leysen, J. E. (1990). Neurotoxic action of veratridine in rat brain neuronal cultures: Mechanism of neuroprotection by Ca++ antagonists nonselective for slow Ca++ channels. *J. Pharmacol. Exp. Ther.* **255,** 1117–1122.

Perez-Pinzon, M. A., Rosenthal, M., Sick, T. J., Lutz, P. L., Pablo, J., and Mash, D. (1992). Downregulation of sodium channels during anoxia: A putative survival strategy of turtle brain. *Am. J. Physiol.* **31,** R712–R715.

Pisani, A., Stefani, A., Siniscalchi, A., Mercuri, N. B., Bernardi, G., and Calabresi, P. (1995). Electrophysiological actions of felbamate on rat striatal neurones. *Br. J. Pharmacol.* **116,** 2053–2061.

Postma, S. W., and Catterall, W. A. (1984). Inhibition of binding of [3H]batrachotoxinin A 20-alpha-benzoate to sodium channels by local anesthetics. *Mol. Pharmacol.* **25,** 219–227.

Potts, J. F., Regan, M. R., Rochelle, J. M., Seldin, M. F., and Agnew, W. S. (1993). A glial-specific voltage-sensitive Na channel gene maps close to clustered genes for neuronal isoforms on mouse chromosome 2. *Biochem. Biophys. Res. Commun.* **197,** 100–104.

Pratt, J., Rataud, J., Bardot, F., Roux, M., Blanchard, J. C., Laduron, P. M., and Stutzmann, J. M. (1992). Neuroprotective actions of riluzole in rodent models of global and focal cerebral ischemia. *Neurosci. Lett.* **140,** 225–230.

Prenen, G. H. M., Gwan, G. K., Postema, F., Zuiderveen, F., and Korf, J. (1988). Cerebral cation shifts in hypoxic-ischemic brain damage are prevented by the sodium channel blocker tetrodotoxin. *Exp. Neurol.* **99,** 118–132.

Quandt, F. N. (1988). Modification of slow inactivation of single sodium channels by phenytoin in neuroblastoma cells. *Mol. Pharmacol.* **34,** 557–565.

Ragsdale, D. S., Scheuer, T., and Catterall, W. A. (1991). Frequency and voltage-dependent inhibition of type IIA Na+ channels, expressed in a mammalian cell line, by local anesthetic, antiarrhythmic, and anticonvulsant drugs. *Mol. Pharmacol.* **40,** 756–765.

Ragsdale, D. S., Numann, R., Catterall, W. A., and Scheuer, T. (1993). Inhibition of Na+ channels by the novel blocker PD85,639. *Mol. Pharmacol.* **43,** 949–954.

Ragsdale, D. S., McPhee, J. C., Scheuer, T., and Catterall, W. A. (1994). Molecular determinants of state-dependent block of Na+ channels by local anesthetics. *Science* **265,** 1724–1728.

Ragsdale, D. S., McPhee, J. C., Scheuer, T., and Catterall, W. A. (1996). Common molecular determinants of local anesthetic, antiarrhythmic and anticonvulsant block of voltage-gated Na^+ channels. *Proc. Natl. Acad. Sci. U. S. A.* **93,** 9270–9275.

Rando, T. A., Wang, G. K., and Strichartz, G. R. (1986). The interaction between the activator agents batrachotoxin and veratridine and the gating processes of neuronal sodium channels. *Mol. Pharmacol.* **29,** 467–477.

Rasool, N., Faroqui, M., and Rubinstein, E. H. (1990). Lidocaine accelerates neuroelectric recovery after incomplete global ischemia in rabbits. *Stroke* **21,** 929–935.

Rataud, J., Debanot, F., Mary, V., Pratt, J., Stutzmann, J. M., Silverstein, F. S., Buchanan, K., Hudson, C., and Johnston, M. V. (1994). Comparative study of voltage-sensitive sodium channel blockers in focal ischaemia and electric convulsions in rodents. *Neurosci. Lett.* **172,** 19–23.

Rock, D. M., McLean, M. J., Macdonald, R. L., Catterall, W. A., and Taylor, C. P. (1991). Ralitoline (CI-946) and CI-953 block sustained repetitive sodium action potentials in cultured mouse spinal cord neurons and displace batrachotoxinin A 20-alpha-benzoate binding in vitro. *Epilepsy Res.* **8,** 197–203.

Rogart, R. B., Cribbs, L. L., Muglia, L. K., Kephart, D. D., and Kaiser, M. W. (1989). Molecular cloning of a putative tetrodotoxin-resistant rat heart Na^+ channel isoform. *Proc. Natl. Acad. Sci. U. S. A.* **86,** 8170–8174.

Rogawski, M. A., and Porter, R.J. (1990). Antiepileptic drugs: Pharmacological mechanisms and clinical efficacy with consideration of promising developmental stage compounds. *Pharmacol. Rev.* **42,** 223–286.

Rostock, A., Rundfeldt, C., Tober, C., and Bartsch, R. (1995). AWD 140–190: A new anticonvulsant with sodium channel blocking properties. *Soc. Neurosci. Abstr.* **21,** 203 (abstr.)

Rothstein, J. D., and Kuncl, R. W. (1995). Neuroprotective strategies in a model of chronic glutamate-mediated motor neuron toxicity. *J. Neurochem.* **65,** 643–651.

Rothstein, J. D., Dykes Hoberg, M., and Kuncl, R. W. (1993). Chronic inhibition of glutamate uptake produces a model of slow neurotoxicity. *Proc. Natl. Acad. Sci. U. S. A.* **90,** 6591–6595.

Rowbotham, M. C., Reisner-Keller, L. A., and Fields, H. L. (1991). Both intravenous lidocaine and morphine reduce the pain of postherpetic neuralgia. *Neurology* **441,** 1024–1028.

Roy, M. L., and Narahashi, T. (1992). Differential properties of tetrodotoxin-sensitive and tetrodotoxin-resistant sodium channels in rat dorsal root ganglion neurons. *J. Neurosci.* **12,** 2104–2111.

Sanchez, D. Y., and Harris, E. W. (1995). The effects of the anticonvulsant remacemide HCl at neuronal sodium channels. *Soc. Neurosci. Abstr.* **21,** 2117.

Sangameswaran, L., Delgado, S. G., Fish, L. M., Koch, B. D., Jakeman, L. B., Stewart, G. R., Sze, P., Hunter, J. C., Eglen, R. M., and Herman, R. C. (1996). Structure and function of a novel voltage-gated, tetrodoxtoxin-resistant sodium channel specific to sensory neurons. *J. Biol. Chem.* **271,** 5953–5956.

Satin, J. J., Kyle, J. W., Chen, M., Bell, P., Cribbs, L. L., and Fozzard, H. A. (1992). A mutatant of TTX-resistant cardiac sodium channels with TTX-sensitive properties. *Science* **256,** 1202–1205.

Schaller, K. L., Krzemien, D. M., Yarowsky, P. J., Krueger, B. K., and Caldwell, J. H. (1995). A novel, abundant sodium channel expressed in neurons and glia. *J. Neurosci.* **15**, 3231–3242.

Schauf, C. L. (1987). Zonisamide enhances slow sodium inactivation in Myxicola. *Brain Res.* **413**, 185–189.

Schleef, M., Werner, K., Satzger, U., Kaupmann, K., and Jockusch, H. (1993). Chromosomal localization and genomic cloning of the mouse alpha-tropomyosin gene Tpm-1. *Genomics* **17**, 519–521.

Schmidt, J. W., and Catterall, W. A. (1986). Biosynthesis and processing of the alpha subunit of the voltage-sensistive sodium channel in rat brain neurons. *Cell (Cambridge, Mass.)* **46**, 437–444.

Schwindt, P. C., and Crill, W. E. (1995). Amplification of synaptic current by persistent sodium conductance in apical dendrite of neocortical neurons. *J. Neurophysiol.* **74**, 2220–2224.

Segal, M. M. (1994). Endogenous bursts underlie seizurelike activity in solitary excitatory hippocampal neurons in microcultures. *J. Neurophysiol.* **72**, 1874–1884.

Segal, M. M., Zurakowski, D., and Douglas, A. F. (1995). Late sodium channel openings underlie ictal epileptiform activity, and are preferentially dimished by the anticonvulsant phenytoin. *Soc. Neurosci. Abstr.* **21**, 777.

Sheldon, R. S., Duff, H. J., Thakore, E., and Hill, R. J. (1994). Class I antiarrhythmic drugs: Allosteric inhibitors of [3H]batrachotoxinin binding to rat cardiac sodium channels. *J. Pharmacol. Exp. Ther.* **268**, 187–194.

Siesjo, B. K. (1988). Historical overview. Calcium, ischemia, and death of brain cells. *Ann. N. Y. Acad. Sci.* **522**, 638–661.

Silverstein, F. S., Buchanan, K., Hudson, C., and Johnston, M. V. (1986). Flunarizine limits hypoxia-ischemia induced morphologic injury in immature rat brain. *Stroke* **17**, 477–482.

Smith, S. E., and Meldrum, B. S. (1995). Cerebroprotective effect of lamotrigine after focal ischemia in rats. *Stroke* **26**, 117–121.

Smith, S. E., Lekieffre, D., Sowinski, P., and Meldrum, B. S. (1993). Cerebroprotective effect of BW619C89 after focal or global cerebral ischaemia in the rat. *NeuroReport* **4**, 1339–1342.

Soares, H. D., Thomas, M., Cloherty, K., and McIntosh, T. K. (1992). Development of prolonged focal cerebral edema and regional cation changes following experimental brain injury in the rat. *J. Neurochem.* **58**, 1845–1852.

Squire, I. B., Lees, K. R., Pryse-Phillips, W., Kertesz, A., and Bamford, J. (1995). Efficacy and tolerability of lifarizine in acute ischemic stroke. A pilot study. *Ann. N. Y. Acad. Sci.* **765**, 317–318.

Staden, R. (1982). An interactive graphic program of comparing and aligning nucleic acid and amino acid sequences. *Nucleic Acids Res.* **10**, 2951–2961.

Stafström, C. E., Schwindt, P. C., Chubb, M. C., and Crill, W. E. (1985). Properties of persistent sodium conductance and calcium conductance of layer V neurons from cat sensorimotor cortex in vitro. *J. Neurophysiol.* **53**, 153–170.

Stanton, P. K., and Moskal, J. R. (1991). Diphenylhydantoin protects against hypoxia-induced impairment of hippocampal synaptic transmission. *Brain Res.* **546**, 351–354.

Steinberg, I.Z. (1990). Computer simulations of electrical bistability in excitable cells due to non-inactivating sodium channels: Space and time-dependent behavior. *J. Theor. Biol.* **144**, 75–92.

Stone, W. E., and Javid, M. J. (1988). Anticonvulsive and convulsive effects of lidocaine: Comparison with those of phenytoin, and implications for mechanism of action concepts. *Neurol. Res* **10**, 161–168.

Striessnig, J., Glossmann, H., and Catterall, W. A. (1990). Identification of a phenylalkylamine binding region within the alpha 1 subunit of skeletal muscle Ca2+ channels. *Proc. Natl. Acad. Sci. U. S. A.* **87**, 9108–9112.

Strijbos, P. J. L. M., Leach, M. J., and Garthwaite, J. (1996). Vicious cycle involving Na^+ channels, glutamate release, and NMDA receptors mediates delayed neurodgeneration through nitric oxide formation. *J Neurosci.* **16**, 5004–5013.

Stuart, G. J., and Sakmann, B. (1994). Active propagation of somatic action potentials into neocortical pyramidal cell dendrites. *Nature (London)* **367,** 69–72.

Stuart, G. J., and Sakmann, B. (1995). Amplification of EPSPs by axosomatic sodium channels. *Neuron* **15,** 1065–1076.

Stuhmer, W., Conti, F., Suzuki, H., Wang, X., Noda, M., Yahadi, N., Kubo, H., and Numa, S. (1989). Structural parts involved in activation and inactivation of the sodium channel. *Nature (London)* **339,** 597–603.

Stys, P. (1995). Protective effects of antiarrhythmic agents against anoxic injury in CNS white matter. *J. Cereb. Blood Flow Metab.* **15,** 425–432.

Stys, P. K., and Lesiuk, H. (1996). Correlation between electrophysiological effects of mexiletine and ischemic protection in CNS white matter. *Neuroscience* **71,** 27–36.

Stys, P., Ransom, B. R., and Waxman, S. G. (1992a). Tertiary and quaternary local anesthetics protect CNS white matter from anoxic injury at concentrations that do not block excitability. *J. Neurophysiol.* **67,** 236–40.

Stys, P., Waxman, S. G., and Ransom, B. R. (1992b). Ionic mechanisms of anoxic injury in mammalian CNS white matter: Role of Na+ channels and Na+-Ca2+ exchanger. *J. Neurosci.* **12,** 430–439.

Stys, P., Sontheimer, H., Ransom, B. R., and Waxman, S. G. (1993). Non-inactivating, TTX-sensitive Na+ conductance in rat optic nerve axons. *Proc. Natl. Acad. Sci. U. S. A.* **90,** 6976–6980.

Sun, F. Y., and Faden, A. I. (1995). Neuroprotective effects of BW619C89, a use-dependent sodium channel blocker, in rat traumatic brain injury. *Brain Res.* **637,** 133–140.

Szatkowski, M., and Attwell, D. (1994). Triggering and execution of neuronal death in brain ischemia: Two phases of glutamate release by different mechanisms. *Trends Neurosci.* **17,** 359–365.

Taft, W. C., Clifton, G. L., Blair, R. E., and DeLorenzo, R. J. (1989). Phenytoin protects against ischemia-produced neuronal cell death. *Brain Res.* **483,** 143–148.

Tagaki, H., Takashima, M., Liou, S.Y., and Kunihara, M. (1994). Effects of KB-2796, a novel Ca2+ channel blocker, on spreading depression and Ca2+ uptake in rat hippocampal slices. *Jpn. J. Pharmacol.* **64,** 302.

Tanelian, D. L., and Brose, W. G. (1991). Neuropathic pain can be relieved by drugs that are use-dependent sodium channel blockers: Lidocaine, carbamazepine and mexiletine. *Anesthesiology* **74,** 949951.

Tang, L., Smith, C. P., Huger, F. P., and Kongsamut, S. (1995). Effects of besipirdine at the voltage-dependent sodium channel. *Br. J. Pharmacol.* **116,** 2468–2472.

Tasker, R. C., Coyle, J. T., and Vornov, J. J. (1992). The regional vulnerability to hypoglycemia-induced neurotoxicity in organotypic hippocampal culture: Protection by early tetrodotoxin or delayed MK-801. *J. Neurosci.* **12,** 4298–4308.

Taylor, C. P. (1993). Na+ currents that fail to inactivate. *Trends Neurosci.* **16,** 455–460.

Taylor, C. P., and Meldrum, B. S. (1995). Na+ channels as targets for neuroprotective drugs. *Trends Pharmacol. Sci.* **16,** 309–316.

Taylor, C. P., Burke, S. P., and Weber, M. L. (1995). Hippocampal slices: Glutamate release and cellular damage from ischemia are reduced by sodium channel blockade. *J. Neurosci. Methods* **59,** 121–128.

Taylor, C. P., Patrylo, P. R., Weber, M. L., Bloomquist, J. L., and Dudek, F. E. (1996). Na^+ Channel blockers reduce prolonged seizure-like activity in low-$[Ca^{2+}]_o$ solutions. *Epilepsia* **37**(Suppl. 5), 21 (Abstract).

Terlau, H., Heinemann, S. H., Stuhmer, W., Pusch, M., Conti, F., Imoto, K., and Numa, S. (1991). Mapping the site of block by tetrodotoxin and saxitoxin of sodium channel II. *FEBS Lett.* **293,** 93–96.

Thompson, M., and Bones, M. (1985). Nontraditional analgesics for the management of postherpetic neuralgia. *Clin. Pharm.* **4,** 170–176.

Thomsen, W. J., Hays, S. J., Hicks, J. L., Schwarz, R. D., and Catterall, W. A. (1993). Specific binding of the novel Na+ channel blocker PD85,639 to the alpha subunit of rat brain Na+ channels. *Mol. Pharmacol.* **43,** 955–964.

Torp, R., Arvin, B., Le Peillet, E., Chapman, A. G., Ottersen, O. P., and Meldrum, B. S. (1993). Effect of ischaemia and reperfusion on the extra- and intracellular distribution of glutamate, glutamine, aspartate and GABA in the rat hippocampus, with a note on the effect of the sodium channel blocker BW1003C87. *Exp. Brain Res.* **96,** 365–376.

Trimmer, J. S., and Agnew, W. S. (1989). Molecular diversity of voltage-sensitive Na channels. *Annu. Rev. Physiol.* **51,** 401–418.

Trimmer, J. S., Cooperman, S. S., Tomiko, S. A., Zhou, J. Y., Crean, S. M., Boyle, M. B., Kallen, R. G., Sheng, Z. H., Barchi, R. L., Sigworth, F. J., Goodman, R. H., Agnew, W. S., and Mandel, G. (1989). Primary structure and functional expression of a mammalian skeletal muscle sodium channel. *Neuron* **3,** 33–49.

Tsuchida, E., Harms, J. F., Woodward, J. J., and Bullock, R. (1996). A use-dependent sodium channel antagonist, 619C89, in reduction of ischemic brain damage and glutamate release after acute subdural hematoma in the rat. *J. Neurosurg.* **85,** 104–111.

Vandenberg, C. A., and Bezanilla, F. (1991). A sodium channel gating model based on single channel, macroscopic ionic, and gating currents in the squid giant axon. *Biophys. J.* **60,** 1511-1533.

Van Reempts, J., Haseldonckx, M., Van Deuren, B., Wouters, L., and Borgers, M. (1986). Structural damage of the ischemic brain: Involvement of calcium and effects of postischemic treatment with calcium entry blockers. *Drug Dev. Res.* **8,** 387–395.

Vassilev, P. M., Scheuer, T., and Catterall, W. A. (1989). Inhibition of inactivation of single sodium channels by a site- directed antibody. *Proc. Natl. Acad. Sci. U. S. A.* **86,** 8147–8151.

Wahl, F., Allix, M., Plotkine, M., and Boulu, R. G. (1993). Effect of riluzole on focal cerebral ischemia in rats. *Eur. J. Pharmacol.* 230, 209-214.

Waldmeier, P. C., Baumann, P. A., Wicki, P., Feldtrauer, J.- J., Stierlin, C., and Schmutz, M. (1995). Similar potency of carbamazepine, oxcarbazepine, and lamotrigine in inhibiting the release of glutamate and other neurotransmitters. *Neurology* **45,** 1907–1913.

Wallis, R. A., and Panizzon, K. L. (1995). Felbamate neuroprotection against CA1 traumatic neuronal injury. *Eur. J. Pharmacol.* **294,** 475–482.

Wallis, R. A., Panizzon, K. L., Fairchild, M. D., and Wasterlain, C.G . (1992). Protective effects of felbamate against hypoxia in the rat hippocampal slices. *Stroke* **23,** 547–551.

Wasterlain, C. G., Adams, L. M., Hattori, H., and Schwartz, P. H. (1992). Felbamate reduces hypoxic-ischemic brain damage in vivo. *Eur. J. Pharmacol.* **212,** 275–278

Wauquier, A., Melis, W., and Janssen, P. A. J. (1989). Long-term neurological assessment of the post-resuscitative effects of flunarizine, verapamil and nimodipine in a new model of global complete ischeamia. *Neuropharmacology* 28, 837-846.

Waxman, S. G., Kocsis, J. D., and Black, J. A. (1994). Type III sodium channel mRNA is expressed in embryonic but not adult spinal sensory neurons, and is reexpressed following axotomy. *J. Neurophysiol.* **72,** 466–470.

Weber, M. L., and Taylor, C. P. (1994). Damage from oxygen and glucose deprivation in hippocampal slices is prevented by tetrodotoxin, lidocaine and phenytoin without blockade of action potentials. *Brain Res.* **664,** 167–177.

West, J. W., Patton, D. E., Scheuer, T., Wang, Y., Goldin, A. L., and Catterall, W. A. (1992a). A cluster of hydrophobic amino acid residues required for fast Na+ channel inactivation. *Proc. Natl. Acad. Sci. U. S. A.* **89,** 10910–10914.

West, J. W., Scheuer, T., Maechler, L., and Catterall, W. A. (1992b). Efficient expression of rat brain type IIA Na+ channel alpha subunits in a somatic cell line. *Neuron* **8,** 59–70.

Westenbroek, R. E., Merrick, D. K., and Catterall, W. A. (1989). Differential subcellular localization of the RI and RII Na+ channel subtypes in central neurons. *Neuron* **3,** 695–704.

White, M. M., Chen, L., Keinfield, R., Kallen, R. G., and Barchi, R. L. (1991). SkM2, a Na^+ Channel cDNA clone from denervated skeletal muscle, encodes a tetrodotoxin-insensitive Na^+ channel. *Mol. Pharmacol.* **39,** 604–608.

Wiard, R. S., Dickerson, M. C., Beek, O., Norton, R., and Cooper, B. R. (1995). Neuroprotective properties of the novel antiepileptic lamotrigine in a gerbil model of global cerebral ischemia. *Stroke* **26,** 466–472.

Willow, M., and Catterall, W. A. (1982). Inhibition of the binding of [3H]batrachotoxinin A 20-α-benzoate to sodium channels by the anticonvulsant drugs diphenylhydantoin and carbamazepine. *Mol. Pharmacol* **22,** 627–635.

Willow, M., Gonoi, T., and Catterall, W. A. (1985). Voltage clamp analysis of the inhibitory actions of diphenylhydantoin and carbamazepine on voltage-sensitive sodium channels in neuroblastoma cells. *Mol. Pharmacol.* **27,** 549–558.

Woolf, C. J., and Wiesenfeld-Hallin, Z. (1985). The systemic administration of local anesthetics produces a selective depression of C-afferent fibre evoked activity in the spinal cord. *Pain* **23,** 361–374.

Xie, Y., Dengler, K., Zacharias, E., Wilffert, B., and Tegtmeier, F. (1994). Effects of the sodium channel blocker tetrodotoxin (TTX) on cellular ion homeostasis in rat brain subjected to complete ischemia. *Brain Res.* **652,** 216–224.

Xie, Y., Lancaster, B., Peakman, T., and Garthwaite, J. (1995a). Interaction ofthe antiepileptic drug lamotrigine with recombinant rat brain type IIA Na^+ channels and with native Na^+ channels in rat hippocampal neurones. *Pfluegers Arch.* **430,** 437–446.

Xie, Y., Zacharias, E., Hoff, P., and Tegtmeier, F. (1995b). Ion channel involvement in anoxic depolarization induced by cardiac arrest in rat brain. *J. Cereb. Blood Flow Metab.* **15,** 587–594.

Yaari, Y., and Devor, M. (1985). Phenytoin suppresses spontaneous ectopic discharge in rat sciatic nerve neuromas. *Neurosci. Lett.* **58,** 117–122.

Yajnik, S., Singh, G. P., Singh, G., and Kumar, M. (1992). Phenytoin as a coanalgesic in cancer pain. *J. Pain Symptom. Manage.* **7,** 209–213.

Yamaguchi, S., and Rogawski, M. A. (1992). Effects of anticonvulsant drugs on 4-aminopyridine-induced seizures in mice. *Epilepsy Res.* **11,** 9–16.

Yamakami, I., and McIntosh, T. K. (1989). Effects of traumatic brain injury on regional cerebral blood flow in rats as measured with radiolabeled microspheres. *J. Cereb. Blood Flow Metab.* **9,** 117–124.

Yamasaki, Y., Kogure, K., Hara, H., Ban, H., and Akaike, N. (1991). The possible involvement of tetrodotoxin-sensitive ion channels in ischemic neuronal damage in the rat hippocampus. *Neurosci. Lett.* **121,** 251–254.

Yang, N., George, A. L. J., and Horn, R. (1996). Molecular basis of charge movement in voltage-gated sodium channels. *Neuron* **16,** 113–122.

Yoshidomi, M., Hayashi, T., Abe, K., and Kogure, K. (1989). Effects of a new calcium channel blocker, KB-2796, on protein synthesis of the CA1 pyramidal cell and delayed neuronal death following transient forebrain ishemia. *J. Neurochem.* **53,** 1589–1594.

Zha, H., Remmers, E. F., Du, Y., Goldmuntz, E. A., Mathern, P., Zhang, H., Cash, J. M., Crofford, L. J., and Wilder, R. L. (1994). A single linkage group comprising 11 polymorphic DNA markers on rat chromosome 3. *Mamm. Genome* **5,** 538–541.

Zhang, Y.-L., and Lipton, P. (1995). Mitochondria and endoplasmic reticulum are major sources of increased cytosolic calcium during ischemia in the rat hippocampus. *Soc. Neurosci. Abstr.* **21,** 217.

Zhu, Y., and Im, W. B. (1992). Block of sodium channel current by anticonvulsant U-54494A in mouse neuroblastoma cells. *J. Pharmacol. Exp. Ther.* **260,** 110–116.

Zimanyi, I., Weiss, S. R. B., Lajtha, A., Post, R. M., and Reith, M. E. A. (1989). Evidence for a common site of action of lidocaine and carbamazepine in voltage-dependent sodium channels. *Eur. J. Pharmacol.* **167,** 419–442.

Carol J. Cornejo*
Robert K. Winn*,†
John M. Harlan‡

*Department of Surgery
†Department of Physiology and Biophysics
‡Department of Medicine
Division of Hematology
University of Washington
Seattle, Washington 98104

Anti-adhesion Therapy

I. Introduction

Leukocytes are an integral component of the host defense system. However, in some disease states their action may instead be deleterious to the host and they may cause a significant amount of tissue damage. For example, in ischemia–reperfusion (I-R) injury an ischemic insult may trigger an inflammatory response during reperfusion that causes more injury than the initial ischemic insult. In other diseases, such as rheumatoid arthritis, leukocytes cause tissue damage without an apparent initial insult. In still other instances, leukocytes may function normally, but it is advantageous to manipulate their function. An example of this would be in allogeneic organ transplantation where leukocytes appropriately recognize the graft as foreign and so try to destroy it, but it is beneficial to curtail this activity.

In order for leukocytes to cause vascular or tissue damage, they must first adhere to the endothelium and then exit the bloodstream to gain access

Advances in Pharmacology, Volume 39

1054-3589/97/$25.00

to extravascular tissue. Leukocyte emigration involves adhesion molecules both on the leukocyte and on the endothelial cell surface. These adhesion molecules are vital not only for adherence but participate in several other leukocyte functions such as signal transduction. Therefore, adherence molecules have emerged as important targets for therapy in a broad spectrum of inflammatory and immune disorders. This chapter reviews the current status of "anti-adhesion" therapy in a number of *in vivo* models of disease states and considers some of the safety concerns associated with anti-adhesion therapy.

II. Leukocyte and Endothelial Adhesion Molecules

The following is intended as only a brief introduction to the adhesion molecule targets. For a detailed consideration of leukocyte and endothelial adhesion molecules, the reader is referred to several reviews (Bevilacqua, 1993; Bevilacqua and Nelson, 1993; Carlos and Harlan, 1994; Springer, 1994; Imhof and Dunon, 1995; Tedder *et al.*, 1995).

A. Selectins

Three classes of adhesion molecules are involved in leukocyte–endothelial interactions: selectins, integrins, and members of the immunoglobulin (Ig-like) superfamily. Selectins mediate the initial, low-affinity adherence of leukocytes to endothelium, manifested by rolling along the endothelial cell surface under conditions of flow. There are three different selectins: L-selectin (CD62L), E-selectin (CD62E), and P-selectin (CD62P). L-selectin is found only on leukocytes, E-selectin is endothelial restricted, and P-selectin is expressed on platelets as well as endothelial cells. All three of these molecules contain an amino-terminal lectin domain, a variable number of complement regulatory repeat sequences, an epidermal growth factor domain, a transmembrane domain, and a cytoplasmic domain (Bevilacqua and Nelson, 1993). The selectins function by binding via their lectin domains to specific carbohydrate moieties on glycoproteins and glycolipids. It has been shown that all three selectins recognize sialylated, fucosylated ligands such as sialyl Lewis^x (SLe^x, CD15s) (Phillips *et al.*, 1990; Walz *et al.*, 1990); some L-selectin ligands are also sulfated. Several glycoproteins bearing selectin ligands have been identified, including PSGL-1 for P- and E-selectin (Sako *et al.*, 1993), ESL-1 for E-selectin (Steegmaier *et al.*, 1995), and CD34 for L-selectin (Baumheter *et al.*, 1993).

L-selectin was first identified as a homing receptor for lymphocyte migration to peripheral lymph nodes and was found to mediate the binding of lymphocytes to high endothelial venules in peripheral lymph nodes (Gallatin *et al.*, 1983). It has since been found to be constitutively expressed on most leukocytes, including lymphocytes, monocytes, neutrophils (PMN), and eosinophils. Leukocytes can be induced to shed L-selectin from their surface by a variety of activating agents such as formyl peptides, phorbol ester, and lipopolysaccharide (LPS).

E-selectin is expressed on the surface of endothelial cells only following stimulation. Tumor necrosis factor-α (TNF-α), interleukin-1 (IL-1), substance P, LPS, and several other stimuli have been found to induce the expression of E-selectin (Bevilacqua *et al.*, 1987, 1989; Bevilacqua and Nelson, 1993; Carlos and Harlan, 1994; Springer, 1994; Imhof and Dunon, 1995; Tedder *et al.*, 1995). E-selectin expression requires *de novo* protein synthesis with transcription and translation resulting in peak surface expression in 4–6 hr following stimulation *in vitro* with a gradual decrease to basal levels by 24 hr (Bevilacqua *et al.*, 1987, 1989).

P-selectin is stored in the Weibel–Palade bodies of endothelial cells and the α granules of platelets (McEver *et al.*, 1989). Its expression on endothelial cells is also induced by a variety of stimuli, including thrombin, histamine, and phorbol esters (Hattori *et al.*, 1989). In response to this stimulation, P-selectin is rapidly redistributed to the cell surface, resulting in expression within minutes. The duration of expression following these stimuli is 15 min or less (Hattori *et al.*, 1989) as a result of reinternalization of the molecule where it is either degraded or recycled back into Weibel–Palade bodies. In some endothelial cells, P-selectin, like E-selectin, is also induced by cytokines or LPS (Gotsch *et al.*, 1994).

B. Integrins

The second class of adhesion molecules involved in leukocyte traffic is the integrin family. Integrins are transmembrane heterodimers consisting of noncovalently linked α and β chains. Integrins are subclassified based on the specific β subunit. The subclasses that have been found to be involved in leukocyte–endothelial cell interactions are the β2-integrins, the β1-integrin, VLA-4 ($\alpha 4\beta 1$, CD49b/CD29), and the β7-integrin, $\alpha 4\beta 7$.

The three β2-integrins are leukocyte restricted and are composed of a common β2 subunit (CD18) that is noncovalently linked to one of three α subunits; CD11a (αL; LFA-1), CD11b (αM; Mac-1, Mo-1), or CD11c (αX; p150,95). CD11a/CD18 is expressed on all leukocytes, whereas CD11b/CD18 is expressed only on PMN, monocytes, and natural killer cells, CD11c/CD18 is expressed only on PMN, monocytes, and some lymphocytes (Arnaout, 1990). In PMN and monocytes there are intracellular stores of CD11b/CD18 and CD11c/CD18, and expression can rapidly be induced by a variety of stimuli, but there are no intracellular stores of CD11a/CD18. Cell surface expression of β2-integrins is not sufficient for adhesion of leukocytes to endothelial cells. Activation of the $\beta2$-integrins due to a change in conformation or postreceptor events (e.g., cytoskeletal association) is required before adhesion occurs (Faull *et al.*, 1994). This activation is induced by soluble agents (cytokines, chemotactic factors, coagulation factors) and by ligation of other cell surface receptors. Ligands for the $\beta2$-integrins include Ig-like surface proteins expressed on endothelial cells such as intercellular adhesion molecule-1 (ICAM-1, CD54) for CD11b/CD18 and ICAM-1 and -2 (CD102) for CD11a/CD18. CD11b/CD18 also recognizes a variety of other proteins such as C3bi, fibrinogen, and factor X. Binding of $\beta2$-integrins to endothelial cell surface proteins occurs *in vivo* at low shear rates or after initial tethering of the leukocytes by selectins, and is responsible for firm adherence (i.e., sticking) of leukocytes to the vessel wall (Lawrence and Springer, 1991; Von-Andrian *et al.*, 1991).

The $\beta1$-integrins consist of a common $\beta1$ subunit (CD29) noncovalently linked to an α subunit and are found on nearly all cell types. However, one $\beta1$-integrin, VLA-4, is found primarily on leukocytes. It is constitutively expressed on all circulating leukocytes except PMN and, like the $\beta2$-integrins, requires activation in order to bind its ligand with high avidity. The endothelial ligand for VLA-4 is vascular cell adhesion molecule-1 (VCAM-1, INCAM-110, CD106), a member of the immunoglobulin superfamily that is induced on endothelial cells following cytokine stimulation. VLA-4 also binds to the CS-1 fragment of fibronectin, which may be expressed on the endothelial luminal surface (Elices *et al.*, 1994).

The $\beta7$-integrin, $\alpha4\beta7$, is expressed on some B and T lymphocytes and functions as the homing receptor for intestinal lymphoid tissue. It binds to the mucosal vascular addressin MAdCAM-1, an Ig-like protein that is found on high endothelial venules in mucosal lymph nodes (Peyer's patches) (Berlin *et al.*, 1993). $\alpha4\beta7$ also binds to VCAM-1 and fibronectin, although to a lesser extent than VLA-4.

C. Immunoglobulin Superfamily

Members of the immunoglobulin superfamily constitute the third class of adhesion molecules. This superfamily consists of cell surface proteins that are involved in antigen recognition and complement binding, as well as cell adhesion. Endothelial members of this superfamily involved in leukocyte–endothelial cell adhesion include ICAM-1, ICAM-2, VCAM-1, MAdCAM-1, and platelet–endothelial cell adhesion molecule-1 (PECAM-1, CD31).

ICAM-1 is expressed on leukocytes, fibroblasts, and epithelial cells, as well as on endothelial cells. It is constitutively expressed at low levels on endothelial cells, but its expression can be increased with stimulation of endothelial cells with cytokines (IL-1, TNF-α, and interferon-γ), LPS, thrombin, and phorbol esters (Pober *et al.*, 1986). Stimulation of endothelial cells induces *de novo* transcription and translation, resulting in peak expression at 12–24 hr which is maintained for up to 72 hr. As stated earlier, ICAM-1 binds both CD11a/CD18 and CD11b/CD18 on leukocytes and mediates the firm adherence of leukocytes to endothelial cells.

ICAM-2 is a ligand for CD11a/CD18. It is constitutively expressed on the surface of endothelial cells. Although its expression is not upregulated by stimulation with cytokines or LPS, ICAM-2 surface expression has been found to be increased on high endothelial venules in malignant versus non-malignant lymph nodes. Therefore, its expression may be upregulated by some other stimuli.

VCAM-1 is variably expressed on endothelial cells. Its expression is upregulated by stimulation with a variety of agents, including IL-4, IL-1, TNF-α, LPS, thrombin, and lysophosphatidylcholine (Carlos and Harlan, 1994; Springer, 1994). Similar to ICAM-1, its upregulation requires *de novo* synthesis, resulting in peak surface expression at 6 hr with a decline in expression to low levels by 48–72 hr. As noted previously, VCAM-1 is the predominant endothelial ligand for VLA-4 found on lymphocytes, monocytes, and eosinophils, but not on PMN.

PECAM-1 is found on endothelial cells, platelets, and some leukocytes. PECAM-1 is constitutively expressed on endothelial cells and its surface expression is not increased by stimulation with TNF-α or IL-1. It is localized to intracellular junctions and has been shown to play a role in the process of PMN and monocyte diapedesis between endothelial cells, both *in vitro* (Muller *et al.*, 1993) and *in vivo* (Vaporciyan *et al.*, 1993).

III. Adhesion Cascade and Inflammation

The sequence of events involved in leukocyte adherence to vascular endothelium and transmigration into tissue is complex and has been termed the adhesion cascade (reviewed in Carlos and Harlan, 1994; Springer, 1994) (Fig. 1). The first step involves a random contact of the leukocyte with the

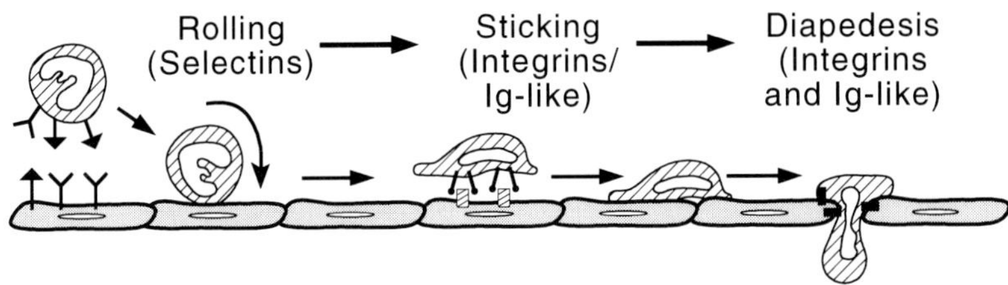

FIGURE 1 The adhesion cascade. After random contact with the endothelium, leukocytes form low-affinity bonds with the endothelium mediated by the selectins. This results in "tethering" of the leukocyte and rolling along the surface of the endothelium. The leukocyte then firmly adheres to the endothelium and subsequently diapedeses between endothelial cells into the extravascular space. The firm adherence and diapedesis are mediated by the interaction of integrins and Ig superfamily adhesion molecules.

endothelial cell surface. After initial contact, relatively weak binding of L-, P-, and/or E-selectin with their carbohydrate ligands occurs. Under conditions of flow, these multiple weak interactions are sufficient to slow the leukocyte down, and the leukocyte is seen to roll along the surface of the endothelial cells. The next step involves further activation of the endothelial cell and leukocyte by cytokines, chemoattractants, and chemokines that are produced locally. This leads to upregulation and/or activation of the leukocyte integrins and the endothelial Ig-like molecules. The interaction of these two classes of adhesion molecules mediates the firm adherence of leukocytes to the endothelial cell surface.

The firmly adherent leukocytes migrate across the endothelial cell surface via integrin–Ig-like interactions, diapedese between endothelial cells utilizing PECAM-1 (or other as yet unidentified adherence molecules), and then migrate to the subendothelial matrix via integrin binding to matrix components. While the adherence cascade functions normally to recruit leukocytes to extravascular sites for host defense and repair, under some circumstances the adhesive interactions may lead to vascular and/or tissue damage. Once leukocytes are firmly adherent to the endothelium, a protected microenvironment is formed. In this microenvironment, inflammatory mediators produced by the leukocyte may potentially reach high concentrations and overcome local and systemic anti-inflammatory protective mechanisms, thereby allowing endothelial cell injury to occur and resulting in an increase in microvascular permeability and hemorrhage. This series of events may initiate and sustain a cycle of inflammation, leading to further leukocyte recruitment and endothelial cell injury. The continued recruitment of leukocytes can lead to occlusion of the microvasculature by leukocyte aggregates, causing local ischemia. The leukocytes may also diapedese between endothelial cells, gaining access to the extravascular space, where they can mediate further tissue damage, producing organ dysfunction.

This cascade of events leading to vascular and tissue injury is dependent on leukocyte–endothelial adhesive interactions, and, thus, interrupting these interactions at the level of rolling, firm adherence, or diapedesis should decrease leukocyte-mediated injury.

IV. Strategies to Inhibit Adhesion

The most basic method to prevent leukocyte-mediated injury is to remove the leukocytes from the bloodstream, thus eliminating the effector cells that do the damage. This approach has been employed in ischemia–reperfusion injury. Ischemia–reperfusion injury is thought to begin with an ischemic insult that, in addition to causing direct ischemic damage, initiates a chain of events leading to a deleterious inflammatory response during reperfusion. The injury that occurs during reperfusion was shown to be mediated in part by PMN in that PMN depletion reduced I-R injury in the heart (Engler *et al.*, 1983; Romson *et al.*, 1983), gut (Smith *et al.*, 1987), and liver (Jaeschke *et al.*, 1990; Langdale *et al.*, 1993). For example, Langdale *et al.* (1993) depleted PMN in rabbits using vinblastine and then induced hepatic ischemia followed by reperfusion. They found that the amount of I-R injury as measured by aminotransferase levels and a histological scoring system of injury severity was less in those rabbits depleted of PMN compared to those rabbits with a normal PMN count. It has also been shown that generalized I-R injury that occurs following hemorrhagic shock can be reduced by PMN depletion (Barroso-Aranda *et al.*, 1988).

A more practical method to inhibit leukocyte adherence to endothelial cells is to block the function of the adhesion molecules that mediate adherence. Two general approaches to adherence blockade are possible (Fig. 2). The first approach targets the receptor–ligand interaction itself and seeks to interfere directly with receptor binding to ligand utilizing monoclonal antibodies (MAb), saccharides, soluble receptors, peptides, or small molecules. The second approach is directed at the intracellular processes involved in controlling the expression or activation of adhesion molecules. The majority of studies of adhesion blockade have utilized MAbs. Monoclonal antibodies have been developed that bind to the adhesion-active epitopes of all the leukocyte and endothelial adhesion molecules, and have been shown to block leukocyte–endothelial adhesive interactions in a variety of *in vitro* assays. These blocking MAbs have been employed in numerous *in vivo* models. In addition to MAbs, the administration of a soluble oligosaccharide ligand for E- and P-selectin has been shown to block selectin-mediated adherence of PMN *in vivo* (Asako *et al.*, 1994; Zimmerman *et al.*, 1994). Soluble chimeric receptors consisting of the extracellular domains of the selectins or Ig-like proteins linked to the CH2 and CH3 domains of human γ-globulin have been used for adhesion blockade (Watson *et al.*, 1991;

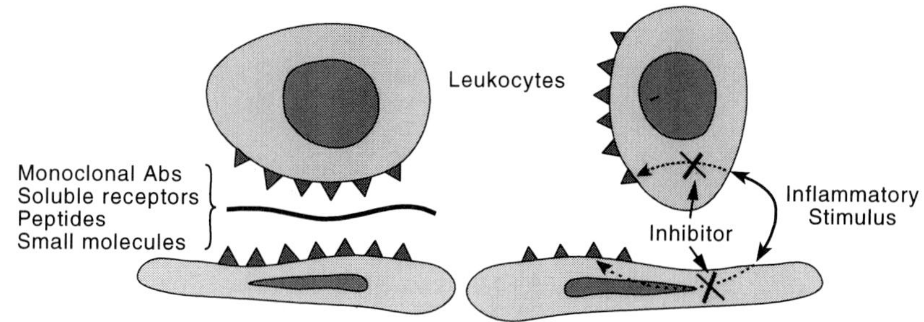

FIGURE 2 Approaches to anti-adhesion therapy. There are two approaches to anti-adhesion therapy. The first approach targets the receptor–ligand interaction itself and interferes with receptor–ligand binding. The second approach targets the intracellular processes involved in controlling the expression or activation of adhesion molecules.

Mulligan *et al.*, 1993b; Lee *et al.*, 1995). Several small peptides that bear homology to the lectin domain of the selectins have been found to reduce leukocyte binding to endothelial cells or recombinant E- and P-selectin *in vitro* and to block the adhesion of lymphocytes expressing L-selectin to high endothelial venules in lymph nodes that express the ligand for L-selectin (Briggs *et al.*, 1995). In addition, peptides from pertussis toxin inhibit PMN adherence and have been found to inhibit PMN recruitment to sites of inflammation *in vivo* (Sandros *et al.*, 1994; Martens *et al.*, 1995). Neutrophil inhibitory factor, a glycoprotein derived from the canine hookworm that functions as an antagonist to CD11b/CD18, has been found to block adhesion of PMN to endothelial cells *in vitro* (Moyle *et al.*, 1994; Muchowski *et al.*, 1994) and to reduce leukocyte adhesion in the liver after hemorrhagic shock (Bauer *et al.*, 1995).

Regarding the second approach to adherence blockade, several leukocyte and endothelial intracellular targets have been identified *in vitro* and some tested *in vivo*. For example, a small molecule, a leumedin, has been found to inhibit leukocyte recruitment into inflammatory lesions *in vivo* (Burch *et al.*, 1993) through its blockade of $\beta 2$-integrin expression and function (Bator *et al.*, 1992; Pou *et al.*, 1993). Another small molecule, gold sodium thiomalate, inhibits cytokine-stimulated expression of VCAM-1 and E-selectin *in vitro* (Newman *et al.*, 1994). Nonsteroidal anti-inflammatory drugs have been found to induce shedding of L-selectin *in vitro*, providing one new potential mechanism for their activity *in vivo* (Díaz-González *et al.*, 1995). Inhibitors of the proteasome reduce the TNF-α-induced expression of E-selectin, VCAM-1, and ICAM-1 *in vitro* (Read *et al.*, 1995). Antisense oligonucleotides that bind to the mRNA of ICAM-1, VCAM-1, and E-selectin have been shown to reduce surface expression of these molecules and to reduce adhesion (Bennett *et al.*, 1994).

All of the strategies just listed target the leukocyte or endothelial cell adhesion molecules and have the potential to reduce leukocyte adherence to endothelium and migration into tissue. However, blockade of the adhesion molecules, particularly the integrins, may interrupt the intracellular signaling that results from the binding of these molecules to their ligands and in this way also modulate the inflammatory response (Clark and Brugge, 1995) (Fig. 3).

The inflammatory stimuli that induce endothelial cell adherence molecules or activate leukocyte integrins also represent potential therapeutic targets, and are thus, indirectly, anti-adhesion therapies. In this regard, inhibition of cytokines such as TNF-α or IL-1 will prevent induction of E-selectin, VCAM-1, or ICAM-1, thereby reducing adherence. Similarly, inhibition of chemokines such as IL-8 or lipid mediators such as platelet-activating factor will prevent the activation of leukocyte integrins. However, a consideration of this indirect approach to adhesion blockade is beyond the scope of this review.

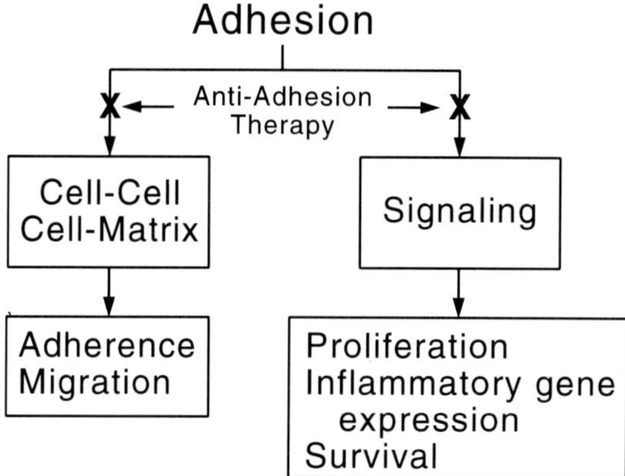

FIGURE 3 Effects of anti-adhesion therapy. Therapy that blocks adhesion molecule binding to its ligand can have two effects. One effect is to inhibit leukocyte–endothelial and leukocyte–matrix interaction which may inhibit leukocyte adherence and migration. The other effect is to inhibit intracellular signaling which may inhibit proliferation, inflammatory gene expression, and cell survival.

V. Ischemia–Reperfusion Injury

Anti-adhesion therapy has been extensively evaluated in reducing I-R injury. Ischemia–reperfusion injury is involved in a wide spectrum of disease processes such as myocardial infarction, stroke, mesenteric and peripheral vascular ischemia, and circulatory shock. Therapy that reduced I-R injury could thus have a significant impact on the eventual outcome of a large number of patients. As stated earlier, a major component of I-R injury is thought to occur during the reperfusion phase as a result of a host inflammatory response and PMN-mediated injury. As discussed earlier, PMN depletion has been shown to reduce I-R injury. With the development of MAbs to adhesion molecules or other agents, targeted anti-adhesion therapy has also been shown to reduce I-R injury.

A. Selectins

As stated earlier, selectins are a family of molecules found on leukocytes (L-selectin) or endothelial cells (P- and E-selectin) that mediate the initial rolling of leukocytes on endothelial cells under conditions of flow. Blocking this initial step would be expected to reduce the subsequent firm adherence of leukocytes to endothelial cells, thereby reducing leukocyte-mediated reperfusion injury. This has been found to be the case for P- and L-selectin which appear to function predominantly in the early phases of the inflammatory response.

1. L-selectin

L-selectin is constitutively expressed on the surface of PMN, lymphocytes, and monocytes. It has been found to mediate PMN recruitment to sites of inflammation, and blocking L-selectin with MAb inhibits PMN accumulation at sites of inflammation (Lewinsohn *et al.*, 1987), presumably by reducing rolling of PMN on endothelial cells. Monoclonal antibody blockade of L-selectin was found to reduce local I-R injury in the heart by Ma *et al.* (1993). In their study, they induced 1.5 hr of myocardial ischemia in cats followed by 4.5 hr of reperfusion and administered a MAb to L-selectin just prior to reperfusion. They noted a significant reduction in myocardial necrosis in the treated animals compared to the untreated animals. This correlated with a reduction in PMN accumulation as measured by the tissue content of myeloperoxidase (MPO). MPO is an enzyme found primarily in PMN and is used as a marker of PMN accumulation. Similarly, Seekamp *et al.* (1994) reported a reduction in rat hind limb I-R injury following treatment with MAb to L-selectin during reperfusion.

Mihelcic *et al.* (1994) studied the effect of L-selectin blockade on I-R injury in the rabbit ear. They induced ischemia in the ears of rabbits by partially amputating the ear at the base, leaving only the central artery and vein intact with an underlying bridge of avascular cartilage. A microvascular clamp was used to occlude the central artery producing complete ischemia. The ears were kept ischemic for 6 hr. The clamp was then removed and the ears allowed to reperfuse. Prior to clamp removal the rabbits were treated systemically with a blocking MAb to L-selectin, a nonblocking MAb to L-selectin, or saline. I-R injury was quantified by measuring ear volume (edema) using water displacement daily for 7 days. There was a significant attenuation in I-R injury (ear edema) in the group treated with the blocking MAb to L-selectin compared to the group treated with either saline or nonblocking MAb to L-selectin (Fig. 4). There was also a decrease in the estimated tissue necrosis at 7 days following ischemia in the rabbits treated with the blocking anti (α)-L-selectin MAb compared to the saline or nonblocking MAb-treated groups. MPO content was measured using a colorimetric assay at 24 hr following ischemia in homogenates of whole ears. The MPO content was significantly less in the ears of the blocking α-L-selectin MAb-treated groups than in the other two groups. L-selectin blockade thus resulted in a reduction in I-R injury and PMN accumulation.

2. P-selectin

P-selectin is found in the Weibel–Palade bodies of endothelial cells and is rapidly redistributed to the cell surface by a variety of stimuli. Blockade of P-selectin by MAbs was found to reduce local I-R injury in the heart (Weyrich *et al.*, 1992), intestine (Davenpeck *et al.*, 1994), skeletal muscle (Jerome *et al.*, 1994), liver (Garcia-Criado *et al.*, 1995), rabbit ear (Winn *et*

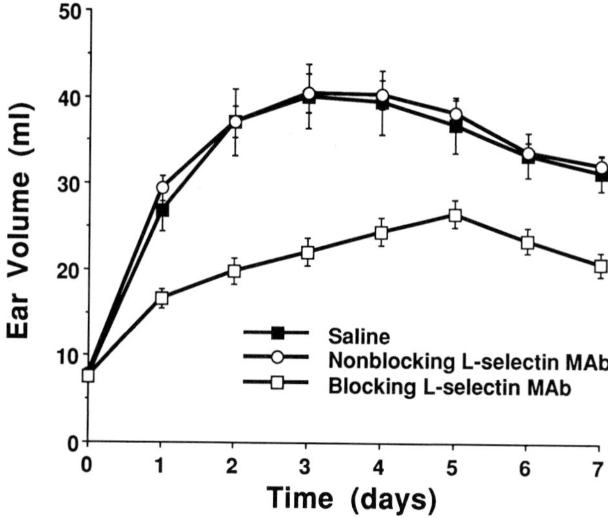

FIGURE 4 Ear edema after 6 hr of ischemia followed by reperfusion in rabbits. Values represent mean ear volume ± SEM for each of the treatment groups for each day following reperfusion. Ear volume was measured using water displacement. Ear volume for the blocking α-L-selectin MAb-treated group was significantly different from the saline and nonblocking α-L-selectin MAb-treated groups. Adapted with permission from Mihelcic *et al.* (1994).

al., 1993), and lung (Moore *et al.*, 1995). Using a feline model of myocardial ischemia and reperfusion, Weyrich *et al.* (1992) found a reduction in myocardial necrosis, expressed as a percentage of the area at risk, in the treated group (15%) compared to the untreated group (35%). Davenpeck *et al.* (1994) studied the effect of α-P-selectin MAb on intestinal I-R injury. They induced I-R in the ileum of rats and administered a MAb to P-selectin just before reperfusion. They noted that blockade of P-selectin significantly reduced leukocyte rolling and adherence in postcapillary venules that correlated with a reduction of MPO content in the intestine. Jerome *et al.* (1994) noted that treatment of rats with α-P-selectin MAb attenuated the postischemic capillary no-reflow seen in hind limbs subjected to 4 hr of ischemia followed by 30 min of reperfusion. Garcia-Criado *et al.* (1995) studied the effect of P-selectin blockade on I-R injury in the liver of rats. A MAb to P-selectin administered prior to reperfusion improved survival (55%) compared to controls (15%) whereas there was no improvement in survival if the MAb was administered after reperfusion. These results correlated with a decrease in liver injury in the α-P-selectin MAb-treated group compared to controls, as measured by an attenuation in the increase of plasma AST, ALT, and LDH levels. They also noted a reduction in PMN accumulation in the treated animals, as measured by MPO. Using the same rabbit ear I-R model just described, Winn *et al.* (1993) found a reduction in tissue injury and MPO content in the ears of rabbits treated with a MAb to P-selectin. In a similar rabbit ear I-R model, treatment with P-selectin IgG chimera resulted in a reduction of ear edema and surface necrosis compared to controls (Lee *et al.*, 1995).

In addition, MAb blockade of P-selectin has been shown to reduce global I-R resulting from hemorrhagic shock (Winn *et al.*, 1994). Winn *et al.* (1994) induced hypovolemic shock in rabbits by withdrawing blood until the cardiac output reached 33% of baseline. This level of shock was maintained for 90 min and the rabbits were then treated with a blocking MAb to P-selectin, a nonblocking MAb to P-selectin, or saline. The rabbits were then resuscitated with infusion of their shed blood, and lactated Ringer's solution was continued as necessary to maintain the cardiac output at 90% of baseline. Resuscitation was continued for 6 hr following shock. Fluid requirements were used as an indicator of global I-R injury and were found to be significantly less in the group treated with the blocking α-P-selectin MAb compared to the control groups (Fig. 5). They concluded that blockade of P-selectin-mediated adherence reduced the global I-R injury that occurs following hemorrhagic shock.

3. E-selectin

E-selectin expression is induced on the surface of endothelial cells following a variety of stimuli. Unlike P-selectin, there are no intracellular stores

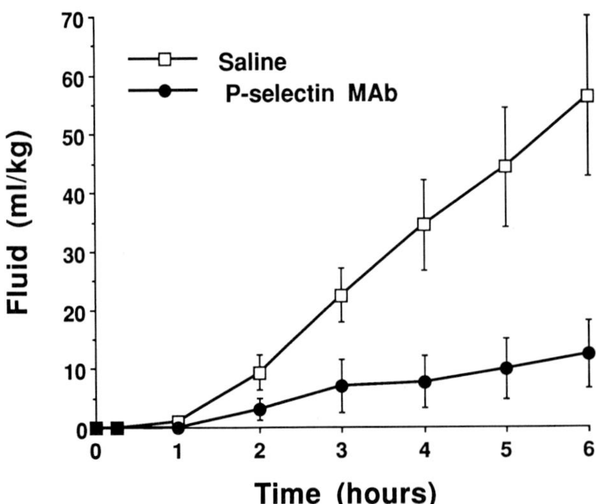

FIGURE 5 Fluid requirements during resuscitation following 90 min of hypovolemic shock in rabbits. Treatment with either α-P-selectin MAb or saline was given at the time of resuscitation. Fluid was administered to maintain cardiac output within 90% of baseline. Values represent mean fluid requirements ± SEM for each treatment group at each hour following the shock period. The fluid requirements for the group treated with α-P-selectin MAb were significantly less than the saline treated group. Adapted with permission from Winn *et al.* (1994).

of E-selectin, and thus E-selectin expression requires *de novo* gene transcription and protein synthesis. Relatively little work has been done on anti-adhesion therapy with MAbs to E-selectin due to the lack of blocking α-E-selectin MAb for most animal species. In rat hind limbs subjected to I-R, E-selectin blockade with MAb failed to reduce vascular permeability, hemorrhage, or PMN accumulation (Seekamp *et al.*, 1994). In contrast, Altavilla *et al.* (1994) found E-selectin blockade reduced local I-R injury in myocardium. They induced myocardial ischemia in rats by temporarily ligating the left main coronary artery. The rats were treated with hyperimmune serum containing antibodies against E-selectin 3 hr before the onset of ischemia. The ligature was removed after 1 hr of ischemia and the hearts were allowed to reperfuse for 1 hr. The group treated with antibodies against E-selectin had a higher survival (80%) compared to the control group (50%). The size of myocardial infarction, expressed as a percentage of the area at risk, was smaller in the E-selectin hyperimmune serum-treated group (26%) compared to the control group (70%). The reduction in infarct size was accompanied by a decrease in myocardial tissue MPO in the group treated with antibodies against E-selectin, indicating a reduction in PMN accumulation. They concluded that E-selectin was involved in PMN accumulation that resulted in myocardial I-R injury and specific antibodies blocking E-selectin may be beneficial in the treatment of myocardial I-R injury.

4. Oligosaccharides

As stated earlier, the ligand for selectins is thought to be a sialylated, fucosylated carbohydrate moiety contained on glycoproteins or glycolipids. Studies *in vitro* have shown that selectins recognize the sialyl Lewis^x oligosaccharide (SLe^x) (Phillips *et al.*, 1990; Walz *et al.*, 1990); the administration of this carbohydrate inhibits selectin-mediated adherence to endothelium (Asako *et al.*, 1994; Zimmerman *et al.*, 1994). Therefore, SLe^x oligosaccharide can act as an anti-adhesion therapy by inhibiting the initial selectin-mediated rolling of PMN on endothelial cells through competitive inhibition. Thus, it is not surprising that the administration of SLe^x oligosaccharide has been found to reduce I-R injury in the heart (Buerke *et al.*, 1994; Lefer *et al.*, 1994), skeletal muscle (Seekamp *et al.*, 1994), and rabbit ear (Han *et al.*, 1995). Seekamp *et al.* (1994) studied the effect of SLe^x oligosaccharide on I-R injury in rats. They induced ischemia in the hind limbs of rats by placing a tourniquet and inflating it at sufficient pressure to block arterial inflow. The tourniquet was left in place for 4 hr of ischemia and then removed and the hind limb allowed to reperfuse. SLe^x oligosaccharide or sialyl-*N*-acetyllactosamine pentasaccharide (SLeN), a nonblocking nonfucosylated oligosaccharide, was administered at 1, 2, and 3 hr after reperfusion. They measured hemorrhage by extravasation of ^{51}Cr-labeled erythrocytes, vascular permeability by leakage of ^{125}I-labeled albumin, and PMN accumulation by MPO content in the hind limb muscle. Hemorrhage was reduced by 47% and vascular permeability by 25% following treatment with SLe^x oligosaccharide compared to SLeN oligosaccharide or phosphate-buffered saline (PBS). These findings correlated with a reduction in PMN accumulation, or MPO content, which was reduced by 46% following treatment with SLe^x oligosaccharide compared to SLeN oligosaccharide or PBS. They concluded that SLe^x oligosaccharide reduced hind limb injury following I-R, presumably by blocking selectin-mediated adherence.

Lefer *et al.* (1994) studied the effect of an SLe^x analog on myocardial I-R in dogs. They induced 1.5 hr of myocardial ischemia followed by 4.5 hr of reperfusion and administered the SLe^x analog, a nonfucosylated analog, or saline 5 min before reperfusion. Myocardial injury, as measured by creatine kinase levels, and myocardial necrosis were reduced in the group treated with the SLe^x analog compared to the nonfucosylated analog or saline group. This correlated with a reduction in PMN accumulation, as measured by myocardial MPO content, in the SLe^x analog-treated group.

B. Integrins

Monoclonal antibodies to both the α and the β subunits of integrins have been found to be protective in reducing I-R injury in a variety of models.

1. CD18

Monoclonal antibody blockade of the common CD18 subunit of the β2-integrins has been found to reduce local I-R injury in the brain (Clark *et al.*, 1991a; del Mori *et al.*, 1992; Matsuo *et al.*, 1994), heart (Ma *et al.*, 1991; Byrne *et al.*, 1992; Lefer *et al.*, 1993; Yamazaki *et al.*, 1993; Aversano *et al.*, 1995), intestine (Hernandez *et al.*, 1987; Schoenberg *et al.*, 1991), kidney (Thornton *et al.*, 1989), lung (Horgan *et al.*, 1990; Bishop *et al.*, 1992; Moore *et al.*, 1995), skeletal muscle (Weselcouch *et al.*, 1991; Jerome *et al.*, 1993; Petrasek *et al.*, 1994), and rabbit ear (Vedder *et al.*, 1990; Sharar *et al.*, 1994). The earliest study on anti-adhesion therapy in I-R injury *in vivo* was published by Hernandez *et al.* in 1987. This study examined the effect of CD18 blockade on intestinal I-R injury in cats. Ischemia was induced in an isolated segment of ileum by reducing arterial blood flow to 15–20% of baseline value and was maintained for 1 hr before reperfusion. One hour prior to ischemia, the animals were treated with either a blocking CD18 MAb or saline. Treatment with CD18 MAb significantly attenuated the increase in microvascular permeability induced by I-R compared to the controls.

Clark *et al.* (1991a) studied the effect of CD18 blockade on spinal cord I-R injury in rabbits. They induced spinal cord ischemia by occluding the abdominal aorta and administering a CD18 MAb 30 min prior to ischemia. The average length of ischemic time to produce permanent paraplegia was longer in the treated group (32 min) compared to the control group

(23 min), indicating that pretreatment with CD18 MAb reduced the ischemic injury. Matsuo *et al.* (1994) studied the effect of CD18 blockade on the brain following transient middle cerebral artery occlusion in rats. They found that treatment with CD18 MAb 15 min before ischemia and again immediately after reperfusion significantly reduced PMN accumulation, as measured by MPO content, and edema formation, as measured by brain water content, and infarct size.

CD18 blockade has also been found to reduce global I-R injury and increase survival following hemorrhagic shock in rabbits when given either prior to (Vedder *et al.,* 1988) or following (Vedder *et al.,* 1989) shock. Mileski *et al.* (1990a) found similar results in rhesus monkeys. Hypovolemic shock was induced by withdrawing blood until the cardiac output was reduced to 30% of baseline for 90 min. Just prior to resuscitation, the animals were treated with a CD18 MAb or saline. Resuscitation was initiated by infusing the animals' shed blood. Resuscitation was continued for 24 hr with a maintenance infusion of lactated Ringer's solution of 4 ml/kg/hr and additional lactated Ringer's solution as needed to maintain the cardiac output at 90% of baseline. Fluid requirements in the CD18 MAb-treated group were significantly less than in the saline-treated group (Fig. 6). In addition, none of the treated animals had hemorrhagic gastritis on endoscopy, whereas all of the control animals exhibited gastritis.

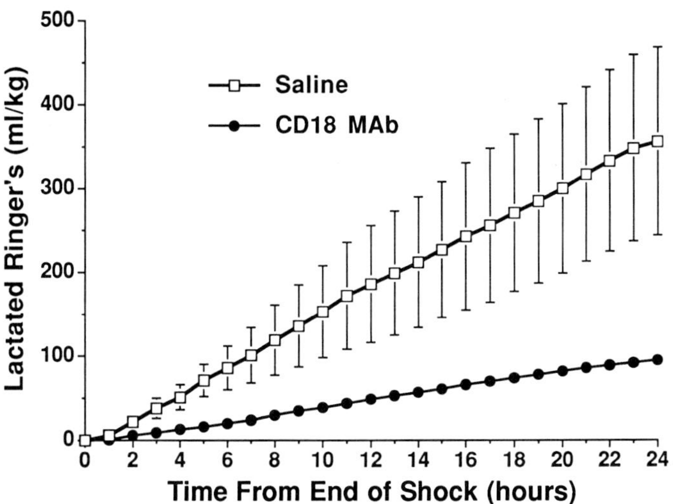

FIGURE 6 Fluid requirements during resuscitation following 90 min of hypovolemic shock in monkeys. Treatment with either CD18 MAb or saline was given at the time of resuscitation. Animals were given maintenance fluids at 4 ml/kg/hr plus additional lactated Ringer's solution as necessary to maintain cardiac output within 90% of baseline. Values represent mean fluid requirements ± SEM for each treatment group at the indicated time following shock. The fluid requirements for the CD18 MAb-treated group were significantly less than that of the saline treated group. Adapted with permission from Mileski *et al.* (1990a).

2. CD11a

Monoclonal antibodies directed at the CD11a subunit have been found to reduce local I-R injury in the heart (Yamazaki *et al.*, 1993) and brain (Matsuo *et al.*, 1994). Yamazaki *et al.* (1993) treated rats with a blocking MAb to CD11a just before 30 min of left coronary artery occlusion. Size of myocardial infarct, expressed as a percentage of area at risk, was significantly less in the treated animals (8%) compared to the untreated animals (34%). Matsuo *et al.* (1994) found protection of cerebral I-R injury in rats treated with MAb to CD11a. They induced cerebral ischemia by transiently occluding the middle cerebral artery for 1 hr. Treatment with CD11a MAb was given 15 min before occlusion and again immediately after reperfusion. The CD11a MAb reduced infarct size and cerebral edema formation at 24 hr after reperfusion and this protection correlated with a reduction in PMN accumulation as measured by histology and MPO content.

3. CD11b

Blockade of the CD11b subunit by MAb has been found to reduce I-R injury in the heart (Simpson *et al.*, 1988, 1990; Yamazaki *et al.*, 1993), liver (Jaeschke *et al.*, 1993), and skeletal muscle (Nolte *et al.*, 1994). Simpson *et al.* (1988) induced 90 min of myocardial ischemia in dogs by occluding the left circumflex artery. Administration of a MAb to CD11b after 45 min of ischemia reduced infarct size in the treated group by 46% compared to the control group. In a later study using the same model, they noted that this reduction in infarct size was sustained after 72 hr following reperfusion (Simpson *et al.*, 1990). Similar results were observed in rats subjected to 30 min of myocardial ischemia (Yamazaki *et al.*, 1993). A CD11b MAb given just prior to ischemia significantly reduced infarct size, expressed as a percentage of the area at risk, in the treated group (10%) compared to the untreated group (34%).

Jaeschke *et al.* (1993) induced 45 min of hepatic ischemia in rats followed by 24 hr of reperfusion. A CD11b MAb was administered 30 min before ischemia and again after 6 hr of reperfusion. There was a reduction in hepatic I-R injury in the CD11b MAb-treated animals compared to the controls as measured by plasma ALT levels and area of hepatic necrosis. This correlated with a 59% decrease in PMN accumulation as seen on histology in the CD11b MAb-treated animals. Similar results were noted when the CD11b MAb was administered following ischemia at 1 and 8 hr after reperfusion, indicating that the protective effect occurred during reperfusion and treatment could be delayed by 1 hr following ischemia.

Nolte *et al.* (1994) studied the effect of CD11b MAb blockade on striated muscle I-R injury in mice. They induced 3 hr of ischemia in striated skin muscle followed by reperfusion, and administered a bolus of CD11b MAb 15 min before reperfusion followed by a continuous infusion of MAb.

Using intravital microscopy, they found that CD11b MAb did not reduce leukocyte rolling in postcapillary venules, but did reduce leukocyte firm adhesion to these venules. In addition, the CD11b MAb attenuated the increase in microvascular permeability and decrease in capillary perfusion seen in postischemic muscle.

C. ICAM-1

Blockade of ICAM-1 with MAb has been found to reduce I-R injury in the brain (Bowes *et al.*, 1993; Matsuo *et al.*, 1994), spinal cord (Clark *et al.*, 1991b), heart (Byrne *et al.*, 1992; Ma *et al.*, 1992; Yamazaki *et al.*, 1993), liver (Suzuki and Toledo-Pereyra, 1993), kidney (Kelly *et al.*, 1994), skeletal muscle (Jerome *et al.*, 1994; Nolte *et al.*, 1994), and lung (Horgan *et al.*, 1991; Moore *et al.*, 1995).

The effect of MAb blockade of ICAM-1 on renal I-R injury in rats was studied by Kelly *et al.* (1994). They induced renal ischemia by transiently occluding the renal artery for 30 or 40 min. An α-ICAM-1 MAb was administered either at the time of ischemia or was delayed until 30, 120, or 480 min after reperfusion. Treatment with α-ICAM-1 MAb at the time of ischemia reduced renal I-R injury as measured by increases in serum creatinine and blood urea nitrogen levels at 24, 48, and 72 hr of reperfusion. Delaying treatment with α-ICAM-1 MAb until after 30 min of reperfusion did not alter the protective effects of the MAb. If treatment was delayed by 120 min after reperfusion, renal I-R injury was reduced at 24 hr, but was not at 48 hr after reperfusion. However, delaying treatment by 480 min was not protective at either 24 or 48 hr.

Suzuki and Toledo-Pereyra (1993) studied the effects of α-ICAM-1 MAb blockade on hepatic I-R in rats. In this study, 90 min of total hepatic ischemia was followed by reperfusion. The MAb to ICAM-1 was administered at the end of the ischemic period and significantly reduced hepatic I-R injury at 360 min after reperfusion as measured by the degree of liver necrosis and plasma ALT and AST levels. Survival at 7 days was increased in the MAb-treated group (63%) compared to the untreated group (16%).

Matsuo *et al.* (1994) examined the effect of ICAM-1 blockade on cerebral I-R in rats. They occluded the middle cerebral artery for 1 hr and administered an α-ICAM-1 MAb 15 min before ischemia and again at reperfusion. They noted a reduction in infarct size in treated animals compared to the untreated animals, which was correlated with a decrease in PMN accumulation and brain edema. Bowes *et al.* (1993) found similar results in rabbits using a cerebral embolism stroke model. In this study, α-ICAM-1 MAb improved the neurological outcome, as measured by an increase in the average size of embolism required to produce permanent neurological damage.

The effect of ICAM-1 blockade on myocardial I-R injury in cats was studied by Ma *et al.* (1992). In this study, they induced myocardial ischemia by occluding the left anterior descending artery for 1.5 hr and administering α-ICAM-1 MAb 10 min before reperfusion. Treatment with α-ICAM-1 MAb reduced the plasma creatine kinase level, the area of myocardial necrosis, and myocardial MPO content in the treated group compared to the control group. Yamazaki *et al.* (1993) found similar results in rats. A reduction in infarct size, expressed as a percentage of the area at risk, was observed in α-ICAM-1 MAb-treated rats (14%) compared to control rats (34%). They also noted a decrease in myocardial MPO content in the treated group.

VI. Atherosclerosis

A. Adhesion Molecule Expression

Atherosclerosis is the most common cause of stroke, myocardial infarction, intestinal ischemia, and gangrene of the extremities. As such, it is the leading cause of death in the United States. Atherosclerotic lesions are thought to begin as a response to various forms of injury to the endothelium or the underlying artery wall (reviewed by Ross, 1993). These insults result in a chronic inflammatory process with dysfunctional endothelium and intimal smooth muscle accumulation. The early lesion in atherosclerosis is called a fatty streak and consists primarily of foam cells and a few T lymphocytes that are located subendothelially. Foam cells in early lesions are predominantly blood monocyte-derived macrophages. Intimal foam cell accumulation in early atherosclerosis thus requires monocyte adherence to and migration across the endothelium. Anti-adhesion therapy directed against this leukocyte–endothelial cell interaction should reduce the initiation and progression of fatty streaks and, perhaps, prevent or retard the formation of the later complicated lesions that are characterized by intimal smooth muscle cell accumulation.

Much attention has been directed at the elucidation of adhesion molecules expressed on endothelium during atherogenesis. VCAM-1, also designated as "athero-ELAM," was shown (Cybulsky and Gimbrone, 1991) by immunohistochemistry to be present on endothelial cells overlying early foam cell lesions induced by dietary hypercholesterolemia in rabbits. Subsequently, they showed that VCAM-1 expression on endothelial cells preceded intimal macrophage accumulation in this model (Li *et al.*, 1993a). More recently, Li *et al.* (1993b) showed that VCAM-1 was not only expressed on endothelial cells overlying regions of intimal thickening in rabbits fed an atherogenic diet, but was also expressed on vascular smooth muscle cells found within these atherosclerotic lesions. VCAM-1 has also been found to be expressed on coronary atherosclerotic lesions in humans by immunohistochemistry (O'Brien *et al.*, 1993). Of note, the majority of VCAM-1 staining appeared to be present in the neovasculature at the base of these plaques and on intimal smooth muscle cells associated with inflammatory cell infiltrates.

Using immunohistochemistry, Poston *et al.* (1992) also found ICAM-1 expression on endothelial cells, macrophages, and smooth muscle cells of human atherosclerotic plaques whereas there was little or no expression on endothelial cells and intimal smooth muscle cells in normal arteries. They postulated that ICAM-1 may enhance monocyte recruitment in the growth of atherosclerotic lesions. Van der Wal *et al.* (1992) examined diffuse intimal thickening and atheromatous plaques in human coronary arteries and abdominal aortas. They found an increase in ICAM-1 expression on endothelial cells that were adjacent to subendothelial infiltrates of macrophages and T lymphocytes, further supporting the proposal that ICAM-1 may play a part in the early recruitment of monocytes and T lymphocytes during atherogenesis.

In the previously mentioned study by van der Wal *et al.* (1992), an increase in E-selectin expression was also observed on endothelial cells that were adjacent to subendothelial inflammatory infiltrates. Johnson-Tidey *et al.* (1994) reported that P-selectin was also expressed on endothelial cells overlying active atherosclerotic plaques in human carotid and coronary arteries, especially on endothelial cells overlying sites of active macrophage infiltration. In this study, a strong correlation was noted between endothelial cells that stained positive for P-selectin and those that stained positive for ICAM-1, indicating that both adhesion molecules may contribute to leukocyte recruitment in atherogenesis.

B. Anti-adhesion Therapy

As cited earlier, several different adhesion molecules have been demonstrated on atherosclerotic plaques and there may be several pathways by which leukocytes adhere to the endothelium. It may be therefore necessary to block several adhesion molecules to reduce leukocyte–endothelial interaction is this setting. Only one study has looked at the use of anti-adhesion therapy to reduce atherogenesis. Molossi *et al.* (1995) examined the effect of blocking the binding of the β1-integrin, VLA-4 (CD49d/CD29), to fibronectin in rabbit cardiac allografts. Allograft arteriopathy is associated with inflammatory cells, increased intimal smooth muscle, and accumulation of extracellular matrix and is a leading cause of cardiac allograft failure. In this study, they performed heterotopic cardiac transplantation without immunosuppression in cholesterol-fed rabbits, which has been shown to accelerate graft arteriopathy. They treated one group of rabbits each day with a synthetic connecting segment-1 (CS-1) peptide from the fibronectin domain that binds to VLA-4. *In vitro* studies have shown that the CS-1 peptide blocks VLA-4 binding to fibronectin and VCAM-1 through competitive inhibition. Another group received a control peptide with no inhibitory activity. At 7–8 days following transplantation, they found a significant decrease in the incidence of intimal thickening in small and medium coronary arteries in the treated group (35%) compared to the control group (87%). The severity of the intimal lesions was also decreased in the treated group (16% of vessel surface area) compared to the control group (36% of vessel surface area). These results correlated with a decrease in T lymphocyte infiltration in the treated group. In addition, treatment with the CS-1 peptide tended to reduce expression of VCAM-1 and ICAM-1 on the allograft coronary artery endothelium. They concluded that blockade of the interaction between VLA-4 and fibronectin reduced accelerated allograft arteriopathy, possibly by interrupting the inflammatory process produced by subendothelial T lymphocytes.

In a somewhat related study by Kling *et al.* (1992), intimal thickening was induced in rabbit carotid arteries using electrical stimulation and a CD18 MAb was administered. In the control animals exposed to electrical stimulation, there was an accumulation of leukocytes including PMN, monocytes, and lymphocytes in the subendothelial space as well as smooth muscle cell migration from the media into the intima. In the treated animals, PMN accumulation in the subendothelial space was abolished, but monocyte and lymphocyte accumulation was only partially inhibited. There was no change in the migration of smooth muscle cells into the intima despite treatment with CD18 MAb. In a subsequent study using the same model, Kling *et al.* (1995) examined the effect of α-VLA-4 MAb alone or in combination with CD18 MAb. They found that α-VLA-4 MAb alone reduced the infiltration of mononuclear cells into the subendothelial space by 70% and abolished the infiltration of eosinophils and basophils, but had no effect on PMN influx. Anti-VLA-4 MAb also reduced the migration of smooth muscle cells into the intima by 50%. The combination of α-VLA-4 and CD18 MAbs abolished the infiltration of all leukocytes and reduced the migration of smooth muscle cells by 70%. They concluded that mononuclear leukocytes are necessary for smooth muscle migration in the formation of intimal thickening.

VII. Thermal Injury

Thermal injury can produce both local and systemic tissue damage. Locally, the initial injury consists of an area of irreversible tissue injury surrounded by an area of injury with reduced blood flow. This surrounding area is termed the zone of stasis and may proceed on to full thickness tissue loss due to ongoing inflammation and microvascular injury. Burns that are >20% total body surface area also often produce a systemic inflammatory response resulting in hypoxia and hypotension. Anti-adhesion therapy in the setting of burns may therefore reduce injury in the zone of stasis and reduce the systemic inflammatory response seen with larger burns.

Mileski *et al.* (1992) studied the effect of ICAM-1 or CD18 blockade on the zone of stasis. In this study, they created full thickness burns on the backs of rabbits separated by zones of stasis. Treatment with either α-ICAM-1 MAb or CD18 MAb was administered either before the burn injury or 30 min after the burn injury. Control animals received saline. Serial measurements of cutaneous blood flow were made using a laser doppler flowmeter for 72 hr. There was no difference among the five groups in cutaneous blood flow in unburned skin (baseline blood flow) or in the full thickness burns (indicating an equivalent degree of burn injury between the groups). However, there was a difference between the groups in cutaneous blood flow in the zone of stasis. The groups that received α-ICAM-1 MAb either before or after the burn injury had a significant increase in blood flow in the zone of stasis (expressed as a percentage of baseline flow) compared to the controls at 4, 24, 48, and 72 hr after the burn injury. The animals that received CD18 MAb before the burn had an initial decrease in blood flow in the zone of stasis comparable to controls at 1, 2, 3, and 4 hr, but then exhibited a gradual recovery in perfusion that was significantly greater than controls by 24, 48, and 72 hr after the burn. The animals that received CD18 MAb 30 min after the burn had significantly greater perfusion in the zone of stasis starting at 1 hr and continuing until 72 hr. The blood flow measurements correlated with the number of zones of stasis that exhibited burn extension to the point of confluence with the burn sites: control, 41%; preburn treatment with CD18 MAb, 15%; postburn treatment with CD18 MAb, 5%; and preburn or postburn treatment with α-ICAM-1 MAb, 5%. In a later study using the same model, Mileski *et al.* (1994) examined the effect of delaying administration of α-ICAM-1 MAb until 3 or 6 hr postburn. They found that even the group with treatment at 6 hr postburn still had an increase in cutaneous blood flow in the zone of stasis compared to the control. However, only the group that received treatment at 3 hr postburn had a decrease in progression of the zone of stasis to full thickness (0%) compared to the controls (41%).

Bucky *et al.* (1994) examined the effect of CD18 blockade on dermal burns in rabbits and found similar results. They created either partial thickness or full thickness burns on the dorsal skin of rabbits and administered a CD18 MAb 30 min after the burn. Grossly, in the partial thickness burns, the CD18 MAb-treated group had less edema, thinner eschars, and earlier elevation of eschars compared to the control group. There was no gross difference with MAb treatment in the full thickness burns. In the partial thickness burns, there was a reduction in the burn surface area by 15% at 24 hr in the CD18 MAb-treated animals. There were also significantly more hair follicles and earlier reepithelialization in the partial thickness burns in the MAb-treated group compared to controls. There was no difference between groups in the full thickness burns.

Mulligan *et al.* (1994a) examined the effect of anti-adhesion therapy on dermal vascular edema and dermal vascular injury developing 4 hr after thermal injury. They also looked at the effect on remote vascular injury in the lung 4 hr following thermal injury. In this study, they induced a 25–30% total body surface area scald burn on rats. Treatment with MAb to CD18, ICAM-1, E-selectin, L-selectin, or P-selectin was administered at 2.5, 3, and 3.5 hr following thermal injury. Another group of rats received treatment with MAb to CD11a just prior to thermal injury or CD11b at the time of thermal injury. Vascular permeability was determined by measuring the leakage of ^{125}I-labeled bovine serum albumin, and hemorrhage was quantified by measuring the leakage of ^{51}Cr-labeled erythrocytes. PMN accumulation in the lung was quantified by measuring tissue MPO content using a colorimetric assay. In the dermis, both vascular permeability and hemorrhage were reduced by treatment with MAb to CD18, CD11b, ICAM-1, E-selectin, and L-selectin. There was no reduction in either dermal vascular permeability or hemorrhage by treatment with MAb to CD11a, VLA-4, or P-selectin. In the lung, both vascular permeability and hemorrhage were reduced by treatment with MAb to CD18, CD11a, CD11b, ICAM-1, E-selectin, and L-selectin. Lung vascular permeability was reduced by treatment with MAb to VLA-4 or P-selectin, but hemorrhage was not reduced. The reduction in lung vascular permeability and hemorrhage correlated with a reduction in MPO content with all MAb tested except mAb to VLA-4. They concluded that dermal vascular injury 4 hr following thermal injury was PMN dependent and required CD11b/CD18, ICAM-1, E-selectin, and L-selectin but did not require participation of CD11a/CD18, VLA-4, or P-selectin. Remote lung vascular injury 4 hr following thermal injury was also PMN dependent and required both CD11a/CD18 and CD11b/CD18 as well as ICAM-1, E-selectin, and L-selectin. Remote lung injury did not appear to consistently require VLA-4 or P-selectin.

The results of these studies provide evidence of the efficacy of anti-adhesion therapy in thermal injury and demonstrate that the blockade of several different adhesion molecules is effective in reducing injury. Currently, there is an ongoing phase II clinical trial examining the effect of treatment with α-ICAM-1 MAb on the outcome of adult patients with thermal injury (Glaser, 1995).

VIII. Arthritis

Rheumatoid arthritis is a chronic, progressive disease that causes significant deformity and debility. It is the result of an ongoing systemic inflammatory process and has been shown to be driven in part by T lymphocyte activity. As such, rheumatoid arthritis may be amenable to treatment with anti-adhesion therapy, especially that aimed at T lymphocytes. Of the many different adhesion molecules, the interactions of ICAM-1 with CD11a/CD18 and VCAM-1 with VLA-4 have best been shown to mediate the emigration of T lymphocytes.

Kavanaugh *et al.* (1994) examined the effect of ICAM-1 blockade in patients with rheumatoid arthritis. In this study, patients with refractory rheumatoid arthritis were treated with α-ICAM-1 MAb daily for 2 or 5 days. Of patients who received 5 days of treatment, 57% had a moderate or marked clinical response at day 8 of follow-up that was sustained for 29 days. At 60 days the clinical response had decreased to 39% and at 90 days to 13% of patients. Treatment with 2 days resulted in a lower response rate of 33% at day 8 which was sustained in only 11% of patients. Currently, a phase II clinical trial is underway to further test the efficacy of ICAM-1 blockade in refractory rheumatoid arthritis.

Barbadillo *et al.* (1995) studied the effects of VLA-4 blockade on adjuvant arthritis in rats. Adjuvant arthritis is produced by the subdermal injection of mycobacterial adjuvant into susceptible rats. These rats develop joint inflammation that is T lymphocyte dependent and thus can be used as an experimental model to test therapies for rheumatoid arthritis. In this study, they injected mycobacterial adjuvant in rats and administered an α-VLA-4 MAb at day 10. In the animals treated with α-VLA-4 MAb, only 10% developed adjuvant arthritis whereas 90% of control animals developed the disease. Anti-VLA-4 MAb treatment thus prevented the development of adjuvant arthritis in rats and, consequently, may be beneficial in the treatment of rheumatoid arthritis.

IX. Asthma

Patients with asthma develop acute airway constriction upon inhalation of allergens. Inhalation of antigen usually causes acute airway obstruction that resolves in 1–2 hr, but can cause late airway obstruction that begins 4–5 hr after antigen inhalation and persists for 24 hr. This airway hypersensitivity is associated with the influx of inflammatory cells into the lung, particularly PMN and eosinophils. Anti-adhesion therapy to block the influx of inflammatory cells may reduce the severity of antigen-induced airway obstruction.

Noonan *et al.* (1991) studied the effect of CD18 blockade on antigen-induced airway obstruction in guinea pigs. Guinea pigs were sensitized to ovalbumin for 2 weeks and were then given an aerosol challenge to ovalbumin. Either acetylcholine or 5-hydroxytryptamine was administered intravenously to provoke airway hyperresponsiveness. Treatment with either CD18 MAb or a nonspecific IgG was administered 1 hr before and 4 hr after ovalbumin aerosol challenge. MAb blockade of CD18 reduced the number of leukocytes recovered on bronchoalveolar lavage (BAL) and reduced the influx of eosinophils compared to the nonspecific IgG. In addition, treatment with CD18 MAb reduced the airway hyperresponsiveness induced by acetylcholine, but not that induced by 5-hydroxytryptamine. They concluded that CD18 plays a role in the emigration of leukocytes in asthma.

In a similar study, Milne and Piper (1994) also used a guinea pig model of antigen-induced airway obstruction and administered two different CD18 MAb intravenously. They noted that both MAbs reduced the number of eosinophils in BAL, but did not reduce the number of eosinophils in lung tissue. Only one of the MAb reduced airway hyperresponsiveness to acetylcholine and histamine, whereas the other MAb had no effect.

Wegner *et al.* (1990) studied the effect of ICAM-1 blockade on asthma in rhesus monkeys. They induced asthma in the monkeys with three alternate day inhalations of antigen and inhaled methacholine. This protocol usually results in a greater than eightfold increase in airway hyperresponsiveness. Daily treatment with α-ICAM-1 MAb attenuated the eosinophil influx in BAL and the airway hyperresponsiveness induced by inhalation of methacholine.

The effect of MAb blockade of E-selectin and ICAM-1 on acute-phase and late-phase antigen-induced asthma in rhesus monkeys was examined by Gundel *et al.* (1991). In this study, animals were treated with α-E-selectin MAb, α-ICAM-1 MAb, or vehicle 1 hr prior to an inhaled antigen challenge. Bronchoalveolar lavage was obtained before antigen challenge and again at the peak late-phase airway hyperresponsiveness. Airway hyperresponsiveness was monitored 1 hr after antigen challenge (acute-phase response) and again at 4, 6, 8, and 10 hr after antigen challenge (late-phase response). Treatment with α-E-selectin MAb significantly decreased the leukocyte infiltration and PMN influx seen on BAL compared to controls. Treatment with α-ICAM-1 MAb did not decrease leukocyte or PMN influx. Treatment with α-E-selectin MAb also reduced the late-phase airway hyperresponsiveness, whereas treatment with α-ICAM-1 MAb had no effect. Neither MAb had an effect on the early phase response.

In another study examining early and late-phase responses of antigen-induced asthma in sheep, Abraham *et al.* (1994) administered an α-VLA-4 MAb. Intravenous or airway administration of α-VLA-4 MAb inhibited the late-phase airway hyperresponsiveness and increase in lung resistance induced by antigen inhalation. Neither method of treatment affected the early phase response. Of note, they did not find a consistent decrease in either total leukocyte or eosinophil count in BAL with α-VLA-4 MAb treatment.

Pretolani *et al.* (1994) studied the effect of VLA-4 blockade on antigen-induced asthma in guinea pigs. Guinea pigs sensitized to ovalbumin were administered an α-VLA-4 MAb 1 hr before and 4 hr after inhalation of ovalbumin. They were then injected intravenously with methacholine. The

α-VLA-4 MAb attenuated the airway hyperresponsiveness, reduced the eosinophil count in BAL and lung tissue, and suppressed the lymphocyte infiltration of the bronchial wall.

Nakajima *et al.* (1994) further studied the role of VLA-4/VCAM-1 and LFA-1/ICAM-1 interactions in antigen-induced asthma in mice by administering MAb to these four adhesion molecules. They noted that treatment with MAb to VLA-4 or VCAM-1 reduced the eosinophil and lymphocyte infiltration into the trachea induced by antigen inhalation, but treatment with MAb to LFA-1 or ICAM-1 did not. They also noted that antigen inhalation induced expression of VCAM-1, but not of ICAM-1, on the endothelium of the trachea. They concluded that VLA-4 and VCAM-1 interactions play a predominant role in eosinophil and lymphocyte recruitment in antigen-induced asthma.

X. Organ Transplantation

Graft rejection remains a major problem in organ transplantation. Early graft rejection is primarily due to T lymphocyte-mediated injury. T lymphocytes attack graft endothelial and parenchymal cells bearing foreign histocompatibility antigens and injure these cells either by direct cytotoxicity or by the release of lymphokines. Recent advances in immunosuppressive therapy such as OKT3 and cyclosporin A have greatly increased graft survival. However, these immunosuppressive tretments result in nonspecific T lymphocyte suppression, which can produce serious infectious complications. Therapy that is directed specifically at T lymphocyte adhesion to graft endothelium has the potential to reduce graft rejection without an increased incidence of infectious complications seen with systemic immunosuppression. This potential benefit has led to a great deal of interest in anti-adhesion therapy in organ transplantation.

MAb blockade of ICAM-1 has been found to reduce rejection in cardiac (Flavin *et al.,* 1991), renal (Cosimi *et al.,* 1990), and small bowel (Yamataka *et al.,* 1993) allografts and in pancreatic islet cell xenografts (Zeng *et al.,* 1994). For example, Flavin *et al.,* (1991) transplanted a cardiac allograft into the abdomen of cynomolgus monkeys. An α-ICAM-1 MAb was administered for 2 days prior to transplantation and was continued for 10 days following transplantation. Mean allograft survival was increased in the treated group (27 days) compared to the untreated group (9 days). In contrast, Komori *et al.* (1993) performed a similar study in which they transplanted a cardiac allograft into the neck of recipients rats. An α-ICAM-1 MAb was administered on the day of transplant and continued for 7 days. There was no increase in graft survival compared to controls (6.4 days versus 6.0 days). However, treatment with α-ICAM-1 MAb and subtherapeutic doses of cyclosporin A did prolong graft survival compared to treatment with subtherapeutic doses of cyclosporin A alone (50 days versus 6.3 days). Therefore, α-ICAM-1 MAb reduced the rejection of cardiac allografts in monkeys. Although α-ICAM-1 MAb alone did not reduce rejection of cardiac allografts in rats, it did reduce rejection when combined with subtherapeutic doses of cyclosporin A which may lead to a decrease in the amount of systemic immunosuppression required and perhaps a reduction in infectious complications.

Cosimi *et al.* (1990) showed that treatment with α-ICAM-1 MAb increased the survival of cynomolgus monkeys subjected to renal allograft transplantation and decreased the allograft leukocyte infiltration seen on histology. A phase I clinical trial was then completed in human renal allograft recipients (Haug *et al.,* 1993). In this study, patients receiving cadaver donor renal transplants who were at high risk for delayed graft function were treated with α-ICAM-1 MAb 1–3 hr before transplant and then received a daily dose for 2 weeks after transplantation. These patients also received conventional immunosuppression consisting of azathioprine and corticosteroids. Cyclosporin A was begun 2 days prior to discontinuing the α-ICAM-1 MAb. Conventionally treated patients who received the contralateral cadaver kidneys were used as controls in this study. There were no instances of primary nonfunction in the 18 patients treated with α-ICAM-1 MAb, and 78% of patients had good to excellent graft function at 16–30 months of follow-up. In contrast, there were three instances of primary nonfunction in the 15 patients (20%) who received the contralateral kidney and conventional immunosuppression, and only 56% of patients had a functioning graft at follow-up. Data from phase II and III clinical trials examining the efficacy of α-ICAM-1 MAb in patients undergoing renal allograft transplantation are currently being evaluated (Glaser, 1995).

Few studies have been done examining the effect of blockade of other adhesion molecules on allograft rejection. In the previously mentioned study by Komori *et al.* (1993) where they examined the effect of α-ICAM-1 MAb on rat cardiac allograft survival, they found similar results with CD11a MAb. The authors found that CD11a MAb alone or in combination with α-ICAM-1 MAb did not increase graft survival compared to controls, but CD11a MAb administered with subtherapeutic doses of cyclosporin A did increase graft survival (88 days) compared to subtherapeutic doses of cyclosporin A alone (6.3 days). Jendrisak *et al.* (1993) studied the effect of blocking a combination of adhesion molecules on mouse cardiac allograft survival. They administered MAb to CD11a, ICAM-1, and CD4 to mice for 14 days and performed heterotopic cardiac transplantations on day 4. Allograft survival was prolonged (59 days) in the treated group compared to the untreated group of mice (15 days). Kameoka *et al.* (1993) observed similar results with cardiac allografts in rats. They administered MAb to CD11a alone, MAbs to CD11a and ICAM-1, and MAbs to CD11a and CD18. They found no significant increase in graft survival with CD11a

MAb alone (26 days) compared to controls (11 days), but there was an increase in graft survival with the combination of MAbs to CD11a and ICAM-1 (48 days) and MAbs to CD11a and CD18 (37 days). Therefore, although ICAM-1 blockade has been shown to reduce allograft rejection and is currently in a phase II clinical trial, in the future it may prove more beneficial to block a combination of adhesion molecules and further reduce rejection.

XI. Acute Lung Injury

Anti-adhesion therapy has been found to be protective in a number of acute lung injury models. For example, Mulligan *et al.* (1992a) induced oxidant-mediated acute lung injury in rats by the rapid infusion of cobra factor venom (CFV) intravascularly. They administered either CD18 or CD11b MAb 10 min before CFV injection. Lung vascular permeability was quantified by the leakage of ^{125}I-labeled bovine serum albumin, and lung hemorrhage was quantified by the extravasation of ^{51}Cr-labeled erythrocytes into lung tissue 30 min after CFV infusion. PMN accumulation was quantified by measuring lung tissue MPO content. They found that pretreatment with either CD18 or CD11b MAb attenuated the increase in vascular permeability and hemorrhage seen with CFV-induced lung injury. This correlated with a decrease in PMN accumulation seen in the treated groups. Using the same model of CFV-induced lung injury, Mulligan *et al.* (1992b) reported that treatment with α-P-selectin MAb also reduced vascular permeability, hemorrhage, and PMN accumulation. In a later study using the same model, they noted that treatment with either P-selectin chimeras or L-selectin chimeras reduced vascular permeability, hemorrhage, and PMN accumulation (Mulligan *et al.*, 1993b). Of note in this study, Mulligan *et al.* (1993b) found that E-selectin chimeras did not attenuate lung injury. The same group (Mulligan *et al.*, 1994b) showed that α-L-selectin MAb also reduced CFV-induced lung injury. Therefore, in the CFV-induced model, acute lung injury appeared to be partly dependent on CD18, CD11b, P-selectin, and L-selectin, but was independent of E-selectin.

Mulligan *et al.* also examined the role of adhesion molecules in a different model of acute lung injury in rats induced by the intrapulmonary deposition of IgG immune complexes. In their initial study, Mulligan *et al.* (1992a) found that pretreatment with CD18 MAb reduced vascular permeability, hemorrhage, and PMN accumulation. Of note, treatment with CD11b MAb did not significantly reduce lung injury. Using the same model of IgG immune complex-induced lung injury, treatment with either L-selectin chimeras or E-selectin chimeras attenuated the increase in vascular permeability, hemorrhage, and PMN accumulation whereas P-selectin chimeras did not reduce lung injury (Mulligan *et al.*, 1993b).

In two different studies, Mulligan *et al.* (1991, 1994b) found that treatment with either α-E- or α-L-selectin MAb reduced lung injury in this model. This model was also used to examine the role of VLA-4 (Mulligan *et al.*, 1993a). They found that an α-VLA-4 MAb reduced lung injury and PMN accumulation. To test the method of MAb administration in this model, MAb to CD11a, CD11b, L-selectin, or ICAM-1 was administered either intravenously or intratracheally (Mulligan *et al.*, 1995). Intravenous administration of MAb to CD11a, L-selectin, or ICAM-1 all reduced lung injury and PMN accumulation, but CD11b MAb was without effect. However, intratracheal treatment with either CD11b or α-ICAM-1 MAb was protective, whereas intratracheal treatment with CD11a or α-L-selectin MAb was without benefit. They concluded that in acute lung injury induced by intrapulmonary deposition of IgG immune complexes, CD18, CD11a, ICAM-1, L-selectin, and E-selectin appear to play important roles in the vascular compartment for PMN recruitment, whereas CD11b and ICAM-1 appear to be involved in the alveolar compartment.

The role of adhesion molecules in acute lung injury induced by IgA immune complexes was also studied. Intravenous treatment with MAb to CD11a, CD11b, VLA-4, or ICAM-1 all reduced vascular permeability and hemorrhage, although CD11a MAb did so to a slightly lesser extent than the other MAbs (Mulligan *et al.*, 1993a). The same group (Mulligan *et al.*, 1992c, 1994b) showed that CD18 MAb was highly protective, but α-L-selectin and α-E-selectin MAb were not protective against IgA immune complex-induced lung injury. Therefore it appears that lung injury induced by intrapulmonary deposition of IgA immune complexes is dependent in part on CD18, CD11a, CD11b, ICAM-1, and VLA-4, but is independent of L- and E-selectin.

The role of adhesion molecules in TNF-induced lung injury has also been studied. Lo *et al.* (1992) examined the role of CD18 and ICAM-1 in TNF-induced lung injury in guinea pig lungs *ex vivo*. They perfused isolated guinea pig lungs with TNF and then with perfusate containing human PMN. In one group they pretreated the PMN with CD18 MAb, and in another group they added α-ICAM-1 MAb to the perfusate. They found a decrease in lung injury with either CD18 or α-ICAM-1 MAb. Using the same isolated guinea pig lung model, Lo *et al.* (1994) found that pretreatment of PMN with SLe^x MAb reduced lung injury and PMN accumulation. Eichacker *et al.* (1992) studied the effect of CD11b MAb on TNF-induced lung injury in dogs. Pretreatment with CD11b MAb reduced early mortality and hypoxemia, but did not have an effect on overall survival or cardiopulmonary function. Therefore, it appears that TNF-induced acute lung injury is dependent in part on CD18, CD11b, ICAM-1, and the selectins.

Barton *et al.* (1989) examined the role of ICAM-1 in phorbol ester-induced lung injury in rabbits. They pretreated rabbits with MAb to ICAM-1, CD18, or CD11a and 2 hr later induced lung injury by an intravenous injection of phorbol ester. They obtained BAL cell counts 20 hr after phorbol ester injection. Pretreatment with CD18 MAb reduced PMN influx by 75% and α-ICAM-1 MAb reduced PMN influx by 63%, but a CD11a MAb was not effective. Thus, it appears that CD18 and ICAM-1, but not CD11a, play a role in phorbol ester-induced lung injury.

Another method of inducing acute lung injury in rats is by inducing I-R in a remote tissue. Both Seekamp *et al.* (1993, 1994) and Hill *et al.* (1992) have examined the role of adhesion molecules in this form of lung injury. In two different studies, Seekamp *et al.* (1993, 1994) studied the role of CD18, CD11a, CD11b, ICAM-1, and the selectins in lung injury following hind limb I-R in rats. They induced 4 hr of hind limb ischemia followed by 4 hr of reperfusion. They administered MAb to CD18, CD11a, CD11b, ICAM-1, VLA-4, P-selectin, E-selectin, or L-selectin during reperfusion. They found that lung vascular permeability, hemorrhage, and PMN accumulation were reduced by treatment with MAb to CD18, CD11a, CD11b, ICAM-1, E-selectin, and L-selectin. An α-VLA-4 MAb did not reduce vascular permeability or hemorrhage but did reduce PMN accumulation. MAb to P-selectin did not reduce vascular permeability, hemorrhage, or PMN accumulation following 4 hr of hind limb ischemia. However, when they shortened the ischemia time to 1 hr and the reperfusion time to 1.5 hr, they found that treatment with MAb to P-selectin did reduce lung injury and PMN infiltration. They concluded that remote lung injury following hind limb I-R is dependent in part on CD11a, CD11b, CD18, ICAM-1, E-selectin, L-selectin, and, to a lesser degree, on P-selectin. VLA-4 appears to play little role in remote lung injury following I-R. Hill *et al.* (1992) examined the role of CD11b in remote lung injury following intestinal I-R in rats. They found that treatment with CD11b reduced lung vascular permeability but did not reduce PMN accumulation.

XII. Multiple Sclerosis

Multiple sclerosis is an inflammatory disease of the central nervous system in which leukocytes penetrate the blood–brain barrier and damage myelin. The progressive demyelination results in impaired nerve conduction and paralysis. Its clinical course is usually characterized by periods of active disease with deterioration of nerve conduction and periods of quiescence in which there is no progression of disease but no improvement either. Prevention of leukocyte penetration of the blood–brain barrier through anti-adhesion therapy may prove beneficial.

Experimental autoimmune encephalomyelitis (EAE) has been used as a model of multiple sclerosis. EAE is an inflammatory disease of the central nervous system in rats that can be either active or passive. The active form of the disease is produced by active immunization with myelin or myelin basic protein. The passive form of the disease is produced by injecting rats with myelin basic protein-specific CD4-positive T cells. Huitinga *et al.* (1993) examined the role of CD11b and CD18 in the pathophysiology of EAE. They found that treatment with MAb to CD18 suppressed clinical signs of EAE, whereas treatment with a MAb to CD11b did not. Archelos *et al.* (1993) studied the effect of ICAM-1 blockade on active and passive EAE. Treatment with an α-ICAM-1 MAb suppressed active EAE symptoms and reduced inflammatory infiltrates of the central nervous system seem on histology. Anti-ICAM-1 MAb had little effect on passive EAE symptoms or pathology. In a similar study, Willenborg *et al.* (1993) reported similar results with an α-ICAM-1 MAb. Of note, they found that treatment with α-ICAM-1 MAb in passive EAE not only did not inhibit disease, but at high doses actually appeared to enhance disease with an earlier onset of symptoms. In a study by Kobayashi *et al.* (1995), administration of MAb to ICAM-1 and CD11a/CD18 together during the induction phase did not reduce disease, but treatment during the effector phase suppressed progression of EAE. Treatment with either MAb alone had no effect. Yednock *et al.* (1992) found that α-VLA-4 MAb prevented the development of passive EAE and reduced the accumulation of leukocytes into the central nervous system. Therefore, in EAE it appears that ICAM-1, CD11a/CD18, and VLA-4 play a role in the recruitment of leukocytes to the central nervous system and blockade of these adhesion molecules may reduce disease. Phase I clinical trials are currently examining the effect of VLA-4 and CD18 MAbs on the progression of disease in multiple sclerosis (Glaser, 1995).

XIII. Miscellaneous

A. Inflammatory Bowel Disease

Inflammatory bowel disease is a chronic inflammatory response that results in tissue injury. Although the exact cause of the disease is unknown, it is apparent that leukocytes play an important role in disease activity and as such are found in affected tissues. Blocking this leukocyte emigration should therefore reduce disease activity. Wong *et al.* (1995) found that MAb to ICAM-1 reduced acetic acid-induced colitis in rats. In a study by Wallace *et al.* (1992), colitis in rats was induced with an intracolonic administration of dinitrobenzene sulfonic acid in 30% ethanol. There was a reduction in MPO content with administration of MAb to CD18. Podolsky *et al.* (1993) examined the effect of either α-E-selectin or α-VLA-4 MAb on colitis in cotton-top tamarin monkeys. These monkeys develop a spontaneous acute and chronic colitis similar to ulcerative colitis. Anti-E-selectin MAb or saline was given every other day for 8 days to monkeys with active colitis. An α-VLA-4 MAb or saline was administered daily for 8 days to a different group of monkeys with active colitis. Colonic mucosal biopsies were obtained every other day for 12 days. They found that treatment with the α-E-selectin MAb had no effect on the colitis whereas treatment with the α-VLA-4 MAb led to a significant improvement in acute colitis.

B. Glomerulonephritis

Autoimmune glomerulonephritis is a disease that results in loss of renal function secondary to chronic inflammation in the kidney. Animal models exist for this disease, and several studies have been done examining the effect of anti-adhesion therapy on glomerulonephritis. Kawasaki *et al.* (1993) examined the effect of MAb to ICAM-1 or CD11a on nephrotoxic serum nephritis in rats. Nephritis was induced by injecting the rats with serum containing anti-glomerular basement membrane (GBM) antibodies and either CD11a or α-ICAM-1 MAb was administered three times per week for 2 weeks. The control animals developed proteinuria by day 8 whereas treatment with either CD11a or α-ICAM-1 MAb prevented proteinuria in a dose-dependent manner. Histologically, control animals developed necrotizing lesions and crescents by day 6. Treatment with either MAb prevented these lesions. Treatment with both CD11a and α-ICAM-1 MAb at suboptimal doses resulted in an additive inhibitory effect on both proteinuria and histologic lesions. Nishikawa *et al.* (1993) found similar results using the same MAbs in the same model. Harning *et al.* (1992) examined the effect of α-ICAM-1 MAb in mice that were born with normal kidneys but then developed progressive, lethal autoimmune nephritis by 8 weeks of age. Treatment with α-ICAM-1 MAb reduced leukocyte infiltration into the kidney and proteinuria. Wu *et al.* (1993) examined the effect of CD11b blockade on nephrotoxic serum nephritis in rats. They pretreated with CD11b MAb 30 min or 16 hr prior to injection with serum containing anti-GBM antibodies. In the animals pretreated 30 min before injection, they found a reduction in proteinuria by 50% but no change in glomerular PMN. In the animals pretreated 16 hr before injection, they found an even greater reduction in proteinuria (80%) which was accompanied by a decrease in glomerular PMN. There was no change in the number of macrophages in either treatment group. Molina *et al.* (1994) induced nephritis in rats by administering mercuric chloride. Mercuric chloride induces the formation of anti-GBM antibodies resulting in glomerular and interstitial nephritis and proteinuria. They found that treatment leukocyte infiltrates, and proteinuria. Tipping *et al.* (1994a) induced nephrotoxic serum nephritis in mice and pretreated with an α-P-selectin MAb. There was a reduction in proteinuria and in glomerular PMN in the MAb-treated group. In an earlier study, Tipping *et al.* (1994b) found that treatment with CD18 MAb in rabbits with anti-GBM-induced nephritis did not reduce proteinuria or glomerular PMN influx. In the same study, rendering rabbits neutropenic markedly reduced proteinuria and decreased PMN glomerular infiltration. It is unclear why Tipping *et al.* (1994b) found no effect with CD18 MAb in rabbits, but the studies just discussed found a protective effect with CD11a, CD11b, and α-ICAM-1 MAb in rats and mice. Despite these differing results, it does appear that autoimmune glomerulonephritis is dependent in part on the β2-integrins, ICAM-1, and P-selectin.

XIV. Safety Concerns

As reviewed earlier, there is strong evidence that anti-adhesion therapy is effective in reducing a variety of diseases. However, because this therapy results in the impairment of the body's own natural defense mechanisms, one must be concerned about the possibility of a higher incidence of infectious complications when using anti-adhesion therapy. There are two genetic deficiencies of adhesion molecules that show that this concern is warranted. They are designated leukocyte adhesion deficiency type I (LAD I) and type II (LAD II) (reviewed by Etzioni, 1994). LAD I patients have a deficiency in expression of the β2-integrins and therefore a defect in firm adherence of leukocytes to endothelial cells. These patients have a defect in phagocyte emigration and fail to form pus at sites of inflammation. Clinically, severely deficient LAD I patients develop recurrent life-threatening bacterial and fungal infections. LAD II patients have a defect in fucose metabolism that results in an absence of SLe^x, the ligand for E- and P-selectin. These patients have a defect in the initial rolling of leukocytes along the endothelial cell surface. Clinically, these LAD II patients also develop recurrent infections, although the infections have not been life-threatening to date. Clinical observations in the LAD patients vividly illustrate the possible increased risk for infectious complications following anti-adhesion therapy. Several studies have been performed to assess the magnitude of this risk.

Rosen *et al.* (1989) found that pretreating mice with MAb to CD11b prior to inoculation of *Listeria monocytogenes* into the liver and spleen significantly increased their mortality compared to controls and converted a sublethal injection into a lethal one. Using a rabbit model of subcutaneous abscess formation, Garcia *et al.* (1994) found that pretreating with CD18 MAb prior to subcutaneous inoculation with *Pseudomonas aeruginosa* significantly increased the incidence and severity of abscess formation. In contrast, several investigators have found no increase in infectious complications following anti-adhesion therapy. In the same study by Garcia *et al.* (1994), there was no increase in subcutaneous abscess severity following *P. aeruginosa* inoculation in rabbits treated with MAb to L-selectin. A similar study by Mileski *et al.* (1993) showed that treatment of rabbits with α-ICAM-1 MAb followed by subcutaneous inoculations of *P. aeruginosa* or *Staphylococcus aureus* did not increase the severity of abscess formation. Sharar *et al.* (1991) reported that treatment with CD18 MAb did not increase the incidence or size of abscesses resulting from clinically relevant subcutaneous inoculations of *S. aureus* ($<10^8$ colony-forming units, CFU) when antibiotics were also given. However, if an inoculation of $>10^8$ CFU was given, CD18 MAb treatment resulted in a higher incidence of abscess formation and a larger size of abscesses compared to controls (Fig. 7). Treatment with an α-P-selectin MAb did not result in a higher incidence of abscess formation in rabbits inoculated with *S. aureus* (Sharar *et al.*, 1993).

Mileski *et al.* (1991) examined the effect of blockade of CD18 on intra-abdominal infection in rabbits. They devascularized the appendix and then removed the appendix 18 hr later. Treatment with CD18 MAb was given at the time of appendiceal devascularization and at the time of removal of the appendix. They followed the rabbits for 10 days and found no increase in mortality or infectious complications with CD18 MAb treatment compared to controls. There was, however, a significant decrease in PMN emigration into the peritoneum at 18 hr in the animals treated with CD18 MAb. Using the same model, Thomas *et al.* (1992) found an increase in survival at 10 days when CD18 MAb was given at the time of appendiceal devascularization and continued every 12 hr for 3 days. In the CD18 MAb-treated group, 90% of the rabbits survived 10 days whereas only 40% of the control rabbits survived. In an *Escherichia coli*-induced peritonitis model in rabbits,

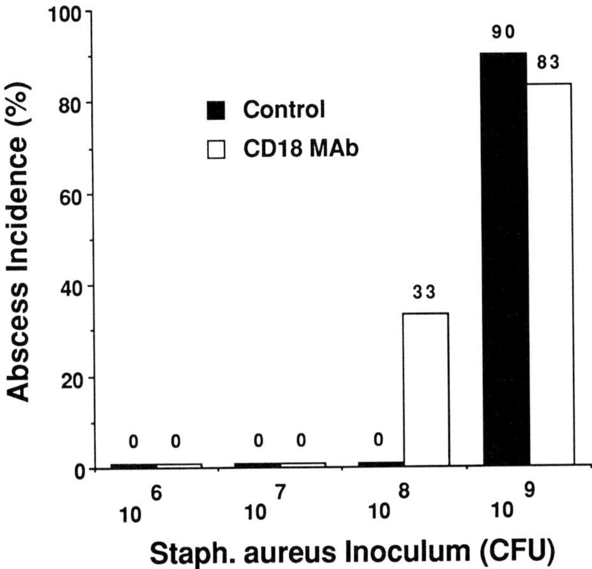

FIGURE 7 Abscess formation following subcutaneous injection with *Staphylococcus aureus* bacteria in rabbits. Values represent the percentage of rabbits who developed abscesses for each amount of bacteria inoculated. Treatment with CD18 MAb or saline was given at the time of inoculation. Adapted with permission from Sharar *et al.* (1991).

PMN emigration into the peritoneum was reduced in animals treated with CD18 MAb (Mileski *et al.*, 1990b). In contrast, P-selectin blockade did not decrease PMN emigration into the peritoneum of rabbits in a similar model of *E. coli*-induced peritonitis (Sharar *et al.*, 1993).

In a rabbit model of bacterial meningitis induced by intrathecal injection of *Streptococcus pneumoniae,* Tuomanen *et al.* (1989) actually found a decrease in mortality with CD18 MAb treatment. Cerebral edema and cerebrospinal fluid protein content were reduced in treated animals due to protection of the blood–brain barrier. The course of bacterial growth in the cerebral spinal fluid was not changed with CD18 MAb treatment, but the course of bacterial growth in the blood was delayed with CD18 MAb treatment. In addition, CD18 MAb treatment reduced the inflammatory response to bacterial lysis induced by ampicillin.

As summarized, there are mixed results in studies regarding the effect of anti-adhesion therapy on infectious complications. CD18 blockade increased the severity of infection following subcutaneous inoculation with *P. aeruginosa,* but ICAM-1 or L-selectin blockade did not. Neither CD18 nor P-selectin blockade increased the severity of infection induced by clinically relevant inoculations with *S. aureus*. However, CD18 blockade did increase the severity of infection produced by a large inoculation with *S. aureus*. Treatment with CD18 MAb did not appear to increase the infectious complications or mortality in intra-abdominal infections, but did decrease PMN emigration into the peritoneum. P-selectin blockade did not decrease PMN emigration into the peritoneum. At this point, the potential benefits of anti-adhesion therapy appear to outweigh the potential increased risk of infectious complications.

XV. Conclusion

Anti-adhesion therapy has been found to be beneficial in animal models of a variety of disease processes. Blocking either the initial rolling of leukocytes along the endothelium or the firm adherence of leukocytes to the endothelium has been found to be effective in reducing leukocyte-mediated injury and leukocyte accumulation. A number of phase I and II clinical trials are already underway examining the effect of anti-adhesion therapy in a variety of disease states. These include clinical trials of SLe^x oligosaccharide in myocardial infarction and chronic pulmonary thrombotic obstruction, CD18 MAb and CD49d MAb in multiple sclerosis, and α-ICAM-1 MAb in renal allograft recipients, burn patients, stroke patients, and patients with refractory rheumatoid arthritis (Glaser, 1995). More such trials are planned. While anti-adhesion therapy directed at leukocyte–endothelial interaction is an exciting field with the potential to benefit a large number of patients, the potential risk of infectious complications will always have to be considered carefully in each disease setting. It is hoped that current and future clinical trials will establish that the benefits of anti-adhesion therapy outweigh any possible complications.

References

Abraham, W. M., Sielczak, M. W., Ahmed, A., Cortes, A., Lauredo, I. T., Kim, J., Pepinsky, B., Benjamin, C. D., Leone, D. R., Lobb, R. R., and Weller, P. F. (1994). Alpha 4-integrins mediate antigen-induced late bronchial responses and prolonged airway hyperresponsiveness in sheep. *J. Clin. Invest.* **93**, 776–787.

Altavilla, D., Squadrito, F., Ioculano, M., Canale, P., Campo, G. M., Zingarelli, B., and Caputi, A. P. (1994). E-selectin in the pathogenesis of experimental myocardial ischemia-reperfusion injury. *Eur. J. Pharmacol.* **270**, 45–51.

Archelos, J. J., Jung, S., Maurer, M., Schmied, M., Lassmann, H., Tamatani, T., Miyasaka, M., Toyka, K. V., and Hartung, H. P. (1993). Inhibition of experimental autoimmune encephalomyelitis by an antibody to the intercellular adhesion molecule ICAM-1. *Ann Neurol.* **34**, 145–154.

Arnaout, M. A. (1990). Structure and function of the leukocyte adhesion molecules CD11/CD18. *Blood* **75**, 1037–1050.

Asako, H., Kurose, I., Wolf, R., DeFrees, S., Zheng, Z. L., Phillips, M. L., Paulson, J. C., and Granger, D. N. (1994). Role of H1 receptors and P-selectin in histamine-induced leukocyte rolling and adhesion in postcapillary venules. *J. Clin. Invest.* **93**, 1508–1515.

Aversano, T., Zhou, W., Nedelman, M., Nakada, M., and Weisman, H. (1995). A chimeric IgG4 monoclonal antibody directed against CD18 reduces infarct size in a primate model of myocardial ischemia and reperfusion. *J. Am. Coll. Cardiol.* **25**, 781–788.

Barbadillo, C., G-Arroyo, A., Salas, C., Mulero, J., Sánchez-Madrid, F., and Andreu, J. L. (1995). Anti-integrin immunotherapy in rheumatoid arthritis: Protective effect of anti-alpha 4 antibody in adjuvant arthritis. *Springer Semin. Immunopathol.* **16**, 427–436.

Barroso-Aranda, J., Schmid-Schonbein, G. W., Zweifach, B. W., and Engler, R. L. (1988). Granulocytes and no-reflow phenomenon in irreversible hemorrhagic shock. *Circ. Res.* **63**, 437–447.

Barton, R. W., Rothlein, R., Ksiazek, J., and Kennedy, C. (1989). The effect of anti-intercellular adhesion molecule-1 on phorbol-ester-induced rabbit lung inflammation. *J. Immunol.* **143**, 1278–1282.

Bator, J. M., Weitzberg, M., and Burch, R. M. (1992). N-[9H-(2,7-dimethylfluorenyl-9-methoxy)carbonyl]-L-leucine, NPC 15669, prevents neutrophil adherence to endothelium and inhibits CD11b/CD18 upregulation. *Immunopharmacology* **23**, 139–149.

Bauer, C., Siaplaouras, S., Soule, H. R., Moyle, M., and Marzi, I. (1995). A natural glycoprotein inhibitor (NIF) of CD11b/CD18 reduces leukocyte adhesion in the liver after hemorrhagic shock. *Shock* **4**, 187–192.

Baumheter, S., Singer, M. S., Henzel, W., Hemmerich, S., Renz, M., Rosen, S. D., and Lasky, L. A. (1993). Binding of L-selectin to the vascular sialomucin CD34. *Science* **262**, 436–438.

Bennett, C. F., Condon, T. P., Grimm, S., Chan, H., and Chiang, M. Y. (1994). Inhibition of endothelial cell adhesion molecule expression with antisense oligonucleotides. *J. Immunol.* **152**, 3530–3540.

Berlin, C., Berg, E. L., Briskin, M. J., Andrew, D. P., Kilshaw, P. J., Holzmann, B., Weissman, I. L., Hamann, A., and Butcher, E. C. (1993). Alpha 4 beta 7 integrin mediates lymphocyte binding to the mucosal vascular addressin MAdCAM-1 Cell (*Cambridge, Mass.*) **74**, 185–195.

Bevilacqua, M. P., Pober, J., Mendrick, D., Cotran, R., and Gimbrone, M. (1987). Identification of an inducible endothelial-leukocyte adhesion molecule. *Proc. Natl. Acad. Sci. U. S. A.* **84,** 9238–9242.

Bevilacqua, M. P., Stenglin, S., Gimbrone, M., Jr., and Seed, B. (1989). An inducible receptor for neutrophils related to complement regulatory proteins and lectins. *Science* **243,** 1160–1165.

Bevilacqua, M. P. (1993). Endothelial-leukocyte adhesion molecules. *Annu. Rev. Immunol.* **11,** 767–804.

Bevilacqua, M. P., and Nelson, R. M. (1993). Selectins. *J. Clin. Invest.* **91,** 379–387.

Bishop, M. J., Kowalski, T. F., Guidotti, S. M., and Harlan, J. M. (1992). Antibody against neutrophil adhesion improves reperfusion and limits alveolar infiltrate following unilateral pulmonary artery occlusion. *J. Surg. Res.* **52,** 199–204.

Bowes, M. P., Zivin, J. A., and Rothlein, R. (1993). Monoclonal antibody to the ICAM-1 adhesion site reduces neurological damage in a rabbit cerebral embolism stroke model. *Exp. Neurol.* **119,** 215–219.

Briggs, J. B., Oda, Y., Gilbert, J. H., Schaefer, M. E., and Maher, B. A. (1995). Peptides inhibit selectin-mediated cell adhesion *in vitro,* and neutrophil influx into inflammatory sites *in vivo. Glycobiology* **5,** 583–588.

Bucky, L. P., Vedder, N. B., Hong, H. Z., Ehrlich, H. P., Winn, R. K., Harlan, J. M., and May, J. W., Jr. (1994). Reduction of burn injury by inhibiting CD18-mediated leukocyte adherence in rabbits. *Plast. Reconstr. Surg.* **93,** 1473–1480.

Buerke, M., Weyrich, A. S., Zheng, Z., Gaeta, F. C. A., Forrest, M. J., and Lefer, A. M. (1994). Sialyl LewisX-containing oligosaccharide attenuates myocardial reperfusion injury in cats. *J. Clin. Invest.* **93,** 1140–1148.

Burch, R. M., Noronha-Blob, L., Bator, J. M., Lowe, V. C., and Sullivan, J. P. (1993). Mice treated with a leumedin or antibody to Mac-1 to inhibit leukocyte sequestration survive endotoxin challenge. *J. Immunol.* **150,** 3397–3403.

Byrne, J. G., Smith, W. J., Murphy, M. P., Couper, G. S., Appleyard, R. F., and Cohn, L. H. (1992). Complete prevention of myocardial stunning, contracture, low-reflow, and edema after heart transplantation by blocking neutrophil adhesion molecules during reperfusion. *J. Thorac Cardiovasc. Surg.* **104,** 1589–1596.

Carlos, T. M., and Harlan, J. M. (1994). Leukocyte-endothelial adhesion molecules. *Blood* **84,** 2068–2101.

Clark, E. A., and Brugge, J. S. (1995). Integrins and signal transduction pathways: The road taken. *Science* **268,** 233–239.

Clark, W. M., Madden, K. P., Rothlein, R., and Zivin, J. A. (1991). Reduction of central nervous systemic ischemic injury by monoclonal antibody to intercellular adhesion molecule. *J. Neurosurg.* **75,** 623–627.

Clark, W. M., Madden, K. P., Rothlein, R., and Zivin, J. A. (1991b). Reduction of central nervous system ischemic injury in rabbits using leukocyte adhesion antibody treatment. *Stroke* **22,** 877–883.

Cosimi, A. B., Conti, D., Delmonico, F. L., Preffer, F. I., Wee, S. L., Rothlein, R., Faanes, R., and Colvin, R. B. (1990). In vivo effects of monoclonal antibody to ICAM-1 (CD54) in nonhuman primates with renal allografts. *J. Immunol.* **144,** 4604–4612.

Cybulsky, M. I., and Gimbrone, M. A., Jr. (1991). Endothelial expression of a mononuclear leukocyte adhesion molecule during atherogenesis. *Science* **251,** 788–791.

Davenpeck, K. L., Gauthier, T. W., Albertine, K. H., and Lefer, A. M. (1994). Role of P-selectin in microvascular leukocyte-endothelial interaction in splanchnic ischemia-reperfusion. *Am. J. Physiol.* **267,** H622–H630.

del Mori, E., Z. G. J., Chambers, J. D., Copeland, B. R., and Arfors, K. E. (1992). Inhibition of polymorphonuclear leukocyte adherence suppresses no-reflow after focal cerebral ischemia in baboons. *Stroke* **23,** 712–718.

Díaz-González, F., González-Alvaro, I., Campanero, M. R., Mollinedo, F., del Pozo, M. A., Munoz, C., Pivel, J. P., and Sánchez-Madrid, F. (1995). Prevention of in vitro neutrophil-endothelial attachment through shedding of L-selectin by nonsteroidal antiinflammatory drugs. *J. Clin. Invest.* **95,** 1756–1765.

Eichacker, P. Q., Farese, A., Hoffman, W. D., Banks, S. M., Mouginis, A., Richmond, S., Kuo, G. C., Macvitte, T. J., and Natanson, C. (1992). Leukocyte CD11b/18 antigen-directed monoclonal antibody improves early survival and decreases hypoxemia in dogs challenged with tumor necrosis factor. *Am. Rev. Respir. Dis.* **145,** 1023–1029.

Elices, M. J., Tsai, V., Strahl, D., Goel, A. S., Tollefson, V., Arrhenius, T., Wayner, E. A., Gaeta, F. C., Fikes, J. D., and Firestein, G. S. (1994). Expression and functional significance of alternatively spliced CS1 fibronectin in rheumatoid arthritis microvasculature. *J. Clin. Invest.* **93,** 405–416.

Engler, R. L., Schmid-Schonbein, G. W., and Pavelec, R. S. (1983). Leukocyte capillary plugging in myocardial ischemia and reperfusion in the dog. *Am. J. Pathol.* **111,** 98–111.

Etzioni, A. (1994). Adhesion molecule deficiencies and their clinical significance. *Cell Adhes. Commun.* **2,** 257–260.

Faull, R. J., Kovach, N. L., Harlan, J. M., and Ginsberg, M. H. (1994). Stimulation of integrin-mediated adhesion of T lymphocytes and monocytes: Two mechanisms with divergent biological consequences. *J. Exp. Med.* **179,** 1307–1316.

Flavin, T., Ivens, K., Rothlein, R., Faanes, R., Clayberger, C., Billingham, M., and Starnes, V. A. (1991). Monoclonal antibodies against intercellular adhesion molecule 1 prolong cardiac allograft survival in cynomolgus monkeys. *Transplant. Proc.* **23,** 533–534.

Gallatin, W. M., Weissman, I. L., and Butcher, E. C. (1983). A cell-surface molecule involved in organ-specific homing of lymphocytes. *Nature (London)* **304,** 30–34.

Garcia, N. M., Mileski, W. J., Sikes, P., Atiles, L., Lightfoot, E., Lipsky, P., and Baxter, C. (1994). Effect of inhibiting leukocyte integrin (CD18) and selectin (L-selectin) on susceptibility to infection with *Pseudomonas aeruginosa*. *J. Trauma* **36,** 714–718.

Garcia-Criado, F. J., Toledo-Pereyra, L. H., Lopez-Niblina, F., Phillips, M. L., Paez-Rollys, A., and Misawa, K. (1995). Role of P-selectin in total hepatic ischemia and reperfusion. *J. Am. Coll. Surg.* **181,** 327–334.

Glaser, V. (1995). Work on cell-adhesion-based interactions beginning to bear fruit. *Genet. Eng. News,* pp. 6–7.

Gotsch, U., Jager, U., Dominis, M., and Vestweber, D. (1994). Expression of P-selectin on endothelial cells is upregulated by LPS and TNF-alpha in vivo. *Cell Adhes. Commun.* **2,** 7–14.

Gundel, R. H., Wegner, C. D., Torcellini, C. A., Clarke, C. C., Haynes, N., Rothlein, R., Smith, C. W., and Letts, L. G. (1991). Endothelial leukocyte adhesion molecule-1 mediates antigen-induced acute airway inflammation and late-phase airway obstruction in monkeys. *J. Clin. Invest.* **88,** 1407–1411.

Han, K. T., Sharar, S. R., Phillips, M. L., Harlan, J. M., and Winn, R. K. (1995). Sialyl Lewis(x) oligosaccharide reduces ischemia-reperfusion injury in the rabbit ear. *J. Immunol.* **155,** 4011–4015.

Harning, R., Pelletier, J., Van, G., Takei, F., and Merluzzi, V. J. (1992). Monoclonal antibody to MALA-2 (ICAM-1) reduces acute autoimmune nephritis in kdkd mice. *Clin. Immunol. Immunopathol.* **64,** 129–34.

Hattori, R., Hamilton, K. K., Fugate, R. D., McEver, R. P., and Sims, P. J. (1989). Stimulated secretion of endothelial von Willebrand factor is accompanied by rapid redistribution to the cell surface of the intracellular granule membrane protein GMP-140. *J. Biol. Chem.* **264,** 7768–7771.

Haug, C. E., Colvin, R. B., Delmonico, F. L., Auchincloss, H., Jr., Tolkoff-Rubin, N., Preffer, F. I., Rothlein, R., Norris, S., Scharschmidt, L., and Cosimi, A. B. (1993). A phase I trial of immunosuppression with anti-ICAM-1 (CD54) mAb in renal allograft recipients. *Transplantation* **55,** 766–772.

Hernandez, L. A., Grisham, M. B., Twohig, B., Arfors, K.-E., Harlan, J. M., and Granger, D. N. (1987). Role of neutrophils in ischemia-reperfusion induced microvascular injury. *Am. J. Physiol.* **253,** H699–H703.

Hill, J., Lindsay, T., Rusche, J., Valeri, C. R., Shepro, D., and Hechtman, H. B. (1992). A Mac-1 antibody reduces liver and lung injury but not neutrophil sequestration after intestinal ischemia-reperfusion. *Surgery (St. Louis)* **112,** 166–172.

Horgan, M. J., Wright, S. D., and Malik, A. B. (1990). Antibody against leukocyte integrin (CD18) prevents reperfusion-induced lung vascular injury. *Am. J. Physiol.* **259,** L315–L319.

Horgan, M. J., Ge, M., Gu, J., Rothlein, R., and Malik, A. B. (1991). Role of ICAM-1 in neutrophil-mediated lung vascular injury after occlusion and reperfusion. *Am. J. Physiol.* **261,** H1578–H1584.

Huitinga, I., Damoiseaux, J. G., Dopp, E. A., and Dijkstra, C. D. (1993). Treatment with anti-CR3 antibodies ED7 and ED8 suppresses experimental allergic encephalomyelitis in Lewis rats. *Eur. J. Immunol.* **23,** 709–715.

Imhof, B. A., and Dunon, D. (1995). Leukocyte migration and adhesion. *Adv. Immunol.* **58,** 345–416.

Jaeschke, H., Farhood, A., and Smith, C. W. (1990). Neutrophils contribute to ischemia/reperfusion injury in rat liver in vivo. *FASEB J.* **4,** 3355–3359.

Jaeschke, H., Farhood, A., Bautista, A. P., Spolarics, Z., Spitzer, J. J., and Smith, C. W. (1993). Functional inactivation of neutrophils with a Mac-1 (CD11b/CD18) monoclonal antibody protects against ischemia-reperfusion injury in rat liver. *Hepatology* **17,** 915–923.

Jendrisak, M., Jendrisak, G., Gamero, J., and Mohanakumar, T. (1993). Prolongation in murine cardiac allograft survival with monoclonal antibodies to LFA-1, ICAM-1, and CD4. *Transplant. Proc.* **25,** 825–827.

Jerome, S. N., Smith, C. W., and Korthuis, R. J. (1993). CD18-dependent adherence reactions play an important role in the development of the no-reflow phenomenon. *Am. J. Physiol.* **264,** H479–H483.

Jerome, S. N., Dore̊, M., Paulson, J. C., Smith, C. W., and Korthuis, R. J. (1994). P-selectin and ICAM-1-dependent adherence reactions: Role in the genesis of postischemic no-reflow. *Am. J. Physiol.* **266,** H1316–H1321.

Johnson-Tidey, R. R., McGregor, J. L., Taylor, P. R., and Poston, R. N. (1994). Increase in the adhesion molecule P-selectin in endothelium overlying atherosclerotic plaques. Coexpression with intercellular adhesion molecule-1. *Am. J. Pathol.* **144,** 952–961.

Kameoka, H., Ishibashi, M., Tamatani, T., Takano, Y., Moutabarrik, A., Jiang, H., Kokado, Y., Takahara, S., Miyasaka, M., Okuyama, A., Kinoshita, T., and Sonoda, T. (1993). Comparative immunosuppressive effect of anti-CD18 and anti-CD11a monoclonal antibodies on rat heart allotransplantation. *Transplant. Proc.* **25,** 833–836.

Kavanaugh, A. F., Davis, L. S., Nichols, L. A., Norris, S. H., Rothlein, R., Scharschmidt, L. A., and Lipsky, P. E. (1994). Treatment of refractory rheumatoid arthritis with a monoclonal antibody to intercellular adhesion molecule-1. *Arthritis Rheum.* **37,** 992–999.

Kawasaki, K., Yaoita, E., Yamamoto, T., Tamatani, T., Miyasaka, M., and Kihara, I. (1993). Antibodies against intercellular adhesion molecule-1 and lymphocyte function-associated antigen-1 prevent glomerular injury in rat experimental crescentic glomerulonephritis. *J. Immunol.* **150,** 1074–1083.

Kelly, K. J., Williams, W. W., Jr., Colvin, R. B., and Bonventre, J. V. (1994). Antibody to intercellular adhesion molecule 1 protects the kidney against ischemic injury. *Proc. Natl. Acad. Sci. U. S. A.* **91,** 812–816.

Kling, D., Fingerle, J., and Harlan, J. M. (1992). Inhibition of leukocyte extravasation with a monoclonal antibody to CD18 during formation of experimental intimal thickening in rabbit carotid arteries. *Arterioscler. Thromb.* **12,** 997–1007.

Kling, D., Fingerle, J., Harlan, J. M., Lobb, R. R., and Lang, F. (1995). Mononuclear leukocytes invade rabbit arterial intima during thickening formation via CD18- and VLA-4-dependent mechanisms and stimulate smooth muscle migration. *Circ. Res.* **77,** 1121–1128.

Kobayashi, Y., Kawai, K., Honda, H., Tomida, S., Niimi, N., Tamatani, T., Miyasaka, M., and Yoshikai, Y. (1995). Antibodies against leukocyte function-associated antigen-1 and against intercellular adhesion molecule-1 together suppress the progression of experimental allergic encephalomyelitis. *Cell. Immunol.* **164,** 295–305.

Komori, A., Nagata, M., Ochiai, T., Nakajima, K., Hori, S., Asano, T., Isono, K., Tamatani, T., and Miyasaka, M. (1993). Role of ICAM-1 and LFA-1 in cardiac allograft rejection of the rat. *Transplant. Proc.* **25,** 831–832.

Langdale, L. A., Flaherty, L. C., Liggitt, H. D., Harlan, J. M., Rice, C. L., and Winn, R. K. (1993). Neutrophils contribute to hepatic ischemia-reperfusion injury by a CD18-independent mechanism. *J. Leukocyte Biol.* **53,** 511–517.

Lawrence, M. B., and Springer, T. A. (1991). Leukocytes roll on a selectin at physiologic flow rates: Distinction from and prerequisite for adhesion through integrins. *Cell (Cambridge, Mass.)* **65,** 859–873.

Lee, W. P., Gribling, P., De Guzman, L., Ehsani, N., and Watson, S. R. (1995). A P-selectin-immunoglobulin G chimera is protective in a rabbit ear model of ischemia-reperfusion. *Surgery (St. Louis)* **117,** 458–465.

Lefer, D. J., Shandelya, S. M., Serrano, C. V., Jr., Becker, L. C., Kuppusamy, P., and Zweier, J. L. (1993). Cardioprotective actions of a monoclonal antibody against CD-18 in myocardial iscehmia-reperfusion injury. *Circulation* **88,** 1779–1787.

Lefer, D. J., Flynn, D. M., Phillips, M. L., Ratcliffe, M., and Buda, A. J. (1994). A novel sialyl LewisX analog attenuates neutrophil accumulation and myocardial necrosis after ischemia and reperfusion. *Circulation* **90,** 2390–2401.

Lewinsohn, D., Bargatze, R., and Butcher, E. (1987). Leukocyte-endothelial cell recognition: Evidence of a common molecular mechanism shared by neutrophils, lymphocytes, and other leukocytes. *J. Immunol.* **138,** 4313–4321.

Li, H., Cybulsky, M. I., Gimbrone, M. A., Jr., and Libby, P. (1993a). An atherogenic diet rapidly induces VCAM-1, a cytokine-regulatable mononuclear leukocyte adhesion molecule, in rabbit aortic endoethlium. *Arterioscler. Thromb.* **13,** 197–204.

Li, H., Cybulsky, M. I., Gimbrone, M. A., Jr., and Libby, P. (1993b). Inducible expression of vascular cell adhesion molecule-1 by vascular smooth muscle cells in vitro and within rabbit atheroma. *Am. J. Pathol.* **143,** 1551–1559.

Lo, S. K., Everitt, J., Gu, J., and Malik, A. B. (1992). Tumor necrosis factor mediated experimental pulmonary edema by ICAM-1 and CD18-dependent mechanism. *J. Clin. Invest.* **89,** 981–988.

Lo, S. K., Bevilacqua, B., and Malik, A. B. (1994). E-selectin ligands mediate tumor necrosis factor-induced neutrophil sequestration and pulmonary edema in guinea pig lungs. *Circ. Res.* **75,** 955–960.

Ma, X. L., Tsao, P. S., and Lefer, A. M. (1991). Antibody to CD18 exerts endoethelial and cardiac protective effects inmyocardial ischemia and reperfusion. *J. Clin. Invest.* **88,** 1237–1243.

Ma, X. L., Lefer, D. J., Lefer, A. M., and Rothlein, R. (1992). Coronary endothelial and cardiac protective effects of a monoclonal antibody to intercellular adhesion molecule-1 in myocardial ischemia and reperfusion. *Circulation* **86,** 937–946.

Ma, X. L., Weyrich, A. S., Lefer, D. J., Buerke, M., Albertine, K. H., Kishimoto, T. K., and Lefer, A. M. (1993). Monoclonal antibody to L-selectin attenuates neutrophil accumulation and protects ischemic reperfused cat myocardium. *Circulation* **88,** 649–658.

Martens, C. L., Cwirla, S. E., Lee, R. Y., Whitehorn, E., Chen, E. Y., Bakker, A., Martin, E. L., Wagström, C., Gopalan, P., Smith, C. W., Tate, E., Koller, K. J., Schatz, P. J., Dower, W. J., and Barrett, R. W. (1995). Peptides which bind to E-selectin and block neutrophil adhesion. *J. Biol. Chem.* **270,** 21129–21136.

Matsuo, Y., Onodera, H., Shiga, Y., Shozuhara, H., Ninomiya, M., Kihara, T., Tamatani, T., Miyasaka, M., and Kogure, K. (1994). Role of cell adhesion molecules in brain injury after transient middle cerebral artery occlusion in the rat. *Brain Res.* **656,** 344–352.

McEver, R. P., Beckstead, J. H., Moore, K. L., Marshall, C. L., and Bainton, D. F. (1989). GMP-140, a platelet alpha-granule membrane protein, is also synthesized by vascular endothelial cells and is localized in Weibel-Palade bodies. *J. Clin. Invest.* **84,** 92–99.

Mihelcic, D., Schleiffenbaum, B., Tedder, T. F., Sharar, S. R., Harlan, J. M., and Winn, R. K. (1994). Inhibition of leukocyte L-selectin function with a monoclonal antibody attenuates reperfusion injury to the rabbit ear. *Blood* **84,** 2322–2328.

Mileski, W. J., Winn, R. K., Vedder, N. V., Pohlman, T. H., Harlan, J. M., and Rice, C. L. (1990a). Inhibition of CD18-dependent neutrophil adherence reduces organ injury after hemorrhagic shock in primates. *Surgery (St. Louis)* **108,** 205–212.

Mileski, W., Harlan, J., Rice, C., and Winn, R. (1990b). Streptococcus pneumoniae-stimulated macrophages induce neutrophils to emigrate by a CD18-independent mechanism of adherence. *Circ. Shock* **31,** 259–267.

Mileski, W. J., Winn, R. K., Harlan, J. M., and Rice, C. L. (1991). Transient inhibition of neutrophil adherence with the anti-CD18 monoclonal antibody 60.3 does not increase mortality rates in abdominal sepsis. *Surgery (St. Louis)* **109,** 497–501.

Mileski, W., Borgström, D., Lightfoot, E., Rothlein, R., Faanes, R., Lipsky, P., and Baxter, C. (1992). Inhibition of leukocyte-endothelial adherence following thermal injury. *J. Surg. Res.* **52,** 334–339.

Mileski, W. J., Sikes, P., Atiles, L., Lightfoot, E., Lipsky, P., and Baxter, C. (1993). Inhibition of leukocyte adherence and susceptibility to infection. *J. Surg. Res.* **54,** 349–354.

Mileski, W. J., Rothlien, R., and Lipsky, P. (1994). Interference with the function of leukocyte adhesion molecules by monoclonal antibodies: A new approach to burn injury. *Eur. J. Pediatr. Surg.* **4,** 225–230.

Milne, A. A., and Piper, P. J. (1994). The effects of two anti-CD18 antibodies on antigen-induced airway hyperresponsiveness and leukocyte accumulation in the guinea pig. *Am. J. Respir. Cell Mol. Biol.* **11,** 337–343.

Molina, A., Sánchez-Madrid, F., Bricio, T., Martín, A., Barat, A., Alvarez, V., and Mampaso, F. (1994). Prevention of mercuric chloride-induced nephritis in the brown Norway rat by treatment with antibodies against the alpha 4 integrin. *J. Immunol.* **153,** 2313–2320.

Molossi, S., Elices, M., Arrhenius, T., Diaz, R., Coulber, C., and Rabinovitch, M. (1995). Blockade of very late antigen-4 integrin binding to fibronectin with connecting segment-1 peptide reduces accelerated coronary arteriopathy in rabbit cardiac allografts. *J. Clin. Invest.* **95,** 2601–2610.

Moore, T. M., Khimenko, P., Adkins, W. K., Miyasaka, M., and Taylor, A. E. (1995). Adhesion molecules contribute to ischemia and reperfusion-induced injury in the isolated rat lung. *J. Appl. Physiol.* **78,** 2245–2252.

Moyle, M., Foster, D. L., McGrath, D. E., Brown, S. M., Laroche, Y., De Meutter, J., Stanssens, P., Bogowitz, C. A., Fried, V. A., Ely, J. A., Soule, H. R., and Vlasuk, G. P. (1994). A hookworm glycoprotein that inhibits neutrophil function is a ligand of the integrin CD11b/CD18. *J. Biol. Chem.* **269,** 10008–10015.

Muchowski, P. J., Zhang, L., Chang, E. R., Soule, H. R., Plow, E. F., and Moyle, M. (1994). Functional interaction between the integrin antagonist neutrophil inhibitory factor and the I domain of CD11b/CD18. *J. Biol. Chem.* **269,** 26419–26423.

Muller, W. A., Weigl, S. A., Deng, X., and Phillips, D. M. (1993). PECAM-1 is required for transendothelial migration of leukocytes. *J. Exp. Med.* **178,** 449–460.

Mulligan, M. S., Varani, J., Dame, M. K., Lane, C. L., Smith, C. W., Anderson, D. C., and Ward, P. A. (1991). Role of endothelial-leukocyte adhesion molecule 1 (ELAM-1) in neutrophil-mediated lung injury in rats. *J. Clin. Invest.* **88,** 1396–1406.

Mulligan, M. S., Varani, J., Warren, J. S., Till, G. O., Smith, C. W., Anderson, D. C., Todd, R. F. I., and Ward, P. A. (1992a). Roles of beta-2 integrins of rat neutrophils in complement- and oxygen radical-mediated acute inflammatory injury. *J. Immunol.* **148,** 1847–1857.

Mulligan, M. S., Polley, M. J., Bayer, R. J., Nunn, M. F., Paulson, J. C., and Ward, P. A. (1992b). Neutrophil-dependent acute lung injury. Requirement for P-selectin (GMP-140). *J. Clin. Invest.* **90,** 1600–1607.

Mulligan, M. S., Warren, J. S., Smith, C. W., Anderson, D. C., Yeh, C. G., Rudolph, A. R., and Ward, P. A. (1992c). Lung injury after depositing of IgA immune complexes. *J. Immunol.* **148,** 3086–3092.

Mulligan, M. S., Wilson, G. P., Todd, R. F., III, Smith, C. W., Anderson, D. C., Varani, J., Issekutz, T. B., Miyasaka, M., Tamatani, T., and Miyasaka, M. (1993a). Role of beta 1, beta 2 integrins and ICAM-1 in lung injury after deposition of IgG and IgA immune complexes. *J. Immunol.* **150,** 2407–2417.

Mulligan, M. S., Watson, S. R., Fennie, C., and Ward, P. A. (1993b). Protective effects of selectin chimeras in neutrophil-mediated lung injury. *J. Immunol.* **151,** 6410–6417.

Mulligan, M. S., Till, G. O., Smith, C. W., Anderson, D. C., Miyasaka, M., Tamatani, T., Todd, R. F., III, Issekutz, T. B., and Ward, P. A. (1994a). Role of leukocyte adhesion molecules in lung and dermal vascular injury after thermal trauma of skin. *Am. J. Pathol.* **144,** 1008–1015.

Mulligan, M. S., Miyasaka, M., Tamatani, T., Jones, M. L., and Ward, P. A. (1994b). Requirements for L-selectin in neutrophil-mediated lung injury in rats. *J. Immunol.* **152,** 832–840.

Mulligan, M. S., Vaporciyan, A. A., Warner, R. L., Jones, M. L., Foreman, K. E., Miyasaka, M., Todd, R. F., III, and Ward, P. A. (1995). Compartmentalized roles for leukocytic adhesion molecules in lung inflammatory injury. *J. Immunol.* **154,** 1350–1363.

Nakajima, H., Sano, H., Nishimura, T., Yoshida, S., and Iwamoto, I. (1994). Role of vascular cell adhesion molecule 1/very late activation antigen 4 and intercellular adhesion molecule 1/lymphocyte function-associated antigen 1 interactions in antigen-induced eosinophil and T cell recruitment into the tissue. *J. Exp. Med.* **179,** 1145–1154.

Newman, P. M., To, S. S., Robinson, B. G., Hyland, V. J., and Schrieber, L. (1994). Effect of gold sodium thiomalate and its thiomalate component on the in vitro expression of endothelial cell adhesion molecules. *J. Clin. Invest.* **94,** 1864–1871.

Nishikawa, K., Guo, Y. J., Miyasaka, M., Tamatani, T., Collins, A. B., Sy, M. S., McCluskey, R. T., and Andres, G. (1993). Antibodies to intercellular adhesion molecule 1/lymphocyte function-associated antigen 1 prevent crescent formation in rat autoimmune glomerulonephritis. *J. Exp. Med.* **177,** 667–677.

Nolte, D., Hecht, R., Schmid, P., Botzlar, A., Menger, M. D., Neumueller, C., Sinowatz, F., Vestweber, D., and Messmer, K. (1994). Role of Mac-1 and ICAM-1 in ischemia-reperfusion injury in a microcirculation model of BALB/C mice. *Am. J. Physiol.* **267,** H1320–H1328.

Noonan, T. C., Gundel, R. H., Desai, S. N., Stearns, C., Barton, R. W., Rothlein, R., Letts, L. G., and Piper, P. J. (1991). The effects of an anti-CD18 antibody (R15.7) in antigen-induced airway hyperresponsiveness (AH) and cell influx in guinea pigs. *Agents Actions* **34,** 211–213.

O'Brien, K. D., Allen, M. D., McDonald, T. O., Chait, A., Harlan, J. M., Fishbein, D., McCarty, J., Ferguson, M., Hudkins, K., Benjamin, C. D., Lobb, R., and Alpers, C. E. (1993). Vascular cell adhesion molecule-1 is expressed in human coronary atherosclerotic plaques. Implications for the mode of progression of advanced coronary atherosclerosis. *J. Clin. Invest.* **92,** 945–951.

Petrasek, P. F., Liauw, S., Romaschin, A. D., and Walker, P. M. (1994). Salvage of postischemic skeletal muscle by monoclonal antibody blockade of neutrophil adhesion molecule CD18. *J. Surg. Res.* **56,** 5–12.

Phillips, M. L., Nudelman, E., Gaeta, F. C., Perez, M., Singhal, A. K., Hakomori, S., and Paulson, J. C. (1990). ELAM-1 mediates cell adhesion by recognition of a carbohydrate ligand, sialyl-Lex. *Science* **250,** 1130–1132.

Pober, J. S., Gimbrone, M. A., Jr., Lapierre, L. A., Mendrick, D. L., Fiers, W., Rothlein, R., and Springer, T. A. (1986). Overlapping patterns of activation of human endothelial cells by interleukin 1, tumor necrosis factor, and immune interferon. *J. Immunol.* **137,** 1893–1896.

Podolsky, D. K., Lobb, R., King, N., Benjamin, C. D., Pepinsky, B., Sehgal, P., and deBeaumont, M. (1993). Attenuation of colitis in the cotton-top tamarin by anti-alpha 4 integrin monoclonal antibody. *J. Clin. Invest.* **92,** 372–380.

Poston, R. N., Haskard, D. O., Coucher, J. R., Gall, N. P., and Johnson-Tidey, R. R. (1992). Expression of intercellular adhesion molecule-1 in atherosclerotic plaques. *Am. J. Pathol.* **140,** 665–673.

Pou, S., Gunther, M. R., Pou, W. S., Cao, G. L., Bator, J. M., Cohen, M. S., Burch, R. M., and Rosen, G. M. (1993). Effect of NPC 15669, an inhibitor of neutrophil recruitment and neutrophil-mediated inflammation, on neutrophil function in vitro. *Biochem. Pharmacol.* **45,** 2123–2127.

Pretolani, M., Ruffié, C., Lapa-e-Silva, J. R., Joseph, D., Lobb, R. R., and Vargaftig, B. B. (1994). Antibody to very late activation antigen 4 prevents antigen-induced bronchial hyperreactivity and cellular infiltration in the guinea pig airways. *J. Exp. Med.* **180,** 795–805.

Read, M. A., Neish, A. S., Luscinskas, F. W., Palombella, V. J., Maniatis, T., and Collins, T. (1995). The proteasome pathway is required for cytokine-induced endothelial-leukocyte adhesion molecule expression. *Immunity* **2,** 493–506.

Romson, J. L., Hook, B. G., Kunkel, S. L., Abrams, G. D., Schork, A., and Lucchesi, B. R. (1983). Reduction of the extent of ischemic myocardial injury by neutrophil depletion in the dog. *Circulation* **67,** 1016–1023.

Rosen, H., Gordon, S., and North, R. J. (1989). Exacerbation of murine listeriosis by a monoclonal antibody specific for the type 3 complement receptor of myelomonocytic cells. Absence of monocytes at infective foci allows Listeria to multiply in nonphagocytic cells. *J. Exp. Med.* **170,** 27–37.

Ross, R. (1993). Rous-Whipple Award Lecture. Atherosclerosis: A defense mechanism gone awry. *Am. J. Pathol.* **143,** 987–1002.

Sako, D., Chang, X. J., Barone, K. M., Vachino, G., White, H. M., Shaw, G., Veldman, G. M., Bean, K. M., Ahern, T. J., Furie, B., Cummings, D. E., and Larsen, G. R. (1993). Expression cloning of a functional glycoprotein ligand for P-selectin. *Cell (Cambridge, Mass.)* **75,** 1179–1186.

Sandros, J., Rozdzinski, E., and Tuomanen, E. (1994). Peptides from pertussis toxin interfere with neutrophil adherence in vitro and counteract inflammation in vivo. *Microb. Pathog.* **16,** 213–220.

Schoenberg, M. H., Poch, B., Younes, M., Schwarz, A., Baczako, K., Lundberg, C., Haglund, U., and Beger, H. G. (1991). Involvement of neutrophils in postischaemic damage to the small intestine. *Gut* **32,** 905–912.

Seekamp, A., Mulligan, M. S., Till, G. O., Smith, C. W., Miyasaka, M., Tamatani, T., Todd, R. F., III, and Ward, P. A. (1993). Role of beta 2 integrins and ICAM-1 in lung injury following ischemia-reperfusion of rat hind limbs. *Am. J. Pathol.* **143,** 464–472.

Seekamp, A., Till, G. O., Mulligan, M. S., Paulson, J. C., Anderson, D. C., Miyasaka, M., and Ward, P. A. (1994). Role of selectins in local and remote tissue injury following ischemia and reperfusion. *Am. J. Pathol.* **144,** 592–598.

Sharar, S., Winn, R., Murry, C., Harlan, J., and Rice, C. (1991). A CD18 monoclonal antibody increases the incidence and severity of subcutaneous abscess formation after high-dose *Staphylococcus aureus* injection in rabbits. *Surgery (St. Louis)* **110,** 213–220.

Sharar, S. R., Sasaki, S. S., Flaherty, L. C., Paulson, J. C., Harlan, J. M., and Winn, R. K. (1993). P-selectin blockade does not impair leukocyte host defense against bacterial peritonitis and soft tissue infection in rabbits. *J. Immunol.* **151,** 4982–4988.

Sharar, S. R., Mihelcic, D. D., Han, K. T., Harlan, J. M., and Winn, R. K. (1994). Ischemia-reperfusion injury in the rabbit ear is reduced by both immediate and delayed CD18 leukocyte adherence blockade. *J. Immunol.* **153,** 2234–2238.

Simpson, P. J., Todd, R. F., III, Fantone, J. C., Mickelson, J. K., Griffin, J. D., and Lucchesi, B. R. (1988). Reduction of experimental canine myocardial reperfusion injury by a monoclonal antibody (Anti-Mo-1, Anti-CD11b) that inhibits leukocyte adhesion. *J. Clin. Invest.* **81**, 624–629.

Simpson, P. J., Todd, R. F., III, Mickelson, J. K., Fantone, J. C., Gallagher, K. P., Lee, K. A., Tamura, Y., Cronin, M., and Lucchesi, B. R. (1990). Sustained limitation of myocardial reperfusion injury by a monoclonal antibody that alters leukocyte function. *Circulation* **81**, 226–237.

Smith, S. M., Holm-Rutili, L., Perry, M. A., Grisham, M. B., Arfors, K.-E., Granger, D. N., and Kvietys, P. R. (1987). Role of neutrophils in hemorrhagic shock-induced gastric mucosal injury in the rat. *Gastroenterology* **93**, 466–471.

Springer, T. A. (1994). Traffic signals for lymphocyte recirculation and leukocyte emigration: The multistep paradigm. *Cell (Cambridge, Mass.)* **76**, 301–314.

Steegmaier, M., Levinovitz, A., Isenmann, S., Borges, E., Lenter, M., Kocher, H. P., Kleuser, B., and Vestweber, D. (1995). The E-selectin-ligand ESL-1 is a variant of a receptor for fibroblast growth factor. *Nature (London)* **373**, 615–620.

Suzuki, S., and Toledo-Pereyra, L. H. (1993). Monoclonal antibody to intercellular adhesion molecule 1 as an effective protection for liver ischemia and reperfusion injury. *Transplant. Proc.* **25**, 3325–3327.

Tedder, T. F., Steeber, D. A., Chen, A., and Engel, P. (1995). The selectins: Vascular adhesion molecules. *Faseb J.* **9**, 866–873.

Thomas, J. R., Harlan, J. M., Rice, C. L., and Winn, R. K. (1992). Role of leukocyte CD11/CD18 complex in endotoxic and septic shock in rabbits. *J. Appl. Physiol.* **73**, 1510–1516.

Thornton, M. A., Winn, R., Alpers, C. E., and Zager, R. A. (1989). An evaluation of the neutrophil as a mediator of in vivo renal ischemic-reperfusion injury. *Am. J. Pathol.* **135**, 509–515.

Tipping, P. G., Huang, X. R., Berndt, M. C., and Holdsworth, S. R. (1994a). A role for P selectin in complement-independent neutrophil-mediated glomerular injury. *Kidney Int.* **46**, 79–88.

Tipping, P. G., Cornthwaite, L. J., and Holdsworth, S. R. (1994b). Beta 2 integrin independent neutrophil recruitment and injury in anti-GBM glomerulonephritis in rabbits. *Immunol. Cell Biol.* **72**, 471–479.

Tuomanem E. I., Saukkonen, K., Sande, S., Cioffe, and C., and Wright, S. D. (1989). Reduction of inflammation, tissue damage, and mortality in bacterial meningitis in rabbits treated with monoclonal antibodies against adhesion-promoting receptors of leukocytes. *J. Exp. Med.* **170**, 959–968.

van der Wal, A. C., Das, P. K., Tigges, A. J., and Becker, A. E. (1992). Adhesion molecules on the endothelium and mononuclear cells in human atherosclerotic lesions. *Am. J. Pathol.* **141**, 1427–1433.

Vaporciyan, A. A., DeLisser, H. M., Yan, H. C., Mendiguren, I. I., Thom, S. R., Jones, M. L., Ward, P. A., and Albelda, S. M. (1993). Involvement of platelet-endothelial cell adhesion molecule-1 in neutrophil recruitment in vivo. *Science* **262**, 1580–1582.

Vedder, N. B., Winn, R. K., Rice, C. L., Chi, E., Arfors, K.-E., and Harlan, J. M. (1988). A monoclonal antibody to the adherence promoting leukocyte glycoprotein CD18 reduces organ injury and improves survival from hemorrhagic shock and resuscitation in rabbits. *J. Clin. Invest.* **81**, 939–944.

Vedder, N. B., Fouty, B. W., Winn, R. K., Harlan, J. M., and Rice, C. L. (1989). Role of neutrophils in generalized reperfusion injury associated with resuscitation from shock. *Surgery (St. Louis)* **106**, 509–516.

Vedder, N. B., Winn, R. K., Rice, C. L., Chi, E., Arfors, K.-E., and Harlan, J. M. (1990). Inhibition of leukocyte adherence by anti-CD18 monoclonal antibody attenuates reperfusion injury in the rabbit ear. *Proc. Natl. Acad. Sci. U. S. A.* **81**, 939–944.

Von-Andrian, U. H., Chambers, J. D., McEvoy, L. M., Bargatze, R. F., Arfors, K. E., and Butcher, E. C. (1991). Two-step model of leukocyte-endothelial cell interaction in inflammation: Distinct roles for LECAM-1 and the leukocyte beta 2 integrins in vivo. *Proc. Natl. Acad. Sci. U. S. A.* **88,** 7538–7542.

Wallace, J. L., Higa, A., McKnight, G. W., and MacIntyre, D. E. (1992). Prevention and reversal of experimental colitis by a monoclonal antibody which inhibits leukocyte adherence. *Inflammation* **16,** 343–354.

Walz, G., Aruffo, A., Kolanus, W., Bevilacqua, M., and Seed, B. (1990). Recognition by ELAM-1 of the sialyl-Lex determinant on myeloid and tumor cells. *Science* **250,** 1132–1135.

Watson, S. R., Fennie, C., and Lasky, L. A. (1991). Neutrophil influx into an inflammatory site inhibited by a soluble homing receptor-IgG chimaera. *Nature* (*London*) **349,** 164–167.

Wegner, C. D., Gundel, R. H., Reoly, P., Haynes, N., Letts, L. G., and Rothlein, R. (1990). Intercellular adhesion molecule-1 (ICAM-1) in the pathogenesis of asthma. *Science* **247,** 456–459.

Weselcouch, E. O., Grove, R. I., Demusz, C. D., and Baird, A. J. (1991). Effect of in vivo inhibition of neutrophil adherence adherence on skeletal muscle function during ischemia in ferrets. *Am. J. Physiol.* **261,** H1178–H1183.

Weyrich, A. S., Ma, S.-L., and Lefer, A. M. (1992). Protective effects of a P-selectin monoclonal antibody in myocardial ischemia and reperfusion. *Circulation* **86,** I80.

Willenborg, D. O., Simmons, R. D., Tamatani, T., and Miyasaka, M. (1993). ICAM-1-dependent pathway is not critically involved in the inflammatory process of autoimmune encephalomyelitis or in cytokine-induced inflammation of the central nervous system. *J. Neuroimmunol.* **45,** 147–154.

Winn, R. K., Liggitt, D., Vedder, N. B., Paulson, J. C., and Harlan, J. M. (1993). Anti-P-selectin monoclonal antibody attenuates reperfusion injury to the rabbit ear. *J. Clin. Invest.* **92,** 2042–2047.

Winn, R. K., Paulson, J. C., and Harlan, J. M. (1994). A monoclonal antibody to P-selectin ameliorates injury associated with hemorrhagic shock in rabbits. *Am. J. Physiol.* **267,** H2391–H2397.

Wong, P. Y., Yue, G., Yin, K., Miyasaka, M., Lane, C. L., Manning, A. M., Anderson, D. C., and Sun, F. F. (1995). Antibodies to intercellular adhesion molecule-1 ameliorate the inflammatory response in acetic acid-induced inflammatory bowel disease. *J. Pharmacol. Exp. Ther.* **274,** 475–480.

Wu, X., Pippin, J., and Lefkowith, J. B. (1993). Attenuation of immune-mediated glomerulonephritis with an anti-CD11b monoclonal antibody. *Am. J. Physiol.* **264,** F715–F7121.

Yamataka, T., Kobayashi, H., Yagita, H., Okumura, K., Tamatani, T., and Miyasaka, M. (1993). The effect of anti-ICAM-1 monoclonal antibody treatment on the transplantation of the small bowel in rats. *J. Pediatr. Surg.* **28,** 1451–1457.

Yamazaki, T., Seko, Y., Tamatani, T., Miyasaka, M., Yagita, H., Ikumura, K., Nagai, R., and Yazaki, T. (1993). Expression of intercellular adhesion molecule-1 in rat heart with ischemia/reperfusion and limitation of infarct size by treatment with antibodies against cell adhesion molecules. *Am. J. Pathol.* **143,** 410–418.

Yednock, T. A., Cannon, C., Fritz, L. C., Sánchez-Madrid, F., Steinman, L., and Karin, N. (1992). Prevention of experimental autoimmune encephalomyelitis by antibodies against alpha 4 beta 1 integrin. *Nature* (*London*) **356,** 63–66.

Zeng, Y., Gage, A., Montag, A., Rothlein, R., Thistlethwaite, J. R., and Bluestone, J. A. (1994). Inhibition of transplant rejection by pretreatment of xenogeneic pancreatic islet cells with anti-ICAM-1 antibodies. *Transplantation* **58,** 681–689.

Zimmerman, B. J., Paulson, J. C., Arrhenius, T. S., Gaeta, F. C., and Granger, D. N. (1994). Thrombin receptor peptide-mediated leukocyte rolling in rat mesenteric venules: Roles of P-selectin and sialyl Lewis X. *Am. J. Physiol.* **267,** H1049–H1053.

Carol A. Kauffman*
Peggy L. Carver†

*Division of Infectious Diseases
Department of Internal Medicine
Department of Veterans Affairs Medical Center
University of Michigan Medical School
Ann Arbor, Michigan 48105

†College of Pharmacy
University of Michigan
Ann Arbor, Michigan 48109-1065

Use of Azoles for Systemic Antifungal Therapy

I. Introduction

The introduction of the azole antifungal agents has rapidly expanded the armamentarium of agents useful in the treatment of systemic fungal infections. Clotrimazole, an early imidazole antifungal, proved inadequate for the treatment of systemic infections as it was found to rapidly induce its own metabolism after oral or intravenous administration. Its use is now confined to topical therapy. Miconazole has been used in a limited fashion because of its toxicity and availability only as an intravenous formulation. Ketoconazole was the first oral imidazole to be developed. It has a broad spectrum of activity and has proved useful for a wide variety of fungal infections. N-substitution of imidazoles resulted in the triazole antifungal agents, itraconazole and fluconazole. These agents have the same mechanism of action and spectrum of activity as the imidazoles, but they appear to

Advances in Pharmacology, Volume 39

1054-3589/97/$25.00

interact much less with human cytochromes P450 and, consequently, have less effect on human sterol metabolism. This review focuses on the use of these four azole agents that have proved beneficial in treating systemic fungal infections.

II. Chemistry

The imidazole compounds contain a five-membered azole ring with two nitrogen atoms. The triazoles have a third nitrogen atom added (Fig. 1). The triazole ring increases tissue penetration, prolongs half-life, and enhances efficacy of the azoles while decreasing the toxicity when compared with imidazole antifungal agents (Fromtling, 1988).

III. Mechanism of Action

The mechanism of action of all azole antifungal agents appears to be similar. Azoles inhibit the biosynthesis of ergosterol, an essential component

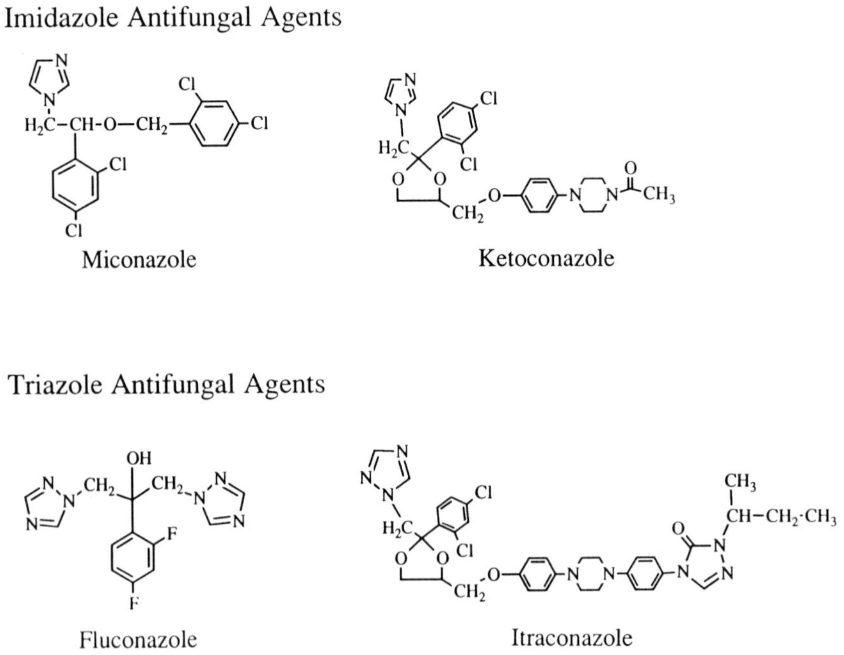

Imidazole Antifungal Agents

Miconazole

Ketoconazole

Triazole Antifungal Agents

Fluconazole

Itraconazole

FIGURE 1 Structures of azole antifungal agents. The imidazole compounds contain a five-membered azole ring with two nitrogen atoms. The triazoles have a third nitrogen atom added. The triazole ring increases tissue penetration, prolongs half-life, and enhances efficacy of the azoles while decreasing the toxicity when compared with imidazole antifungal agents.

of fungal cell membranes, via inhibition of the cytochromes P450-dependent enzyme lanosterol 14-α-demethylase (Fig. 2). Lanosterol 14-α-demethylase is necessary for the conversion of lanosterol to ergosterol. Depletion of ergosterol in the fungal cell membrane results in altered membrane fluidity, thereby reducing the activity of membrane-associated enzymes. This leads to increased permeability and subsequent inhibition of cell growth and replication (Como and Dismukes, 1994). In addition, azoles may exhibit other direct effects on cell membrane fatty acids and oxidative enzyme systems and appear to inhibit the formation of pseudohyphae in *Candida* species (Uno *et al.,* 1982).

The relative binding efficiency of azole antifungal agents to cytochromes P450 differs, resulting in differences in antifungal activity, toxicity of the agents, and the relative likelihood of drug interactions with other cytochrome P450-metabolized drugs (Vanden Bossche, 1987). Cytochromes P450, ubiquitous heme-containing proteins found throughout the plant and animal kingdom, act as terminal mono-oxygenases in an electron transport chain mediated via NADPH reductase. The major role of cytochromes P450 is to insert oxygen via electrophilic attack of lipophilic substrates (Groves and Gross, 1995) (Fig. 3).

The binding of lipophilic azoles to cytochromes P450 is very tight and can be stoichiometric. However, the use of classic binding plots to characterize the relative affinities of azoles for cytochromes P450 can be misleading. Several different methods have been utilized to measure the binding of azoles to cyto-

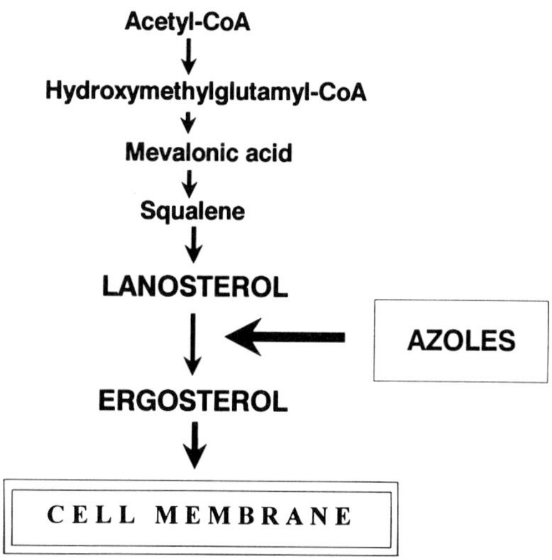

FIGURE 2 Mechanism of action of azole antifungal agents. Azoles inhibit the biosynthesis of ergosterol, an essential component of fungal cell membranes, via inhibition of the cytochrome P450-dependent enzyme lanosterol 14-α-demethylase, which is necessary for the conversion of lanosterol to ergosterol.

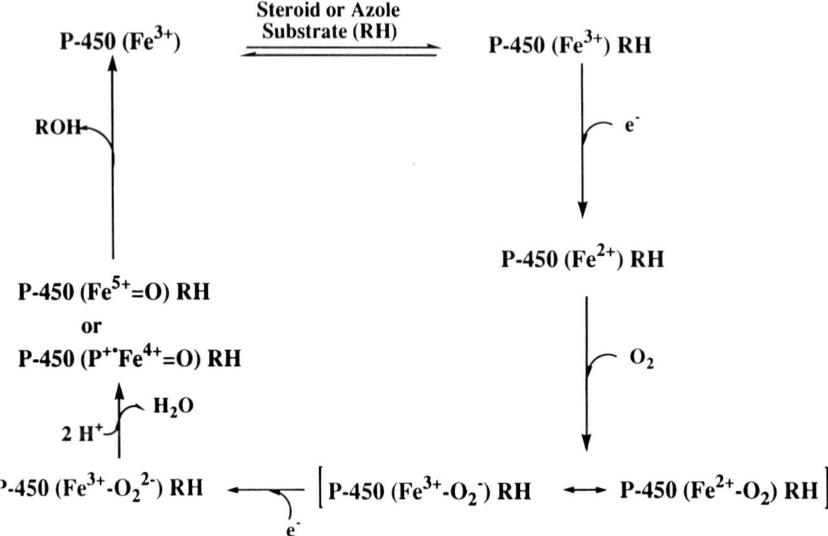

FIGURE 3 The catalytic cycle for cytochromes P450 as adapted from Groves and Gross (1995). The first step is binding of substrate to the ferric form (Fe^{3+}) of the enzyme allowing reduction to the ferrous form (Fe^{2+}). Dioxygen binds to form a complex that may be described either as an [Fe^{2+} dioxygen species] or as an [Fe^{3+} superoxide species]. Further reduction of the enzyme generates an Fe^{3+} peroxide species that subsequently releases water and forms the activated catalyst. This catalyst can be described as either an $Fe^{5+} = O$ or, probably more correctly, an $P^{+\cdot}$ $Fe^{4+} = O$ (where $P^{+\cdot}$ is an oxidized porphyrin radical). Oxidation of the substrate gives ROH, regenerating the resting form of the enzyme.

chromes P450. Schenkman *et al.* (1967) described the characteristic "type II" difference spectrum which indicates the formation of an inhibitory ligand complex between the "lone pair" nitrogen of the azole moiety and the heme component of the enzyme, and conversion of the enzyme to a low spin or deactivated form. Several investigators have attempted to quantify apparent binding affinity constants of azoles by titration of azole drug concentrations against the size of their difference spectra. However, differences in binding affinities to different hepatic cytochromes P450 have resulted in nonlinear plots, and some binding curves are curvilinear, suggesting the presence of more than one binding site on the enzyme. At low drug concentrations, all of the drug may be bound to the enzyme so that an equilibrium between bound and unbound drug may not exist, invalidating an inherent assumption in binding analysis plots. Investigators have utilized a competition assay that compares the rates of formation of a characteristic carbon monoxide–cytochromes P450 complex to measure azole binding affinity. For example, itraconazole appears to delay binding of carbon monoxide to fungal cytochromes P450 significantly longer than does ketoconazole, indicating a higher affinity of itraconazole for the fungal protein, consistent with the differences in their relative antifungal potency. Although the optimal determinants of the relative affinities of azoles for different cytochromes P450 remain unknown, studies suggest that the relative field strength of the lone pair nitrogen in the heterocycle, the overall lipophilicity of the molecule, and the relative steric hindrance around the liganding nitrogen are important determinants (Tarbit *et al.*, 1990).

IV. Spectrum of Antifungal Activity

All of the azoles have a wide spectrum of *in vitro* antifungal activity that generally includes dermatophytes; yeast-like opportunists, such as *Candida* and *Cryptococcus;* various filamentous fungi; and the dimorphic fungi, including *Histoplasma capsulatum, Blastomyces dermatitidis,* and *Coccidioides immitis* (Shadomy *et al.*, 1977, 1985; Heel *et al.*, 1982; Dixon *et al.*, 1978; Rogers and Galgiani, 1986). None of the azoles has activity against the *Mucorales* (*Rhizopus, Mucor,* etc.) (Eng *et al.*, 1981). Itraconazole, but not the other azoles, has activity against *Aspergillus* species and *Sporothrix schenckii* (Espinel-Ingroff *et al.*, 1984; Odds *et al.*, 1984). Dematiaceous fungi, such as *Exophiala, Phialophora,* and *Wangiella,* are inhibited to a variable extent by the different azoles. There are several clinically important fungi that are resistant to fluconazole. These include several yeast species that are innately resistant, such as *Candida krusei* (Wingard *et al.*, 1991), and others relatively resistant, such as C. *glabrata* (Wingard *et al.*, 1993; Tiballi *et al.*, 1995; Rex *et al.*, 1995).

V. Use of Specific Azole Antifungal Agents

A. Miconazole

1. Overview

Intravenous miconazole was released for use in the United States in 1978. Although miconazole is active against many fungi, its use has been limited, primarily because of toxicity associated with intravenous administration. Intravenous miconazole is now a drug of mostly historical interest; there are very few indications for its use. However, local formulations of miconazole (creams, powders, vaginal suppositories) are widely used for the treatment of dermatophyte infections, intertrigenous candidiasis, and vaginitis.

2. Pharmacology

Miconazole is poorly absorbed from the gastrointestinal tract (Table I). Peak serum concentrations are achieved 4 hr after oral administration (Brugmans *et al.*, 1972). Following oral administration of 200-mg and 1-g

TABLE I Pharmacology of Azole Antifungal Agents[a]

Feature	*Miconazole*	*Ketoconazole*	*Itraconazole*	*Fluconazole*
Molecular weight	416	531	706	306
Water solubility	Poor	Poor	Poor	Excellent
Protein binding (%)	High	High	High	Low
	90	99	99.8	12
Cerebrospinal fluid (CSF) penetration	Poor	Poor	Poor	Excellent
(CSF/serum)	(<10%)	(<10%)	(<10%)	(>80%)
Affinity for mammalian cytochrome P450	High	High	Low	Low
Elimination half-life (hr)	20	8	21–64	30
Excretion in urine (%)	<5	<5	<1	80
Reduction of dose in renal failure	Not necessary	Not necessary	Not necessary	>50 ml/min: no reduction 20–50 ml/min: ↓ by 50% 10–20 ml/min: ↓ by 75%
Oral bioavailability (%)	<10	~75[b]		90[c]
With meal		(see text)	99.8[b]	
			40[b]	
Without meal				
Influence of food on oral bioavailability	Not applicable	Variable	Increase	None
Effect of ↑ gastric pH on oral bioavailability	Not applicable	Decrease	Decrease	None
Dosage formulations	IV	Oral	Oral	IV/oral
	20 mg/ml IV solution in 1% Cremophor EL	200-mg tabs	100-mg caps	50-, 100-, 150-, 200-mg tablets, 2 mg/ml IV solution, 50 or 200 mg/5 ml suspension
Usual daily dose	200 to 2400 mg	200 to 800 mg	100 to 400 mg	100 to 800 mg
Dosing regimen	Every 8 hr	Once daily	≤200 mg: once daily >200 mg: twice daily	Once daily

[a] Compiled from Barone *et al.* (1993); Brammer *et al.* (1990); Brass *et al.* (1982); Brugmans *et al.* (1972); Carlson *et al.* (1983); Daneshmend *et al.* (1983, 1984); Debruyne *et al.* (1990); Hardin *et al.* (1988); Heel *et al.* (1980, 1982); Heykants *et al.* (1989); Hoeprich and Goldstein (1974); Houang *et al.* (1990); Mannisto *et al.* (1982); Toon *et al.* (1990).

[b] As compared to oral solution.

[c] As compared to intravenous solution.

doses, respectively, serum concentrations of 0.07 to 0.1 μg/ml and 0.5 to 1.0 μg/ml are achieved. Following administration of a 200-mg intravenous dose over 1 hr, peak serum concentrations of about 1.6 μg/ml are achieved, followed by a rapid early decay period with a half-life of approximately 30 min and a slower decay period with a serum half-life of about 20 hr. Penetration of miconazole into sputum and cerebrospinal fluid (CSF) is poor, although penetration into vitreous body and infected joints appears to be adequate (Heel *et al.*, 1980).

The serum protein binding of miconazole is approximately 90%. Miconazole is inactivated in the body to produce a number of O-dealkylated and oxidative N-dealklylated metabolites. Metabolism of the drug or possible excretion in the feces appears to account for most of the removal of drug from the body. Miconazole, unlike clotrimazole, does not cause induction of liver enzymes following prolonged intravenous administration. Hoeprich and Goldstein (1974) reported that no active drug was recovered in the urine of four volunteers given a 200-mg intravenous dose, but that 25% of the dose was present as inactive metabolites. Miconazole plasma concentrations do not accumulate in patients with renal failure, and the drug is only minimally removed by hemo- or peritoneal dialysis.

3. *Clinical Use*

Currently, the major indication for the use of intravenous miconazole is serious life-threatening illness due to *Pseudallescheria boydii* (Bodey, 1992; Dworzack *et al.*, 1989; Walsh *et al.*, 1995). There is more experience with micronazole than the newer azoles for this rare infection (Patterson *et al.*, 1990; Goldberg *et al.*, 1993). It seems feasible to treat with miconazole until the patient's condition has stabilized and then an oral azole agent, such as itraconazole or fluconazole, can be substituted. For localized *P. boydii* infections, such as skin and subcutaneous nodules or osteoarticular infections, itraconazole or fluconazole may be as effective as miconazole and should be tried first (Patterson *et al.*, 1990; Lopes *et al.*, 1994; Piper *et al.*, 1990).

Prior to the introduction of the newer azole antifungal agents, miconazole had been shown to be modestly successful for the treatment of cryptococcosis (Weinstein and Jacoby, 1980; Graybill and Levine, 1978), coccidioidomycosis (Stevens *et al.*, 1976; Deresinski *et al.*, 1977), and blastomycosis (Rose and Varkey, 1978). However, relapse rates were high and the drug was poorly tolerated (Bennett and Remington, 1981). Currently, there are more effective and less toxic drugs that should be used to treat these infections.

There are two other uncommon uses of the intravenous formulation of miconazole. Bladder irrigation has been used for treatment of *Candida* cystitis (Wise *et al.*, 1987). The usual dosage recommended is 50 mg/liter. Intraperitoneal administration has proved useful for treating *Candida* peritonitis associated with chronic ambulatory peritoneal dialysis (Cheng *et al.*, 1989). Generally, a concentration of 50–100 mg/liter has been used.

4. *Side Effects*

The vehicle in which miconazole is administered appears to be responsible for many of the adverse effects associated with intravenous micronazole therapy: phlebitis and pruritus have been noted in over 20% of patients; nausea, fever, and chills in 10 to 20%; and vomiting and anemia in approximately 5% (Heel *et al.*, 1980). With higher dosages of the drug, thrombocytosis, rouleaux formation of erythrocytes, and hyperlipidemias have been reported (Bagnarello *et al.*, 1977; Bennett and Remington, 1981; Stevens, 1977). Jordan *et al.* (1979) reported central nervous system side effects, such as tremors, confusion, dizziness, hallucinations, and occasionally grand mal seizures in 16% of patients. Rapid infusions of miconazole have resulted in cardiorespiratory arrest and anaphylactoid reactions that are theorized to result from massive histamine release triggered by the solvent vehicle.

5. *Administration*

Miconazole is poorly soluble in aqueous solutions and is therefore administered in a polyethoxylated castor oil vehicle (Cremaphor EL) for intravenous administration. Miconazole is available as a 200-mg base in a 20-ml solution containing 1% Cremophor EL. The daily dosage of miconazole varies from 200 to 2400 mg, given in divided doses every 8 hr via a slow (100 mg/hr) intravenous infusion. Rapid infusion should be avoided due to its association with arrhythmias and cardiac and respiratory arrest. The dosage of miconazole does not need to be decreased in patients with renal insufficiency.

B. Ketoconazole

1. *Overview*

Ketoconazole was the first oral azole agent developed for use in treating systemic mycoses. After its introduction in 1981, it became the drug of choice for treating patients who had nonlife-threatening, nonmeningeal histoplasmosis, blastomycosis, and coccidioidomycosis. Ketoconazole tablets have been used widely for the treatment of *Candida* vaginitis, thrush, and esophagitis, and cutaneous and nail infections caused by either dermatophytes or *Candida*. In addition to the oral formulation, a cream and a shampoo are available for the treatment of seborrhea, tinea versicolor, and other cutaneous fungal infections.

The use of ketoconazole is somewhat problematic given its drug interactions and problems with absorption. For many infections, ketoconazole has been superseded by the newer azoles, itraconazole and fluconazole, which appear to be more effective with fewer side effects (Kauffman, 1996). However, since ketoconazole remains the least expensive oral azole, it continues to be used widely.

2. *Pharmacology*

Ketoconazole, a dibasic imidazole antifungal agent with a pK_{a_1} of 2.94 and a pK_{a_1} of 6.94, is insoluble in water except at a pH <3 (Carlson *et al.*, 1983) (Table I). In humans, the presence of gastric acid is required for dissolution and subsequent oral absorption of ketoconazole. In achlorhydric patients, ketoconazole may be dissolved in 0.1 *N* HCl and the solution sipped through a straw (to avoid erosion of tooth enamel). Alternatively, administration of oral glutamic acid capsules (1360 mg) may be employed to increase absorption (Knapp *et al.*, 1991; Lelawongs *et al.*, 1988). Concomitant administration of agents known to increase gastric pH should be avoided as they will decrease the bioavailability of ketoconazole. Ketoconazole should be administered at least 2 hr prior to administration of agents such as histamine receptor antagonists, proton-pump inhibitors, and antacids, which increase gastric pH. Similarly, although administration of sucralfate does not significantly alter gastric pH, concomitant administration with ketoconazole will also decrease the absorption of ketoconazole via a chelation interaction (Carver *et al.*, 1994; Hoeschele *et al.*, 1994). Doses of ketoconazole and sucralfate should be separated by at least 2 hr.

Studies examining the effect of food on the oral bioavailability of ketoconazole have provided conflicting results. Because ketoconazole is a lipophilic drug, some authors have suggested that administration of drug with a high fat meal can improve oral bioavailability. However, Mannisto *et al.* (1982) reported that the absorption of ketoconazole was decreased when given with a standardized breakfast, and Brass *et al.* (1982) and Daneshmend *et al.* (1984) reported variable effects of meals over a wide dosage range (200 to 800 mg) of ketoconazole administered to patients in the fasting state and following a standardized breakfast. Although administration of food increased the time to peak plasma concentrations (t_{max}), it did not reduce peak plasma concentrations (Cp_{max}) or the oral bioavailability of ketoconazole. Food appeared to enhance the absorption of 400- and 600-mg, but not 800-mg doses. The oral bioavailability of ketoconazole appears to be markedly decreased in bone marrow transplant patients immediately post-transplantation, probably due to chemotherapy-induced alterations in the gastric mucosa (Maksymiuk *et al.*, 1982; Vu Van *et al.*, 1983).

Plasma concentrations of ketoconazole very widely among individuals, even in the absence of factors known to alter gastric pH. Following administration of a single 200-mg oral dose of ketoconazole, mean peak serum concentrations (Cp_{max}) are achieved in 1 to 2 hr and range from 2.75 to 4.5 μg/ml (Daneshmend *et al.*, 1983; Daneshmend and Warnock, 1988; Heel *et al.*, 1982; Brass *et al.*, 1982). Serum concentrations of ketoconazole appear to decline in biexponential fashion, with an initial rapid elimination phase with a half-life of 1.7 to 2.2 hr following single oral dosages of 200 or 400 mg, respectively. The slower, terminal elimination phase, which occurs at serum concentrations less than 0.1 μg/ml, has a half-life of approximately 8 hr (Heel *et al.*, 1982).

Ketoconazole is highly protein bound (~99%) and distributes poorly into various body compartments. Minimal concentrations are detected in CSF, urine, aqueous humor and vitreous body, and peritoneal fluid. In patients with meningeal disease, CSF concentrations of ketoconazole ranged from 0 to 0.24 μg/ml following a 200-mg oral dose, and from 0 to 0.85 μg/ml following a 400-mg oral dose (Heel *et al.*, 1982). Higher and more prolonged concentrations of ketoconazole have been reported in lumbar and ventricular CSF of patients with coccidioidal meningitis receiving large doses of ketoconazole. Following an 800-mg dose, mean ventricular fluid concentrations of 0.2 μg/ml were reported at 2 and 4 hr postdose, with lumbar CSF concentrations of 0.25 μg/ml detectable at 8 hr (Craven *et al.*, 1983).

Ketoconazole is extensively metabolized in the liver by oxidation, O-dealkylation, and aromatic hydroxylation and is excreted primarily in the bile as inactive drug. Approximately 57% of the dose is eliminated in the feces, 20 to 65% as unchanged drug, and the remainder as metabolites. As less than 5% of an oral dosage is excreted as unchanged drug in the urine, dosage adjustments are not necessary in patients with renal dysfunction. Due to the high degree of plasma protein binding and high metabolic clearance, clearance of drug by hemodialysis or peritoneal dialysis is minimal and supplemental dosages following dialysis are not necessary (Brass *et al.*, 1982).

There are few data regarding the effect of liver dysfunction on plasma concentrations of ketoconazole. Although Heel *et al.* (1982) reported no change in serum concentrations of ketoconazole in a few patients with liver dysfunction compared with normal patients, Brass *et al.* (1982) reported that a patient with hepatic insufficiency demonstrated persistently high serum concentrations of drug.

3. Clinical Use

a. Blastomycosis Ketoconazole has been shown to be effective for the treatment of blastomycosis. In two open treatment trials, the overall rate of response was 76% among 46 patients treated with 400 mg ketoconazole daily (Bradsher *et al.*, 1985) and 77% among 80 patients treated with either 400 or 800 mg daily (Dismukes *et al.*, 1985). Patients treated with 800 mg had a higher cure rate (85%) than those receiving 400 mg (70% cured).

b. Histoplasmosis In the 1980s, several Mycoses Study Group trials established the effectiveness of ketoconazole for the treatment of endemic mycoses (Dismukes *et al.*, 1983, 1985). In a randomized trial of two different dosages, the overall response rate for 54 patients with histoplasmosis was 63%; in those patients that had been treated for at least 6 months, the success rate was 85%. A low dose (400 mg) was shown to be as effective as a higher dose (800 mg) (Dismukes *et al.,* 1985). For 31 patients with disseminated histoplasmosis, ketoconazole was efficacious in 55% overall and in 85% of those treated at least 6 months. For 23 patients with chronic cavitary pulmonary histoplasmosis, the response rate was 74% overall and 84% in those receiving at least 6 months of ketoconazole.

Ketoconazole has not proved effective in the treatment of histoplasmosis in AIDS patients (Wheat *et al.,* 1990). The high failure rate may be due to poor absorption of the drug by AIDS patients (Lake-Bakaar *et al.,* 1988).

c. Coccidioidomycosis Ketoconazole has been shown to be moderately efficacious for the treatment of a variety of different forms of coccidioidomycosis. Using stringent criteria to establish efficacy, the Mycoses Study Group trial reported by Galgiani *et al.* (1988) showed response rates of 23 to 32%. These results reflect the chronic relapsing nature of this infection and the strict criteria for response used in this study (Galgiani, 1993). Most studies of treatment of coccidioidomycosis used 400 mg ketoconazole daily (Ross *et al.,* 1982; Catanzaro *et al.,* 1982; de Felice *et al.,* 1982), but for many patients, 800 mg or higher doses may be required (Galgiani *et al.,* 1988). Doses as high as 1600 mg daily have been used, but significant toxicity is routinely seen at doses above 800 mg daily (Galgiani *et al.,* 1988).

It should be noted that for all of the just-described studies of histoplasmosis, blastomycosis, and coccidioidomycosis, with the exception of the trial reported by de Felice *et al.* (1982), patients were excluded from study if they had meningeal involvement or a serious life-threatening infection. Thus, patients with severe disease or meningeal involvement should not be treated with ketoconazole.

d. Sporotrichosis Ketoconazole has been shown to be only modestly effective in the treatment of sporotrichosis. In one study of osteoarticular fungal infections, patients with sporotrichosis failed ketoconazole therapy (Horsburgh *et al.,* 1983), but higher dose of ketoconazole were shown to be more effective in another study (Calhoun *et al.,* 1991). Patients with pulmonary sporotrichosis treated with ketoconazole generally have had a poor outcome (Dall and Salzman, 1987; Pluss and Opal, 1986).

e. Mucocutaneous Candidiasis Before the release of fluconazole, ketoconazole was widely used for treating localized candidiasis, including thrush, denture stomatitis, esophagitis, and vaginitis. It was the first systemic antifungal agent that could be given chronically to treat patients with the rare syndrome chronic mucocutaneous candidiasis, a disease for which previously there had been no effective long-term treatment (Petersen *et al.,* 1980).

Although still useful for these indications, ketoconazole appears to be less effective than fluconazole for thrush (Meunier *et al.*, 1990; de Wit *et al.*, 1989) and esophagitis (Laine *et al.*, 1992), and has been used less frequently for *Candida* vaginitis since the approval of single-dose fluconazole therapy (Sobel, 1993). The usual dosage regimen for thrush has been 200 mg daily for 5–10 days; for esophagitis, 400 mg daily for 10–14 days; and for vaginitis, 400 mg daily for 5 days. For women with recurrent vaginitis, maintenance therapy with ketoconazole using 100 mg daily for 6 months has proved to be effective in preventing relapses (Sobel, 1986), but this regimen also will likely be supplanted by fluconazole maintenance therapy.

f. Invasive Candidiasis Early open treatment trials of candidiasis showed benefit in approximately 70% of patients receiving ketoconazole (Drouhet and Dupont, 1983). However, anecdotal case reports showed failure of ketoconazole to cure visceral candidiasis (Brooks *et al.*, 1982; Morris *et al.*, 1990). Ketoconazole is not excreted as an active drug in the urine and thus has been only minimally effective for the treatment of *Candida* urinary tract infections (Graybill *et al.*, 1983). Although administered to a few patients with several different types of fungal meningitis, the dosages required were high (800–1200 mg daily) and relapses occurred in a significant number of patients (Craven *et al.*, 1983). In general, fluconazole is more effective for the just described fungal infections, and ketoconazole should not be used for these indications.

g. Dermatophyte Infections In situations in which local creams have not proved beneficial, oral ketoconazole is an effective drug for dermatophyte infections. *Tinea corporis, pedis,* and *cruris* usually respond promptly to 200 mg ketoconazole daily (Symoens *et al.*, 1980; Heel *et al.*, 1982; Rezabek and Friedman, 1992). Onychomycosis has been effectively treated with ketoconazole, but therapy usually must be continued for at least 6 months.

4. Side Effects

The most common adverse effect of ketoconazole is dose-related gastrointestinal discomfort (Heel *et al.*, 1982). Nausea, vomiting, and anorexia have been reported in over 20% of patients receiving 200 mg daily; the incidence rises to >50% of patients when the dosage is increased to ≥400 mg daily (Dismukes *et al.*, 1985). Because many patients experience gastrointestinal discomfort with ketoconazole, administration with food is generally recommended. Asymptomatic, reversible elevations in hepatic transaminases have been observed in 5 to 10% of patients, regardless of the dosage of ketoconazole administered (Heel *et al.*, 1982). Hepatitis is estimated to occur in 1 in 15,000 patients (Janssen and Symoens, 1983; Lewis *et al.*, 1984). Hepatic necrosis has been reported, but is rare, and hepatic enlargement with fatty infiltration has been reported in one patient

(Gradon and Sepkowitz, 1990). Allergic reactions, including urticaria, rash, and pruritis, are infrequent and anaphylaxis and anaphylactoid reactions are very rare (Heel *et al.,* 1982).

Ketoconazole inhibits adrenal steroid synthesis by reversible, dose-dependent inhibition of the cytochromes P450-dependent 11-β-hydroxylation of steroids (Pont *et al.,* 1982). Although precipitation of adrenal crisis is exceedingly rare (Tucker *et al.,* 1985), patients should be considered potentially unable to mount an adrenal stress response. Administration of ketoconazole as a single (rather than multiple) daily dose appears to minimize adrenal axis suppression. Gynecomastia, decreased libido, oligospermia, azospermia, and impotence secondary to decreased testosterone synthesis have been reported in men following high (>600 mg) daily dosages and during prolonged administration of lower dosages (Pont *et al.,* 1982b, 1984; Dismukes *et al.,* 1985). Ketoconazole is teratogenic in rats (Heel *et al.,* 1982) and should not be used in pregnant women.

5. Administration

Ketoconazole is available for systemic use in a 200-mg oral tablet. The usual daily dosage is 200 mg daily for localized infections, such as tinea or thrush, and 400 to 800 mg daily for serious systemic infections, although dosages as high as 1200 mg daily may be required. Despite conflicting studies regarding the effects of a meal on oral absorption, ketoconazole is usually administered with a meal in order to minimize gastric upset. Patients should avoid concomitant administration of histamine receptor antagonists, proton-pump inhibitors, antacids, and sucralfate, which markedly decrease the oral bioavailability of ketoconazole. In patients with increased gastric pH, administration of oral glutamic acid (1360 mg) or an acidic beverage (Coca-Cola Classic) may increase the bioavailability of ketoconazole (Chin *et al.,* 1995; Knapp *et al.,* 1991; Lelawongs *et al.,* 1988). In order to minimize the suppressive effects of the drug on the adrenal axis, once daily dosing is preferred. If large daily doses cannot be tolerated, the dose should be split into two portions. The dosage of ketoconazole does not need adjustment in patients with renal insufficiency. Although there are no guidelines for decreasing the dosage in patients with severe hepatic dysfunction, it is prudent to not use ketoconazole in this situation unless absolutely required.

C. Itraconazole

1. Overview

Itraconazole was released for use in the United States in 1992. Currently, it is available only as an oral capsule formulation. Itraconazole has fewer toxicities than ketoconazole and appears to be more effective in treating endemic mycoses (Kauffman, 1996). Thus, it has become the drug of choice for treating nonlife-threatening histoplasmosis and blastomycosis and has found widespread use in the treatment of sporotrichosis, coccidioidomycosis, and infections due to dematiaceous fungi (Kauffman, 1994; Como and Dismukes, 1994). Itraconazole is also approved for use in treating aspergillosis in patients who cannot tolerate or who have failed amphotericin B therapy. Recently, approval has been granted by the FDA for the use of itraconazole in treating onychomycosis.

One major drawback to the use of itraconazole is its poor bioavailability. A solution of itraconazole in cyclodextrin has better bioavailibility and is likely to be released in 1997 for use in the treatment of localized forms of candidiasis. Additionally, there is a newly developed intravenous itraconazole formulation. If this proves effective and nontoxic, the use of itraconazole will most likely expand, especially in the treatment of opportunistic mycoses and serious endemic mycoses.

2. *Pharmacology*

Despite its marked structural similarity to ketoconazole, itraconazole differs in several important respects (Table I). Itraconazole appears to have greater specificity against fungal versus mammalian cytochromes P450, resulting in greater potency and a decrease in cytochromes P450-mediated side effects and drug interactions.

Like ketoconazole, itraconazole depends on the availability of low gastric pH for dissolution and absorption (Heykants *et al.*, 1989). Administration with food appears to significantly enhance the oral bioavailability of itraconazole (Saag and Dismukes, 1988). Because itraconazole exhibits pH-dependent dissolution and absorption, absorption is impaired in patients receiving antacids or H2-receptor antagonists and in patients with achlorhydria (Lim *et al.*, 1993). Plasma concentrations of itraconazole following a single oral dose in HIV-infected patients are approximately 50% lower than concentrations observed in healthy volunteers (Smith *et al.*, 1992). The oral bioavailability of itraconazole appears to be markedly decreased in bone marrow transplant patients immediately posttransplantation (Kintzel *et al.*, 1995; Prentice *et al.*, 1994).

Itraconazole is extensively (>99%) bound to plasma proteins, but the unbound drug distributes well throughout tissues, including adipose tissue, endometrium, cervical and vaginal mucus, skin, and nails (Heykants *et al.*, 1989; Cleary *et al.*, 1992; Como and Dismukes, 1994). However, the drug penetrates poorly into the cerebrospinal fluid (Perfect and Durack, 1985), and active drug is not found in the urine (Hardin *et al.*, 1988).

The terminal elimination half-life of itraconazole at steady state following oral doses of 200 mg daily is 24 to 42 hr, but the half-life increases as the dosage is increased from 100 to 400 mg daily, suggesting the presence of saturable metabolic pathways. Itraconazole is extensively metabolized in the liver to more than 30 metabolites and is excreted almost exclusively in the feces and urine. To date, hydroxyitraconazole is the only metabolite identified with antifungal activity. Hydroxyitraconazole is eliminated more rapidly than itraconazole, but its volume of distribution is much smaller, resulting in plasma concentrations at steady state that are approximately twice those of the parent drug (Barone *et al.*, 1993). Similar to ketoconazole, clearance of itraconazole by hemodialysis or peritoneal dialysis is minimal, and supplemental dosages following dialysis are not necessary (Boelaert *et al.*, 1988).

3. Clinical Use

a. Blastomycosis A Mycoses Study Group trial using 200–400 mg daily established that itraconazole was effective for the treatment of blastomycosis (Dismukes *et al.*, 1992). Among 40 patients who had received therapy for at least 2 months, 38 (95%) were cured. For the entire group of 45 patients, the overall response rate was 90%. Most patients were treated with 200 mg daily. For those with a successful outcome, the median time treated was 6.2 months. These results were improved over those previously noted with ketoconazole (Bradsher *et al.*, 1985; Dismukes *et al.*, 1985). Few side effects were noted in this trial, and only 1 patient relapsed.

b. Histoplasmosis The use of itraconazole for the treatment of histoplasmosis was also established by a Mycoses Study Group trial that enrolled 35 patients, 10 of whom had disseminated disease and 25 of whom had pulmonary disease (Dismukes *et al.*, 1992). The response rate was 86% in those patients who received at least 2 months of treatment with 200–400 mg itraconazole daily. All patients with disseminated histoplasmosis responded, but only 72% of those with pulmonary histoplasmosis responded. These rates of response are similar to or slightly better than those previously noted with ketoconazole (Dismukes *et al.*, 1985). Most patients received 200 mg daily, and the median treatment time for those who were cured was 9 months. Patients who had chronic cavitary or chronic progressive disseminated histoplasmosis received the longest courses of therapy.

Itraconazole has also found widespread use in the treatment of histoplasmosis in AIDS patients. Most patients with HIV infection have disseminated forms of histoplasmosis. Although some patients have a subacute illness, many have severe life-threatening infection with adult respiratory distress syndrome, central nervous system involvement, disseminated intravascular coagulation, pancytopenia, and fungemia (Johnson *et al.*, 1988; Wheat *et al.*, 1990).

Several treatment trials of histoplasmosis have been carried out by the AIDS Clinical Trials Group (ACTG), in conjunction with the Mycoses Study Group. For primary treatment of patients with mild-to-moderate histoplasmosis, the overall response rate with 200 mg itraconazole twice daily was 85% (Wheat *et al.*, 1995). Similar results were obtained by Negroni *et al.* (1992), but most of their 27 patients were treated with lower dosages of itraconazole. In another trial of maintenance itraconazole following induction therapy with amphotericin B, 200 mg twice daily prevented relapse in 95% of patients (Wheat *et al.*, 1993); thus, itraconazole was as effective or more effective as preventing relapse than amphotericin B (McKinsey *et al.*, 1992; Wheat *et al.*, 1990).

The standard therapy of histoplasmosis in AIDS patients has become itraconazole for mild-to-moderate infection not involving the central nervous system. Patients with life-threatening disease or central nervous system infection should be treated initially with amphotericin B, and when stabilized, therapy can be changed to 200 mg of itraconazole twice daily. Therapy must be continued for life as the relapse rate is extraordinarily high in this population.

c. Coccidioidomycosis Coccidioidomycosis can be effectively treated with itraconazole (Tucker, *et al.*, 1990a; Graybill *et al.*, 1990; Diaz *et al.*, 1991; Galgiani, 1993; Stevens, 1995). The usual dosage that has been used is 400 mg, given as two daily doses, although higher amounts have been required in some patients. In the most recent Mycoses Study Group trial, 57% of patients responded to itraconazole treatment, a response rate not significantly different from those noted with fluconazole and better than those noted with similar doses of ketoconazole (Graybill *et al.*, 1990). A blinded, randomized trial comparing fluconazole with itraconazole for the treatment of coccidioidomycosis is being conducted; no results are available at this time.

Although itraconazole achieves very poor cerebrospinal fluid levels, the drug has been shown to be effective for the treatment of coccidioidal meningitis (Tucker *et al.*, 1990b). At this point, with so little data available, itraconazole should be considered second-line therapy and fluconazole the preferred treatment for coccidioidal meningitis (Galgiani *et al.*, 1993).

d. Sporotrichosis Prior to the release of itrazonazole, the most effective therapy for lymphocutaneous or cutaneous sporotrichosis was saturated solution of potassium iodide (SSKI). Amphotericin B was generally required for osteoarticular, pulmonary, or visceral involvement. Itraconazole is not approved by the FDA for the treatment of sporotrichosis, but is commonly used for this fungal infection based on several studies (Kauffman, 1995b; Conti Diaz *et al.*, 1992; Restrepo *et al.*, 1986). Restrepo *et al.* (1986) showed a cure rate of 100% for 26 patients with lymphocutaneous or cutaneous sporotrichosis treated with only 100 mg itraconazole daily for 3–6 months.

An evaluation by the Mycoses Study Group showed effectiveness of itraconazole in 22 of 27 patients with a variety of forms of sporotrichosis treated with doses varying from 200 to 600 mg daily (Sharkey-Mathis *et al.*, 1993). Of the 22 patients who responded, 6 later relapsed and had to be retreated. Patients with lymphocutaneous or cutaneous sporotrichosis had a 90% response rate; the 1 patient who failed therapy was cured after he was retreated with itraconazole. Most of the failures had osteoarticular or pulmonary disease. The overall response rate seen with osteoarticular infections was 73%, similar to the 80% response noted by Winn *et al.* (1993). Pulmonary sporotrichosis has been particularly difficult to treat (Pluss and Opal, 1986). Itraconazole was effective in only 1 of 3 patients, but this compares with similar cure rates with amphotericin B, ketoconazole, and fluconazole (Pluss and Opal, 1986).

e. Dematiaceous Fungi Itraconazole has been used for treating recalcitrant subcutaneous and other localized infections due to a variety of different dematiaceous fungi (Duggan *et al.*, 1995; Yu, 1995; Whittle and Kominos, 1995). Much of the data consists of single case reports, although Sharkey *et al.* (1990) reported a series of 17 patients treated with itraconazole. Most of the patients had failed prior treatment with other antifungal drugs, including amphotericin B. The 65% response rate is similar to that noted with amphotericin B (Adam *et al.*, 1986).

f. Aspergillosis Itraconazole has become an effective second-line treatment for aspergillosis (Denning *et al.*, 1989b, 1994; Dupont, 1990; Viviani *et al.*, 1990; De Beule *et al.*, 1988). In a open study of treatment of this infection with itraconazole, the overall success rate was shown to be 39% (Denning *et al.*, 1994). A randomized study comparing itraconazole with amphotericin B for culture-proved aspergillosis has not been carried out, but the response rate noted historically with amphotericin B was about the same as that noted with itraconazole (Denning and Stevens, 1990). For aspergillosis, the major determinant of outcome is the host's ability to eliminate the organism. For example, patients with solid organ transplants appear to respond better than those with bone marrow transplants; patients who are neutropenic respond after resolution of neutropenia (Denning *et al.*, 1994). AIDS patients, who almost always develop aspergillosis during the late stage of advanced HIV infection (Lortholary *et al.*, 1993), have not responded well to itraconazole.

The current approach to the treatment of invasive aspergillosis is to use amphotericin B for patients who are immunosuppressed and/or severely ill. Itraconazole then can be used as consolidation therapy after an initial response to amphotericin B is obtained. Itraconazole can be used as primary therapy for patients with more subacute forms of aspergillosis, such as chronic necrotizing cavitary pulmonary aspergillosis (Binder *et al.*, 1982). Trials are currently underway to determine whether itraconazole has a role in the treatment of allergic bronchopulmonary aspergillosis. The hope is that use of the drug in these atopic individuals or in cystic fibrosis patients who have a similar syndrome will decrease the requirement for corticosteroids. Itraconazole has been used for aspergillomas in open treatment trials

(De Beule *et al.*, 1988; Viviani *et al.*, 1990; Dupont, 1990), but it has not been clearly shown if the drug has an impact on the disease. A placebo-controlled trial will soon be underway to determine if itraconazole has a role to play in the therapy of this disease.

g. Candidiasis Itraconazole appears to be effective therapy for *Candida* vaginitis (Stein and Mummaw, 1993; Tobin *et al.*, 1992; Beyer and Voorhoeve-den Hartog, 1992), but it does not have FDA approval for this indication. It appears likely that fluconazole will remain the drug of choice for this infection.

Little experience has been reported using itraconazole for the treatment of oral or esophageal candidiasis. Although itraconazole capsules have been shown in AIDS patients to be as good as or superior to clotrimazole troches and ketoconazole tablets, they generally are not as efficacious as fluconazole (Blatchford, 1990; Smith *et al.*, 1991; Barbaro *et al.*, 1995). A new oral formulation of itraconazole in cyclodextrin solution has proved to be effective in early clinical trials, several of which have included patients with fluconazole-refractory *C. albicans* thrush (Graybill *et al.*, 1995; Cartledge *et al.*, 1994).

h. Cryptococcosis Itraconazole was shown to be effective in several open-treatment trials of cryptococcal meningitis in AIDS patients (Denning *et al.*, 1989a; Cauwenbergh, 1993; de Gans *et al.*, 1992; Viviani *et al.*, 1990). However, the success rate has been less than that noted with fluconazole. Preliminary results from two studies comparing itraconazole with fluconazole for the treatment of cryptococcal meningitis have been reported (van der Horst *et al.*, 1995; Saag *et al.*, 1995a,b). In a very large trial of cryptococcal meningitis in AIDS patients (381 patients), 400 mg itraconazole daily was less efficacious than 400 mg fluconazole daily when given as consolidation therapy; all patients had received an initial 2 weeks of therapy with amphotericin B, with or without flucytosine (Saag *et al.*, 1995a; van der Horst *et al.*, 1995). Another smaller trial (108 patients) using itraconazole for maintenance therapy after primary treatment had cleared *C. neoformans* from the cerebrospinal fluid showed a less than optimal response with itraconazole (Saag *et al.*, 1995b). Thus, fluconazole remains the drug of choice for both consolidation and maintenance therapy in AIDS patients who have received primary treatment with amphotericin B and flucytosine for cryptococcal meningitis.

i. Dermatophyte Infections Itraconazole was released in late 1995 for the treatment of onychomycosis, but the drug does not have an indication for treatment of cutaneous *Candida* or dermatophyte infections. However, a large number of studies have shown itraconazole to be as effective as ketoconazole or griseofulvin for a variety of cutaneous fungal infections (reviewed in Zuckerman and Tunkel, 1994). For onychomycosis, treatment can be given for 1 week out of every month at a dose of 200 mg daily for a total of 3–6 months. This regimen is an effective as daily treatment because of the persistence of itraconazole in the nail for weeks after the drug is stopped (Heykants *et al.,* 1989). The response rate in several studies of onychomycosis has been greater than 80% (Hay *et al.,* 1988; Piepponen *et al.,* 1992).

4. Side Effects

Adverse effects of itraconazole appear to be similar to those observed with ketoconazole, but occur with lower frequency. Gastrointestinal disturbances (primarily nausea, vomiting, epigastric pain, and diarrhea) have been the most common complaints, occurring in up to 20% of patients (Tucker *et al.,* 1990c). Transient elevation of liver function tests occurs in ~5% of patients; symptomatic hepatitis has been rarely reported (Lavrijsen *et al.,* 1992). Sexual impotence despite normal testosterone levels has been reported in a small number of patients (Como and Dismukes, 1994). Sharkey *et al.* (1991) noted reversible adrenal insufficiency in one patient treated with 600 mg itraconazole daily for 5 months. Hypokalemia, hypertension, and edema may occur. The incidence of these side effects is unknown, and the mechanism has not been elucidated. These effects may be severe enough to warrant stopping the drug. Although there are no data in humans, itraconazole, similar to the other azoles, is potentially teratogenic and should be avoided in pregnant women.

5. Administration

Itraconazole is currently available in 100-mg oral capsules. The usual dosage is 100 or 200 mg daily for less serious infections and 400 mg daily for serious systemic mycotic infections. The oral bioavailability of itraconazole is markedly increased by the administration of food with each dose. Daily dosages larger than 200 mg should be administered in divided dosages because the absorption of itraconazole decreases as larger single doses are administered (i.e., it exhibits nonlinear absorption). A study done on AIDS patients suggested that administration of 8 oz of a cola beverage will increase the oral bioavailability of a 200-mg dose of itraconazole by 38% (Hardin *et al.,* 1995a). All the caveats regarding gastric absorption noted for ketoconazole apply to itraconazole as well. The dosage of itraconazole does not need to be decreased in patients with renal insufficiency. There are no dosage recommendations for patients with severe hepatic dysfunction, but it would be prudent to avoid the use of the drug in these patients.

A new formulation of itraconazole in cyclodextrin solution has been used in clinical trials (Graybill *et al.,* 1995). This preparation has proved useful in treating fluconazole-refractory thrush. The drug appears to be better absorbed in this formulation and achieves very high oral mucosal concentrations, which is probably beneficial in eradicating fluconazole-refractory candidiasis. An intravenous preparation formulated in cyclodextrin is also under evaluation and should prove useful in seriously ill patients who are unable to absorb itraconazole capsules. (De Beule *et al.*, 1995).

D. Fluconazole

1. Overview

Fluconazole was released for use in the United States in 1990 based on treatment studies for cryptococcal meningitis in AIDS patients. Several randomized trials comparing amphotericin B with fluconazole have been reported and have clearly shown the role of this drug in the treatment of yeast infections in both immunocompromised hosts and hospitalized patients. Fluconazole appears to have fewer drug interactions, and its pharmacology is markedly different from that of itraconazole and ketoconazole (Como and Dismukes, 1994). It is available as an IV formulation, as well as tablets and an oral suspension. This drug has enjoyed widespread use since its release (Kauffman, 1996; Zervos *et al.*, 1994) In part, this great use is probably responsible for the emergence of resistance to fluconazole among strains of *C. albicans*.

2. Pharmacology

The small molecular weight, low protein binding, and increased water solubility of fluconazole result in rapid, essentially complete absorption of drug following oral administration (Table I). Peak plasma concentrations are achieved 2 to 4 hr after oral administration and range from 1.4 μg/ml following a 50-mg dose to 2.8 μg/ml following a 150-mg oral dose. The absorption of drug in patients undergoing bone marrow transplantation and in AIDS patients is not significantly different from healthy subjects (Milliken *et al.*, 1989; Tett *et al.*, 1995; Akkerman *et al.*, 1993). The amount of fluconazole absorbed appears to be linearly proportional to the dose, whereas urinary excretion data indicate that the oral bioavailability of fluconazole is greater than 90%. Absorption is not affected by food or gastric pH (Lim *et al.*, 1993; Blum *et al.*, 1991a; Zimmermann *et al.*, 1994).

Administration of 50- and 100-mg intravenous doses of fluconazole daily for 7 days results in no substantial change in half-life, total body or renal clearance, or volume of distribution from day 1 to day 7. Fluconazole has a steady-state volume of distribution of 0.6 to 0.8 liter/kg, a terminal elimination half-life ranging from 28 to 32 hr, and a total body clearance ranging from 15 to 24 ml/min (Brammer *et al.*, 1990; Houang *et al.*, 1990; Humphrey *et al.*, 1985). The half-life of fluconazole is prolonged to 50 hr in HIV-infected patients with CD4 counts $<200/\mu$l (Tett *et al.*, 1995). Fluconazole distributes widely to tissues and body fluids achieving excellent concentrations in aqueous humor and vitreous body, cerebrospinal fluid, cerebral parenchyma, bile, and urine (Bozzette *et al.*, 1992; Arndt *et al.*,

1988; Perfect and Durack, 1985; Tucker *et al.*, 1988; Thaler *et al.*, 1995; Walsh *et al.*, 1989; Foulds *et al.*, 1988).

Fluconazole is only minimally metabolized; more than 80% of the drug is excreted as unchanged drug in the urine, with the remainder of the dose excreted as glucuronide and N-oxide metabolites in the urine and as unchanged drug in the feces (Humphrey *et al.*, 1985). Like itraconazole, fluconazole appears to have only minimal effects on steroid metabolism (Hanger *et al.*, 1988; Touchette *et al.*, 1992). The terminal elimination half-life increases from approximately 30 hr in patients with normal renal function to 98 hr in patients with severe renal impairment (<20 ml/min) (Toon *et al.*, 1990). Fluconazole is effectively removed (38% of a 50-mg dose in a 3-hr session) during hemodialysis and to a lesser extent (18% recovery of a 100-mg oral dose in dialysate over a 48-hr period) during peritoneal dialysis (Debruyne *et al.*, 1990; Toon *et al.*, 1990). Systemic absorption of intraperitoneal fluconazole is slow (time to peak, 7 hr) but nearly complete (87% of a dose).

3. Clinical Use

a. Localized Candidiasis Fluconazole has proved very useful in the treatment of oropharyngeal, vaginal, and esophageal candidiasis. Several open-treatment and placebo-controlled studies have shown the benefit of fluconazole for treating thrush (Dupont and Drouhet, 1988; Budtz-Jorgensen *et al.*, 1988); fluconazole appears to be more effective than ketoconazole (de Wit *et al.*, 1989) and clotrimazole troches (Sangeorzan *et al.*, 1994; Koletar *et al.*, 1990) in AIDS patients. The usual dosage for treating thrush is 100 mg daily. Laine *et al.* (1992) showed that therapy with 100 mg fluconazole daily was superior to 200 mg ketoconazole daily in treating AIDS patients with *Candida* esophagitis. Fluconazole has been released for the treatment of vaginal candidiasis. A single dose of 150 mg has been shown to be as effective as multiple doses of other azoles for treatment of vaginal candidiasis (Lebech *et al.*, 1988; Sobel, 1993; Houang *et al.*, 1990).

Fluconazole is used widely for the treatment of *Candida* urinary tract infections (Fisher *et al.*, 1995; Voss *et al.*, 1994). Only recently have controlled studies been performed showing the benefits of therapy for this form of candidiasis. Studies on *Candida* urinary tract infections are difficult to perform because of the difficulty in differentiating colonization from infection and controlling for the role played by indwelling catheters. Depending on the end points evaluated and the patient groups enrolled, investigators have found fluconazole (100–200 mg daily for 4–7 days) to be superior (Leu and Huang, 1995), equivalent (Fan-Havard *et al.*, 1995), or inferior (Jacobs *et al.*, 1996) to amphotericin B bladder washes for eradication of candiduria.

Other localized *Candida* infections have been successfully treated with fluconazole, but most of the reported experience consists of anecdotal reports of individual cases of meningitis (Voice *et al.*, 1994), cholecystitis (Bozzette *et al.*, 1992), and endophthalmitis (Akler *et al.*, 1995; del Palacio *et al.*, 1993; Tunkel *et al.*, 1993; Kauffman *et al.*, 1993). However, failures have also been reported (Nomura and Ruskin, 1993; White and Goetz, 1995; Dan and Priel, 1994; Kauffman *et al.*, 1993).

b. Invasive Candidiasis Until the report by Rex *et al.* (1994), almost all reports of the use of fluconazole for treating invasive candidiasis were open-treatment trials. Most of these reports documented the effectiveness of fluconazole in patients with intraperitoneal or visceral candidiasis or candidemia (Milatovic and Voss, 1992; Kujath and Lerch, 1989; Ikemoto, 1989; Viscoli *et al.*, 1991; de Pauw *et al.*, 1995; Graninger *et al.*, 1993), but some noted failure (McIlroy, 1991; Evans *et al.*, 1991). The study by Rex *et al.* (1994) documented an equivalent response rate for fluconazole (400 mg daily) and amphotericin B (0.5–0.6 mg/kg daily) in patients with candidemia. This study was conducted in nonneutropenic patients, and 75% of those enrolled had catheter-associated candidemia. Preliminary results from a similar study from Canada confirm the results noted by Rex *et al.* (Phillips *et al.*, 1995) and a prospective observational study and a retrospective matched cohort study provide similar data for fluconazole efficacy for treating candidemia (Nguyen *et al.*, 1995; Anaissie *et al.*, 1996).

Chronic disseminated or hepatosplenic candidiasis has been successfully treated with fluconazole (Kauffman *et al.*, 1991; Anaissie *et al.*, 1991; de Pauw *et al.*, 1995), although most patients had received prior amphotericin B therapy, which could have played a role in the favorable outcome noted with fluconazole (Kauffman *et al.*, 1991; Anaissie *et al.*, 1991). In addition, several case reports describe successful treatment of *Candida* prosthetic valve endocarditis with chronic fluconazole therapy (Wallbridge *et al.*, 1993; Czwerwiec *et al.*, 1993; Castiglia *et al.*, 1994). Thus, fluconazole is an effective and frequently used antifungal agent for patients with a variety of different forms of candidiasis.

c. Cryptococcosis In 1992, several studies reported the benefit of fluconazole for both acute and chronic maintenance therapy for cryptococcal meningitis. Saag *et al.* (1992) showed that fluconazole (200 mg daily) was equivalent to amphotericin B (0.4–0.5 mg/kg daily) in the treatment of cryptococcal meningitis in AIDS patients. Although the outcomes were not statistically significantly different in the two treatment regimens, deaths in the first 2 weeks of therapy were higher in the fluconazole group than in the amphotericin B group, and in the fluconazole group the time until the cerebrospinal fluid became culture negative was significantly longer than in the amphotericin B group. A smaller study performed at the same time showed the superiority of amphotericin B combined with flucytosine over fluconazole (Larsen *et al.*, 1990).

Later trials sought more effective therapy for cryptococcal meningitis in patients with HIV infection. Saag *et al.* (1995a) and van der Horst *et al.* (1995) reported that an initial 2-week treatment period with amphotericin B, with or without flucytosine, followed by consolidation therapy with either itraconazole or fluconazole led to markedly improved outcomes in comparison to the results noted in the earlier study by Saag *et al.* (1992). In the later study, the dosages of both fluconazole and amphotericin B were almost twice the amounts used in the prior study. This study also confirmed the benefit of flucytosine added to amphotericin B for induction therapy and the slight superiority of fluconazole over itraconazole for consolidation therapy.

Another approach used in the treatment of cryptococcal meningitis in AIDS patients is to add flucytosine to fluconazole. Larsen *et al.* (1994) found that CSF became culture negative more quickly in patients treated with 400 mg fluconazole plus 150 mg/kg daily of flucytosine than the trial that used 200 mg fluconazole as primary therapy (Saag *et al.*, 1992). Several studies have shown that fluconazole is clearly the drug of choice for maintenance therapy in preventing the relapse of cryptococcal meningitis in AIDS patients (Powderly *et al.*, 1992; Saag *et al.*, 1995b).

d. Antifungal Prophylaxis Fluconazole has become a very useful drug for prophylaxis against fungal infections in immunocompromised hosts (Reents *et al.*, 1993). Because fluconazole has no activity against *Aspergillus* species, its primary prophylactic role is prevention of *Candida* and *Cryptococcus* infections. Goodman *et al.* (1992) reported that 400 mg of fluconazole daily (as compared with placebo) significantly prevented both systemic and local *Candida* infections in patients undergoing bone marrow transplantation; Slavin *et al.* (1995) confirmed this and showed for the first time that use of prophylactic fluconazole was associated with improved survival. Neither of these studies showed a significant increase in infections with fluconazole-resistant yeast species, as noted by Wingard *et al.* (1991, 1993).

Winston *et al.* (1993) showed a significant decrease in local, but not systemic yeast infections when 400 mg fluconazole daily was compared with placebo in neutropenic patients with acute leukemia. Similarly, Schaffner and Schaffner (1995) noted that prophylaxis in neutropenic leukemics was associated with prolonged neutropenia and there was no benefit on long-term outcome. It is possible that if these latter two studies had included more patients, a significant difference from placebo might have been detected.

Among AIDS patients, fluconazole has been shown to prevent cryptococcosis and local *Candida* infections, including esophagitis, but overall mortality was not improved (Powderly *et al.*, 1995). Because of the high costs of long-term prophylaxis, the improved therapeutic regimens available for treating cryptococcal meningitis, and increasing reports of fluconazole resistance among *Candida* isolates from AIDS patients, many clinicians prefer not to use fluconazole prophylaxis in AIDS patients. However, for some patients with very low CD4 counts, some clinicians feel it is cost effective to use fluconazole prophylaxis to prevent cryptococcosis.

e. *Endemic Mycoses* Fluconazole has been studied for the treatment of histoplasmosis, blastomycosis, and sporotrichosis. All of these studies have been open-treatment trials and have generally shown fluconazole to be less efficacious than the results noted with itraconazole in prior studies (Kauffman *et al.*, 1996; Pappas *et al.*, 1995a; Diaz *et al.*, 1992; McKinsey *et al.*, 1996). For coccidioidomycosis, fluconazole has proved to be effective, but it has not been established which of the three oral azoles currently available is most efficacious (Galgiani, 1993; Catanzaro *et al.*, 1995). It is clear, however, that fluconazole has become the drug of choice for treating coccidioidal meningitis (Galgiani *et al.*, 1993; Classen *et al.*, 1988; Perez *et al.*, 1995). A minimum daily dose of 400 mg leads to a clinical response in most patients and has been shown to obviate the need for intrathecal amphotericin B (Galgiani *et al.*, 1993). However, it is also clear that fluconazole only leads to remission rather than curing the infection and thus suppressive therapy must be continued for life (Dewsnup *et al.*, 1996).

4. *Side Effects*

Side effects of fluconazole suggest that the drug is well tolerated in most patients. Gastrointestinal complaints are the most frequently reported, followed by headaches and rash (Zervos *et al.*, 1994). Transient elevations of liver function tests occur in 1–7% of patients, and fatal hepatic necrosis has been rarely reported (Jacobson *et al.*, 1994; Franklin *et al.*, 1990; Gearhart, 1994). Unlike ketoconazole, fluconazole does not inhibit testicular or adrenal steroidogenesis in healthy volunteers or in hospitalized patients (Michaelis *et al.*, 1993). Stevens–Johnson syndrome has been noted in one patient (Gussenhoven *et al.*, 1991). Reversible alopecia occurs infrequently and usually appears after several months of treatment with higher doses of fluconazole (Pappas *et al.*, 1995b). Fluconazole has been associated with several well-described cases of fetal malformations (Lee *et al.*, 1992; Pursley *et al.*, 1996) and should not be used in pregnant women.

5. *Administration*

Fluconazole is available as 50-, 100-, 150-, and 200-mg tablets; as an oral suspension, containing either 50 or 200 mg/5 ml; and as an intravenous preparation at a concentration of 2 mg/ml. Because fluconazole absorption is rapid and complete in almost all patients, fluconazole should be administered orally unless the patient is vomiting or unable to absorb oral medications. Absorption is excellent when fluconazole is administered via a feeding tube into stomach, duodenum, or jejunum (Nicolau *et al.*, 1995). The dosage of fluconazole is generally 50 to 200 mg daily (as a single dose) for minor infections. For serious systemic infections, the usual dose is 400 to 800 mg daily. Although doses greater than 800 mg have been utilized in experimental studies, they are not currently approved or recommended at this time. The dosage of fluconazole should be reduced in patients with renal insufficiency as follows: reduce by 50% in patients with a creatinine clearance of 20 to 50 ml/min; reduce the dosage by an additional 50% (i.e., reduce initial dose by 75%) in patients with a creatinine clearance less than 10 to 20 ml/min.

VI. Drug Interactions

Drug interactions with azole antifungals can generally be placed into two broad categories: (1) decreases in azole bioavailability due to chelation or secondary to increases in gastric pH and (2) interactions with other cytochrome P450-metabolized drugs. Drug interactions in the second category may result in increases or decreases in the azole antifungal, in the interacting drug, or in both drugs.

The high water solubility of fluconazole results in high bioavailability regardless of alterations in gastric pH. However, ketoconazole and itraconazole are poorly soluble except in acidic (pH <3) media (Carlson *et al.*, 1983; Cleary *et al.*, 1992). Patients with elevated gastric pH due to drugs (antacids, H2-receptor antagonists, proton-pump inhibitors, or the excipients in didanosine) or disease (AIDS patients) may not adequately absorb ketoconazole or itraconazole (Knupp *et al.*, 1993; Lake-Bakaar *et al.*, 1988; Lim *et al.*, 1993; May *et al.*, 1994; Smith *et al.*, 1992).

The simultaneous administration of sucralfate and ketoconazole (and probably itraconazole, but not fluconazole) results in a significant decrease in oral bioavailability, probably via a chelation interaction at acidic pHs. This interaction can be avoided by separation of doses by 2 hr.

The interaction of azole antifungal agents with other cytochrome P450-metabolized drugs is well recognized. The azoles appear to be metabolized almost entirely via the cytochrome P450 IIIA4 subfamily. As expected, they interact with other drugs metabolized partly or wholly via this enzyme pathway (Gillum *et al.*, 1993). Decreases in the metabolism of warfarin and cyclosporine due to the administration of intravenous miconazole result in increased plasma concentrations and toxicity of both drugs (O'Reilly *et al.*, 1992; Horton *et al.*, 1992). Although older agents such as miconazole have been poorly studied, numerous clinically significant interactions have been documented with ketoconazole, itraconazole, and fluconazole with a variety of other drugs (Tables II and III). In most cases, the azole interferes with the metabolism of the other cytochrome P450-metabolized drug.

Particularly noteworthy are the interactions between azoles and cisapride, terfenadine, astemizole, or loratidine. Cisapride, terfenadine, and astemizole are metabolized almost entirely via the cytochrome P450 IIIA4

TABLE II Effects of Concomitantly Administered Drugs on Azole Antifungal Drug Concentrations[a]

Drug affecting azole concentration	*Azole antifungal drug concentration*[b]		
	Ketoconazole	*Itraconazole*	*Fluconazole*
Alterations in cytochromes P450			
Carbamazepine	None known[c]	↓	None known
Phenytoin	↓	↓	None known
Isoniazid	↓	None known	None known
Rifampin	↓	↓	↓
Rifabutin	None known	↓	No effect[d]
Indinavir	None known	None known	No effect
Saquinavir	No effect	None known	None known
Ritonavir	None known	None known	None known
Inhibition of absorption from the gastrointestinal tract			
Sucralfate	↓	None known	No effect
Histamine 2 receptor antagonists	↓	↓	No effect
Omeprazole	↓	↓	No effect
Antacids	↓	↓	No effect
Didanosine (DDI)	None known	↓	None known

[a] Tables II and III are compiled from Alderman and Jersmann, (1993); Apseloff *et al.* (1991); Assan *et al.* (1994); Baciewicz and Baciewicz (1993); Baciewicz *et al.* (1994); Back *et al.* (1989); Back and Tjia (1991); Blum *et al.* (1991a,b); Bruzzese *et al.* (1995); Cadle *et al.* (1994); Canafax *et al.* (1991); Carver *et al.* (1994); Coker *et al.* (1990); Crane and Shih (1993); Crussell-Porter *et al.* (1993); Doble *et al.* (1988); Drayton *et al.* (1994); Ducharme, (1995); Gericke (1993); Gomez *et al.* (1995); Hardin *et al.* (1995b); Hoeschele *et al.* (1994); Honig *et al.* (1993a,b,c); Horton *et al.* (1992); Karlix *et al.* (1993); Kauffman and Bagnasco (1992); Keogh *et al.* (1995); Knupp *et al.* (1993); Kramer *et al.* (1990); Krishnaiah *et al.* (1994); Lees and Lees (1995); Lopez-Gil (1993); May *et al.* (1994); McClean and Sheehan (1994); McNulty *et al.* (1989); Mitra, (1996); Monahan *et al.* (1990); Narang *et al.* (1993, 1994); Neuvonen and Jalava (1996); Olkkola *et al.* (1994); Olkkola, (1996) Patton *et al.* (1994); Piscitelli *et al.* (1991); Pohjola-Sintonen *et al.* (1993); Rex (1992); Sachs *et al.* (1993); Seaton *et al.* (1990); Smith (1984); Sugar *et al.* (1989); Thorpe *et al.* (1990); Touchette *et al.* (1992); Trapnell *et al.* (1993); Tucker *et al.* (1992); Varhe *et al.* (1994); Varhe (1996); Vincent *et al.* (1995); von Moltke *et al.* (1994a,b,c); Wahllander and Paumgartner (1989); White *et al.* (1984); Yeh, *et al.* (1990); Zimmermann *et al.* (1992, 1994).

[b] Reductions in plasma azole concentrations have led to therapeutic failure for some fungal infections.

[c] Interaction has not been studied in human subjects; however, caution should be used in using this combination until further information is available.

[d] Drug combination has been studied in human subjects and no clinically significant pharmacokinetic or pharmacodynamic interaction was detected.

subfamily; inhibition of metabolism by azoles results in the accumulation of the cardiotoxic parent drug. Torsades de pointes and fatal arrhythmias have been described as consequences of the interactions between azoles (ketoconazole and itraconazole) and terfenadine (Crane and Shih, 1993;

TABLE III Effects of Azole Antifungal Drugs on Serum Concentrations of Concomitantly Administered Drugs

	Azole antifungal drug		
Drug affected by azole	*Ketoconazole*	*Itraconazole*	*Fluconazole*
Alterations in cytochromes P450			
Warfarin	↑[a]	↑	↑[a]
Cyclosporine	↑[a]	↑[a]	↑[a]
Phenytoin	↑[a]	None known[c]	↑[a]
Triazolam, alprazolam, midazolam	↑	↑	↑
Diltiazem	↑	None known	None known
Lovastatin	None known	↑	None known
Zidovudine	None known	None known	↑
Carbamazepine	None known	None known	↑[a]
Terfenadine	↑[b]	↑[b]	No effect[d]
Astemizole	↑[b]	↑[b]	None known
Loratidine	↑	None known	None known
Cisapride	↑[b]	↑[b]	↑
Prednisone/ Methylprednisolone	↑	None known	None known
Sulfamethoxazole	None known	None known	↑
Indinavir	↑	None known	↓
Saquinavir	None known	None known	↑
Ritonavir	↑	None known	None known
Oral hypoglycemics	↑	None known	↑
Isoniazid	↓[a]	None known	None known
Rifampin	↓[a]	None known	None known
Rifabutin	None known	None known	↑
FK 506	None known	None known	↑[a]
Quinidine	↑	None known	None known
Unknown mechanisms			
Digoxin	None known	↑[a]	None known

[a] Clinically significant interaction; serum concentrations of drug and/or clinical status of patient should be monitored.
[b] Life-threatening interaction causing arrhythmias; avoid use of combination.
[c] Interaction has not been studied in human subjects; however, caution should be used in using this combination until further information is available.
[d] Drug combination has been studied in human subjects and no clinically significant pharmacokinetic or pharmacodynamic interaction was detected.

Pohjola-Sintonen *et al.*, 1993; Zimmermann *et al.*, 1992). Although no published reports are available at this time, the manufacturer reports similar toxicities in patients receiving cisapride and itraconazole, ketoconazole, fluconazole, or miconazole (manufacturer's package insert for cisapride, September 1995). Syncope and torsades de pointes has been reported in a patient receiving erythromycin (which also inhibits cytochrome P450 IIIA4), ketoconazole, and astemizole (manufacturer's package insert for astemizole, July 1993). Honig *et al.* (1993b) reported that the addition of 200 mg oral fluconazole daily to a regimen of 60 mg terfenadine every 12 hr for 7 days did not increase concentrations of unmetabolized terfenadine, and cardiac repolarization was not significantly changed from baseline, suggesting that a clinically significant interaction is unlikely with this relatively low dosage of fluconazole. FDA "box warnings" have been added to the package inserts for terfenadine and astemizole warning clinicians of the potential for interactions with itraconazole and ketoconazole.

Currently, there are no published case reports documenting toxicities due to an interaction between loratidine and an azole antifungal agent, and the manufacturer's package insert (1995) does not contain a "box warning" for azoles. However, the package insert states that coadministration of ketoconazole and loratidine in healthy volunteers results in a 307% increase in the area under the curve (AUC) for loratidine without any clinically relevant effects on QT_c intervals. Loratidine is extensively metabolized by cytochrome P450 IIIA4 and, to a less extent, by cytochrome P450 IID6. In the presence of a cytochrome P450 IIIA4 inhibitor such as ketoconazole, loratidine is metabolized primarily by cytochrome P450 IID6. Concurrent administration of loratidine with both ketoconazole and cimetidine (which inhibits both cytochrome P450 IIIA4 and cytochrome P450 IID6) results in significantly increased plasma concentrations of loratidine (manufacturer's package insert for loratidine, 1995).

Perhaps the most prudent approach for the H1 antagonists is to follow the recommendations in the package insert "box warning" for cisapride, which cautions clinicians of the potential for interactions with all four systemically administered azoles. The lack of reported interactions between miconazole and H1 antagonists likely reflects the minimal systemic usage of this drug; it would be prudent to assume that similar interactions would occur with intravenous administration of this agent.

The interaction between ketoconazole and cyclosporine has been exploited in order to reduce drug costs associated with the administration of cyclosporine following organ transplantation (First *et al.*, 1989, 1991, 1993; Keogh *et al.*, 1995; Patton *et al.*, 1994). Relative to ketoconazole and itraconazole, fluconazole appears to be intermediate in its ability to inhibit human cytochromes P450. However, the magnitude of fluconazole-induced inhibition of cyclosporine metabolism appears to depend on the dosage of fluconazole (Lopez-Gil, 1993). As increasingly larger dosages of fluconazole are employed for the treatment of fungal infections, an increase in the number of clinically significant interactions may be expected with fluconazole and H1 antagonists, as well as other cytochrome P450-metabolized drugs.

Predictably, drugs such as rifampin, rifabutin, isoniazid, phenytoin, and carbamazepine, which are known to induce the activity of cytochromes P450, result in increased metabolism of the azole antifungals and may result in therapeutic failures (Apseloff *et al.*, 1991; Tucker *et al.*, 1992). Increased dosages of azole antifungals may be required in patients receiving these combinations of drugs.

VII. Resistance to Azoles

Resistance to azole antifungal agents has been intensively studied due in part to the increase in the number of fluconazole-resistant *Candida* strains isolated from AIDS patients. This issue has been reviewed by Rex *et al.* (1995), White and Goetz (1994), and Vanden Bossche *et al.* (1994), and is too extensive to be reviewed in detail in this chapter.

Resistance to miconazole was noted only rarely. A single case report documented resistance in a strain of *C. albicans* isolated from a patient who had received miconazole per nephrostomy tube for 2 months for chronic *Candida* urinary tract infection (Holt and Azmi, 1978).

Even though ketoconazole was used widely for the treatment of mucocutaneous candidiasis, resistant strains appeared very rarely. However, in patients with the uncommon syndrome of chronic mucocutaneous candidiasis, the chronic use of ketoconazole was associated with the emergence of ketoconazole-resistant *C. albicans* (Horsburgh and Kirkpatrick, 1983; Odds, 1993). It appears likely that resistance developed in this specific population of patients because of two factors: the chronic use of ketoconazole and the inability of patients with this syndrome to eradicate the organism by normal host defense mechanisms. The development of resistance to ketoconazole in patients on long-term therapy for chronic mucocutanenous candidiasis presaged the current problem with fluconazole-resistant *C. albicans* in patients with AIDS. These two clinical situations are similar in regard to long-term azole use and defective host immune mechanisms allowing long-term colonization with the same organism.

Fluconazole-resistant *C. albicans* have been noted almost entirely in AIDS patients and usually only after CD4 counts are $<50/\mu l$ and after fluconazole has been used chronically for repeated episodes of thrush over months to years (Sangeorzan *et al.*, 1994; White and Goetz, 1994; Rex *et al.*, 1995; Bart-Delabesse *et al.*, 1993). It appears that resistance develops in a stepwise progression in patients who have repeated episodes of thrush with one or several persisting strains of *C. albicans* (Sangeorzan *et al.*, 1994). *In vitro* susceptibility testing shows a progressive decrease in susceptibility to fluconazole, and this has been correlated with clinical failure. To date, this type of resistance has not become a problem in hospitalized patients treated with short courses of fluconazole or in those in whom fluconazole has been used for prophylaxis (Rex *et al.*, 1995).

A separate, but equally important, issue is the selection of more inherently resistant species of *Candida* in patients treated with fluconazole. It has been found among hospitalized patients that there is increasing evidence for a shift toward isolation of those species, such as *C. glabrata* and *C. krusei*, that have moderate or high-level resistance to fluconazole (Price *et al.*, 1994). This phenomenon has been especially common among patients in whom fluconazole has been used extensively (Wingard *et al.*, 1991, 1993). However, this has not been noticed in other similar units that have high rates of fluconazole utilization (Goodman *et al.*, 1992; Winston *et al.*, 1993). Although described in AIDS patients, in this population, selection of resistant species appears to be less common than development of resistance among strains of *C. albicans* (Sangeorzan *et al.*, 1994; White and Goetz, 1994; Rex *et al.*, 1995).

Resistance has not been described widely with itraconazole. This may be partly related to the fact that the drug has been used primarily for the treatment of endemic mycoses and not candidiasis. However, even in patients never treated with itraconazole, *C. albicans* strains that are resistant to fluconazole also show decreased susceptibility to itraconazole (He *et al.*, 1994; Rex *et al.*, 1995). The decrease in susceptibility is modest in comparison to the larger decreases noted with fluconazole. The relevance of decreased susceptibility to itraconazole for the treatment of clinical infections is not yet clear. In AIDS patients, a poor clinical response to itraconazole could be related to diminished absorption of the drug (Smith *et al.*, 1992), as well as increasing resistance of the organism. Decreased susceptibility to itraconazole among other species of *Candida* has also been described and appears to occur more often in AIDS patients (Tiballi *et al.*, 1995).

The most commonly reported mechanisms of azole resistance among *C. albicans* isolates include reduced permeability of the fungal cell membrane to azoles, alteration in the target fungal enzymes (cytochromes P450) resulting in decreased binding of the azole to the target site, and overproduction of the fungal cytochrome P450 enzymes (Odds, 1993; Vanden Bossche *et al.*, 1994; Hitchcock, 1993). Studies have also suggested the presence of efflux pumps capable of actively pumping azoles from the target pathogen, conferring multidrug resistance to azole antifungals (Goldway *et al.*, 1995; Sanglard *et al.*, 1995).

C. glabrata is intrinsically more resistant than *C. albicans* to ketoconazole. Several strains of *C. glabrata* have been well characterized in terms of the mechanisms of ketoconazole resistance (Hitchcock *et al.*, 1993; Vanden Bossche *et al.*, 1992). Decreased permeability to azoles has been described, but other strains show enhanced activity of the P450 cell membrane enzymes as well. *C. krusei* is inherently resistant to fluconazole, but appears to be more susceptible to the other azoles. Decreased uptake of fluconazole into the fungal cell has been noted for several *C. krusei* strains (Vanden Bossche *et al.*, 1994).

Acknowledgment

This work was supported by National Institute of Allergy and Infectious Diseases N01-AI-15082.

References

Adam, R. D., Paquin, M. L., Petersen, E. A., Saubolle, M. A., Rinaldi, M. G., Corcoran, J. G., Galgiani, J. N., and Sobonya, R. E. (1986). Phaeohyphomycosis caused by the fungal genera *Bipolaris* and *Exserohilum*. A report of 9 cases and review of the literature. *Medicine (Baltimore)* **65**, 203–217.

Akkerman, S., Lampasona, V., Dix, S., Zhang, H., Wingard, J., and Saral, R. (1993). Pharmacokinetics of fluconazole in autologous bone marrow transplant patients prior to and after the development of chemotherapy-induced mucositis. *Intersci. Conf. Antimicrob. Agents Chemother., 33rd,* New Orleans, Abstr. No. 1434.

Akler, M. E., Vellend, H., McNeely, D. M., Walmsley, S. L., and Gold, W. L. (1995). Use of fluconazole in the treatment of candidal endophthalmitis. *Clin. Infect. Dis.* **20**, 657–664.

Alderman, C. P., and Jersmann, H. P. (1993). Digoxin-itraconazole interaction (letter). *Med. J. Aust.* **159**, 838–839.

Anaissie, E., Bodey, G. P., Kantarjian, H., David, C., Barnett, K., Bow, E., de Felice, R., Downs, N., File, T., Karam, G., Potts, D., Shelton, M., and Sugar, A. (1991). Fluconazole therapy for chronic disseminated candidiasis in patients with leukemia and prior amphotericin B therapy. *Am. J. Med.* **91**, 142–150.

Anaissie, E. J., Vartivarian, S. E., Abi-said, D., Uzun, O., Pinczowski, H., Kontoyiannis, D. P., Khoury, P., Papadakis, K., Gardner, A., Raad, I. I., Gilbreath, J. and Bodey, G. P. (1996). Fluconazole versus amphotericin B in the treatment of hematogenous candidiasis: a matched cohort study. *Am. J. Med.* **101**, 170–176.

Apseloff, G., Hilligoss, D. M., Gardner, M. J., Henry, E. B., Inskeep, P. B., Gerber, N., and Lazar, J. D. (1991). Induction of fluconazole metabolism by rifampin: *In vivo* study in humans. *J. Clin. Pharmacol.* **31**, 358–361.

Arndt, C. A., Walsh, T. J., McCulley, C. L., Balis, F. M., Pizzo, P. A., and Poplack, D. G. (1988). Fluconazole penetration into cerebrospinal fluid: Implications for treating fungal infections of the central nervous system. *J. Infect. Dis.* **157**, 178–180.

Assan, R., Fredj, G., Larger, E., Feutren, G., and Bismuth, H. (1994). FK 506/fluconazole interaction enhances FK 506 nephrotoxicity. *Diabete Metab.* **20**, 49–52.

Baciewicz, A. M., and Baciewicz, F. A., Jr. (1993). Ketoconazole and fluconazole drug interactions. *Arch. Intern. Med.* **153**, 1970–1976.

Baciewicz, A. M., Menke, J. J., Bokar, J. A., and Baud, E. B. (1994). Fluconazole-warfarin interaction (letter). *Ann. Pharmacother.* **28**, 1111.

Back, D. J., and Tjia, J. F. (1991). Comparative effects of the antimycotic drugs ketoconazole, fluconazole, itraconazole and terbinafine on the metabolism of cyclosporin by human liver microsomes. *Br. J. Clin. Pharmacol.* **32**, 624–626.

Back, D. J., Stevenson, P., and Tjia, J. F. (1989). Comparative effects of two antimycotic agents, ketoconazole and terbinafine on the metabolism of tolbutamide, ethinyloestradiol, cyclosporin and ethoxycoumarin by human liver microsomes in vitro. *Br. J. Clin. Pharmacol.* **28**, 166–170.

Bagnarello, A. G., Lewis, L. A., McHenry, M. C., Weinstein, A. J., Naito, H. K., McCullough, A. J., Lederman, R. J., and Gavan, T. L. (1977). Unusual serum lipoprotein abnormality induced by the vehicle of miconazole. *N. Engl. J. Med.* **296**, 497–499.

Barbaro, G., Barbarini, G., and di Lorenzo, G. (1995). Fluconazole compared with itraconazole in the treatment of esophageal candidiasis in AIDS patients: A double-blind, randomized, controlled clinical study. *Scand. J. Infect. Dis.*, **27**, 613–617.

Barone, J. A., Koh, J. G., Bierman, R. H., Colaizzi, J. L., Swanson, K. A., Gaffar, M. C., Moskovitz, B. L., Mechlinski, W., and van de Velde, V. (1993). Food interaction and steady-state pharmacokinetics of itraconazole capsules in healthy male volunteers. *Antimicrob. Agents Chemother.* **37**, 778–784.

Bart-Delabesse, E., Boiron, P., Carlotti, A., and Dupont, B. (1993). *Candida albicans* genotyping in studies with patients with AIDS developing resistance to fluconazole. *J. Clin. Microbiol.* **31**, 2933–2937.

Bennett, J. E., and Remington, J. S. (1981). Miconazole in cryptococcosis and systemic candidiasis: A word of caution. *Ann. Intern. Med.* **94**, 708–709.

Beyer, G. P. J., and Voorhoeve-den Hartog, H. J. (1992). Day-to-day follow-up after a short oral treatment of acute vaginal candidosis with itraconazole. *Mycoses* **35**, 99–101.

Binder, R. E., Faling, J., Pugatch, R. D., Mahasaen, C., and Snider, G. L. (1982). Chronic necrotizing pulmonary aspergillosis: A discrete clinical entity. *Medicine* (*Baltimore*) **61**, 109–124.

Blatchford, N. R. (1990). Treatment of oral candidosis with itraconazole: A review. *J. Am. Acad. Dermatol.* **23**, 565–567.

Blum, R. A., D'Andrea, D. T., Florentino, B. M., Wilton, J. H., Hilligoss, D. M., Gardner, M. J., Henry, E. B., Goldstein, H., and Schentag, J. J. (1991a). Increased gastric pH and the bioavailability of fluconazole and ketoconazole. *Ann. Intern. Med.* **114**, 755–757.

Blum, R. A., Wilton, J. H., Hilligoss, D. M., Gardner, M. J., Henry, E. B., Harrison, N. J., and Schentag, J. J. (1991b). Effect of fluconazole on the disposition of phenytoin. *Clin. Pharmacol. Ther.* **49**, 420–425.

Bodey, G. P. (1992). Azole antifungal agents. *Clin. Infect. Dis.* **14**, Suppl. 1, S161–S169.

Boelaert, J., Schurgers, M., Matthys, E., Daneels, R., Van Peer, A., De Beule, K., Woestenborghs, R., and Heykants, J. (1988). Itraconazole pharmacokinetics in patients with renal dysfunction. *Antimicrob. Agents Chemother.* **32**, 1595–1597.

Bozzette, S. A., Gordon, R. L., Yen, A., Rinaldi, M., Ito, M. K., and Fierer, J. (1992). Biliary concentrations of fluconazole in a patient with candidal cholecystitis: Case report. *Clin. Infect. Dis.* **15**, 701–703.

Bradsher, R. W., Rice, D. C., and Abernathy, R. S. (1985). Ketoconazole therapy for endemic blastomycosis. *Ann. Intern. Med.* **103**, 872–879.

Brammer, K. W., Farrow, P. R., and Faulkner, J. W. (1990). Pharmacokinetics and tissue penetration of fluconazole in humans. *Rev. Infect. Dis.* **12**, Suppl. 3, S318–S326.

Brass, C., Galgiani, J. N., Blaschke, T. F., de Felice, R., O'Reilly, R. A., and Stevens, D. A. (1982). Disposition of ketoconazole, an oral antifungal, in humans. *Antimicrob. Agents Chemother.* **21**, 151–158.

Brooks, B. J., Williams, W. L., Sanders, C. V., and Marier, R. L. (1982). Apparent ketoconazole failure in candidal cholecystitis. *Arch. Intern. Med.* **142**, 1934–1935.

Brugmans, J., Van Cutsem, J., Heykants, J., Schuermans, V., and Thienpont, D. (1972). Systemic antifungal potential, safety, biotransport, and transformation of miconazole nitrate. *Eur. J. Clin. Pharmacol.* **5**, 93–99.

Bruzzese, V. L., Gillum, J. G., Israel, D. S., Johnson, G. L., Kaplowitz, L. G., and Polk, R. E. (1995). Effect of fluconazole on pharmacokinetics of 2′,3′-dideoxyinosine in persons seropositive for human immunodeficiency virus. *Antimicrob. Agents Chemother.* **39**, 1050–1053.

Budtz-Jorgensen, E., Holmstrup, P., and Krogh, P. (1988). Fluconazole in the treatment of *Candida*-associated denture stomatitis. *Antimicrob. Agents Chemother.* **32**, 1859–1863.

Cadle, R. M., Zenon, G. J., Rodriguez-Barradas, M. C., and Hamill, R. J. (1994). Fluconazole-induced symptomatic phenytoin toxicity. *Ann. Pharmacother.* **28**, 191–195.

Calhoun, D. L., Waskin, H., White, M. P., Bonner, J. R., Mulholland, J. H., Rumans, L. W., Stevens, D. A., and Galgiani, J. N. (1991). Treatment of systemic sporotrichosis with ketoconazole. *Rev. Infect. Dis.* **13,** 47–51.

Canafax, D. M., Graves, N. M., Hilligoss, D. M., Carleton, B. C., Gardner, M. J., and Matas, A. J. (1991). Interaction between cyclosporine and fluconazole in renal allograft recipients. *Transplantation* **51,** 1014–1018.

Carlson, J. A., Mann, H. J., and Canafax, D. M. (1983). Effect of pH on disintegration and dissolution of ketoconazole tablets. *Am. J. Hosp. Pharm.* **40,** 1334–1336.

Cartledge, J., Midgley, J., Youle, M., Gazzard, B. (1994). Itraconazole cyclodextrin solution—effective treatment for HIV-related candidosis unresponsive to other azole therapy. *J. Antimicrob. Chemother.* **33,** 1071–1073.

Carver, P. L., Berardi, R. R., Knapp, M. J., Rider, J. M., Kauffman, C. A., Bradley, S. F., and Atassi, M. (1994). In vivo interaction of ketoconazole and sucralfate in healthy volunteers. *Antimicrob. Agents Chemother.* **38,** 326–329.

Castiglia, M., Smego, R. A., and Sames, E. L. (1994). Candida endocarditis and amphotericin B intolerance: Potential role for fluconazole. *Infect. Dis. Clin. Pract.* **3,** 248–253.

Catanzaro, A., Einstein, H., Levine, B., Ross, J. B., Schillaci, R., Fierer, J., and Friedman, P. J. (1982). Ketoconazole for treatment of disseminated coccidioidomycosis. *Ann. Intern. Med.* **96,** 436–440.

Catanzaro, A., Galgiani, J. N., Levine, B. E., Sharkey-Mathis, P. K., Fierer, J., Stevens, D. A., Chapman, S. W., Cloud, G., and the NIAID Mycoses Study Group (1995). Fluconazole in the treatment of chronic pulmonary and nonmeningeal disseminated coccidioidomycosis. *Am. J. Med.* **98,** 249–256.

Cauwenbergh, G. (1993). Cryptococcal meningitis: The place of itraconazole. *Mycoses* **36,** 221–228.

Cheng, I. K. P., Fang, G.-X., Chan, T.-M., Chan, P. C. K., and Chan, M.-K. (1989). Fungal peritonitis complicating peritoneal dialysis: Report of 27 cases and review of treatment. *Q. J. Med.* **71,** 407–416.

Chin, T. W., Loeb, M., and Fong, I. W. (1995). Effects of an acidic beverage (Coca-Cola) on absorption of ketoconazole. *Antimicrob. Agents Chemother.* **39,** 1671–1675.

Classen, D. C., Burke, J. P., and Smith, C. B. (1988). Treatment of coccidioidal meningitis with fluconazole. *J. Infect. Dis.* **158,** 903–904.

Cleary, J. D., Taylor, J. W., and Chapman, S. W. (1992). Itraconazole in antifungal therapy. *Ann. Pharmacother.* **26,** 502–509.

Coker, R. J., Tomlinson, D. R., Parkin, J., Harris, J. R., and Pinching, A. J. (1990). Interaction between fluconazole and rifampicin. *Br. Med. J.* **301,** 818.

Como, J. A., and Dismukes, W. E. (1994). Oral azole drugs as systemic antifungal therapy. *N. Engl. J. Med.* **330,** 263–272.

Conti Diaz, I. A., Civila, E., Gezuele, E., Lowinger, M., Calegari, L., Sanabria, D., Fuentes, L., de Rosa, D., and Alzueta, G. (1992). Treatment of human cutaneous sporotrichosis with itraconazole. *Mycoses* **35,** 153–156.

Crane, J. K., and Shih, H. T. (1993). Syncope and cardiac arrhythmia due to an interaction between itraconazole and terfenadine. *Am. J. Med.* **95,** 445–446.

Craven, P. C., Graybill, J. R., Jorgensen, J. H., Dismukes, W. E., and Levine, B. E. (1983). High-dose ketoconazole for treatment of fungal infections of the central nervous system. *Ann. Intern. Med.* **98,** 160–167.

Crussell-Porter, L. L., Rindone, J. P., Ford, M. A., and Jaskar, D. W. (1993). Low-dose fluconazole therapy potentiates the hypoprothrombinemic response of warfarin sodium. *Arch. Intern. Med.* **153,** 102–104.

Czwerwiec, F. S., Bilsker, M. S., Kamerman, M. L., and Bisno, A. L. (1993). Long-term survival after fluconazole therapy of candidal prosthetic valve endocarditis. *Am. J. Med.* **94,** 545–546.

Dall, I., and Salzman, G. (1987). Treatment of pulmonary sporotrichosis with ketoconzole. *Rev. Infect. Dis.* **9**, 795–798.

Dan, M., and Priel, I. (1994). Failure of fluconazole therapy for sternal osteomyelitis due to *Candida albicans. Clin. Infect. Dis.* **18**, 126–127.

Daneshmend, T. K., and Warnock, D. W. (1988). Clinical pharmacokinetics of ketoconazole. *Clin. Pharmacokinet.* **14**, 13–34.

Daneshmend, T. K., Warnock, D. W., Ene, M. D., Johnson, E. M., Parker, G., Richardson, M. D., and Roberts, C. J. (1983). Multiple dose pharmacokinetics of ketoconazole and their effects on antipyrine kinetics in man. *J. Antimicrob. Chemother.* **12**, 185–188.

Daneshmend, T. K., Warnock, D. W., Ene, M. D., Johnson, E. M., Potten, M. R., Richardson, M. D., and Williamson, P. J. (1984). Influence of food on the pharmacokinetics of ketoconazole. *Antimicrob. Agents Chemother.* **25**, 1–3.

De Beule, K., De Doncker, P., Cauwenbergh, G., Koster, M., Legendre, R., Blatchford, N., Daunas, J., and Chwetzoff, E. (1988). The treatment of aspergillosis and aspergilloma with itraconazole, clinical results of an open international study (1982–1987). *Mycoses* **31**, 476–485.

De Beule, K., Jacqmin, P. H., Van Peer, A., Stoffels, P., and Heykants, J. (1995). The pharmacokinetic rationale behind intravenous itraconazole. *Intersci. Conf. Antimicrob. Agents Chemother. 35th,* San Francisco, Abstr. No. A75.

Debruyne, D., Ryckelynck, J.-P., Moulin, M., Hurault de Ligny, B. H., Levaltier, B., and Bigot, M. C. (1990). Pharmacokinetics of fluconazole in patients undergoing continuous ambulatory peritoneal dialysis. *Clin. Pharmacokinet.* **18**, 491–498.

de Felice, R., Galgiani, J. N., Campbell, S. C., Palpant, S. D., Friedman, B. A., Dodge, R. R., Weinberg, M. G., Lincoln, L. J., Tennican, P. O., and Barbee, R. A. (1982). Ketoconazole treatment of nonprimary coccidioidomycosis. Evaluation of 60 patients during three years of study. *Am. J. Med.* **72**, 681–687.

de Gans, J., Portegies, P., Tiessens, G., Eeftinck Schattenkerk, J. K., van Boxtel, C. J., van Ketel, R. J., and Stam, J. (1992). Itraconazole compared with amphotericin B plus flucytosine in AIDS patients with cryptococcal meningitis. *AIDS* **6**, 185–190.

del Palacio, A., Cuetara, M. S., Ferro, M., Perez-Blazquez, E., Lopez-Sana, J. A., Roiz, M. P., Carnevali, D., and Noriega, A. R. (1993). Fluconazole in the management of endophthalmitis in disseminated candidosis of heroin addicts. *Mycoses* **36**, 193–199.

Denning, D. W., and Stevens, D. A. (1990). Antifungal and surgical treatment of invasive aspergillosis: Review of 2121 published cases. *Rev. Infect. Dis.* **12**, 1147–1201.

Denning, D. W., Tucker, R. M., Hanson, L. H., Hamilton, J. R., and Stevens, D. A. (1989a). Itraconazole therapy for cryptococcal meningitis and cryptococcosis. *Arch. Intern. Med.* **149**, 2301–2308.

Denning, D. W., Tucker, R. M., Hanson, L. H., and Stevens, D. A. (1989b). Treatment of invasive aspergillosis with itraconazole. *Am. J. Med.* **86**, 791–800.

Denning, D. W., Lee, J. Y., Hostetler, J. S., Pappas, P., Kauffman, C. A., Dewsnup, D. H., Galgiani, J. N., Graybill, J. R., Sugar, A. M., Catanzaro, A., Gallis, H., Perfect, J. R., Dockery, B., Dismukes, W. E., and Stevens, D. A. (1994). NIAID Mycoses Study Group multicenter trial of oral itraconazole therapy of invasive aspergillosis. *Am. J. Med.* **97**, 135–144.

de Pauw, B. E., Raemaekers, J. M. M., Donnelly, J. P., Kullberg, B. J., and Meis, J. F. G. M. (1995). An open study on the safety and efficacy of fluconazole in the treatment of disseminated Candida infections in patients treated for hematological malignancy. *Ann. Hematol.* **70**, 83–87.

Deresinski, S. C., Lilly, R. B., Levine, H. B., Galgiani, J. N., and Stevens, D. A. (1977). Treatment of fungal meningitis with miconazole. *Arch. Intern. Med.* **137**, 1180–1185.

de Wit, S. D., Weerts, D., Goossens, H., and Clumeck, N. (1989). Comparison of fluconazole and ketoconazole for oropharyngeal candidiasis in AIDS. *Lancet* **1**, 746–748.

Dewsnup, D. H., Galgiani, J. N., Graybill, J. R., Diaz, M., Rendon, A., Cloud, G. A., and Stevens, D. A. (1996). Is it ever safe to stop azole therapy for *Coccidioides immitis* meningitis? *Ann. Intern. Med.* **124,** 305–310.

Diaz, M., Puente, R., de Hoyos, L. A., and Cruz, S. (1991). Itraconazole in the treatment of coccidioidomycosis. *Chest* **100,** 682–684.

Diaz, M., Negroni, R., Montero-Gei, F., Castro, L. G. M., Sampaio, S. A. P., Borelli, D., Restrepo, A., Franco, L., Bran, J. L., Arathoon, E. G., and Stevens, D. A. (1992). A Pan-American 5-year study of fluconazole therapy for deep mycoses in the immunocompetent host. *Clin. Infect. Dis.* **14,** Suppl. 1, S68–S76.

Dismukes, W. E., Stamm, A. M., Graybill, J. R., Craven, P. C., Stevens, D. A., Stiller, R. L., Sarosi, G. A., Medoff, G., Gregg, C. R., Gallis, H. A., Fields, B. T., Marier, R. L., Kerkering, T. A., Kaplowitz, L. G., Cloud, G., Bowles, C., and Shadomy, S. (1983). Treatment of systemic mycoses with ketoconazole: Emphasis on toxicity and clinical response in 52 patients. *Ann. Intern. Med.* **98,** 13–20.

Dismukes, W. E., and the NIAID Mycoses Study Group (1985). Treatment of blastomycosis and histoplasmosis with ketoconazole: Results of a prospective randomized clinical trial. *Ann. Intern. Med.* **103,** 861–872.

Dismukes, W. E., Bradsher, R. W., Cloud, G. C., Kauffman, C. A., Chapman, S. W., George, R. B., Stevens, D. A., Girard, W. M., Saag, M. S., Bowles-Patton, C., and the NIAID Mycoses Study Group (1992). Itraconazole therapy for blastomycosis and histoplasmosis. *Am. J. Med.* **93,** 489–497.

Dixon, D. M., Shadomy, H. J., Espinel-Ingroff, A., and Kerkering, T. M. (1978). Comparison of the *in vitro* antifungal activities of miconazole and a new imidazole, R41,400. *J. Infect. Dis.* **138,** 245–248.

Doble, N., Shaw, R., Rowland-Hill, C., Lusk, M., Warnock, D. W., and Keal, E. E. (1988). Pharmacokinetic study of the interaction between rifampin and ketoconazole. *J. Antimicrob. Chemother.* **21,** 633–635.

Drayton, J., Dickinson, G., and Rinaldi, M. G. (1994). Coadministration of rifampin and itraconazole leads to undetectable levels of serum itraconazole (letter). *Clin. Infect. Dis.* **18,** 266.

Drouhet, E., and Dupont, B. (1983). Laboratory and clinical assessment of ketoconazole in deep-seated mycoses. *Am. J. Med.* **74,** Suppl. 1B, 30–47.

Ducharme, M. P., Slaughter, R. L., Warbasse, L. H., Chandrasekar, P. H., van de Velde, V., Mannens, G., Edwards, D. J. (1995). Itraconazole and hydroxyitraconazole serum concentrations are reduced more than tenfold by phenytoin. *Clin. Pharmacol. Ther.* **58,** 617–624.

Duggan, J. M., Wolf, M. D., and Kauffman, C. A. (1995). *Phialophora verrucosa* infection in an AIDS patient. *Mycoses* **38,** 215–218.

Dupont, B. (1990). Itraconazole therapy in aspergillosis: Study in 49 patients. *J. Am. Acad. Dermatol.* **23,** 607–614.

Dupont, B., and Drouhet, E. (1988). Fluconazole in the management of oropharyngeal candidosis in a predominantly HIV antibody-positive group of patients. *J. Med. Vet. Mycol.* **26,** 67–71.

Dworzack, D. L., Clark, R. B., Borkowski, W. J., Smith, D. L., Dykstra, M., Pugsley, M. P., Horowitz, E. A., Connolly, T. L., McKinney, D. L., Hostetler, M. K., Fitzgibbons, J. F., and Galant, M. (1989). *Pseudallescheria boydii* brain abscess: Association with near-drowning and efficacy of high-dose prolonged miconazole therapy in patients with multiple abscesses. *Medicine (Baltimore)* **68,** 218–224.

Eng, R. H. K., Person, A., Mangura, C., Chmel, H., and Corrado, M. (1981). Susceptibility of zygomycetes to amphotericin B, miconazole, and ketoconazole. *Antimicrob. Agents Chemother.* **20,** 688–690.

Espinel-Ingroff, A., Shadomy, S., and Gebhart, R. J. (1984). In vitro studies with R51,211 (Itraconazole). *Antimicrob. Agents Chemother.* **26,** 5–9.

Evans, T. G., Mayer, J., Cohen, S., Classen, D., and Carroll, K. (1991). Fluconazole failure in the treatment of invasive mycoses. *J. Infect. Dis.* **164,** 1232–1235.

Fan-Havard, P., O'Donovan, C., Smith, S. M., Oh, J., Bamberger, M., and Eng, R. H. K. (1995). Oral fluconazole versus amphotericin B bladder irrigation for treatment of candidal funguria. *Clin. Infect. Dis.* **21,** 960–965.

First, M. R., Schroeder, T. J., Weiskittel, P., Myre, S. A., Alexander, J. W., and Pesce, A. J. (1989). Concomitant administration of cyclosporin and ketoconazole in renal transplant recipients. *Lancet* **2,** 1198–1201.

First, M. R., Schroeder, T. J., Alexander, J. W., Stephens, G. W., Weiskittel, P., Myre, S. A., and Pesce, A. J. (1991). Cyclosporine dose reduction by ketoconazole administration in renal transplant recipients. *Transplantation* **51,** 365–370.

First, M. R., Schroeder, T. J., Michael, A. Hariharan, S., Weiskittel, P., and Alexander, J. W. (1993). Cyclosporine-ketoconazole interaction. Long-term follow-up and preliminary results of a randomized trial. *Transplantation* **55,** 1000–1004.

Fisher, J. F., Newman, C. L., and Sobel, J. D. (1995). Yeast in the urine: Solution for a budding problem. *Clin. Infect. Dis.* **20,** 183–189.

Foulds, G., Brennan, D. R., Wajszczuk, C., Cantanzaro, A., Garg, D. C., Knopf, W., Rinaldi, M., and Weidler, D. J. (1988). Fluconazole penetration into cerebrospinal fluid in humans. *J. Clin. Pharmacol.* **28,** 363–366.

Franklin, I. M., Elias, E., and Hirsch, C. (1990). Fluconazole-induced jaundice (letter). *Lancet* **336,** 565.

Fromtling, R. A. (1988). Overview of medically important antifungal azole derivatives. *Clin. Microbiol. Rev.* **1,** 187–217.

Galgiani, J. N. (1993). Coccidioidomycosis. *West. J. Med.* **159,** 153–171.

Galgiani, J. N., Stevens, D. A., Graybill, J. R., Dismukes, W. E., Cloud, G. A., and the NIAID Mycoses Study Group (1988). Ketoconazole therapy of progressive coccidioidomycosis: Comparison of 400 and 800 mg doses and observations at higher doses. *Am. J. Med.* **84,** 603–610.

Galgiani, J. N., Catanzaro, A., Cloud, G. A., Higgs, J., Friedman, B. A., Larsen, R. A., Graybill, J. R., and the NIAID Mycoses Study Group (1993). Fluconazole therapy for coccidiodal meningitis. *Ann. Intern. Med.* **119,** 28–35.

Gearhart, M. O. (1994). Worsening of liver function with fluconazole and review of azole antifungal hepatotoxicity. *Ann. Pharmacother.* **28,** 1177–1181.

Gericke, K. R. (1993). Possible interaction between warfarin and fluconazole. *Pharmacotherapy* **13,** 508–509.

Gillum, J. G., Israel, D. S., and Polk, R. E. (1993). Pharmacokinetic drug interactions with antimicrobial agents. *Clin. Pharmacokinet.* **25,** 450–482.

Goldberg, S. L., Geha, D. J., Marshall, W. F., Inwards, D. J., and Hoagland, H. C. (1993). Successful treatment of simultaneous pulmonary *Pseudallescheria boydii* and *Aspergillus terreus* infection with oral itraconazole. *Clin. Infect. Dis.* **16,** 803–805.

Goldway, M., Teff, D., Schmidt, R., Oppenheim, A. B., and Koltin, Y. (1995). Multidrug resistance in *Candida albicans:* Disruption of the *BEN*^{R} gene. *Antimicrob. Agents Chemother.* **39,** 422–426.

Gomez, D. Y., Wacher, V. J., Tomlanovich, S. J., Hebert, M. F., and Benet, L. Z. (1995). The effects of ketoconazole on the intestinal metabolism and bioavailability of cyclosporine. *Clin. Pharmacol. Ther.* **58,** 15–19.

Goodman, J. L., Winston, D. J., Greenfield, R. A., Chandrasekar, P. H., Fox, B., Kaizer, H., Shadduck, R. K., Shea, T. C., Stiff, P., Friedman, D. J., Powderly, W. G., Silber, J. L., Horowitz, H., Lichtin, A., Wolff, S. N., Mangan, K. F., Silver, S. M., Weisdorf, D., Ho, W. G., Gilbert, G., and Buell, D. (1992). A controlled trial of fluconazole to prevent fungal infections in patients undergoing bone marrow transplantation. *N. Engl. J. Med.* **326,** 845–851.

Gradon, J. D., and Sepkowitz, D. V. (1990). Massive hepatic enlargement with fatty change associated with ketoconazole. *DICP* **24,** 1175–1176.

Graninger, W., Presteril, E., Schneeweiss, B., Teleky, B., and Georgopoulos, A. (1993). Treatment of *Candida albicans* fungaemia with fluconazole. *J. Infect.* **26,** 133–146.

Graybill, J. R., and Levine, H. B. (1978). Successful treatment of cryptococcal meningitis with intraventricular miconazole. *Arch. Intern. Med.* **138,** 814–816.

Graybill, J. R., Galgiani, J. N., Jorgensen, J. H., and Strandberg, D. A. (1983). Ketoconazole therapy for fungal urinary tract infections. *J. Urol.* **129,** 68–70.

Graybill, J. R., Stevens, D. A., Galgiani, J. N., Dismukes, W. E., Cloud, G. A., and the NIAID Mycoses Study Group (1990). Itraconazole treatment of coccidioidomycosis. *Am. J. Med.* **89,** 282–290.

Graybill, J. R., Vazquez, J., Darouiche, R. O., Morhart, R., Moskovitz, B. L., and Mallegol, I. (1995). Itraconazole oral solution versus fluconazole treatment of oropharyngeal candidiasis. *Intersci. Conf. Antimicrob. Agents Chemother., 35th,* San Francisco, Abstr. No. I220.

Groves, J. T., and Gross, Z. (1995). On the mechanism of epoxidation and hydroxylation catalyzed by iron porphyrins. Evidence for non-intersecting reaction pathways. *In* "Bioinorganic Chemistry: An Inorganic Perspective of Life" (D. P. Kessissoglou, ed.), NATO ASI Ser., pp. 39–47. Kluwer Academic Publishers, Dordrecht, The Netherlands.

Gussenhoven, M. J. E., Haak, A., Peereboom-Wynia, J. D. R., and Van't Wout, J. W. (1991). Stevens-Johnson syndrome after fluconazole. *Lancet* **338,** 120.

Hanger, D. P., Jevons, S., and Shaw, J. T. (1988). Fluconazole and testosterone: In vivo and in vitro studies. *Antimicrob. Agents Chemother.* **32,** 646–648.

Hardin, J., Lange, D., Heykants, J., Ding, C., Van De Velde, V., Slusser, C., and Klausner, M. (1995a). The effect of co-administration of a cola beverage on the bioavailability of itraconazole in AIDS patients. *Intersci. Conf. Antimicrob. Agents Chemother., 35th,* San Francisco, Abstr. No. A21.

Hardin, T. C., Graybill, J. R., Fetchick, R., Woestenborghs, R., Rinaldi, M. G., and Kuhn, J. G. (1988). Pharmacokinetics of itraconazole following oral administration to normal volunteers. *Antimicrob. Agents Chemother.* **32,** 1310–1313.

Hardin, T. C., Sharkey-Mathis, P. K., Rinaldi, M. G., and Graybill, J. R. (1995b). Evaluation of the pharmacokinetic interaction between itraconazole and didanosine in HIV-infected subjects. *Intersci. Conf. Antimicrob. Agents Chemother., 35th,* San Francisco, Abstr. No. A29.

Hay, R. J., Clayton, Y. M., Moore, M. K., and Midgley, G. (1988). An evaluation of itraconazole in the management of onychomycosis. *Br. J. Dermatol.* **119,** 359–366.

He, X., Tiballi, R. N., Zarins, L. T., Bradley, S. F., Sangeorzan, J. A., and Kauffman, C. A. (1994). Azole resistance in oropharyngeal *Candida albicans* strains isolated from patients with HIV infection. *Antimicrob. Agents Chemother.* **38,** 2495–2497.

Heel, R. C., Brogden, R. N., Pakes, G. E., Speight, T. M., and Avery, G. S. (1980). Miconazole: A preliminary review of its therapeutic efficacy in systemic fungal infections. *Drugs* **19,** 7–30.

Heel, R. C., Brogden, R. N., Carmine, A, Morley, P. A., Speight, T. M., and Avery, G. S. (1982). Ketoconazole: A review of its therapeutic efficacy in superficial and systemic fungal infections. *Drugs* **38,** 1–36.

Heykants, J., Van Peer, A., Van de Velde, V., Van Rooy, P., Meuldermans, W., Lavrijsen, K., Woestenborghs, R., Van Cutsem, J., and Cauwenbergh, G. (1989). The clinical pharmacokinetics of itraconazole: An overview. *Mycoses* **32,** Suppl. 1, 67–87.

Hitchcock, C. A. (1993). Resistance of *Candida albicans* to azole antifungal agents. *Biochem. Soc. Trans.* **21,** 1039–1047.

Hitchcock, C. A., Pye, G. W., Troke, P. F., Johnson, E. M., and Warnock, D. W. (1993). Fluconazole resistance in *Candida glabrata. Antimicrob. Agents Chemother.* **37,** 1962–1965.

Hoeprich, P., and Goldstein, E. (1974). Miconazole therapy for coccidioidomycosis. *J. Am. Med. Assoc.* **230,** 1153–1157.

Hoeschele, J. D., Roy, A. K., Pecoraro, V. L., and Carver, P. L. (1994). In vitro analysis of the interaction between sucralfate and ketoconazole. *Antimicrob. Agents Chemother.* **38,** 319–325.

Holt, R. J., and Azmi, A. (1978). Miconazole-resistant *Candida. Lancet* **1,** 50–51.

Honig, P. K., Wortham, D. C., Zamani, K., Conner, D. P., Mullin, J. C., and Cantilena, L. R. (1993a). Terfenadine-ketoconazole interaction. Pharmacokinetic and electrocardiographic consequences. *J. Am. Med. Assoc.* **269,** 1513–1518.

Honig, P. K., Wortham, D. C., Zamani, K., Mullin, J. C., Conner, D. P., and Cantilena, L. R. (1993b). The effect of fluconazole on the steady-state pharmacokinetics and electrocardiographic pharmacodynamics of terfenadine in humans. *Clin. Pharmacol. Ther.* **53,** 630–636.

Honig, P. K., Wortham, D. C., Hull, R., Zamani, K., Smith, J. E., and Cantilena, L. R. (1993c). Itraconazole affects single-dose terfenadine pharmacokinetics and cardiac repolarization pharmacodynamics. *J. Clin. Pharmacol.* **33,** 1201–1206.

Horsburgh, C. R., and Kirkpatrick, C. H. (1983). Long-term therapy of chronic mucocutaneous candidiasis and ketoconazole: experience with twenty-one patients. *Am. J. Med.* **74,** Suppl. 1B, 23–29.

Horsburgh, C. R., Jr., Cannady, P. B., Jr., and Kirkpatrick, C. H. (1983). Treatment of fungal infections in the bones and joints with ketoconazole. *J. Infect. Dis.* **147,** 1064–1069.

Horton, C. M., Freeman, C. D., Nolan, P. E., Jr., and Copeland, J. G. (1992). Cyclosporine interactions with miconazole and other azole-antimycotics: A case report and review of the literature. *J. Heart Lung Transplant.* **11,** 1127–1132.

Houang, E. T., Chappatte, O., Byrne, D., Macrae, P. V., and Thorpe, J. E. (1990). Fluconazole levels in plasma and vaginal secretions of patients after a 150-milligram single oral dose and rate of eradication of infection in vaginal candidiasis. *Antimicrob. Agents. Chemother.* **34,** 909–910.

Humphrey, M. J., Jevons, S., and Tarbit, M. H. (1985). Pharmacokinetic evaluation of UK-49,858, a metabolically stable triazole antifungal drug, in animals and humans. *Antimicrob. Agents Chemother.* **28,** 648–653.

Ikemoto, H. (1989). A clinical study of fluconazole for the treatment of deep mycoses. *Diagn. Microbiol. Infect. Dis.* **12,** 239S–247S.

Jacobs, L. G., Skidmore, E. A., Freeman, K., Lipshultz, D., and Fox, N. (1996). Oral fluconazole compared with bladder irrigation with amphotericin B for treatment of fungal urinary tract infections in elderly patients. *Clin. Infect. Dis.* **22,** 30–35.

Jacobson, M. A., Hanks, D. K., and Ferrell, L. D. (1994). Fatal hepatic necrosis due to fluconazole. *Am. J. Med.* **96,** 188–190.

Janssen, P. A. J., and Symoens, J. E. (1983). Hepatic reactions during ketoconazole treatment. *Am. J. Med.* **74,** Suppl. 1B, 80–85.

Johnson, P. C., Khardori, N., Najjar, A. F., Butt, F., Mansell, P. W. A., and Sarosi, G. A. (1988). Progressive disseminated histoplasmosis in patients with acquired immunodeficiency syndrome. *Am. J. Med.* **85,** 152–158.

Jordan, W. M., Bodey, G. P., Rodriguez, J., Ketchel, S. J., and Henney, J. (1979). Miconazole therapy for treatment of fungal infections in cancer patients. *Antimicrob. Agents Chemother.* **16,** 792–797.

Karlix, J. L., Cheng, M. A., Brunson, M. E., Ramos, E. L., Howard, R. J., Peterson, J. C., Patton, P. R., and Pfaff, W. W. (1993). Decreased cyclosporine concentrations with the addition of an H2-receptor antagonist in a patient on ketoconazole. *Transplantation* **56,** 1554–1555.

Kauffman, C. A. (1994). Newer developments in therapy for endemic mycoses. *Clin. Infect. Dis.* **19,** Suppl. 1, S28–S32.

Kauffman, C. A. (1995). Old and new therapies for sporotrichosis. *Clin. Infect. Dis.* **21**, 981–985.

Kauffman, C. A., and Bagnasco, F. A. (1992). Digoxin toxicity associated with itraconazole therapy. *Clin. Infect. Dis.* **15**, 886.

Kauffman, C. A., Bradley, S. F., Ross, S. C., and Weber, D. R. (1991). Hepatosplenic candidasis: Successful treatment with fluconazole. *Am. J. Med.* **91**, 137–141.

Kauffman, C. A., Bradley, S. F., and Vine, A. K. (1993). Candida endophthalmitis associated with intraocular lens implantation. Efficacy of fluconazole therapy. *Mycoses* **36**, 13–17.

Kauffman, C. A. (1996). Role of Azoles in antifungal therapy. *Clin. Infect. Dis.* **22**, (Suppl. 2), S148–S153.

Kauffman, C. A., Pappas, P. G., McKinsey, D. S., Greenfield, R. A., Perfect, J. R., Cloud, G. A., Thomas, C. J., Dismukes, W. E., and the NIAID Mycoses Study Group (1996). Treatment of lymphocutaneous and visceral sporotrichosis with fluconazole. *Clin. Infect. Dis.* **22**, 46–50.

Keogh, A., Spratt, P., McCosker, C., Macdonald, P., Mundy, J., and Kann, A. (1995). Ketoconazole to reduce the need for cyclosporine after cardiac transplantation. *N. Engl. J. Med.* **333**, 628–633.

Kintzel, P. E., Rollins, C. J., Yee, W. J., and List, A. F. (1995). Low itraconazole serum concentrations following administration of itraconazole suspension to critically ill allogeneic bone marrow transplant recipients. *Ann. Pharmacother.* **29**, 140–143.

Knapp, M. J., Berardi, R. R., Dressman, J. B., Rider, J. M., and Carver, P. L. (1991). Modification of gastric pH with oral glutamic acid hydrochloride. *Clin. Pharm.* **10**, 866–869.

Knupp, C. A., Brater, D. C., Relue, J., and Barbhaiya, R. H. (1993). Pharmacokinetics of didanosine and ketoconazole after coadministration to patients seropositive for the human immunodeficiency virus. *J. Clin. Pharmacol.* **33**, 912–917.

Koletar, S. L., Russell, J. A., Fass, R. J., and Plouffe, J. F. (1990). Comparison of oral fluconazole and clotrimazole troches as treatment for oral candidiasis in patients infected with human immunodeficiency virus. *Antimicrob. Agents Chemother.* **34**, 2267–2268.

Kramer, M. R., Marshall, S. E., Denning, D. W., Keogh, A. M., Tucker, R. M., Galgiani, J. N., Lewiston, N. J., Stevens, D. A., and Theodore, J. (1990). Cyclosporine and itraconazole interactions in heart and lung transplant recipients. *Ann. Intern. Med.* **113**, 327–329.

Krishnaiah, Y. S., Satyanarayana, S., and Visweswaram, D. (1994). Interaction between tolbutamide and ketoconazole in healthy subjects. *Br. J. Clin. Pharmacol.* **37**, 205–207.

Kujath, P., and Lerch, K. (1989). Secondary mycosis in surgery: Treatment with fluconazole. *Infection* **17**, 111–117.

Laine, L., Dretler, R. H., Conteas, C., Tuazon, C., Koster, F. M., Sattler, F., Squires, K., and Islam, M. Z. (1992). Fluconazole compared with ketoconazole for the treatment of *Candida* esophagitis in AIDS. A randomized trial. *Ann. Intern. Med.* **117**, 655–660.

Lake-Bakaar, G., Tom, W., Lake-Bakaar, D., Gupta, N., Beidas, S., Elsakr, M., and Straus, E. (1988). Gastropathy and ketoconazole malabsorption in the acquired immunodeficiency syndrome (AIDS). *Ann. Intern. Med.* **109**, 471–473.

Larsen, R. A., Leal, M. A. E., and Chan, L. S. (1990). Fluconazole compared with amphotericin B plus flucytosine for cryptococcal meningitis in AIDS: A randomized trial. *Ann. Intern. Med.* **113**, 183–187.

Larsen, R. A., Bozzette, S. A., Jones, B. E., Haghighat, D., Leal, M. A., Forthal, D., Bauer, M., Tilles, J. G., McCutchan, J. A., and Leedom, J. M. (1994). Fluconazole combined with flucytosine for treatment of cryptococcal meningitis in patients with AIDS. *Clin. Infect. Dis.* **19**, 741–745.

Lavrijsen, A. P. M., Balmus, K. J., Nugteren-Huying, W. M., Roldaan, A. C., Van't Wout, J. W., and Stricker, B. H. C. (1992). Hepatic injury associated with itraconazole. *Lancet* **340**, 251–252.

Lebech, P. E., and the Multicenter Study Group (1988). Treatment of vaginal candidiasis with a single dose of fluconazole. *Eur. J. Clin. Microbiol. Infect. Dis.* **7**, 364–367.

Lee, B. E., Feinberg, M., Abraham, J. J., and Murthy, A. R. K. (1992). Congenital malformation in an infant born to a woman treated with fluconazole. *Pediatr. Infect. Dis. J.* **11**, 1062–1064.

Lees, R. S., and Lees, A. M. (1995). Rhabdomyolysis from the coadministration of lovastatin and the antifungal agent itraconazole (letter). *N. Engl. J. Med.* **333**, 664–665.

Lelawongs, P., Barone, J. A., Colaizzi, J. L., Hsuan, A. T., Mechlinski, W., Legendre, R., and Guarnieri, J. (1988). Effect of food and gastric acidity on absorption of orally administered ketoconazole. *Clin. Pharm.* **7**, 228–235.

Leu, H.-S., and Huang, C.-T. (1995). Clearance of funguria with short-course antifungal regimens: A prospective randomized, controlled study. *Clin. Infect. Dis.* **20**, 1152–1157.

Lewis, J. H., Zimmerman, H. J., Benson, G. D., and Ishak, K. G. (1984). Hepatic injury associated with ketoconazole therapy. *Gastroenterology* **86**, 503–513.

Lim, S. G., Sawyeer, A. M., Hudson, M., Sercombe, J., and Pounder, R. E. (1993). Short report: The absorption of fluconazole and itraconazole under conditions of low intragastric acidity. *Aliment. Pharmacol. Ther.* **3**, 317–321.

Lopes, J. O., Alves, S. H., Benevenga, J. P., Salla, A., Khmohan, C., and Silva, C. B. (1994). Subcutaneous pseudallescheriasis in a renal transplant recipient. *Mycopathologia* **125**, 153–156.

Lopez-Gil, J. A. (1993). Fluconazole-cyclosporine interaction: a dose-dependent effect? *Ann. Pharmacother.* **27**, 427–430.

Lortholary, O., Meyohas, M.-C., Dupont B., Cadranel, J., Salmon-Ceron, D., Peyramond, D., and Simonin, D. (1993). Invasive aspergillosis in patients with acquired immunodeficiency syndrome: Report of 33 cases. *Am. J. Med.* **95**, 177–187.

Maksymiuk, A. W., Levine, H. B., and Bodey, G. P. (1982). Pharmacokinetics of ketoconazole in patients with neoplastic diseases. *Antimicrob. Agents Chemother.* **22**, 43–46.

Mannisto, P. T., Mantyla, R., Nykanen, S., Lamminsivu, U., and Ottoila, P. (1982). Impairing effect of food on ketoconazole absorption. *Antimicrob. Agents Chemother.* **21**, 730–733.

May, D. B., Drew, R. H., Yedinak, K. C., and Bartlett, J. A. (1994). Effect of simultaneous didanosine administration on itraconazole absorption in healthy volunteers. *Pharmacotherapy* **14**, 509–513.

McClean, K. L., and Sheehan, G. J. (1994). Interaction between itraconazole and digoxin (letter). *Clin. Infect. Dis.* **18**, 259–260.

McIlroy, M. A. (1991). Failure of fluconazole to suppress fungemia in a patient with fever, neutropenia, and typhlitis. *J. Infect. Dis.* **163**, 420–421.

McKinsey, D. S., Gupta, M. R., Driks, M. R., Smith, D. L., and O'Connor, M. (1992). Histoplasmosis in patients with AIDS: Efficacy of maintenance amphotericin B therapy. *Am. J. Med.* **92**, 225–227.

McKinsey, D. S., Kauffman, C. A., Pappas, P. G., Cloud, G. A., Girard, W. M., Sharkey, P. K., Hamill, R. J., Thomas, C. J., Dismukes, W. E., and the NIAID Mycoses Study Group (1996). Fluconazole therapy for histoplasmosis. *Clin. Infect. Dis.* **23**, 996–1001.

McNulty, R. M., Lazor, J. A., and Sketch, M. (1989). Transient increase in plasma quinidine concentrations during ketoconazole-quinidine therapy. *Clin. Pharm.* **8**, 222–225.

Meunier, F., Aoun, M., and Gerard, M. (1990). Therapy for oropharyngeal candidiasis in the immunocompromised host: A randomized double-blind study of fluconazole vs. ketoconazole. *Rev. Infect. Dis.* **12**, Suppl. 3, S364–S368.

Michaelis, G., Zeiler, D., Biscoping, J., Fussle, R., Hempelmann, G. (1993). Function of the adrenal cortex during therapy with fluconazole in intensive care patients. *Mycoses* **36**, 117–123.

Milatovic, D., and Voss, A. (1992). Efficacy of fluconazole in the treatment of systemic fungal infections. *Eur. J. Clin. Microbiol. Infect. Dis.* **11**, 395–402.

Milliken, S., Powles, R., Jones, A., and Helenglass, G. (1989). Pharmacokinetics of oral fluconazole in autologous bone marrow transplantation recipients given TBI and high-dose melphalan. *Transplant. Proc.* **21**, 3067.

Mitra, A. K., Thummel, K. E., Kalhorn, T. F., Kharasch, E. D., Unadkat, J. D., Slattery, J. T. (1996). Inhibition of sulfamethoxazole hydroxylamine formation by fluconazole in human liver microsomes and healthy volunteers. *Clin. Pharmacol. Ther.* **59**, 332–340.

Monahan, B. P., Ferguson, C. L., Killeavy, E. S., Lloyd, B. K., Troy, J., and Cantilena, J. R., Jr. (1990). Torsades de pointes occurring in association with terfenadine use. *J. Am. Med. Assoc.* **264**, 2788–2790.

Morris, A. B., Sands, M. L., Shiraki, M., Brown, R. B., and Ryczak, M. (1990). Gallbladder and biliary tract candidiasis: Nine cases and review. *Rev. Infect. Dis.* **12**, 483–489.

Narang, P. K., Schoenfelder, J., Lavelle, J., Trapnell, C. B., Wynne, B. A., and Bianchine, J. R. (1993). Lower incidence of MAC in AIDS patients on rifabutin prophylaxis with concomitant fluconazole. *Natl. Conf. Hum. Retroviruses Relat. Infect., 1st,* p. 106.

Narang, P. K., Trapnell, C. B., Schoenfelder, J. R., Lavelle, J. P., and Bianchine, J. R. (1994). Fluconazole and enhanced effect of rifabutin prophylaxis. *N. Engl. J. Med.* **330**, 1316–1317.

Negroni, R., Taborda, A., Robies, A. M., and Archevala, A. (1992). Itraconazole in the treatment of histoplasmosis associated with AIDS. *Mycoses* **35**, 281–287.

Neuvonen, P. J. and Jalava, K. M. (1996). Itraconazole drastically increases plasma concentrations of lovastatin and lovastatin acid. *Clin. Pharmacol. Ther.* **60**, 54–61.

Nguyen, M. H., Peacock, J. E., Tanner, D. C., Morris, A. J., Nguyen, M. L. Snydman, D. R., Wagener, M. M., Yu, V. L. (1995). Therapeutic approaches in patients with candidemia. *Arch. Intern. Med.* **155**, 2429–2435.

Nicolau, D. P., Crowe, H., Nightingale, C. H., and Quintiliani, R. (1995). Bioavailability of fluconazole administered via a feeding tube in intensive care unit patients. *J. Antimicrob. Chemother.* **36**, 395–401.

Nomura, J., and Ruskin, J. (1993). Failure of therapy with fluconazole for candidal endophthalmitis. *Clin. Infect. Dis.* **17**, 888–889.

Odds, F. C. (1993). Resistance of yeasts to azole-derivative antifungals. *J. Antimicrob. Chemother.* **31**, 463–471.

Odds, F. C., Webster, C. E., and Abbott, A. B. (1984). Antifungal relative inhibition factors: BAY1-9139, bifonazole, butoconazole, isoconazole, itraconazole (R51211), oxiconazole, Ro 14-4767/002, sulconazole, terconazole and vibunazole (BAY n-7133) compared *in vitro* with nine established antifungal agents. *J. Antimicrob. Chemother.* **14**, 105–114.

Olkkola, K. T., Backman, J. T., and Neuvonen, P. J. (1994). Midazolam should be avoided in patients receiving the systemic antimycotics ketoconazole or itraconazole. *Clin. Pharmacol. Ther.* **55**, 481–485.

Olkkola, K. T., Ahonen, J., Neuvonen, P. J. (1996). The effects of the systemic antimycotics, itraconazole and fluconazole, on the pharmacokinetics and pharmacodynamics of intravenous and oral midazolam. Anesth. Analg. **82**, 511–516.

O'Reilly, R. A., Goulart, D. A., Kunze, K. L., Neal, J., Gibaldi, M., Eddy, A. C., and Trager, W. F. (1992). Mechanisms of the stereoselective interaction between miconazole and racemic warfarin in human subjects. *Clin. Pharmacol. Ther.* **51**, 656–667.

Pappas, P. G., Bradsher, R. W., Chapman, S. W., Kauffman, C. A., Dine, A., Cloud, G. A., Dismukes, W. E., and the NIAID Mycoses Study Group (1995a). Treatment of blastomycosis with fluconazole. A pilot study. *Clin. Infect. Dis.* **20**, 267–271.

Pappas, P. G., Kauffman, C. A., Perfect, J., Johnson, P. C., McKinsey, D. S., Bamberger, D. M., Hamill, R., Sharkey, P. K., Chapman, W. S., and Sobel, J. D. (1995b). Alopecia associated with fluconazole therapy. *Ann. Intern. Med.* **123**, 354–357.

Patterson, T. F., Andriole, V. T., Zervos, M. J., and Kauffman, C. A. (1990). The epidemiology of pseudallescheriasis complicating transplantation: Nosocomial and community-acquired infection. *Mycoses* **33**, 297–302.

Patton, P. R., Brunson, M. E., Pfaff, W. W., Howard, R. J., Peterson, J. C., Ramos, E. L., and Karlix, J. L. (1994). A preliminary report of diltiazem and ketoconazole. Their cyclosporine-sparing effect and impact on transplant outcome. *Transplantation* **57,** 889–892.

Perez, J. A., Johnson, R. H., Caldwell, J. W., Arsura, E. L., and Nemecheck, P. (1995). Fluconazole therapy in coccidioidal meningitis maintained with intrathecal amphotericin B. *Arch. Intern. Med.* **155,** 1665–1668.

Perfect, J., and Durack, D. T. (1985). Penetration of imidazoles and triazoles into cerebrospinal fluid of rabbits. *J. Antimicrob. Chemother.* **16,** 81–86.

Petersen, E. A., Alling, D. W., and Kirkpatrick, C. H. (1980). Treatment of chronic mucocutaneous candidiasis with ketoconazole. A controlled clinical trial. *Ann. Intern. Med.* **93,** 791–795.

Phillips, P., Shafran, S., Garber, G., Rotstein, C., Smaill, F., Williams, K., Singer, J., Ioannou, S., and the Canadian Candidemia Study Group (1995). Fluconazole versus amphotericin B for candidemia in non-neutropenic patients: A multicenter randomized trial. *Intersci. Conf. Antimicrob. Agents Chemother., 35th.* San Francisco, Abstr. No. LM20.

Piepponen, T., Blomqvist, K., Brandt, H., Havu, V., Hollmen, A., Kohtamäki, K., Lehtonen, L., and Turjanmaa, K. (1992). Efficacy and safety of itraconazole in the long-term treatment of onychomycosis. *J. Antimicrob. Chemother.* **29,** 195–205.

Piper, J. P., Golden, J., Brown, D., and Broestler, J. (1990). Successful treatment of *Scedosporium apiospermum* suppurative arthritis with itraconazole. *Pediatr. Infect. Dis. J.* **9,** 674–675.

Piscitelli, S. C., Goss, T. F., Wilton, J. H., D'Andrea, D. T., Goldstein, H., and Schentag, J. J. (1991). Effects of ranitidine and sucralfate on ketoconazole bioavailability. *Antimicrob. Agents Chemother.* **35,** 1765–1771.

Pluss, J. L., and Opal, S. M. (1986). Pulmonary sporotrichosis: Review of treatment and outcome. *Medicine (Baltimore)* **65,** 143–153.

Pohjola-Sintonen, S., Viitasalo, M., Toivonen, L., and Neuvonen, P. (1993). Itraconazole prevents terfenadine metabolism and increases risk of torsades de pointes ventricular tachycardia. *Eur. J. Clin. Pharmacol.* **45,** 191–193.

Pont, A., Williams, P. L., Loose, D. S., Feldman D., Reitz, R. E., Bochra, C., and Stevens, D. A. (1982a). Ketoconazole inhibits adrenal steroid synthesis. *Ann. Intern. Med.* **97,** 370–372.

Pont, A., Williams, P. L., Azhar, S., Reitz, R. E., Bochra, C., Smith, E. R., and Stevens, D. A. (1982b). Ketoconazole blocks testosterone synthesis. *Arch. Intern. Med.* **142,** 2137–2140.

Pont, A., Graybill, J. R., Craven, P. C., Galgiani, J. N., Dismukes, W. E., Reitz, R. E., and Stevens, D. A. (1984). High-dose ketoconazole therapy and adrenal and testicular function in humans. *Arch. Intern. Med.* **144,** 2150–2153.

Powderly, W. G., Saag, M. S., Cloud, G. A., Robinson, P., Meyer, R. D., Jacobson, J. M., Graybill, J. R., Sugar, A. M., McAuliffe, V. J., Follansbee, S. E., Tuazon, C. U., Stern, J. J., Feinberg, J., Hafner, R., Dismukes, W. E., the NIAIDS AIDS Clinical Trials Group, and the NIAID Mycoses Study Group (1992). A controlled trial of fluconazole or amphotericin B to prevent relapse of cryptococcal meningitis in patients with the acquired immunodeficiency syndrome. *N. Engl. J. Med.* **326,** 793–798.

Powderly, W. G., Finkelstein, D. M., Feinberg, J., Frame, P., He, W., van der Horst, C., Koletar, S. L., Eyster, M. E., Carey, J., Waskin, H., Hooton, T. M., Hyslop, N., Spector, S. A., Bozzette, S. A., and the NIAIDS AIDS Clinical Trials Group (1995). A randomized trial comparing fluconazole with clotrimazole troches for the prevention of fungal infections in patients with advanced human immunodeficiency virus infection. *N. Engl. J. Med.* **332,** 700–705.

Prentice, A. G., Warnock, D. W., Johnson, S. A., Phillips, M. J., and Oliver, D. A. (1994). Multiple dose pharmacokinetics of an oral solution of itraconazole in autologous bone marrow transplant recipients. *J. Antimicrob. Chemother.* **34,** 247–252.

Price, M. F., LaRocco, M. T., and Gentry, L. O. (1994). Fluconazole susceptibilities of *Candida* species and distribution of species recovered from blood cultures over a 5-year period. *Antimicrob. Agents Chemother.* **38,** 1422–1424.

Pursley, T. J., Blomquist, I. K., Abraham, J., Andersen, H. F., and Bartley, J. A. (1996). Fluconazole-induced congenital anomalies in three infants. *Clin. Infect. Dis.* **22,** 336–340.

Reents, S., Goodwin, S. D., and Singh, V. (1993). Antifungal prophylaxis in immunocompromised patients. *Ann. Pharmacother.* **27,** 53–60.

Restrepo, A., Robledo, J., Gomez, I., Tabares, A. M., and Gutierrez, R. (1986). Itraconazole therapy in lymphagitic and cutaneous sporotrichosis. *Arch. Dermatol.* **122,** 413–417.

Rex, J. (1992). Itraconazole-digoxin interaction. *Ann. Intern. Med.* **116,** 525.

Rex, J., Rinaldi, M. G., and Pfaller, M. A. (1995). Resistance of *Candida* species to fluconazole. *Antimicrob. Agents Chemother.* **39,** 1–8.

Rex, J. H., Bennett, J. E., Sugar, A. M., Pappas, P. G., van der Horst, C. M., Edwards, J. E., Washburn, R. G., Scheld, W. M., Karchmer, A. W., Dine, A. P., Levenstein, M. J., and Webb, C. D. (1994). A randomized trial comparing fluconazole with amphotericin B for the treatment of candidemia in patients without neutropenia. *N. Engl. J. Med.* **331,** 1325–1330.

Rezabek, G. H., and Friedman, A. D. (1992). Superficial fungal infections of the skin. Diagnosis and current treatment recommendations. *Drugs* **43,** 674–682.

Rogers, T. E., and Galgiani, J. N. (1986). Activity of fluconazole (UK 49,858) and ketoconazole against *Candida albicans* in vitro and in vivo. *Antimicrob. Agents Chemother.* **30,** 418–422.

Rose, H. D., and Varkey, B. (1978). Miconazole treatment of relapsed pulmonary blastomycosis. *Am. Rev. Respir. Dis.* **118,** 403–408.

Ross, J. B., Levine, B., Catanzaro, A., Einstein, H., Schillaci, R., and Friedman, P. J. (1982). Ketoconazole for treatment of chronic pulmonary coccidioidomycosis. *Ann. Intern. Med.* **96,** 440–443.

Saag, M. S., and Dismukes, W. E. (1988). Azole antifungal agents: Emphasis on new triazoles. *Antimicrob. Agents Chemother.* **32,** 1–8.

Saag, M. S., Powderly, W. G., Cloud, G. A., Robinson, P., Grieco, M. H., Sharkey, P. K., Thompson, S. E., Sugar, A. M., Tuazon, C. U., Fisher, J. F., Hyslop, N., Jacobson, J. M., Hafner, R., Dismukes, W. E., the NIAID Mycoses Study Group, and the AIDS Clinical Trials Group (1992). Comparison of amphotericin B with fluconazole in the treatment of acute AIDS-associated cryptococcal meningitis. *N. Engl. J. Med.* **326,** 83–89.

Saag, M., van der Horst, C., Cloud, G., Hamill, R., Graybill, R., Sobel, J., Johnson, P., Tuazon, C., Kerkering, T., Fisher, J., Henderson, H., Stansell, J., Mildvan, D., Riser, L., Schneider, D., Hafner, R., Thomas, C., Weisinger, B., Moskovitz, B., the NIAID AIDS Clinical Trials Group, and the Mycoses Study Group (1995a). (Part 2) Randomized double blind comparison of amphotericin B plus flucytosine to amphotericin B alone (Step 1) followed by a comparison of fluconazole to itraconazole (Step 2) in the treatment of cryptococcal meningitis in patients with AIDS. *Intersci. Conf. Antimicrob. Agents Chemother. 35th,* San Francisco, Abstr. No. I217.

Saag, M., Cloud, G. C., Graybill, R., Sobel, J., Tuazon, C., Wiesinger, B., Riser, L., Moskovitz, B. L., Dismukes, W. E., and the NIAID Mycoses Study Group (1995b). Camparison of fluconazole vs. itraconazole as maintenance therapy of AIDS-associated cryptococal meningitis. *Intersci. Conf. Antimicrob. Agents Chemother. 35th,* San Francisco, Abstr. No. I218.

Sachs, M. K., Blanchard, L. M., and Green, P. J. (1993). Interaction of itraconazole and digoxin. *Clin. Infect. Dis.* **16,** 400–403.

Sangeorzan, J. A., Bradley, S. F., He, X., Zarins, L. T., Ridenour, G. L., Tiballi, R. N., and Kauffman, C. A. (1994). Epidemiology of oral candidiasis in HIV infected patients: Colonization, infection, treatment, and emergence of fluconazole resistance. *Am. J. Med.* **97,** 339–347.

Sanglard, D., Kuchler, K., Ischer, F., Pagani, J. L., Monod, M., Bille, J. (1995) Mechanisms of resistance to azole antifungal agents in *Candida albicans* isolates from AIDS patients involve specific multidrug transporters. *Antimicrob. Agents Chemother.* **39,** 2378–2386.

Schaffner, A., and Schaffner, M. (1995). Effect of prophylactic fluconazole on the frequency of fungal infections, amphotericin B use, and health care costs in patients undergoing intensive chemotherapy for hematologic neoplasias. *J. Infect. Dis.* **172,** 1035–1041.

Schenkman, J. B., Remmer, H., and Estabrook, R. W. (1967). Spectral studies of drug interaction with hepatic microsomal cytochrome. *Mol. Pharmacol.* **3,** 113–123.

Seaton, T. L., Celum, C. L., and Black, D. L. (1990). Possible potentiation of warfarin by fluconazole. *DICP* **24,** 1777–1778.

Shadomy, S., Paxton, L., Espinel-Ingroff, A., and Shadomy, J. (1977). *In vitro* studies with miconazole and miconazole nitrate. *J. Antimicrob. Chemother.* **3,** 147–152.

Shadomy, S., White, S. C., Yu, H. P., Dismukes, W. E., and the NIAID Mycoses Study Group (1985). Treatment of systemic mycoses with ketoconazole: In vitro susceptibilities of clinical isolates of systemic and pathogenic fungi to ketoconazole. *J. Infect. Dis.* **152,** 1249–1256.

Sharkey, P. K., Graybill, J. R., Rinaldi, M. G., Stevens, D. A., Tucker, R. M., Peterie, J. D., Hoeprich, P. D., Greer, D. L., Frenkel, L., Counts, G. W., Goodrich, J., Zellner, S., Bradsher, R. W., van der Horst, C. M., Israel, K., Pankey, G. W., and Barranco, C. P. (1990). Itraconazole treatment of phaeohyphomycosis. *J. Am. Acad. Dermatol.* **23,** 577–586.

Sharkey, P. K., Rinaldi, M. G., Dunn, J. F., Hardin, T. C., Fetchick, R. J., and Graybill, J. R. (1991). High-dose itraconazole in the treatment of the severe mycoses. *Antimicrob. Agents Chemother.* **35,** 707–713.

Sharkey-Mathis, P. K., Kauffman, C. A., Graybill, J. R., Stevens, D. A., Hostetler, J. S., Cloud, G., Dismukes, W. E., and the NIAID Mycoses Study Group (1993). Treatment of sporotrichosis with itraconazole. *Am. J. Med.* **95,** 279–285.

Slavin, M. A., Osborne, B., Adams, R., Levenstein, M. J., Schoch, H. G., Feldman, A. R., Meyers, J. D., and Bowden, R. A. (1995). Efficacy and safety of fluconazole prophylaxis for fungal infections after marrow transplantation—a prospective, randomized, double-blind study. *Clin. Infect. Dis.* **171,** 1545–1552.

Smith, A. G. (1984). Potentiation of oral anticoagulants by ketoconazole. *Br. Med. J.* **288,** 188–189.

Smith, D. E., Midgley, J., Allan, M., Connolly, G. M., and Gazzard, B. G. (1991). Itraconazole versus ketoconazole in the treatment of oral and oesophageal candidosis in patients infected with HIV. *AIDS* **5,** 1367–1371.

Smith, D. E., Van de Velde, V., Woestenborghs, R., and Gazzard, B. G. (1992). The pharmacokinetics of oral itraconazole in AIDS patients. *J. Pharm. Pharmacol.* **44,** 618–619.

Sobel, J. D. (1986). Recurrent vulvovaginal candidiasis. A prospective study of the efficacy of maintenance ketoconazole therapy. *N. Engl. J. Med.* **315,** 1455–1458.

Sobel, J. D. (1993). Candidal vulvovaginitis. *Clin. Obstet. Gynecol.* **36,** 153–165.

Stein, G. E., and Mummaw, N. (1993). Placebo-controlled trial of itraconazole for treatment of acute vaginal candidiasis. *Antimicrob. Agents Chemother.* **36,** 89–92.

Stevens, D. A. (1977). Miconazole in the treatment of systemic fungal infections. *Am. Rev. Respir. Dis.* **116,** 801–806.

Stevens, D. A. (1995). Coccidioidomycosis. *N. Engl. J. Med.* **332,** 1077–1092.

Stevens, D. A., Levine, H. B., and Deresinski, S. C. (1976). Miconazole in coccididioidomycosis. II. Therapeutic and pharmacologic studies in man. *Am. J. Med.* **60,** 191–202.

Sugar, A. M., Saunders, C., Idelson, B. A., and Bernard, D. B. (1989). Interaction of fluconazole and cyclosporine. *Ann. Intern. Med.* **110,** 844.

Symoens, J., Moens, M., Dom, J., Scheijgrond, H., Dony, J., Schuermans, V., Legendre, R., and Finestine, N. (1980). An evaluation of two years of clinical experience with ketoconazole. *Rev. Infect. Dis.* **2,** 674–687.

Tarbit, M. H., Robertson, W. R., and Lambert, A. (1990). Hepatic and endocrine effects of azole antifungal agents. *In* "Chemotherapy of Fungal Diseases" (J. F. Ryley, ed.), pp. 205–229. Springer-Verlag, New York.

Tett, S., Moore, S., and Ray, J. (1995). Pharmacokinetics and bioavailability of fluconazole in two groups of males with human immunodeficiency virus (HIV) infection compared with those in a group of males without HIV infection. *Antimicrob. Agents Chemother.* **39,** 1835–1841.

Thaler, F., Bernard, B., Tod, M., Jedynak, C. P., Petitjean, D., Derome, P., and Loirat, P. (1995). Fluconazole penetration in cerebral parenchyma in humans at steady state. *Antimicrob. Agents Chemother.* **39,** 1154–1156.

Thorpe, J. E., Baker, N., and Bromet-Petit, M. (1990). Effect of oral antacid administration on the pharmacokinetics of oral fluconazole. *Antimicrob. Agents Chemother.* **34,** 2032–2033.

Tiballi, R. N., Zarins, L. T., He, X., and Kauffman, C. A. (1995). *Torulopsis glabrata:* Azole susceptibilities by microdilution colorimetric and macrodilution broth assays. *J. Clin. Microbiol.* **33,** 2612–2615.

Tobin, J. M., Loo, P., and Granger, S. E. (1992). Treatment of vaginal candidosis: A comparative study of the efficacy and acceptability of itraconazole and clotrimazole. *Genitourin. Med.* **68,** 36–38.

Toon, S., Ross, C. E., Gokal, R., and Rowland, M. (1990). An assessment of the effects of impaired renal function and haemodialysis on the pharmacokinetics of fluconazole. *Br. J. Clin. Pharmacol.* **29,** 221–226.

Touchette, M. A., Chandrasekar, P. H., Milad, M. A., and Edwards, D. J. (1992). Contrasting effects of fluconazole and ketoconazole on phenytoin and testosterone disposition in man. *Br. J. Clin. Pharmacol.* **34,** 75–78.

Trapnell, C. B., Narang, P. K., Li, R., Lewis, R., Colborn, D., and Lavelle, J. (1993). Fluconazole increases rifabutin absorption in HIV (+) patients on stable zidovudine therapy. *Int. Conf. AIDS* **9,** 504 (Abstr. No. PO-B31–2212).

Tucker, R. M., Williams, P. L., Arathoon, E. G., Levine, B. E., Hartstein, A. I., Hanson, L. H., and Stevens, D. A. (1988). Pharmacokinetics of fluconazole in cerebrospinal fluid and serum in human coccidioidal meningitis. *Antimicrob. Agents Chemother.* **32,** 369–373.

Tucker, R. M., Denning, D. W., Arathoon, E. G., Rinaldi, M. G., and Stevens, D. A. (1990a). Itraconazole therapy for nonmeningeal coccidioidomycosis: Clinical and laboratory observations. *J. Am. Acad. Dermatol.* **23,** 593–601.

Tucker, R. M., Denning, D. W., Dupont, B., and Stevens, D. A. (1990b). Itraconazole therapy for chronic coccidioidal meningitis. *Ann. Intern. Med.* **112,** 108–112.

Tucker, R. M., Haq, Y., Denning, D. W., and Stevens, D. A. (1990c). Adverse events associated with itraconazole in 189 patients on chronic therapy. *J. Antimicrob. Chemother.* **26,** 561–566.

Tucker, R. M., Denning, D. W., Hanson, L. H., Rinaldi, M. G., Graybill, J. R., Sharkey, P. K., Pappagianis, D., and Stevens, D. A. (1992). Interaction of azoles with rifampin, phenytoin, and carbamazepine: In vitro and clinical observations. *Clin. Infect. Dis.* **14,** 165–174.

Tucker, W. S., Snell B. B., Island, D. P., and Gregg, C. R. (1985). Reversible adrenal insufficiency induced by ketoconazole. *J. Am. Med. Assoc.* **253,** 2413–2414.

Tunkel, A. R., Thomas, C. Y., and Wispelway, B. (1993). Candida prosthetic arthritis: Report of a case treated with fluconazole and review of the literature. *Am. J. Med.* **94,** 100–103.

Uno, J., Shigematsu, M. L., and Arai, T. (1982). Primary site of action of ketoconazole on *Candida albicans. Antimicrob. Agents Chemother.* **21,** 912–918.

Vanden Bossche, H. (1987). Itraconazole: A selective inhibitor of the cytochrome P-450 dependent ergosterol biosynthesis. *In* "Recent Trends in the Discovery, Development and Evaluation of Antifungal Agents" (R. A. Fromtling, ed.), pp. 207–221. J. R. Prous, Barcelona.

Vanden Bossche, H., Marichal, P., Odds, F., Lejeune, L., and Coene, M. C. (1992). Characterization of an azole-resistant *Candida glabrata* isolate. *Antimicrob. Agents. Chemother.* **36,** 2602–2610.

Vanden Bossche, H., Warnock, D. W., Dupont, B., Kerridge, D., Gupta, S. S., Improvisi, L., Marichal, P., Odds, F. C., Provost, F., and Ronin, O. (1994). Mechanisms and clinical impact of antifungal drug resistance. *J. Med. Vet. Mycol.* **32,** 189–202.

van der Horst, C., Saag, M., Cloud, G., Hamill, R., Graybill, R., Sobel, J., Johnson, P., Tuazon, C., Kerkering, T., Fisher, J., Henderson, H., Stansell, J., Mildvan, D., Riser, L., Schneider, D., Hafner, R., Thomas C., Weisinger, B., Moskovitz, B., The NIAID AIDS Clinical Trials Group, and the Mycoses Study Group (1995). (Part 1) Randomized double blind comparison of amphotericin B plus flucytosine to amphotericin B alone (Step 1) followed by a comparison of fluconazole to itraconazole (Step 2) in the treatment of cryptococcal meningitis in patients with AIDS. *Intersc. Conf. Antimicrob. Agents Chemother., 35th,* San Francisco, Abstr. No. I216.

Varhe, A., Olkkola, K. T., and Neuvonen, P. J. (1994). Oral triazolam is potentially hazardous to patients receiving systemic antimycotics ketoconazole or itraconazole. *Clin. Pharmacol. Ther.* **56,** 601–607.

Varhe, A., Olkkola, K. T., and Neuvonen, P. J. (1996). Fluconazole, but not terbinafine, enhances the effects of triazolam by inhibiting its metabolism. *Br. J. Clin. Pharmacol.* **41,** 319–323.

Vincent, I., Furlan, V., Debray, D., Jacquemin, E., and Taburet, A. M. (1995). Effects of antifungal agents on the pharmacokinetics and nephrotoxicity of FK506 in paediatric liver transplant recipients. *Intersc. Conf. Antimicrob. Agents Chemother., 35th,* San Francisco, Abstr. No. A24.

Viscoli, C., Castagnola, E., Fioredda, F., Ciravegna, B., Barigione, G., and Terragna, A. (1991). Fluconazole in the treatment of candidiasis in immunocompromised children. *Antimicrob. Agents Chemother.* **35,** 365–367.

Viviani, M. A., Tortorano, A. M., Pagano, A., Vigevani, G. M., Gubertini, G., Cristina, S., Assaisso, M. L., Suter, F., Farina, C., Minetti, R., Faggian, G., Caretta, M., Di Fabrizio, N., and Vaglia, A. (1991). European experience with itraconazole in systemic mycoses. *J. Am. Acad. Dermatol.* **23,** 587–593.

Voice, R. A., Bradley, S. F., Sangeorzan, J. A., and Kauffman, C. A. (1994). Chronic candidal meningitis: An uncommon manifestation of candidiasis. *Clin. Infect. Dis.* **19,** 60–66.

von Moltke, L. L., Greenblatt, D. J., Cotreau-Bibbo, M. M., Harmatz, J. S., and Shader, R. I. (1994a). Inhibitors of alprazolam metabolism in vitro: Effect of serotonin-reuptake-inhibitor antidepressants, ketoconazole and quinidine. *Br. J. Clin. Pharmacol.* **38,** 23–31.

von Moltke, L. L., Greenblatt, D. J., Duan, S. X., Harmatz, J. S., and Shader, R. I. (1994b). In vitro prediction of the terfenadine-ketoconazole pharmacokinetic interaction. *J. Clin. Pharmacol.* **34,** 1222–1227.

von Moltke, L. L., Greenblatt, D. J., Cotreau-Bibbo, M. M., Duan, S. X., Harmatz, J. S., and Shader, R. I. (1994c). Inhibition of desipramine hydroxylation in vitro by serotonin-reuptake-inhibitor antidepressants, and by quinidine and ketoconazole: A model system to predict drug interactions in vivo. *J. Pharmacol. Exp. Ther.* **268,** 1278–1283.

Voss, A., Meis, J. F. G. M., and Hoogkamp-Korstanje, J. A. A. (1994). Fluconazole in the management of fungal urinary tract infection. *Infection* **22,** 247–251.

Vu Van, H., Piens, M. A., Archimbaud, E., Monier, M. F., Guyotat, D., Mojon, M., and Fiere, D. (1983). Serum levels of ketoconazole in bone marrow transplanted patients. *Nouv. Rev. Fr. Hematol.* **25,** 241–244.

Wahllander, A., and Paumgartner, G. (1989). Effect of ketoconazole and terbinafine on the pharmacokinetics of caffeine in healthy volunteers. *Eur. J. Clin. Pharmacol.* **37,** 79–83.

Wallbridge, D. R., McCartney, A. C., and Richardson, M. D. (1993). Fluconazole in the treatment of *Candida* prosthetic valve endocarditis. *Mycoses* **36,** 259–261.

Walsh, T. J., Foulds, G., and Pizzo, P. A. (1989). Pharmacokinetics and tissue penetration of fluconazole in rabbits. *Antimicrob. Agents Chemother.* **33,** 467–469.

Walsh, T. J., Peter, J., McGough, D. A., Fothergill, A. W., Rinaldi, M. G., and Pizzo, P. A. (1995). Activities of amphotericin B and antifungal azoles alone and in combination against *Pseudallescheria boydii. Antimicrob. Agents Chemother.* **39,** 1361–1364.

Weinstein, L., and Jacoby, I. (1980). Successful treatment of cerebral cryptococcoma and meningitis with miconazole. *Ann. Intern. Med.* **93,** 569–571.

Wheat, L. J., Connolly-Stringfield, P. A., Baker, R. L., Curfman, M. F., Eads, M. E., Israel, K. S., Norris, S. A., Webb, D. H., and Zeckel, M. L. (1990). Disseminated histoplasmosis in the acquired immune deficiency syndrome: Clinical findings, diagnosis and treatment, and review of the literature. *Medicine (Baltimore)* **69**, 361–374.

Wheat, L. J., Hafner, R., Wulfsohn, M., Spencer, P., Squires, K., Powderly, W., Wong, B., Rinaldi, M., Saag, M., Hamill, R., Murphy, R., Connolly-Stringfield, P., Briggs, N., Owens, S., and the NIAID Mycoses Study Group (1993). Prevention of relapse of histoplasmosis with itraconazole in patients with acquired immunodeficiency syndrome. *Ann. Intern. Med.* **118**, 610–616.

Wheat, J., Hafner, R., Korzun, A. H., Limjoco, M. T., Spencer P., Larsen, R. A., Hecht, F. M., Powderly, W., and the AIDS Clinical Trials Group (1995). Itraconazole treatment of disseminated histoplasmosis in patients with the acquired immunodeficiency syndrome. *Am. J. Med.* **98**, 336–342.

White, A., and Goetz, M. B. (1994). Azole-resistant *Candida albicans:* Report of two cases of resistance to fluconazole and review. *Clin. Infect. Dis.* **19**, 687–692.

White, A., and Goetz, M. B. (1995). *Candida parapsilosis* prosthetic joint infection unresponsive to treatment with fluconazole. *Clin. Infect. Dis.* **20**, 1068– 1069.

White, D. J., Blatchford, N. R., and Cauwenbergh, G. (1984). Cyclosporine and ketoconazole. *Transplantation* **37**, 214–215.

Whittle, D. I., and Kominos, S. (1995). Use of itraconazole for treating subcutaneous phaeohyphomycosis caused by *Exophiala jeanselmei. Clin. Infect. Dis.* **21**, 1068.

Wingard, J. R., Merz, W. G., Rinaldi, M. G., Johnson, T. R., Karp, J. E., and Saral, R. (1991). Increase in *Candida krusei* infection among patients with bone marrow transplantation and neutropenia treated prophylactically with fluconazole. *N. Engl. J. Med.* **325**, 1274–1277.

Wingard, J. R., Merz, W. G., Rinaldi, M. G., Miller, C. B., Karp, J. E., and Saral, R. (1993). Association of *Torulopsis glabrata* infections with fluconazole prophylaxis in neutropenic bone marrow transplant patients. *Antimicrob. Agents Chemother.* **37**, 1847–1849.

Winn, R. E., Anderson, J., Piper, J., Aronson, N. E., and Pluss, J. (1993). Systemic sporotrichosis treated with itraconazole. *Clin. Infect. Dis.* **17**, 210–217.

Winston, D. J. Chandrasekar, P. H., Lazarus, H. M., Goodman, J. L., Silber, J. L., Horowitz, H., Shadduck, R. K., Rosenfeld, C. S., Ho., W. G., Islam, M. Z., and Buell, D. N. (1993). Fluconazole prophylaxis of fungal infections in patients with acute leukemia: Results of a randomized placebo-controlled, double-blind, multicenter trial. *Ann. Intern. Med.* **118**, 495–503.

Wise, G. J., Goldman, W. M., Goldberg, P. E., and Rothenberg, R. G. (1987). Miconazole: A cost-effective antifungal genitourinary irrigant. *J. Urol.* **138**, 1413–1415.

Yeh, J., Soo, S. C., Summerton, C., Richardson, C. (1990). Potentiation of action of warfarin by itraconazole. *Br. Med. J.* **301**, 669.

Yu, R. (1995). Successful treatment of chromoblastomycosis with itraconazole. *Mycoses* **38**, 79–83.

Zervos, M., Silverman, J., and Meunier, F. (1994). Fluconazole in fungal infection: A review. *Infect. Dis. Clin. Pract.* **3**, 94–101.

Zimmermann, M., Duruz, H., Guinand, O., Broccard, O., Levy, P., Lacatis, D., and Bloch, A. (1992). Torsades de Pointes after treatment with terfenadine and ketoconazole. *Eur. Heart J.* **13**, 1002–1003.

Zimmermann, T., Yeates, R. A., Riedel, K. D., Lach, P., and Laufen, H. (1994). The influence of gastric pH on the pharmacokinetics of fluconazole: The effect of omeprazole. *Int. J. Clin. Pharmacol. Ther.* **32**, 491–496.

Zuckerman, J. M., and Tunkel, A. R. (1994). Itraconazole: A new triazole antifungal agent. *Infect. Control Hosp. Epidemiol.* **15**, 397–410.

Lorna M. Colquhoun
James W. Patrick

Division of Neuroscience
Baylor College of Medicine
Houston, Texas 77030

Pharmacology of Neuronal Nicotinic Acetylcholine Receptor Subtypes

I. Introduction

Drugs provide tools for both manipulating behavior and studying the structure and function of the brain. Drugs can help reveal the cellular and molecular mechanisms that contribute to specific behaviors. An important concern is specificity, i.e., the extent to which any drug can be thought to act at a single well-defined site. Early biochemical data supported the idea that the sites of action of drugs were homogeneous: Studies of drug binding to whole brain extracts generally generated linear Scatchard plots, most easily interpreted as representing single classes of binding sites. However, regional brain-binding studies most often showed that this homogeneous population of binding sites was expressed in many different nuclei throughout the brain, suggesting that most drugs would exert multiple effects. The apparent homogeneity of drug-binding sites facilitated biochemical and

Advances in Pharmacology, Volume 39

1054-3589/97/$25.00

binding studies, but moved our explanations of drug action from the drug and its interactions with its receptor to some more complex, interactive, but ill-defined aspect of the nervous system. The potential for critical analysis of drug function and the design of drugs that would help understand the brain were essentially limited to those few cases in which the drug-binding sites were restricted to one or a few specific brain nuclei or cell types. Only under these conditions could the actions of a drug be associated with the function of specific central nervous system nuclei.

It is now known that the diversity of drug/receptor interactions far exceeds earlier estimates. This diversity is seen at two levels. First, populations of binding sites previously thought to be homogeneous are now known to be heterogeneous (for reviews, see Schofield *et al.,* 1990; Betz, 1990). For example, nicotine, once thought to bind to a homogeneous class of binding sites in brain, is now known to interact with many different oligomeric receptors (for reviews, see Karlin and Akabas, 1995; McGehee and Role, 1995; Sargent, 1993; Galzi *et al.,* 1991; Patrick *et al.,* 1993). Likewise, drugs that bind to $GABA_A$ receptors in brain extracts are now known to distinguish dozens of functionally different GABA receptors (for reviews, see Stephenson, 1995; Macdonald and Olsen, 1994). Second, some drugs are now known to bind to specific identified receptors that were not previously thought to bear the appropriate binding sites. For example, curare, a drug that was once thought to bind exclusively to, and be diagnostic for, nicotinic acetylcholine receptors, is now known to have its highest affinity for serotonin ($5HT_3$) receptors (Andres *et al.,* 1991). Phencyclidines were thought to be receptor specific but now have been shown to block a wide variety of ligand-gated ion channels (Amador and Dani, 1991). Even glycine is no longer considered specific for glycine receptors in that it is required for activation of one class of the glutamate receptors (Johnson and Ascher, 1987). Both the diversity of receptor types and the cross-modality of drug–receptor interactions are likely to become more significant as more is learned.

The diversity of drug–receptor interactions requires a change in our view of the actions of drugs and the consequences of both licit and illicit drug use. We know that the prolonged use of drugs results in changes in the number of specific binding sites, changes in the efficacy of the drug inactivation or uptake mechanisms, and perhaps changes in the abundance of endogenous ligands (for reviews, see Korenman and Barchas, 1993). However, the diversity of drug–receptors now also requires consideration of changes in the composition of the receptor or changes in the distribution of these molecules on the surface of a neuron. Drug use may also have long-term effects that result from the expression of specific genes that are activated as a consequence of the action of a drug on one of its many different receptors. We also appreciate more fully the potential for long-term, activity-dependent modification of synaptic function and the roles these mechanisms play in mature and developing animals.

Nicotine is an official drug of abuse that acts in the central and peripheral nervous systems, most likely through its interaction with the neuronal nicotinic acetylcholine receptors. There have been many elegant studies of nicotine-binding sites in the central nervous system, both in extracts and in brain slices (Marks and Collins, 1982; Schwartz *et al.*, 1982, 1984; Rainbow *et al.*, 1984; Clarke *et al.*, 1984; Clarke and Pert, 1985; Marks *et al.*, 1986; Lippiello and Fernandes, 1986; Baneerjee *et al.*, 1990). These studies show that both high- and low-affinity-binding sites are abundant and that they are widely distributed in the brain (Clarke and Pert, 1985; Meeker *et al.*, 1986; Pauly *et al.*, 1991). A key observation in these studies is that the number of binding sites changes with chronic exposure to nicotine (Norbert *et al.*, 1993; Marks *et al.*, 1985, 1992; Marks and Collins, 1983; Pauly *et al.*, 1991; Schwartz and Kellar, 1983, 1985). In addition, α-bungarotoxin also binds to brain membrane preparations and to cells known to contain neuronal nicotinic acetylcholine receptors (Greene *et al.*, 1973; Patrick and Stallcup, 1977a,b; Carbonetto *et al.*, 1978; Brown and Funmagalli, 1977; Duggan *et al.*, 1976; Jacob and Berg, 1983). A second toxin, neuronal bungarotoxin, isolated from the venom of the same species of snake (Ravdin and Berg, 1979; Loring and Zigmond, 1987, 1988; Chiappinelli, 1985) also binds and blocks the function of neuronal nicotinic acetylcholine receptors in the brain (Loring and Zigmond, 1987; Halvorsen and Berg, 1987; Sah *et al.*, 1987).

The specific sites to which nicotine and these two toxins bind are neuronal nicotinic acetylcholine receptors, which are members of the family of ligand-gated ion channels. These receptors, like those found at the neuromuscular junction, contain five subunits (Cooper *et al.*, 1991). The number of different neuronal nicotinic receptors is not known, but 11 different genes encoding receptor subunit-like proteins have been identified (for reviews, see Deneris *et al.*, 1991; Lindström, 1994). Some of these proteins have been shown to participate in the formation of acetylcholine-gated ion channels; others are included in the gene family simply on the basis of their similarities in sequence. Receptors that differ in their subunit composition differ in their physiological and pharmacological properties. Currently, 11 different functional receptors have been identified, and it seems likely that insights into the roles of subunits not yet shown to function will increase this number. Additionally, it is likely that receptors will be found that are composed of more than one kind of α or β subunit. This review discusses the diversity of the neuronal nicotinic acetylcholine receptors with emphasis on their pharmacological properties.

Members of the neuronal nicotinic receptor gene family have been divided into two groups based on their sequences (for reviews, see Karlin and Akabas, 1995; McGehee and Role, 1995; Sargent, 1993; Galzi *et al.*, 1991; Patrick *et al.*, 1993), Members of one group are considered β subunits (1) because they lack the two vicinal cysteines that form part of the ligand-binding site on the muscle α subunit and (2) because the two functional members of this group can actually substitute for the muscle nicotinic acetylcholine receptor β subunit (but cannot substitute for muscle γ or δ subunit) to form a functional receptor. This group contains three subunits: $\beta 2$, $\beta 3$, and $\beta 4$. Only $\beta 2$ and $\beta 4$ have been shown to participate in the formation of an acetylcholine-gated ion channel. A second group of eight subunits are classified as α subunits because they possess two vicinal cysteines. Three of these subunits, $\alpha 2$, $\alpha 3$, and $\alpha 4$, have been shown to form functional receptors when expressed in combination with either a $\beta 2$ or a $\beta 4$ subunit. Three other α subunits, $\alpha 7$, $\alpha 8$, and $\alpha 9$, have been shown to form functional receptors when expressed alone and thus presumably form homooligomeric receptors. An $\alpha 5$ subunit has been shown to coassemble with $\alpha 3$ and $\beta 4$ and thus probably contributes to the function of this receptor, although the $\alpha 3/\beta 4$ combination itself is functional in oocytes. An $\alpha 6$ subunit identified on the basis of homology has yet to be shown to contribute to function in oocytes or to coassemble with other receptor subunits.

The initial demonstration of functional combinations of receptor subunits was done in the *Xenopus* oocyte expression system using rat cDNA clones (Boulter *et al.*, 1987). Although expression in the oocyte has limitations, it is currently the only viable system in which the composition of the expressed receptors can be varied. Consequently, this review begins with the properties of receptors expressed in the oocyte. Less is known of the properties of neuronal nicotinic acetylcholine receptors expressed in neuronal cells largely because transient expression has yet to function reliably in these systems. However, considerable data exist on the properties of neuronal nicotinic receptors in cells isolated from both rat and chick peripheral ganglia or specific brain nuclei. Unfortunately, less is known of the composition of the receptors expressed in these cells. The remainder of the review considers the problem of associating specific properties with known combinations of receptor subunits. Emphasis will be placed on the neuronal nicotinic receptors found in rat and chick.

II. Neuronal Nicotinic Receptors Expressed in Oocytes

A. Introduction

Although genes can be included in gene families on the basis of their similarities to other members of the family, the most compelling test of relatedness is function. The *Xenopus* oocyte has provided a convenient and powerful means of assessing the function of proteins thought to be subunits of ligand-gated ion channels. Injection of RNA transcribed from cDNA clones encoding the appropriate receptor subunits or injection of the cDNA in which the coding sequence is placed downstream of a promoter, such as SV40 (simian virus) or CMV (cytomegalovirus), results in the appearance of functional ligand-gated ion channels on the surface of the oocyte. This expression system has been particularly useful in studying the neuronal nicotinic acetylcholine receptors. Oocytes do not express an endogenous functional nicotinic receptor, although it has been reported that they express receptor coding sequences (Buller and White, 1990). Oocytes do, however, express a calcium-gated chloride channel (Miledi and Parker, 1984) that can confound analysis. Some neuronal nicotinic receptors have a significant permeability to calcium (Vernino *et al.,* 1991; Mulle *et al.,* 1992b; Sands and Barish, 1992; Elgoyhen *et al.,* 1994) and could activate these chloride channels. In the oocyte the chloride reversal potential is around -35 mV so at holding potentials more negative than this, the calcium-gated chloride current is outward and appears to add to inward cationic currents such as those generated by nicotinic receptors.

B. Rat Neuronal Nicotinic Receptors

Pairwise combinations of some α and β subunits produce functional nicotinic acetylcholine receptors in *Xenopus* oocytes. In the case of the rat neuronal nicotinic acetylcholine receptors, injection of oocytes with sequences encoding either the $\beta2$ or the $\beta4$ subunit, in pairwise combination with sequences encoding $\alpha2$, $\alpha3$, or $\alpha4$, results in the formation of a nicotine-gated ion channel. Each of these six pairwise combinations can be distinguished on the basis of the ligands that either activate or block receptor function (Luetje *et al.,* 1990; Luetje and Patrick, 1991). The fact that there are six different pharmacological profiles proves that both the α and the β subunits determine pharmacology and probably contribute to the ligand-binding site. Although many pharmacological differences are subtle, some large differences also exist between these pairwise combinations. For example, the ligand cytisine is a most effective agonist on all receptors containing a $\beta4$ subunit, but is the least effective agonist on receptors containing a $\beta2$ subunit. In fact, cytisine can block the activation of receptors containing the $\beta2$ subunit (Luetje and Patrick, 1991). Furthermore, while some $\beta2$-containing receptors are blocked by neuronal bungarotoxin, all of the $\beta4$-containing receptors are resistant to neuronal bungarotoxin (Duvoisin *et al.,* 1989; Luetje *et al.,* 1990; Wada *et al.,* 1990). Differential activation by cytisine and blockade by neuronal bungarotoxin thus provide potentially powerful tools with which to distinguish $\beta2$-containing receptors from $\beta4$-containing receptors. If the type of β subunit is held constant, the receptors formed by the addition of an $\alpha2$, an $\alpha3$, or an $\alpha4$ subunit differ in their sensitivity to agonists, but not as dramatically. For example, there is roughly a 100-fold difference in the ability of nicotine to activate an $\alpha3/\beta2$ receptor compared to an $\alpha2/\beta2$ receptor. Antagonist sensitivity also varies with the type of α subunit present. In the presence of a $\beta2$ subunit, the substitution of $\alpha4$ for $\alpha3$ renders the receptor 10-fold less sensitive to inhibition by neuronal bungarotoxin whereas the substitution of an $\alpha2$ subunit renders the receptor 100-fold less sensitive (Luetje and Patrick, 1991). The response to the antagonist tubocurarine also depends on the subunit composition (Cachelin and Rust, 1994). $\beta2$-containing receptors are blocked by tubocurarine with $\alpha2$-containing receptors more sensitive than $\alpha3$-containing receptors. In contrast, tubocurarine enhances the peak current elicited by low concentrations of acetylcholine in receptors containing $\beta4$.

Some of the rat α subunits form ligand-gated ion channels when expressed in the oocyte in the absence of β subunits. Both $\alpha7$ and $\alpha9$ (a rat $\alpha8$ gene has not been found) generate acetylcholine-gated currents in the oocyte, presumably functioning as homooligomeric receptors. These homooligomeric receptors are pharmacologically distinguishable from the heterooligomeric receptors in several ways. Both the $\alpha7$ and the $\alpha9$ homooligomeric receptors are blocked by α-bungarotoxin, whereas none of the heterooligomeric receptors are affected by this toxin. These receptors have additional unusual properties. Both are highly permeable to calcium ions (Seguela *et al.,* 1993; Elgoyhen *et al.,* 1994) and $\alpha7$ is blocked by strychnine (Seguela *et al.,* 1993), normally thought of as a glycine-receptor antagonist. $\alpha9$, whose expression is largely limited to the cochlea (Elgoyhen *et al.,* 1994), is unusual in that nicotine acts as an antagonist rather than as an agonist of $\alpha9$ homooligomeric receptors.

It is clear that neuronal nicotinic receptors can be formed from pairwise combinations of α and β subunits and as homooligomeric receptors composed of a subclass of the α subunits. It is also the case that receptors can include three different subunits. Expression of $\alpha3$, $\beta4$, and $\alpha5$ in the oocyte results in the formation of a receptor that is pharmacologically distinguishable from the $\alpha3/\beta4$ receptor (Ramirez-Latorre and Role, 1995), suggesting that additional diversity may result from the addition or nonaddition of the $\alpha5$ subunit to other α/β combinations. Evidence also shows that this combination is formed in the chick ciliary ganglion (Conroy *et al.,* 1992), lending support to the idea that we will have to consider greater than pairwise combinations of subunits.

Neither the $\beta3$ nor the $\alpha6$ subunits have been shown to participate in the formation of a functional receptor in the oocyte, and no pharmacological differences have been reported for receptors formed upon coinjection of these subunits in combination with any of the pairwise combinations described earlier. However, the genes encoding these subunits are clearly expressed in the rat central and peripheral nervous systems and probably contribute to the function of receptors *in vivo*.

C. Chick Neuronal Nicotinic Receptors

The chick offers many experimental advantages, including a rich history of developmental studies, easy access to developing animals, and a convenient source of neural tissue. Much of the original identification of the neuronal nicotinic acetylcholine receptor subunits was done in the chick (Nef *et al.*, 1988; Couturier *et al.*, 1990a,b), and clones encoding all but the $\alpha 9$ subunit are available from chick. Additionally, there is a gene encoding an $\alpha 8$ (Schoepfer *et al.*, 1990) subunit that is found in the chick but has not yet been identified in the rat. Although there are extensive studies of the pharmacology of the chick receptors, the ligands used do not completely overlap with those used in the rat. However, some generalizations and some specific differences are apparent.

It is clear that both α and β subunits contribute to the pharmacology of the chick neuronal nicotinic acetylcholine receptors expressed in oocytes (Bertrand *et al.*, 1990; Gross *et al.*, 1991; Charnet *et al.*, 1992; Ballivet *et al.*, 1988). The responses to acetylcholine and nicotine vary with both the α and the β subunits. Unfortunately, the response of these receptors to cytisine and neuronal bungarotoxin is not known so the specific contribution of the β subunit to these properties cannot be compared with the rat. Desensitization has been shown to vary, and receptors containing an $\alpha 3$ desensitize much more rapidly than do those containing an $\alpha 4$ (Gross *et al.*, 1991). No data exist in the oocyte for any chick receptors containing more than two different subunits.

In the chick, the $\alpha 7$ and $\alpha 8$ subunits can both form homooligomers and heterooligomers composed of both $\alpha 7$ and $\alpha 8$ subunits (Anand *et al.*, 1993a,b). The chick $\alpha 7$ homooligomer expressed in the oocyte differs from the rat clone expressed in the oocyte in that it is not activated by dimethylphenylpiperazinium (DMPP) (Bertrand *et al.*, 1992), although it is similar to rat in other properties reported. This is also in contrast to the chick $\alpha 7$ homooligomer immunopurified from chick brain which appears to bind DMPP. The pharmacology of the chick $\alpha 7$ and $\alpha 8$ homooligomers expressed in the oocyte has been compared (Gerzanich *et al.*, 1993; Amar *et al.*, 1993). These two differ by about 10-fold in sensitivity to all of the ligands tested except for DMPP, which activates the $\alpha 8$ but not the $\alpha 7$ homooligomer. The differences in sensitivity to antagonists are less striking.

III. Properties of Receptors *in Vivo*

It seems that diversity is the rule rather than the exception for ligand-gated ion channels in the brain. To begin with, there are many different genes that encode subunits of the various ligand-gated ion channels. Any one of these genes may produce several different proteins as a result of differential splicing of the primary gene transcript (Padgett *et al.*, 1986; Seeburg, 1996). In some instances the transcript is altered by editing mechanisms that change the coding sequence and the structure of the expressed protein. The complexity increases rapidly as each differentially spliced or edited gene product produces a protein that can form heterooligomeric receptors in an as yet unknown combination with numerous other subunits. This combinatorial complexity magnifies the transcript diversity to produce a large number of possible receptors.

In what ways might this receptor diversity be manifested? For example, different receptors clearly have different patterns of expression in the adult brain and might also might differ with respect to ion permeabilities, desensitization profiles, or single channel properties. *In situ* hybridization has shown that even though the expression of genes coding for nicotinic receptors is widespread, individual members of the gene family are expressed in discrete but overlapping sets of nuclei (Wada *et al.*, 1989, 1990; Dineley-Miller and Patrick, 1992; Seguela *et al.*, 1993; Morris *et al.*, 1990). It also seems likely that temporal differences in the pattern of expression of genes encoding receptor subunits (Brussard *et al.*, 1994) may be important developmentally. Finally, diversity might be manifest in the differential targeting of receptors to specific neuronal domains. For example, specific subtypes might be directed to the axonal or presynaptic domain whereas others might be targeted to the dendrites or cell soma.

This review is interested in pharmacological diversity in part because it provides a tool that can be used to selectively modify the function of certain receptors and in part because the various pharmacological profiles might reflect differences in sensitivity to the transmitter acetylcholine. In fact, there are clear differences in the action of acetylcholine on different subunit combinations which might be exploited to probe function. One specific area in which a difference in agonist sensitivity is striking is in the sensitivity of pre- and postsynaptic receptors. Although categorizing nicotinic receptors based on location (pre or postsynaptic) is not clear cut, for clarity the remainder of this review has been divided into descriptions of pre- and postsynaptic receptors.

A. Presynaptic Receptors

1. Introduction

A long history of experiments suggests that neuronal nicotinic acetylcholine receptors modulate the release of neurotransmitters (reviewed in Chesselet, 1984; see also Hall and Turner, 1972; Goodman and Weiss, 1973; Goodman, 1974; Giorguieff *et al.*, 1977; De Belleroche and Bradford, 1978). Although effects of acetylcholine on release were clear, the demonstration of nicotinic pharmacology was often questionable (reviewed in Balfour, 1982). However, more recent studies have benefited from better ligands and more information and are more convincing. It is now clear that activation of nicotinic receptors on innervating axons can affect the release of a number of neurotransmitters.

Three areas in particular have been examined in detail: the nigrostriatal system, the hippocampus, and the habenulo-interpeduncular pathway. Each of these regions possesses cholinergic input and a high density of [^{3}H]nicotine-binding sites, [^{125}I]α-bungarotoxin-binding sites, or both (Clarke *et al.*, 1984, 1985; Hamill *et al.*, 1986; Schwartz *et al.*, 1984). Here then are three areas where the properties of presynaptic receptors can be examined to see if this population defines a specific subtype of neuronal nicotinic acetylcholine receptors.

2. *Striatum*

In general, most of the evidence cited in support of a presynaptic location for nicotinic acetylcholine receptors is based on lesion studies. The observation is that lesioning of specific inputs to a nucleus leads to a loss of nicotinic-binding sites in that nucleus. This implies that the binding sites were on the innervating axons and their loss is due to degeneration of these innervating axons. In many cases, however, it is difficult to rule out that the receptors are postsynaptic and their maintenance requires the presence of the innervating axons. This argument is unlikely to be the case in the striatum, however, which receives dopaminergic innervation from the substantia nigra. Lesioning of nigrostriatal neurons with 6-hydroxy-dopamine causes a significant decrease (approximately 30%) in the number of [^{3}H]nicotine-binding sites in the striatum (Hamill *et al.*, 1986; Schwartz *et al.*, 1984). Because striatal neurons do not express nicotinic genes at detectable levels (Wada *et al.*, 1989, 1990; Dineley-Miller and Patrick, 1992; Seguela *et al.*, 1993; Deneris *et al.*, 1989), it is unlikely that the decrease in nicotine-binding sites is due to the loss of receptors on these striatal neurons. In this case the simplest conclusion is that the disappearance of sites is due to the loss of presynaptic nicotinic acetylcholine receptors on innervating nigral axons. Substantia nigral efferents to the striatum express $\alpha 3$, $\alpha 4$, $\alpha 5$, $\alpha 6$, $\beta 2$, and $\beta 3$ subunits (Wada *et al.*, 1989, 1990; Dineley-Miller and Patrick, 1992; Seguela *et al.*, 1993; Deneris *et al.*, 1989). The dorsal raphe, which expresses nicotinic receptor genes, provides a serotonergic input to the striatum (for review, see Kawaguchi *et al.*, 1995). Specific lesioning of this pathway results in a further 30% loss of nicotinic receptors (Schwartz *et al.*, 1984). Because few physiological studies have focused on the serotonergic input, this will not be considered further.

The lesion studies are consistent with the idea that activation of nicotinic receptors on nigrostriatal neurons modulates transmitter release. In striatal slices, low concentrations of nicotine or acetylcholine potentiate spontaneous dopamine release in a calcium-dependent manner (Giorguieff *et al.*, 1976, 1979). Furthermore, in the slice these receptors are activated by the definitive nicotinic agonists cytisine, DMPP, and nicotine (Table I) and are blocked by mecamylamine and dihydro-β-erythroidine but not by *d*-tubocurarine (Sacaan *et al.*, 1995).

TABLE I Pharmacology of Pre- and Postsynaptic Receptors

			Presynaptic				*Postsynaptic*				
	[³H]-Nicotine binding	*[¹²⁵I]-BTX binding*	*mRNA expression*	*Preparation*	*αBTX block*	*nBTX block*	*Preparation*	*Agonist pharmacology*	*αBTX block*	*nBTX block*	*Ref.[a]*
Striatum	Moderate	Low	None	Rat: synaptosomes	No	50%					1,2,3,4, 5,6
				synaptosomes slice	No	N.D.					
				Mouse: synaptosomes	No	Yes					
					No	Yes					
Hippocampus	Low	High	α3,α5,(α2),β2,(β4)	Rat: synaptosomes-ACh	No	N.D.	Rat: cultured neurons	Type: 1: D>N>C>A	Yes	Yes	4,6,7
			α7 CA1 and CA3	synaptosomes-GABA	N.D.	N.D.		Type 2: A>N>D>C	No	Yes	
				slice-NE	N.D.	N.D.					
mHB	High	Low	Dorsal α4,α6,α7,β2,β3,β4	Rat: slice (rel-GABA)	No	No	Rat: isolated neurons	N>C>A>D	No	No	9,10,11
			Ventral α3,α4,α7,β2,β3,β4	slice (volley)	No	No					
				Chick: culture (rel-glut)	Yes	No					
IPN	High	High	α2,α3,α4,α5,α7,β2,β4				Rat: isolated neurons	C>A>N>D	No	No	10
Sympathetic ganglion		High	α3,α5,α7,β2,β4				Rat: isolated neurons chick (E10)	N>C>=D>A D>N>A	No	Yes	12,13
Parasympathetic ganglion		High	α3,α5,α7,β2,β4				Chick: isolated neurons	Slow	No	Yes	14,15, 16
								Fast	Yes	N.D	

[a] Pharmacology references: 1, Rapier *et al.* (1987); 2, Rapier *et al.* (1988); 3, Rapier *et al.* (1990); 4, Clarke and Reuben (1997); 5, Grady *et al.* (1992); 6, Sacaan *et al.* (1995); 7, Wonnacott *et al.* (1995); 8, Alkondon and Albuquerque (1991); 9, Lena *et al.* (1993); 10, Mulle *et al.* (1991); 11, McGehee *et al.* (1995); 12, Mandelzys *et al.* (1995); 13, Moss *et al.* (1989); 14, Vijayaragháván *et al.* (1992); 15, Chiappinelli (1983); 16, Loring *et al.* (1984). Expression references: Mandelzys *et al.* (1995); Rust *et al.* (1994); Corriveau and Berg (1993); Wada *et al.* (1989, 1990); Dineley-Miller and Patrick (1992); Seguela *et al.* (1993); Morris *et al.* (1990).

Pharmacological characterization is more readily obtained from isolated nerve terminals known as synaptosomes. Synaptosomes are loaded with an isotopically labeled neurotransmitter that can be quantified directly. It has been clearly demonstrated that the activation of nicotinic receptors on synaptosomes prepared from striatum causes release of dopamine in a concentration-dependent manner (Rapier *et al.*, 1987, 1988, 1990; Grady *et al.*, 1992). Because the dopamine release is assayed, these nicotinic receptors are likely to originate from innervating nigral axons. The pharmacology of the receptors assayed in this manner has been extensively characterized (Table I). The results from the rat striatal slice preparation and rat striatal synaptosomes correlate well in terms of agonist profile (Sacaan *et al.*, 1995; Wonnacott *et al.*, 1989, 1995). However, there are differences in antagonist pharmacology between the two preparations: *d*-tubocurarine blocks the modulation of dopamine release in synaptosomes, but has no effect on slice preparations (Clarke and Reuben, 1996). In rat striatal synaptosomal preparations, neuronal bungarotoxin only partially blocks the nicotinic modulation of dopamine release, whereas in the rat striatal slice preparation the same concentration almost completely blocks the response. In contrast, the IC_{50} for the neuronal bungarotoxin block of nicotine-induced dopamine release in mouse striatal synaptosomes is close to that measured in rat striatal slice (Wonnacott and Drasdo, 1991; Schultz and Zigmond, 1989; Grady *et al.*, 1992). Neuronal bungarotoxin is a potent antagonist in two of the studies of striatal nicotinic receptors described earlier, despite the fact that one study used mouse striatum and one used rat striatum; the partial block seen in rat synaptosome preparations might be explained by differences in the efficacy of toxin batches.

The pharmacology of the nigrostriatal nicotinic receptors does not equate to any of the known pairwise subunit combinations in oocytes. For example, there is no evidence for $\beta 4$ or $\alpha 7$ expression in either striatum or substantia nigra, yet cytisine (to date, an agonist apparently specific for receptors containing $\beta 4$ or $\alpha 7$) effectively induces dopamine release from striatal synaptosomes (Rapier *et al.*, 1990; Grady *et al.*, 1992). Cytisine is not an effective agonist on $\beta 2$-containing receptors expressed in oocytes (Luetje and Patrick, 1991). It is unlikely that there is an $\alpha 7$ component to the nicotinic receptors in striatum. There is no α-bungarotoxin binding in the rat striatum, nor does α-bungarotoxin antagonize the nicotine-induced release of dopamine in rat synaptosomes (Clarke and Pert, 1985; Wonnacott *et al.*, 1995). This is consistent with the absence of $\alpha 7$ message in either the rat striatum or the rat substantia nigra (Seguela *et al.*, 1993). However, in mouse there is α-bungarotoxin binding in the striatum (Marks *et al.*, 1986; Pauly *et al.*, 1989), although there is no evidence that these sites are located on dopaminergic terminals. Furthermore, α-bungarotoxin does not block the nicotine-induced release of dopamine from mouse striatal synaptosomes (Grady *et al.*, 1992).

There are at least three explanations for why the pharmacology is not comparable. First, these receptors might have a subunit composition not yet tested in oocytes; second, receptors may exhibit different properties when expressed in a neuron as opposed to an amphibian egg; or third, heterogeneity of receptors in the slice or synaptosome preparations confounds comparison. The fact that there are a large number of different receptor genes expressed in the nigrostriatal efferents is consistent with the idea that receptor heterogeneity is one factor complicating the comparison of pharmacologies. Detailed examination of the concentration dependence of nicotine-induced dopamine release suggests that there may be more than one type of nicotinic receptor controlling release (Wonnacott *et al.*, 1995). Moreover, both in the slice and in synaptosomes about 50% of the nicotine-induced release is sensitive to tetrodotoxin (Giorguieff *et al.*, 1979; Wonnacott *et al.*, 1995; Wonnacott and Soliakov, 1995). One explanation is that there are two (or more) subtypes of nicotinic receptor on nigral axons, possibly presynaptic and preterminal, as has been demonstrated in the medial habenula (see Section III, A, 4).

In summary, dopaminergic neurons innervating the striatum have presynaptic nicotinic receptors that can modulate transmitter release. A subtype cannot be assigned to the receptor responsible for this effect, and more than one type of receptor may contribute to the response. There are both cholinergic interneurons and cholinergic input to the striatum, which might provide an endogenous source of acetylcholine that could modulate dopamine release *in vivo*.

3. *Hippocampus*

Hippocampal slice preparations and synaptosomes prepared from hippocampus have both been used to show modulation of neurotransmitter release by nicotine. Although there is a noticeable paucity of [^{3}H]nicotine binding in the hippocampal formation (Clarke *et al.*, 1984), α-bungarotoxin binding is readily detectable (Clarke *et al.*, 1985; Barrantes *et al.*, 1995) and $\alpha 7$ message is abundant in the pyramidal cell layer of the hippocampus and in the granule cell layer of the dentate gyrus (Seguela *et al.*, 1993). $\beta 2$ message is also abundant in these cells but there is substantially less message for $\alpha 4$, $\alpha 5$, or $\beta 4$, and neither $\alpha 2$ nor $\alpha 3$ message is detectable. Moreover, $\beta 2$ (Hill *et al.*, 1993) and $\alpha 7$ (Dominiguez del Toro *et al.*, 1994) protein have been shown to be present in the locations predicted by the *in situ* hybridization studies. There are no controlled lesion studies that deplete nicotine-binding sites from the hippocampus. Hippocampal synaptosomes do, however, show nicotinic modulation of neurotransmitter release consistent with the presence of presynaptic nicotinic receptors.

Both hippocampal slice and synaptosome preparations have been used to examine the nicotinic receptor-mediated release of acetylcholine, GABA, and norepinephrine. Micromolar concentrations of nicotine stimulate the release of GABA (Rapier *et al.*, 1987; Wonnacott *et al.*, 1989) and acetylcholine from synaptosomes (Rapier *et al.*, 1987). Neither response is blocked by α-bungarotoxin. The nicotine-induced release of acetylcholine is calcium dependent and is largely tetrodotoxin insensitive, consistent with a presynaptic location of nicotinic receptors. Nicotinic modulation of norepinephrine release has been the most extensively studied. Nicotine, cytisine, and DMPP are all more potent at eliciting norepinephrine release than acetylcholine (Table I). The effect of nicotine on norepinephrine release is blocked by mecamylamine and dihydro-β-erythroidine (Clarke and Reuben, 1996). Again tetrodotoxin had no effect on nicotine-stimulated transmitter release.

Hippocampal slices do not demonstrate the same characteristics of release as synaptosomes. For example, the nicotine-induced release of norepinephrine is blocked approximately 70% by tetrodotoxin in the slice, whereas tetrodotoxin has little effect in the synaptosome preparation. Further, the pharmacology of nicotine-induced norepinephrine release in the hippocampal slice differs from that in the synaptosome preparation (Table I). In both hippocampal slices and synaptosomes, mecamylamine blocks the nicotine-induced release. In contrast, *d*-tubocurarine blocks nicotine-induced release in the slice but not in synaptosomes, and dihydro-β-erythroidine blocks nicotine-induced release in synaptosomes and not in the slice (Sacaan *et al.*, 1995). Here again, as in striatum, the results from both preparations may be confounded by the presence of multiple types of nicotinic receptors. However, the striking difference in antagonist pharmacology between the two preparations suggests that a separate subtype is being activated in each case.

The locus coeruleus is the major noradrenergic input to the hippocampus (Aston-Jones *et al.*, 1995) and is likely to be the source of the nicotinic receptors described earlier. However, as there are no studies correlating locus coeruleus lesions with loss of nicotine-binding sites, we cannot be sure that the receptors affecting norepinephrine release are on those axons. The locus coeruleus expresses $\alpha3$, $\alpha6$, $\beta2$, $\beta4$, and traces of $\alpha4$. The pharmacology described for synaptosomes is consistent with that of oocytes expressing either $\alpha3/\beta4$ (Luetje and Patrick, 1991) or $\alpha3/\beta2/\beta4$ (Colquhoun *et al.*, 1993). Unfortunately, block by neuronal bungarotoxin, which could distinguish between the two possibilities, was not determined.

The primary excitatory neurotransmitter in hippocampus is glutamate. Its release can also be modulated by nicotinic receptors. Activation of nicotinic receptors in cultures of hippocampal neurons increases the frequency of glutamate miniature end plate potentials in a tetrodotoxin-insensitive fashion (Radcliffe and Dani, 1995). Similarly, in the hippocampal slice, activation of nicotinic receptors on mossy fiber terminals not only increases the frequency of minis, but also increases the amplitude of the evoked postsynaptic glutamate current and results in calcium entry into the presynaptic terminal (R. Gray, personal communication). There is no pharmacology available for either of these phenomena as yet.

The cholinergic input to the hippocampus is mainly from the medial septal nucleus or the nucleus of the tractus diagonalis (Jacobovitz and Creed, 1983). Despite the presence of this innervation, it has not been demonstrated that activation of any cholinergic efferents affects neurotransmitter release. The physiological relevance of this modulation has therefore yet to be defined.

4. *Interpeduncular Nucleus*

In the search for central nicotinic function, the habenulo-interpeduncular pathway is probably the most thoroughly studied. Neurons in the medial habenula send their axons through the fasciculus retroflexus to the interpeduncular nucleus. Lesioning the medial habenula causes a differential loss of [^{3}H]nicotine-binding sites and ^{125}I-labeled α-bungarotoxin-binding sites in the various subnuclei of the interpeduncular nucleus (Clarke *et al.,* 1986). Because both the medial habenula and the interpeduncular nucleus express a broad spectrum of nicotinic genes, we cannot determine whether the binding sites lost after lesioning were from the pre- or postsynaptic neuron.

The medial habenula has both excitatory and inhibitory projections to the interpeduncular nucleus; the excitatory transmission is glutamatergic (Brown *et al.,* 1983; McGehee *et al.,* 1995) and the inhibitory transmission is GABAergic (Brown *et al.,* 1983). Both types of transmission are enhanced by low doses of nicotine, but the pharmacology of nicotinic enhancement of inhibitory transmission differs from the pharmacology of nicotinic enhancement of excitatory transmission. Unfortunately, all the studies on enhancement of inhibitory transmission have been done in the rat, and all those on exitatory enhancement have been done in the chick, making direct comparison problematic.

In rat medial habenula-interpeduncular nucleus preparations (slices or dissociated cells), low doses of nicotine increase the frequency of GABA postsynaptic potentials (Brown *et al.,* 1984; Lena *et al.,* 1993). The concentrations required for this effect are submicromolar, whereas the activation of somatic receptors requires much higher concentrations (Lena *et al.,* 1993). The nicotinic modulation of GABA release is markedly decreased by tetrodotoxin, suggesting a preterminal location (Lena *et al.,* 1993). The preterminal receptor on the GABAergic neurons is pharmacologically distinct from a presynaptic receptor on the same set of neurons, as determined by direct measurement of the nicotinic effect on the presynaptic volley (Mulle and Changeux, 1990; Mulle *et al.,* 1991). Both nicotinic receptor populations have the same agonist profile. However, the antagonist profiles vary, but neither are blocked by α-bungarotoxin (Mulle *et al.,* 1991; Vidal and Changeux, 1993). This is a clear example of heterogenous populations of receptors residing on the same set of neurons.

In cocultures of chick medial habenula-interpeduncular nucleus neurons, nicotine enhances glutamatergic neurotransmission. Nicotine potentiates both amplitude of evoked currents and frequency of spontaneous excitatory postsynaptic currents in a calcium-dependent manner (McGehee *et al.*, 1995). Here, the modulation is not affected by the presence of tetrodotoxin, which suggests a presynaptic rather than a preterminal location. The nicotinic modulation is blocked by α-bungarotoxin; this sensitivity to α-bungarotoxin is abolished in cell cultures treated with antisense oligonucleotides to the $\alpha7$ gene. The nicotinic potentiation of transmitter release, however, is still seen, which may be due to a substitution of another nicotinic gene product (McGehee *et al.*, 1995).

In both the rat and the chick almost all the known nicotinic gene products are transcribed in the medial habenula ($\alpha3$, $\alpha4$, $\beta2$, $\beta3$, $\beta4$, and $\alpha7$) and interpeduncular nucleus ($\alpha2$, $\alpha3$, $\alpha4$, $\alpha5$, $\beta2$, $\beta4$, and $\alpha7$) so perhaps the diversity is not surprising. Once again we can only speculate about the composition of these receptors. On GABAergic neurons in rat, the nicotine-induced release is insensitive to block by α-bungarotoxin, therefore the receptor responsible for this effect seems unlikely to have an $\alpha7$ component. The response to cytisine implicates $\alpha7$ or $\beta4$; because $\alpha7$ involvement is not possible and $\beta4$ is present, it is not unreasonable to propose a $\beta4$-containing receptor. In the chick, the habenular presynaptic nicotinic receptor affecting glutamate release is sensitive to α-bungarotoxin and the $\alpha7$ antisense experiments are consistent with the suggestion that the receptor contains $\alpha7$. However, the nicotinic modulation of release is less sensitive to α-bungarotoxin than an $\alpha7$ homooligomer expressed in oocytes, suggesting that the receptor responsible for the effect of nicotine may not be a homooligomer.

Heterogeneity exists among nicotinic receptors modulating release. Data available for the medial habenula do not allow distinction between pharmacological differences between receptors on different classes of neurons or a species difference. It will be interesting to see the effect of α-bungarotoxin on glutamate release in rat medial habenula and also the pharmacology of nicotinic receptors affecting GABA release in chick medial habenula.

5. Summary

The nigrostriatal system, the hippocampus, and the habenulo-interpeduncular pathway in vertebrate brain clearly possess presynaptic nicotinic receptors that can modulate the release of several different neurotransmitters. Pharmacologies reveal that the presynaptic receptor population is heterogeneous. There may be at least two subtypes in the striatum. In rat medial habenular neurons, there are two subtypes on GABAergic neurons: one preterminal and one presynaptic. One hypothesis that could account for the heterogeneity is that the subtype of nicotinic receptor is dependent on more than one factor. For example, the subtype could be dependent on location (presynaptic or preterminal) and the type of neuron, i.e., the subtype of receptor might depend on the neurotransmitter produced by the neuron. There is not sufficient information to be sure at present. One fact is unequivocal though: There is diversity of nicotinic receptors, even at the presynaptic level.

B. Postsynaptic Receptors

1. Introduction

Ligand-gated ion channels have generally been thought to gate fast synaptic transmission and their location is then by definition postsynaptic. In the case of nicotinic receptors, the best evidence is for a presynaptic function in the central nervous system; this does not, however, preclude a postsynaptic role. For example, lesion studies show that although there is a significant decrease in the number of receptors after loss of innervating axons, in most cases at least 70% of binding sites remain. Some of the remaining sites might be on neurons projecting from other areas. For example, in the striatum, 30% of binding sites are lost after removal of the nigral input and a further 30% reduction of nicotinic receptors can be incurred by lesion of the serotonergic neurons from the dorsal raphe (Schwartz *et al.*, 1984). This leaves 40% of binding sites unaccounted for. It may be the case that some of the denervation-resistant receptors are expressed on the axon terminals of interneurons. However, none of the lesion studies rule out the existence of a population of postsynaptic for nicotinic receptors. The following section discusses some experiments that address a postsynaptic role for nicotinic receptors.

2. Central Nervous System

Binding and electrophysiological studies have demonstrated nicotinic receptors on cell somata (reviewed in Clarke, 1990). The function of the somatic receptors is not clear. Both the medial habenula and the interpeduncular nucleus are likely candidates to contain nicotinic synapses. Both areas receive cholinergic input and have somatic nicotinic receptors (McCormick and Prince, 1987). However, in neither case is there evidence to show that nicotinic receptors mediate transmission from the afferent neurons. Direct stimulation of the inputs to the medial habenula show that neurotransmission at medial habenular synapses is glutamatergic, purinergic, and GABAergic (Gottesfeld and Jacobovitz, 1979; Edwards *et al.*, 1992), whereas at the retroflexus interpeduncular nucleus synapses, transmission is clearly glutamatergic and GABAergic (Brown *et al.*, 1983, 1984; Mulle *et al.*, 1991; McGehee *et al.*, 1995). Although there is cholinergic input to both these regions, evoked postsynaptic responses are not blocked by nicotinic antagonists, demonstrating that their postsynaptic role in synaptic transmission is minimal at most. If somatic nicotinic receptors are extrasynaptic, then what is their function? These receptors may be in transit to their final destination or they may possess an as yet unknown somatic function, no evidence is available supporting these or other possibilities.

The somatic nicotinic receptors appear to be neither pre- nor postsynaptic; however, they are experimentally accessible in the slice or in culture so some knowledge of their pharmacology exists. One consideration to bear in mind is that patching on the cell soma may sample a mixture of receptor populations, which may obfuscate analysis of the pharmacology. The most intensively studied somatic nicotinic responses from the central nervous system are those recorded in the hippocampus and the medial habenula-interpeduncular nuclei.

a. Hippocampus Primary cultures of hippocampal neurons have yielded at least two to three pharmacologically and physiologically distinct nicotinic responses (Alkondon and Albuquerque, 1991, 1993; Zorumski *et al.,* 1992). The most frequently observed current is denoted type 1 and is rapidly desensitizing and blocked by both α-bungarotoxin and neuronal bungarotoxin. The type 2 current is observed only in a small percentage of cells, is neuronal bungarotoxin sensitive but α-bungarotoxin insensitive, and has much slower decay characteristics. The two current types can also be defined by their agonist pharmacologies (Table I).

The pharmacology available allows some limited comparison to oocyte experiments. The type 1 receptor closely resembles the $\alpha7$ type of receptor expressed in oocytes in both agonist profile and toxin sensitivity. Furthermore, like the $\alpha7$ receptor, the type 1 receptor is highly permeable to calcium (Castro and Albuquerque, 1995). The type 2 receptor has pharmacological properties that are not equivalent to any pairwise combination of subunits expressed in oocytes. Neuronal bungarotoxin (100 nM) partially blocks the type 2 response to acetylcholine, which is indicative of receptors containing $\beta2$ subunits, possibly in combination with $\alpha3$ (the $\alpha4$ message is not detectable in the hippocampus). However, the fact that cytisine activates type 2 receptors suggests a role for $\beta4$. These data can be explained by postulating either that more than one pairwise receptor combination underlies type 2 currents or that type 2 receptors contain more than two types of subunits. Experiments have been done which could distinguish between these two possibilities, e.g., if neuronal bungarotoxin blocks the response to cytisine, the simplest explanation is that the nicotinic receptor responsible for the cytisine response contains both $\beta2$ and $\beta4$ subunits.

b. Medial Habenula and Interpeduncular Nucleus Pharmacologies of the somatic nicotinic receptors in the medial habenula and the interpeduncular nucleus have been compared by patch clamp recordings from acutely isolated neurons (Mulle *et al.,* 1991). The medial habenula is a target for cholinergic projections from the basal forebrain, and habenular neurons express message for a number of different subtypes of nicotinic receptors (Wada *et al.,* 1989, 1990; Dineley-Miller and Patrick, 1992; Seguela *et al.,* 1993; Deneris *et al.,*

1989). Receptors on neurons isolated from medial habenula are activated by nicotinic agonists as are receptors on neurons isolated from interpeduncular nucleus; however, each shows a different profile of sensitivity to agonists (see Table I for profile). Despite the diversity of transcript types in each region, only one major single channel class has been described in neurons isolated from the medial habenula and only one major single channel class has been described in neurons isolated from interpeduncular nucleus (Mulle *et al.*, 1991, 1992a; Lester and Dani, 1994). In contrast, there is a heterogenous population of single channels in patches recorded in thin slices of medial habenula (Connolly *et al.*, 1995). The difference may result from the dissociation procedure causing loss of axons and dendritic arbors which express nicotinic channels. There are multiple nicotinic receptor subtypes on neurons from both medial habenula and interpeduncular nucleus; however, recordings from isolated somata that show only one major channel class allow comparisons of pharmacology to known subunit combinations.

Despite the presence of transcripts coding for $\alpha7$ in the medial habenula and the interpeduncular nucleus, there is no indication of an $\alpha7$-like current on neurons isolated from either nucleus. The currents recorded are slowly desensitizing and in neither case is the current blocked by either α-bungarotoxin or neuronal bungarotoxin. $\alpha7$ therefore probably does not contribute to receptors on the soma of neurons of the medial habenula or interpeduncular nucleus. Receptors in both areas are activated by cytisine which suggests a $\beta4$ component. Similarly, currents recorded from neurons isolated from either area are not blocked by neuronal bungarotoxin, which, due to the presence of almost all types of transcripts, only rules out the contribution of $\beta2$. Again, the pharmacology of the native receptors does not match any of the pairwise combinations expressed in oocytes. That fact, the presence of multiple transcripts coding for nicotinic receptor subunits in these areas, and the fact that single channel properties of native and heterologously expressed pairwise receptors are not the same once again suggest that native nicotinic receptors contain more than the minimum number of subunits required for function in oocytes.

c. Summary of CNS Pharmacological diversity exists between somatic nicotinic receptors. The nicotinic responses recorded from hippocampal neurons are pharmacologically distinct from those recorded from medial habenular neurons or interpeduncular neurons. Many other regions in vertebrate brain have been demonstrated to have nicotinic responses, including the cerebral cortex, ventral tegmental area, thalamus, dentate gyrus, and cerebellum (see Clarke, 1990, for review), although these are less thoroughly characterized. The snake neurotoxins α-bungarotoxin and neuronal bungarotoxin are valuable tools that discriminate among three different classes of nicotinic receptor in the hippocampus alone. Of those nicotinic responses that have been carefully delineated, it is clear that, like presynaptic receptors, it is difficult to use presently available pharmacological tools to define the subunit composition. One exception to this is in cultured hippocampal neurons where there is a nicotinic response that is closely mimicked by a heterologous receptor; α7 expressed in oocytes.

The best evidence still for a physiological role for nicotinic receptors is that they play a presynaptic role. There are undoubtedly postsynaptic nicotinic receptors on neurons in many areas of the brain, but these as yet have no definable role. Furthermore, the subunit composition of central nicotinic receptors is, for the most part, still unclear.

3. *Peripheral Nervous System*

Fast nicotinic synaptic transmission has been demonstrated unequivocally in the peripheral nervous system (reviewed in Sargent, 1993). Experiments carried out in the autonomic ganglia have helped define the pharmacology of these nicotinic receptors which participate in neurotransmission. Two of the most popular preparations are the chick ciliary ganglion (parasympathetic) and the rat superior cervical ganglion (sympathetic). Both ganglia express the same complement of nicotinic genes: α3, α5, α7, β2, and β4 subunit genes (Mandelzys *et al.*, 1995; Corriveau and Berg, 1993).

a. Chick Ciliary Ganglion Binding of ^{125}I-labeled neuronal bungarotoxin in the chick ciliary ganglion has identified two classes of nicotinic-binding sites: one binding only neuronal bungarotoxin and the other binding both neuronal bungarotoxin and α-bungarotoxin. The sites that bind only neuronal bungarotoxin are thought to be synaptic, whereas the other sites, which also bind α-bungarotoxin, are extrasynaptic (Loring and Zigmond, 1988). Experiments using monoclonal antibodies confirm this observation and extend it to show that the α-bungarotoxin sites are located perisynaptically (Jacob *et al.*, 1984; Wilson Horch and Sargent, 1995).

The neuronal bungarotoxin-labeled sites are responsible for synaptic transmission at the chick ciliary ganglion: They are located at the synapse and neuronal bungarotoxin rapidly and completely blocks ganglionic transmission (Chiappinelli, 1983; Loring *et al.*, 1984). Despite the abundance of α-bungarotoxin-binding sites, α-bungarotoxin itself has no effect on transmission. Two types of current have been recorded from neurons isolated from the chick ciliary ganglion. One is slowly desensitizing, blocked by neuronal bungarotoxin, and has been attributed to a receptor containing α3, β4, and α5 gene products based on experiments employing sequential immunoprecipitations (Vernallis *et al.*, 1993). The second type of current is rapidly desensitizing and is blocked by α-bungarotoxin (Zhang *et al.*, 1994). This current is only revealed by using a very fast agonist application. Like α7 homooligomers expressed in oocytes, the α-bungarotoxin-sensitive receptor on chick ciliary ganglia is highly permeable to calcium (Vijayaraghavan *et al.*, 1992) and probably corresponds to the extrasynaptic sites that are labeled by α-bungarotoxin.

b. Rat Superior Cervical Ganglion The rat superior cervical ganglion expresses the same transcripts coding for nicotinic receptor genes as the chick ciliary ganglion (Rust *et al.*, 1994; Mandelzys *et al.*, 1995). As seen in the chick ciliary ganglion, the rat superior cervical ganglion also possesses two classes of nicotinic-binding sites; one group binding both snake toxins and one solely binding neuronal bungarotoxin (Loring *et al.*, 1985). The α-bungarotoxin sites again appear to be extrasynaptic. Transmission in the rat superior cervical ganglion is substantially blocked by neuronal bungarotoxin, although the concentrations required for block of transmission are significantly higher than those required in the chick cervical ganglion (Chiappinelli and Dryer, 1984).

More data are available on the pharmacology of the postsynaptic current in rat superior cervical ganglion than in the chick ciliary ganglion. Only one type of current can be observed on isolated ganglion neurons, even when a fast application of agonist is employed (Covernton *et al.*, 1994; Mandelzys *et al.*, 1995). The postsynaptic response to an exogenous application of nicotinic agonists is not blocked by α-bungarotoxin, but is partially blocked by neuronal bungarotoxin, with the degree of block depending on the agonist used to elicit the response (Mandelzys *et al.*, 1995). When the exogenous agonist is acetylcholine, 500 n*M* neuronal bungarotoxin completely blocks the response to the agonist; when cytisine is used, however, the same concentration of neuronal bungarotoxin blocked the response by 30% (Mandelzys *et al.*, 1995). As mentioned earlier, there is no α7-like fast current corresponding to that observed in the chick. Furthermore, α-bungarotoxin has no effect on either the nicotinic current recorded from isolated neurons or the nicotine-induced increase in intracellular calcium, in isolated cervical ganglion neurons (Rogers M., pers. comm).

The currents recorded from the postsynaptic cell have pharmacological properties that cannot be explained by comparison with pairwise expression of subunits in oocytes. For example, the fact that the response to cytisine can be blocked by neuronal bungarotoxin is inconsistent with the properties of either $\alpha3/\beta4$ or $\alpha3/\beta2$ combinations (Mandelzys *et al.*, 1995; Covernton *et al.*, 1994): $\alpha3/\beta4$ receptors are activated by cytisine but are resistant to neuronal bungarotoxin, whereas $\alpha3/\beta2$ receptors are blocked by neuronal bungarotoxin but are barely activated by cytisine (Luetje *et al.*, 1990; Luetje and Patrick,1991). On a whole cell level, the pharmacology of rat sympathetic ganglion cells can be closely mimicked in oocytes by injection of $\alpha3$, $\beta2$, and $\beta4$ subunits cDNAs (Colquhoun and Patrick, 1997).

Despite the fact that the pharmacology of the receptors on rat superior cervical ganglion cells can be satisfactorily accounted for by a single population of receptors, single channel recordings reveal a heterogenous population of channels (Mathie *et al.*, 1991). There is a large variation in conductances which may be attributed to an existence of more than one channel subtype or variation in behavior of a single type. Unfortunately, no pharmacological data are yet available to distinguish between the two. Single channel recordings from oocytes expressing nicotinic receptors show that an injection of pairwise or triplet combinations of cDNA is insufficient to reproduce the single channel properties of the native rat superior cervical nicotinic receptors (Sivilotti *et al.*, 1995).

c. Summary of Peripheral Nervous System In summary, the peripheral nervous system is (with one exception) still the only place in the nervous system where fast nicotinic synaptic transmission has been observed. In addition to the two ganglion preparations mentioned earlier, fast transmission has also been observed in the frog cardiac ganglion and in the chick lumbar ganglion. Even in the ganglia there is diversity of nicotinic receptors. It was once thought that there was only one neuronal type of nicotinic receptors and receptors were divided into ganglion-like (C6) and muscle-like (C10) based on their sensitivity to bismethonium compounds. Now it is clear that there are at least two types of nicotinic receptors in all the ganglia investigated, even if in some cases identification of function of α-bungarotoxin receptors has yet to be shown.

IV. Summary

The search for the physiological function of nicotinic receptors on neurons in the brain began with their discovery. It was initially assumed that, as in ganglia and at the neuromuscular junction, nicotinic receptors would gate fast synaptic transmission in the brain. The best functional evidence now, however, points to a role in modifying the release of other transmitters. This does not preclude a postsynaptic role in transmission for nicotinic receptors in the brain, but attempts to locate such a synapse have not been successful. If fast nicotinic synapses are present in the brain, they are probably low in number and may be masked by other more prevalent synapses (such as glutamatergic) so identification will not be easy.

The extent of diversity of nicotinic receptors is substantial. At the molecular level this is reflected in the number of different genes that encode receptor subunits and the multiple possible combinations of subunits that function in expression systems. From the cellular level there is a broad diversity of properties of native receptors in neurons. Some useful pharmacological tools allow the limited identification of subunits in native receptors. For example, block by α-bungarotoxin identifies $\alpha7$, $\alpha8$, or $\alpha9$ subunits; activation of a receptor by cytisine indicates an $\alpha7$ or $\beta4$ subunit; and neuronal bungarotoxin block identifies a $\beta2$ subunit. Despite the clues to identity gained by careful use of these agents, we have not been able to identify all the components of any native receptor based on pharmacological properties assessed from expression studies. When both pharmacological and biophysical properties of a receptor are taken into consideration, none of the combinations tested in oocytes mimics native receptors exactly. The reason for this discrepancy has been debated at length; it is possible that oocytes do not faithfully manufacture neuronal nicotinic receptors. For example, they may not correctly modify the protein after translation or they may allow a combination of subunits that do not occur *in vivo*. Another possibility is that correct combinations of subunits have not yet been tested in oocytes. Data from immunoprecipitation experiments suggest that many receptors contain three or more different subunits. Results from further experiments injecting combinations of three or more subunits into oocytes may be enlightening.

The diversity of receptors may allow targeting of subtypes to specific locations. Nicotinic receptors are located presynaptically, preterminally, and on the cell soma. The function of the nicotinic receptors located on innervating axons is presumably to modify the release of other neurotransmitters. It is an attractive hypothesis that nicotinic receptors might be involved in modifying the weight of central synapses; however, in none of the regions where this phenomenon has been described is there any evidence for axo-axonal contacts. The presynaptic receptors described so far are pharmacologically unique; therefore, if there are different subtypes of nicotinic receptors modifying the release of different transmitters, they may provide a means of exogenously modifying the release of a particular transmitter with drugs.

There are still many basic unanswered questions about nicotinic receptors in the brain. What are the compositions of native nicotinic receptors? What is their purpose on neurons? Although there is clearly a role presynaptically, what is the function of those located on the soma? Neuronal nicotinic receptors are highly permeable to calcium, unlike muscle nicotinic receptors, and this may have important implications for roles in synaptic plasticity and development. Finally, why is there such diversity? Despite documenting many differences in the characteristics of both native receptors and receptors expressed from cloned sequences, such as pharmacology, single channel properties, ion permeability, desensitization, and sensitivity to agonists, little is still known about how these properties determine neuronal function.

Acknowledgment

This work was supported in part by grants from NINDS (NS13546) and NIDA (DA04077).

References

Alkondon, M., and Albuquerque, E. X. (1991). Initial characterization of the nicotinic acetylcholine receptors in rat hippocampal neurons. *J. Recept. Res.* **11**, 1001–1021.

Alkondon, M., and Albuquerque, E. X. (1993). Diversity of nicotinic acetylcholine receptors in rat hippocampal neurons. I. Pharmacological and functional evidence for distinct structural subtypes. *J. Pharmacol. Exp. Ther.* **265,** 1455–1473.

Amador, M., and Dani, J. A. (1991). MK-801 inhibits nicotinic acetylcholine-induced currents. *Synapse* **7,** 207–215.

Amar, M., Thomas, P., Johnson, C., Lunt, G. G., and Wonnacott, S. (1993). Agonist pharmacology of the neuronal $\alpha 7$ nicotinic receptor expressed in *Xenopus* oocytes. *FEBS Lett.* **327,** 284–288.

Anand, R., Peng, X., Ballesta, J. J., and Lindström, J. (1993a). Pharmacological characterization of α-bungarotoxin-sensitive acetylcholine receptors immunoisolated from chick retina: Contrasting properties of $\alpha 7$ and $\alpha 8$ subunit-containing subtypes. *Mol. Pharmocol.* **44,** 1046–1050.

Anand, R., Peng, X., and Lindström, J. (1993b). Homomeric and native $\alpha 7$ acetylcholine receptors exhibit remarkably similar but non-identical pharmacological properties, suggesting that the native receptor is a heteromeric protein complex. *FEBS Lett.* **327** (2), 241–246.

Andres, V. M., Peterson, A. S., Brake, A. J., Myers, R. M., and Julius, D. (1991). Primary structure and functional expression of the $5HT_3$ receptor, a serotonin-gated ion channel. *Science* **254,** 432–437.

Aston-Jones, G., Shipley, M. T., and Grzanna, R. (1995). The Locus coeruleus, A5 and A7 noradrenergic cell groups. *In* "The Rat Nervous System" (G. Paxinos, ed.), pp. 183–213. Academic Press, San Diego, CA.

Balfour, D. J. K. (1982). The effect of nicotine on brain neurotransmitter systems. *Biochem. Pharmacol.* **16,** 269–282.

Ballivet, M., Nef, P., Couturier, S., Rungger, D., Bader, C. R., Bertrand, D., and Cooper, E. (1988). Electrophysiology of a chick neuronal nicotinic acetylcholine receptor expressed in *Xenopus* oocytes after cDNA injection. *Neuron* **1,** 847–852.

Baneerjee, S., Punzi, J. S., Kreilick, K., and Abood, L. G. (1990). [^{3}H] mecamylamine binding to rat brain membranes. Studies with mecamylamine and nicotine analogues. *Biochem. Pharmacol.* **40,** 1205–1210.

Barrantes, G. E., Rogers, A. T., Lindström, J., and Wonnacott, S. (1995). α-bungarotoxin binding sites in rat hippocampal and cortical cultures: Initial characterization, colocalization with $\alpha 7$ subunits and upregulation by chronic nicotine treatment. *Brain Res.* **672,** 228–236.

Bertrand, D., Ballivet, M., and Rungger, D. (1990). Activation and clocking of neuronal nicotinic acetylcholine receptor reconstituted in *Xenopus* oocytes. *Proc. Natl. Acad. Sci. U.S.A.* **87,** 1993–1997.

Bertrand, D., Bertrand, S., and Ballivet, M. (1992). Pharmacological properties of the homomeric $\alpha 7$ receptor. *Neurosci. Lett.* **146,** 87–90.

Betz, H. (1990). Ligand-gated ion channels in the brain: The amino acid receptor super family. *Neuron* **5,** 383–392.

Boulter, J., Connolly, J., Deneris, E., Goldman, D., Heinemann, S., and Patrick, J. (1987). Functional expression of two neuronal nicotinic acetylcholine receptors from cDNA clones identifies a gene family. *Proc. Natl. Acad. Sci. U.S.A.* **84,** 7763–7767.

Brown, D. A., and Fumagalli, L. (1977). Dissociation of alpha-bungarotoxin binding and receptor block in the rat superior cervical ganglion. *Brain Res.* **129,** 165–168.

Brown, D. A., Docherty, R. J., and Halliwell, J. V. (1983). Chemical transmission in the rat interpeduncular nucleus in vitro. *J. Physiol.* (*London*) **341,** 655–670.

Brown, D. A., Docherty, R. J., and Halliwell, J. V. (1984). The action of cholinomimetic substances in the habenulointerpeduncular pathway of the rat in vitro. *J. Physiol.* (*London*) **353,** 101–109.

Brussard, A. B., Yang, X., Doyle, J. P., Huck, S., and Role, L. W. (1994). Developmental regulation of multiple nicotinic AChR channel subtypes in embryonic chick habenula neurons: Contributions of both the $\alpha 2$ and $\alpha 4$ subunit genes. *Pfluegers Arch.* **429,** 27–43.

Buller, A. L., and White, M. M. (1990). Functional acetylcholine receptors expressed in *Xenopus* oocytes after injection of Torpedo b, g and d subunit mRNAs are a consequence of endogenous oocyte gene expression. *Mol. Pharmacol.* **37,** 423–428.

Cachelin, A. B., and Rust, G. (1994). Unusual pharmacology of (+)-tubocurarine with rat neuronal nicotinic acetylcholine receptors containing β4 subunits. *Mol. Pharmacol.* **46,** 1168–1174.

Carbonetto, S. T., Fambrough, D. M., and Moller, K. J. (1978). Nonequivalence of alpha-bungarotoxin receptors and acetylcholine receptors in chick sympathetic neurons. *Proc. Natl. Acad. Sci. U.S.A.* **72,**1016–1028.

Castro, N. G., and Albuquerque, S. X. (1995). α-bungarotoxin-sensitive hippocampal nicotinic receptor channel has a high calcium permeability. *Biophys. J.* **68,** 516–524.

Charnet, P., Labarca, C., Cohen, B. N., Davidson, N., Lester, H. A., and Pilar, G. (1992). Pharmacological and kinetic properties of a4/b2 neuronal nicotinic acetylcholine receptors expressed in *Xenopus* oocytes. *J. Physiol.* (*London*) **450,** 375–394.

Chesselet, M. F. (1984). Presynaptic regulation of neurotransmitter release in the brain: Facts and hypothesis. *Neuroscience* **12,** 347–375.

Chiappinelli, V. A. (1983). Kappa-Bungarotoxin: A probe for the neuronal nicotinic receptor in the Avian ciliary ganglion. *Brain Res.* **277,** 9–21.

Chiappinelli, V. A. (1985). Actions of snake venom toxins on neuronal nicotinic receptors and other neuronal receptors. *Pharmacol. Ther.* **31,** 1–32.

Chiappinelli, V. A., and Dryer, S. E. (1984). Nicotinic transmission in sympathetic ganglia: Blockade by the snake venom neurotoxin kappa-bungarotoxin. *Neurosci. Lett.* **50,** 239–244.

Clarke, P. B. S. (1990). The central pharmacology of nicotine: Electrophysiological approaches. *In* "Nicotinic Psychopharmacology, Molecular, Cellular and Behavioural Aspects" (S. Wonnacott, M. A. H. Russell, and I. P. Stolerman, eds.), pp. 158–193. Oxford Science Publications, Oxford.

Clarke, P. B. S., and Pert, A. (1985). Autoradiographic evidence for nicotinic receptors on nigrostriatal and mesolimbic dopaminergic neurons. *Brain Res.* **348,** 355–358.

Clarke, P. B. S., and Reuben, M. (1996). Release of [3H] Noradrenaline from rat hippocampal synaptosomes by nicotine: Pharmacological comparison with striatal [3H]Dopamine release indicates mediation by different nicotinic receptor subtypes. *Br. J. Pharmacol.* **117,** 595–606.

Clarke, P. B. S., Pert, C. B., and Pert, A. (1984). Autoradiographic distribution of nicotinic receptors in rat brain. *Brain Res.* **323,** 390–395.

Clarke, P. B. S., Schwartz, R. D., Paul, S. M., Pert, C. B., and Pert, A. (1985). Nicotinic binding in rat brain: Autoradiographic comparison of [^{3}H] acetylcholine, [^{3}H] nicotine, and [^{125}I]-alpha-bungarotoxin. *J. Neurosci.* **5,** 1307–1315.

Clarke, P. B. S., Hamill, G. S., Nadi, N. S., Jacobovitz, D. M., and Pert, A. (1986). 3H-nicotine and 125I-a-bungarotoxin-labelled nicotinic receptors in the interpeduncular nucleus. II. Effects of habenular deafferentation. *J. Comp. Neurol.* **251,** 407–413.

Colquhoun, L., and Patrick, J. (1997). α_3, β_2 and β_4 form heterotrimeric neuronal nicotinic receptors in *Xenopus* oocytes. *J. Neurochem.* (submitted)

Colquhoun, L., Dineley, K., and Patrick, J. (1993). A heterobeta neuronal nicotinic receptor expressed in *Xenopus* oocytes. *Soc. Neurosci. Abstr.* **19,** 1533.

Connolly, J., G., Gibb, A. J., and Colquhoun, D. (1995). Heterogeneity of neuronal nicotinic acetylcholine receptors in thin slices of rat medial habenula. *J. Physiol.* (*London*) **481,** 87–105.

Conroy, W. G., Vernallis, A. B., and Berg, D. K. (1992). The a5 gene product assembles with multiple acetylcholine receptor subunits to form distinctive receptor subtypes in brain. *Neuron* **9,** 1–20.

Cooper, E., Couturier, S., and Ballivet, M. (1991). Pentameric structure and subunit stoichiometry of a neuronal nicotinic acetylcholine receptor. *Nature* (*London*) **350,** 235–238.

Corriveau, R. A., and Berg, D. K. (1993). Coexpression of multiple acetylcholine receptor genes in neurons: Quantification of transcripts during development *J. Neurosci.* **13,** 2662–2671.

Couturier, S., Erkman, L., Valera, S., Rungger, D., Bertrand, S., Boulter, J., Ballivet, M., and Bertrand, D. (1990a). $\alpha5$, $\alpha3$, and Non-$\alpha3$: Three clustered avian genes encoding neuronal nicotinic acetylcholine receptor related subunits. *J. Biol. Chem.* **265,** 17560–17567.

Couturier, S., Bertrand, D., Matter, J., Hernandez, M., Bertrand, S., Nillar, N., Soledad, V., Barkas, T., and Ballivet, M. (1990b). A neuronal nicotinic acetylcholine receptor subunit ($\alpha7$) is developmentally regulated and forms a homooligomerhomooligomeric channel blocked by α-BTX. *Neuron* **6,** 847–856.

Covernton, P. J. O., Kojima, H., Sivilotti, L. G., Gibb, A. J., and Colquhoun, D. (1994). Comparison of neuronal nicotinic receptors in rat sympathetic neurons with subunit pairs expressed in xenopus oocytes. *J. Physiol. (London)* **481,** 27–34.

De Belleroche, J., and Bradford, H. F. (1978). Biochemical evidence for the presence of presynaptic receptors on dopaminergic nerve terminals. *Brain Res.* **142,** 53–68.

Deneris, E. S., Boulter, J., Swanson, L. W., Patrick, J., and Heinemann, S. (1989). $\beta3$: A new member of nicotinic acetylcholine receptor gene family is expressed in brain. *J. Biol. Chem.* **264,** 6268–6272.

Deneris, E. S., Connolly, J., and Rogers, S. W. (1991). Pharmacological and functional diversity of neuronal nicotinic acetylcholine receptors. *Trends Pharmacol. Sci.* **2,** 34–40.

Dineley-Miller, K., and Patrick, J. (1992). Gene transcripts for the nicotinic acetylcholine receptor subunit Beta4, are distributed in multiple areas of the rat central nervous system. *Mol. Brain Res.* **16,** 339–344.

Dominiguez del Toro, E., Juiz, J. M., Peng, X., Lindström, J., and Criado, M. (1994). Immunocytochemical localization of the alpha7 subunit of the nicotinic receptor in the rat central nervous system. *J. Comp. Neurol.* **349,** 325–342

Duggan, A. W., Hall, J. G., and Lee, C. Y. (1976). Alpha-bungarotoxin, cobra neurotoxin and excitation of Renshaw cells by acetylcholine. *Brain Res.* **107,** 166–170.

Duvoisin, R. M., Deneris, E. S., Boulter, J., Patrick, J., and Heinemann, S. (1989). The functional diversity of the neuronal nicotinic acetylcholine receptors is increased by a novel subunit: $\beta4$. *Neuron* **3,** 487–496.

Edwards, F. A., Gibb, A. J., and Colquhoun, D. (1992). ATP receptor mediated synaptic currents in the central nervous system. *Nature (London)* **359,** 144–147.

Elgoyhen, A. B., Johnson, D. S., Boulter, J., Vetter, D. E., and Heinemann, S. (1994). *a*9: An acetylcholine receptor with novel pharmacological properties expressed in rat cochlear hair cells. *Cell (Cambridge, Mass.)* **79,** 705–715.

Galzi, J.-L., Revah, F., Bessis, A., and Changeux, J.-P. (1991). Functional architecture of the nicotinic acetylcholine receptor: from electric organ to brain. *Annu. Rev. Pharmacol.* **31,** 37–72.

Gerzanich, V., Anand, R., and Lindström, J. (1993). Homomers of *a*8 and *a*7 subunits of nicotinic receptors exhibit similar channel but contrasting binding site properties. *Mol. Pharmacol.* **45,** 212–220.

Giorguieff, M. F., Le Floc'h, M. L., Westfall, T. C., Glowinski, J., and Besson, M. J. (1976). Nicotinic effect of acetylcholine on the release of newly synthesized [^{3}H] dopamine in rat striatal slices and cat caudate nucleus. *Brain Res.* **106,** 117–131.

Giorguieff, M. F., Le Floc'h, M. L., Glowinski, J., and Besson, M. J. (1977). Involvement of cholinergic presynaptic receptors of nicotinic and muscarinic types in the control of the spontaneous release of dopamine from striatal dopaminergic terminals in the rat[1]. *J. Pharmacol. Exp. Ther.* **200,** 535–544.

Giorguieff-Chesselet, M. F., Kemel, M. L., Wandscheer, D., and Glowinski, J. (1979). Regulation of dopamine release by presynaptic nicotinic receptors in rat striatal slices: Effect of nicotine in a low concentration. *Life Sci.* **25,** 1257–1262.

Goodman, F. R. (1974). Effects of nicotine on distribution and release of ^{14}C-norepinephrine and ^{14}C-dopamine in rat brain striatum and hypothalamus slices. *Neuropharmacology* **13,** 1025–1032.

Goodman, F. R., and Weiss, G. B. (1973). Alteration of 5-hydroxytryptamine-^{14}C efflux by nicotine in rat brain area slices. *Neuropharmacology* **12,** 955–965.

Gottesfeld, Z., and Jacobovitz, D. M. (1979). Cholinergic projections from the septal-diagonal band to the habenular nuclei. *Brain Res.* **176,** 291–394.

Grady, S., Marks, M. J., Wonnacott, S., and Collins, A. C. (1992). Characterisation of nicotinic receptor mediated [3H]dopamine release from synaptosomes prepared from mouse striatum. *J. Neurochem.,* **59,** 848–856.

Greene, L. A., Sytkowski, A. J., Vogel, Z., and Nirenberg, M. W. (1973). α-bungarotoxin used as a probe for acetylcholine receptors on cultured neurons. *Nature* (*London*) **243,** 163–166.

Gross, A., Ballivet, M., Rungger, D., and Bertrand, D. (1991). Neuronal nicotinic acetylcholine receptors expressed in *Xenopus* oocytes: Role of the a subunit in agonist sensitivity and desensitization. *Pfluegers Arch.* **419,** 545–551.

Hall, G. H., and Turner, D. M. (1972). Effects of nicotine on the release of ^{3}H-noradrenaline from the hypothalamus. *Biochem. Pharmacol.* **21,** 1829–1838.

Halvorsen, S. W., and Berg, D. K. (1987). Affinity labeling of neuronal acetylcholine receptor subunits with an α-toxin that blocks receptor function. *J. Neurosci.* **7,** 2547–2555.

Hamill, G. S., Clarke, P. B. S., Pert, A., and Jacobowitz, D. M. (1986). 3H-nicotine and 125I-alpha bun-garotoxin-labelled nicotinic receptors in the interpeduncular nucleus of rats. I. Subnuclear distribution. *J. Comp. Neurol.* **251,** 398–406.

Hill, J. A., Jr., Zoli, M., Bourgeois, J.-P., and Changeux, J.-P. (1993). Immunocytochemical localization of a neuronal nicotinic receptor: The beta2 subunit. *J. Neurosci.* **13,** 1551–1568.

Jacob, M. H., and Berg, D. K. (1983). The ultrastructural localization of alpha-bungarotoxin binding sites in relation to synapses on chick ciliary ganglion neurons. *J. Neurosci.* **3,** 260–271.

Jacob, M. H., Berg, D. K., and Lindström, J. M. (1984). Shared antigenic determinants between electrophorus acetylcholine receptor and a synaptic component on chicken ciliary ganglion neurons. *Proc. Natl. Acad. Sci. U.S.A.* **81,** 3223–3227.

Jacobovitz, D. M., and Creed, G. J. (1983). Cholinergic projection sites of the nucleus of tractus diagonalis. *Br. Res. Bull.* **10,** 365–371.

Johnson, J. W., and Ascher, P. (1987). Glycine potentiates the NMDA response in cultured mouse brain neurons. *Nature* (*London*) **325,** 529–531.

Karlin, A., and Akabas, M. H. (1995). Toward a structural basis for the function of nicotinic acetylcholine receptors and their cousins. *Neuron* **15,** 1231–1244.

Kawaguchi, Y., Wilson, C. S., Augwood, S. J., and Emson, P. C. (1995). Striatal interneurones: Chemical, physiological and morphological characterization. *Trends Neurosci.* **18,** 527–535.

Korenman, S. G., and Barchas, J. D., eds. (1993). "Biological Basis of Substance Abuse." Oxford University Press, Oxford.

Lena, C., Changeux, J.-P., and Mulle, C. (1993). Evidence for "preterminal" nicotinic receptors on GABAergic axons in the rat interpeduncular nucleus. *J. Neurosci.* **13**(6), 2680–2688.

Lester, R. A. J., and Dani, J. A. (1994). Time dependent changes in central nicotinic acetylcholine channel kinetics in excised patches. *Neuropharmacology* **33,** 27–34.

Lindström, J. M. (1994). Nicotinic acetylcholine receptors. In "Handbook of Receptors and Channels" (R. Alan North, ed.), pp 153–175. CRC Press, Boca Raton, FL.

Lippiello, P. M., and Fernandes, K. G. (1986). The binding of [^{3}H]nicotine to a single class of high affinity sites in rat brain membranes. *Mol. Pharmacol.* **29,** 448–454.

Loring, R. H., and Zigmond, R. E. (1987). Ultrastructural distribution of ^{125}I-toxin F binding sites on chick ciliary neurons: Synaptic localization of a toxin that blocks ganglionic nicotinic receptors. *J. Neurosci.* **7,** 2153–2162.

Loring, R. H., and Zigmond, R. E. (1988). Characterization of neuronal nicotinic receptors by snake neurotoxins. *Trends Neurosci.* **11,** 73–78.

Loring, R. H., Chiappinelli, V. A., Zigmond, R. E., and Cohen, J. B. (1984). Characterization of a snake venom neurotoxin which blocks nicotinic transmission in the avian ciliary ganglion. *Neuroscience* **11**, 989–999.

Loring, R. H., Dahm, L. M., and Zigmond, R. E. (1985). Localization of alpha-bungarotoxin binding sites in the ciliary ganglion of the embryonic chick: An autoradiographic study at the light and electron microscope level. *Neuroscience* **14**, 645–660.

Luetje, C. W., and Patrick, J. (1991). Both alpha and beta subunits contribute to the agonist sensitivity of neuronal nicotinic acetylcholine receptors. *J. Neurosci.* **11**, 837–845.

Luetje, C. W., Wada, K., Rogers, S., Abramson, S., Tsuji, K., Heinemann, S., and Patrick, J. (1990). Neurotoxins distinguish between different neuronal nicotinic acetylcholine receptor subunit combinations. *J. Neurochem.* **55**, 632–640.

Macdonald, R. L., and Olsen, R. W. (1994). $GABA_A$ receptor channels. *Annu. Rev. Neurosci.* **17**, 569–602.

Mandelzys, A., De Koninck, P., and Cooper, E. (1995). Agonist and toxin sensitivities of ACh-evoked currents on neurons expressing multiple nicotinic ACh receptor subunits. *J. Neurophysiol.* **7**, 1212–1221.

Marks, M. J., and Collins, A. C. (1982). Characterization of nicotine binding in mouse brain and comparison with the binding of alpha-bungarotoxin and quinuclidinyl benzilate. *Mol. Pharmacol.* **22**, 554–564.

Marks, M. J., and Collins, A. C. (1983). Effects of chronic nicotine infusion on tolerance development and nicotine receptors. *J. Pharmacol. Exp. Ther.* **226**, 283–291.

Marks, M. J., Stitzel, J. A., and Collins, A. C. (1985). Time course study of the effects of chronic nicotine infusion on the drug response and brain receptors. *J. Pharmacol. Exp. Ther.* **235**, 619–628.

Marks, M. J., Stitzel, J. A., Romm, E., Wehner, J. M., and Collins, A. C. (1986). Nicotinic binding sites in rat and mouse brain: Comparison of acetylcholione, nicotine and α-bungarotoxin. *Mol. Pharmacol.* **30**, 427–436.

Marks, M. J., Pauly, J. R., Gross, S. D., Deneris, E. S., Hermans-Borgmeyer, I., Heinemann, S. F., and Collins, A. C. (1992). Nicotine binding and nicotine receptor subunits RNA after chronic nicotine treatment. *J. Neurosci.* **12**, 2756–2784.

Mathie, A., Cull Candy, S. G., and Colquhoun, D. (1991). Conductance and kinetic properties of single nicotinic acetylcholine channels in rat sympathetic neurones. *J. Physiol.* (*London*) **439**, 717–750.

McCormick, D. A., and Prince, D. A. (1987). Acetylcholine causes rapid nicotinic excitation in the medial habenular nucleus of guinea pig, in vitro. *J. Neurosci.* **7**, 742–752.

McGehee, D. S., and Role, L. W. (1995). Physiological diversity of nicotinic acetylcholine receptors expressed by vertebrate neurons. *Annu. Rev. Physiol.* **57**, 521–546.

McGehee, D. S., Heath, M. J. S., Gelber, S., Devay, P., and Role, L. W. (1995). Nicotine enhancement of fast excitatory synaptic transmission in CNS by presynaptic receptors. *Science* **269**, 1692–1696.

Meeker, R. B., Michels, K. M., Libber, M. T., and Hayward, J. N. (1986). Characteristics and distribution of high- and low-affinity alpha bungaotoxin binding sites in the rat hypothalmus. *J. Neurosci.* **6**, 1866–1875.

Miledi, R., and Parker, I. (1984). Chloride current induced by injection of calcium into *Xenopus* oocytes. *J. Physiol.* (*London*) **357**, 173–183.

Morris, B. J., Hicks, A. A., Wisden, W., Darlison, M. G., Hunt, S. P., and Barnard, E. A. (1990). District regional expression of nicotinic acetylcholine subunit receptor genes in chick brain. *Mol. Brain Res.* **7**, 306–315.

Moss, B. L., Schuetze, S. M., and Role, L. W. (1989). Functional properties and developmental regulation of nicotinic acetylcholine receptors on embryonic chicken sympathetic neurons. *Neuron* **3**, 597–607.

Mulle, C., and Changeux, J.-P. (1990). A novel type of nicotinic receptor in the rat cental nervous system characterized by patch clamp techniques. *J. Neurosci.* **10**, 169–175.

Mulle, C., Choquet, D., Korn, H., and Changeux, J.-P. (1992a). Calcium influx through nicotinic receptor in rat central neurons: Relevance to cellular regulation. *Neuron* **8**, 135–143.

Mulle, C., Lena, C., and Changeux, J.-P. (1992b). Potentiation of nicotinic receptor response by external calcium in rat central neurons. *Neuron* **8**, 937–945.

Mulle, C., Vidal, C., Benoit, P., and Changeux, J.-P. (1991). Existence of different subtypes of nicotinic acetylcholine receptors in the rat habenulo-interpeduncular system. *J. Neurosci.* **11**(8), 2588–2597.

Nef, P., Oneyser, C., Alliod, C., Couturier, S., and Ballivet, M. (1988). Genes expressed in the brain define three distinct neuronal nicotinic acetylcholine receptors. *EMBO J.* **7**, 595–601.

Norbert, A., Wahlström, G., Arnelo, U., and Larsson, C. (1983). Effect of long-term nicotine treatment on [^{3}H]nicotine binding sites in the rat brain. *Drug Alcohol Depend.* **16**, 9–17.

Padgett, R. A., Grabowski, P. J., Konarska, M. M., Seiler, S., and Sharp, P. A. (1986). Splicing of messenger RNA precursors. *Annu. Rev. Biochem.* **55**, 1119–1150.

Patrick, J., and Stallcup, W. (1977a). Alpha-bungarotoxin binding and cholinergic receptor function on a rat sympathetic nerve line. *J. Biol. Chem.* **252**, 8629.

Patrick, J., and Stallcup, W. (1977b). Immunological distinction between acetylcholine receptor and the alpha-bungarotoxin-binding component on sympathetic neurons. *Proc. Natl. Acad. Sci. U.S.A.* **74**, 4689–4692.

Patrick, J., Sequela, P., Vernino, S., Amador, M., Luetje, C., and Dani, J. A. (1993). Functional diversity of neuronal nicotinic acetylcholine receptors. *Prog. Brain Res.* **98**, 113–120.

Pauly, J. R., Stitzel, J. A., Marks, M. J., and Collins, A. C. (1989). An autoradiographic analysis of cholinergic receptors in mouse brain. *Brain Res. Bull.* **22**, 453–459.

Pauly, J. R., Marks, M. J., Gross, S. D., and Collins, C. (1991). An autoradiographic analysis of cholinergic receptors in mouse brain after chronic nicotine treatment. *J. Pharmacol. Exp. Ther.* **258**, 1127–1135.

Radcliffe, K. A., and Dani, J. A. (1995). Nicotinic receptor activation potentiates glutamatergic synaptic transmission in cultured hippocampal neurones. *Soc. Neurosci. Abstr.* **21**, 526.1.

Rainbow, T. C., Schwartz, R. D., Parsons, B., and Kellar, K. J. (1984). Quantitative autoradiography of [3H]acetylcholine binding sites in rat brain. *Neuroscience* **50**, 193–196.

Ramirez-Latorre, J. A., and Role, L. (1995). Potentiation of acetylcholine-evoked currents through $\alpha 1 + \beta 2$ and $\alpha 5 + \alpha 4 + \beta 2$ nAChRs: Localization of the Ca^{+2} regulatory site. *Soc. Neurosci. Abstr.* **21**, 527.3.

Rapier, C., Wonnacott, S., Lunt, G. G., and Albuquerque, E. X. (1987). The neurotoxin histrionic-otoxin interacts with the putative ion channel of the nicotinic acetylcholine receptors in the central nervous system. *FEBS Lett.* **212**, 292–296.

Rapier, C., Lunt, G. G., and Wonnacott, S. (1988). Stereoselective nicotine-induced release of dopamine from striatal synaptosomes: Concentration dependence and repetitive stimulation. *J. Neurochem.* **50**, 1123–1130.

Rapier, C., Lunt, G. G., and Wonnacott, S. (1990). Nicotinic modulation of [3H]Dopamine release from striatal synaptosomes: Pharmacological characterization. *J. Neurochem.* **54**, 937–945.

Ravdin, P., and Berg, D. K. (1979). Inhibition of neuronal acetylcholine sensitivity by alpha toxins from *Bungarus multicinctus* venom. *Proc. Natl. Acad. Sci. U.S.A.* **76**, 2072–2076.

Rust, G., Burgunder, J.-M., Lauterberger, T. E., and Cachelin, A. B. (1994). Expression of neuronal nicotinic acetylcholine receptor genes in the rat autonomic nervous system. *Eur. J. Neurosci.* **6**, 478–485.

Sacaan, A. I., Dunlop, J. L., and Lloyd, G. K. (1995). Pharmacological characterization of neuronal acetylcholine gated ion channel receptor-mediated hippocampal norepinephrine and striatal dopamine release from rat brain slices. *J. Pharmacol. Exp. Ther.* **274**, 224–230.

Sah, D. W. Y., Loring, R. H., and Zigmond, R. E. (1987). Long-term blockade by toxin F of nicotinic synaptic potentials in cultured sympathetic neurons. *Neuroscience* **20**, 867–874.

Sands, S. B., and Barish, M. E. (1992). Neuronal nicotinic acetylcholine receptor currents in pheochromocytoma (PC12) cells: Dual mechanisms of rectification. *J. Physiol. (London)* **447,** 467–487.

Sargent, P. B. (1993). The diversity of neuronal nicotinic acetylcholine receptors. *Annu. Rev. Neurosci.* **16,** 403–443.

Schoepfer, R., Conroy, W. G., Whiting, P., Gore, M., and Lindström, J. (1990). Brain α-bungarotoxin binding protein cDNAs and MAbs reveal subtypes of this branch of the ligand-gated ion channel gene superfamily. *Neuron* **5,** 35–48.

Schofield, P. R., Shivers, B. D., and Seeburg, P. H. (1990). The role of receptor subtype diversity in the CNS. *Trends Neurosci.* **13,** 8–11.

Schultz, D. W., and Zigmond, R. E. (1989). Neuronal bungarotoxin blocks the nicotinic stimulation of endogenous dopamine release from rat striatum. *Neurosci. Lett.* **98,** 310–316.

Schwartz, R. D., and Kellar, K. J. (1983). Nicotinic cholinergic receptor binding sites in the brain: regulation in vivo. *Science* **220,** 214–220.

Schwartz, R. D., and Kellar, K. J. (1985). In vivo regulation of [^{3}H]acetylcholine recognition sites in the brain by nicotinic cholinergic drugs. *J. Neurochem.* **45,** 427–433.

Schwartz, R. D., McGee, R., and Kellar, K. J. (1982). Nicotinic cholinergic receptors labeled by [3H]acetylcholine in rat brain. *Mol. Pharmacol.* **22,** 56–62.

Schwartz, R. D., Lehmann, J., and Kellar, K. J. (1984). Presynaptic nicotinic cholinergic receptors labeled by [^{3}H]acetylcholine on catecholamine and serotonin axons in brain. *J. Neurochem.* **42,** 1495–1498.

Seeburg, P. H. (1996). The role of RNA editing in controlling glutamate receptor channel properties. *J. Neurochem.* **66,** 1–5.

Seguela, P., Wadiche, J., Miller, K., Dani, J., and Patrick, J. (1993). Molecular cloning, functional expression and distribution of rat brain α7: A nicotinic cation channel highly permeable to calcium. *J. Neurosci.* **13,** 596–604.

Sivilotti, L. G., McNeil, D. K., Lewis, T. M., Nassar, M., Schoepfer, R., and Colquhoun, D. (1995). a3b4 expressed in oocytes does not reproduce the single channel properties of rat superior cervical ganglion nicotinic receptors. *Soc. Neurosci. Abstr.* **21,** 36.3.

Stephenson, F. A. (1995). The $GABA_A$ receptors. *Biochem. J.* **310,** 1–9.

Vernallis, A. B., Conroy, W. B., and Berg, DF. K. (1993). Neurons assemble acetylcholine receptors with as many as three kinds of subunit while maintaining subunit seggregation among receptor subtypes. *Neuron* **12,** 451–464.

Vernino, S., Amador, M., Luetje, C. W., Patrick, J., and Dani, J. (1991). Calcium modulation and high calcium permeability of neuronal nicotinic acetylcholine receptors. *Neuron* **8,** 127–134.

Vidal, C., and Changeux, J.-P. (1993). Nicotinic and muscarinic modulations of excitatory synaptic transmission in the rat prefrontal cortex *in vitro*. *Neuroscience* **56,** 23–32.

Vijayaraghavan, S., Pugh, P. C., Zhang, Z., Rathouz, M. M., and Berg, D. K. (1992). Nicotinic receptors that bind alpha-bungarotoxin on neurons raise intracellular free calcium. *Neuron* **8,** 352–363.

Wada, E., Wada, K., Boulter, J., Deneris, E., Heinemann, S., Patrick, J., and Swanson, L. W. (1989). Distribution of alpha2, alpha3, alpha4, and beta2 in the rat central nervous system: A hybridization histochemical study in the rat. *J. Comp. Neurol.* **284,** 314–335.

Wada, E., McKinnon, D., Heinemann, S., Patrick, J., and Swanson, L. W. (1990). The distribution of mrna encoded by a new member of the neuronal nicotinic receptor gene family (Alpha5) in the rat central nervous system. *Brain Res.* **526,** 45–53.

Westfall, T. C. (1974). Effect of nicotine and other drugs on the release of ^{3}H-norepinephrine and ^{3}H-dopamine from rat brain slices. *Neuropharmacology* **13,** 693–700.

Wilson Horch, H. L., and Sargent, P. (1995). Perisynaptic surface distribution of multiple classes of nicotinic acetylcholine receptors on neurons in the chicken ciliary ganglion. *J. Neurosci.* **15,** 7778–7795.

Wonnacott, S., and Drasdo, A. L. (1991). Presynaptic actions of nicotine in the CNS. *In* "Effects of Nicotine on Biological Systems," pp. 295–306. (eds Adklofer, F. & Thurau, K.) Birkhauser Verlag, Basel.

Wonnacott, S., and Soliakov, L. (1995). Presynaptic nicotinic receptors evoke [^{3}H] dopamine release from striatal synaptosomes by activation of voltage sensitive calcium channels. *Soc. Neurosci. Abstr.* **21**, 143.3.

Wonnacott, S., Irons, J., Rapier, C., Thorne, B., and Lunt, G. (1989). Presynaptic modulation of transmitter release by nicotinic receptors. *Prog. Brain Res.* **79**, 157–163.

Wonnacott, S., Wilkie, G., Soliakov, L., and Whiteaker, P. (1995). Presynaptic nicotinic autoreceptors and heteroreceptors in the CNS. *In* "Effects of Nicotine on Biological Systems II," Adv. Pharmacol. Sci., pp. 87–94. (eds Clarke, P. B. S., Quik, M., Adklofer, F. & Thurau, K.) Birkhaeuser Verlag, Basel.

Zhang, Z., Vijayaraghavan, S., and Berg, D. K. (1994). Neuronal acetylcholine receptors that bind alpha-bungarotoxin with high affinity function as ligand-gated ion channels. *Neuron* **12**, 167–177.

Zorumski, C. F., Thio, L. L., Isenberg, K. E., and Clifford, D. B. (1992). Nicotinic acetylcholine currents in cultured postnatal rat hippocampal neurons. *Mol. Pharmacol.* **41**, 931–936.

Richard D. Ye*
François Boulay

*Department of Immunology
The Scripps Research Institute
La Jolla, California 92037

†DBMS/Biochimie (CNRS/URA 1130)
CEA/Grenoble
38054 Grenoble Cedex 9
France

Structure and Function of Leukocyte Chemoattractant Receptors

I. Introduction

Leukocytes are capable of migrating along a chemical gradient, a phenomenon known as chemotaxis. Although chemotaxis is not unique to leukocytes, the accumulation of phagocytic leukocytes (phagocytes) at sites of inflammation is of particular importance for host defense against invading microorganisms and for wound healing. Migration of lymphocytes is believed to be essential for T-cell development and maturation. In several pathological conditions, the local accumulation of phagocytes and the subsequent release of superoxide anions and proteolytic enzymes are responsible for tissue damage associated with inflammatory disorders. Understanding the function of leukocyte chemoattractant and its underlying mechanisms is therefore of particular interest and clinical relevance.

Advances in Pharmacology, Volume 39

1054-3589/97/$25.00

Despite the fact that chemotaxis of phagocytes was observed more than a hundred years ago, it was not until the invention of the Boyden chamber that the systematic study of leukocyte chemotaxis began (Boyden, 1962). The finding of N-formylated peptides and the activated component of C5 (C5a) as potent leukocyte chemoattractants led to the pharmacological characterization of the cellular binding sites for these and other chemotactic agents, including the platelet-activating factor (PAF) and leukotriene B_4 (LTB_4). These studies were expanded to include the biochemical characterization of the signaling events following binding of the chemoattractants to their specific receptors. It is generally accepted that the same receptor that mediates leukocyte chemotaxis to a particular chemoattractant can also transduce signals leading to oxidative burst and degranulation, although there may be exceptions (see later). A new surge of research activities on chemoattractants and their receptors began in the mid-1980s with the discovery of a large family of chemotactic cytokines (chemokines) that attract various leukocyte subsets. The broad application of molecular cloning techniques has led to the delineation of the primary structures of many chemoattractant receptors. These leukocyte chemoattractant receptors share significant sequence homology and structural features, and together they constitute a subfamily within the G protein-coupled receptor (GPCR) superfamily.

This review is intended to briefly summarize the current understanding of the structure and function of G protein-coupled leukocyte chemoattractant receptors. These receptors represent specific cell surface binding sites for the classical chemoattractants (N-formyl peptides, C5a, PAF, LTB_4), as well as the α and β chemokines. The reader is referred to several review articles that discuss in more detail the molecular cloning and other aspects of chemoattractant receptors (Allen *et al.*, 1990; Murphy, 1994; Gerard and Gerard, 1994; Ben-Baruch *et al.*, 1995b). Leukocyte activation during inflammation has been discussed in great detail in a review by Snyderman and Uhing (1992).

II. Chemoattractant-Induced Leukocyte Functions

Chemoattractants induce a variety of leukocyte functions (Fig. 1). These functions may be divided into three broad categories. The first category includes cellular responses associated with leukocyte migration. All leukocyte chemoattractants induce directed movement of the cells, although the exact type of leukocytes that can respond to individual chemoattractants is determined by the cell surface expression of the chemoattractant receptors. Chemoattractants can regulate the change of cell shape, chemotaxis, chemokinesis, and leukocyte adhesion. This latter function is believed to correlate with the transendothelial migration of the leukocytes. The N-formyl peptide fMet-Leu-Phe (fMLF) has been shown to cause the shedding of L-selectin

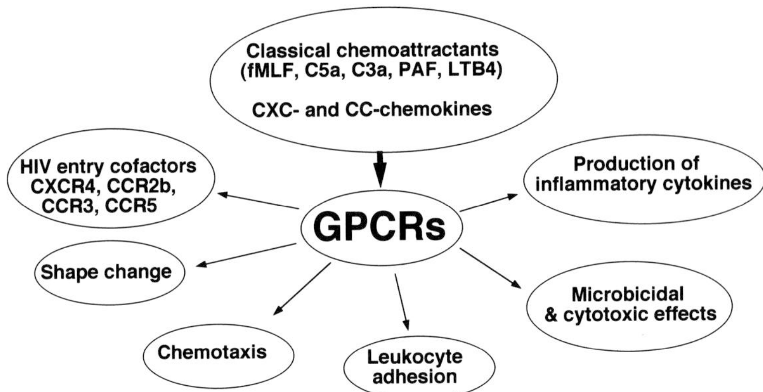

FIGURE 1 Schematic drawing depicting the many functions of leukocyte chemoattractant receptors. GPCRs, G protein-coupled receptors.

(Kishimoto *et al.*, 1989), presumably facilitating further interaction of leukocytes with endothelial cells. In general, the concentrations required for chemoattractant-induced cell movement are relatively low, usually in the nanomolar or subnanomolar range.

The second category includes chemoattractant induction of leukocyte microbicidal functions and cytotoxic effects. Phagocytes treated with fMLF and C5a generate superoxide anions as a result of activation of the NADPH oxidase system. Granulocytes release the contents of granules in response to chemoattractant stimulation. These substances are bactericidal and together constitute the first line of defense against invading pathogenic microorganisms. However, the inappropriate release of the superoxide anions and proteolytic enzymes is responsible for tissue damage associated with ischemic–reperfusion injury and many inflammatory diseases. These leukocyte functions are evoked at higher chemoattractant concentrations, usually 10- to 100-fold higher than the concentrations required for chemotaxis. It has been noted that the capability of chemoattractants to activate the NADPH oxidase system varies widely, with fMLF and C5a being the most potent activators (Snyderman and Uhing, 1992).

In addition to these well-characterized functions, leukocyte chemoattractants also stimulate other important cellular functions that can be grouped into the third category. C5a, fMLF, and PAF have been shown to stimulate the production of inflammatory cytokines at nanomolar concentrations (Goodman *et al.*, 1982; Cassatella *et al.*, 1992; Weyrich *et al.*, 1995). It has been found that these chemoattractants can induce the activation of the transcription factor NF-κB, which regulates the expression of a variety of immediate-early genes (Pan *et al.*, 1995; Kravchenko *et al.*, 1995; Ye *et al.*, 1996). The PAF receptor has been shown to mediate the adhesion of *Streptococcus pneumoniae* to endothelial and epithelial cells (Cundell *et al.*,

1995). Experiments with target deletion of the mouse C5a receptor suggested that it is essential in mice for protection against infection by *Pseudomonas aeruginosa* (Höpken *et al.,* 1996). The C-C chemokine RANTES (*R*egulated on *A*ctivation, *N*ormal *T* cell *E*xpressed and *S*ecreted) is capable of activating T cells (Bacon *et al.,* 1995). More recently, MIP-1α, MIP-1β, and RANTES have been shown to possess anti-HIV activity associated with the activation of $CD8^+$ T lymphocytes (Cocchi *et al.,* 1995). This new finding triggered a tremendous effort to characterized the role of chemokines and chemokine receptors in HIV-1 infection.

Based on previous observations that a cofactor is necessary for efficient entry of HIV-1 into host cells, Berger and colleagues devised a novel functional cloning method to study fusion between cells expressing the HIV-1 envelope glycoprotein and $CD4^+$ cells. Their work resulted in the cloning of a cDNA encoding a cell surface protein named "fusin," which serves as a cofactor for entry of T-cell line-tropic HIV-1 isolates into $CD4^+$ cells (Feng *et al.,* 1996). Fusin is identical in sequence to a previously isolated chemokine receptor homolog, now known as a receptor for stromal cell-derived factor 1 (SDF-1; see Section III for more detail). Other studies identified that the chemokine receptor CCR5[1] mediates the entry of macrophage-tropic isolates of HIV-1 (Dragic *et al.,* 1996; Alkhatib *et al.,* 1996; Deng *et al.,* Choe *et al.,* 1996; Doranz *et al.,* 1996), whereas CCR3 (Choe *et al.,* 1996; Doranz *et al.,* 1996) and CCR2b (Doranz *et al.,* 1996) were found to facilitate the entry of dual-tropic primary HIV-1 isolates. Several studies demonstrated that binding of the agonists to these receptors inhibited viral fusion (see Section III). These important discoveries suggested a new function of chemokine receptors in viral infection and raised the possibility of using chemokines or their homologues for blocking virus entry into the host cells.

Binding of a chemoattractant to its receptor generates signals that are further amplified and regulated at several levels, therefore contributing to the diverse functions of leukocytes. Chemoattractant receptors are functionally coupled to heterotrimeric G proteins. The G_{i2} and G_{i3} proteins have been shown to be the major G protein α subunits that interact with chemoattractant receptors (Gierschik *et al.,* 1989). Pertussis toxin, which ADP-ribosylates the G_i and G_o classes of G_α proteins, abolishes the majority of leukocyte functions (Bokoch and Gilman, 1984; Snyderman and Uhing, 1992). Although the G_{16} and G_z classes of G protein α subunits have been shown to couple to chemoattractant receptors in transfected cells, their role

[1] A new nomenclature for chemokine receptors was recommended at the Gordon Conference on Chemokines in New Hampshire, June 23–27, 1996. According to the new nomenclature, CXC (α) chemokine receptors are named CXCRs, and CC (β) chemokine receptors are termed CCRs. The names of these receptors appear in Table I. While the previous names are used frequently in this review when referring existing data, the new nomenclature is adopted whenever possible.

in leukocyte function remains to be established (Amatruda *et al.*, 1993; Tsu *et al.*, 1995). Chemoattractant binding stimulates the GTPase activity of the G protein α subunits and the dissociation of the α subunits from the $\beta\gamma$ subunits. The latter then activates the phospholipase $C_{\beta 2}$ isoform in leukocytes (Camps *et al.*, 1992a,b; Blank *et al.*, 1992; Katz *et al.*, 1992). The subsequent breakdown of phospatidylinositol 4,5-bisphosphate (PIP_2) leads to the formation of the secondary messengers inositol trisphosphate (IP_3) and diacylglycerol (DAG), which regulate the mobilization of Ca^{2+} from intracellular stores and the activation of protein kinase C (PKC), respectively. Various neutrophil functions can be triggered as a result of phosphorylation by PKC and other kinases (Thelen and Wirthmueller, 1994). In addition, chemoattractants also stimulate phospholipase A_2 and phospholipase D, although the regulatory mechanisms have not been fully appreciated (Cockroft, 1992; Billah, 1993; Thelen and Wirthmueller, 1994).

In addition to the heterotrimeric G proteins, a group of low molecular weight GTPases are activated by chemoattractants and are essential for many neutrophil functions. Members of these Ras-like monomeric proteins participate in the regulation of the NADPH oxidase system (Quinn, 1995), cell shape change (Hall, 1992), and leukocyte adhesion (Laudanna *et al.*, 1996). GTPases serve as molecular switches: "on" in a GTP-bound state and "off" when GDP is bound. The GTPase activity is further regulated by a number of proteins including the GTPase-activating proteins (GAP), guanine nucleotide exchange factors (GEF), and GDP dissociation stimulators and inhibitors (GDS, GDI). Several review articles have covered this topic as well as a large body of related literature in detail (Hall, 1992; Bokoch and Der, 1993; Quinn, 1995).

Other protein kinases are involved in chemoattractant signaling. In neutrophils, stimulation with fMLF induces tyrosine phosphorylation of several polypeptides, as seen with *in vitro* kinase renaturation assays (Grinstein and Furuya, 1992). One of the peptides identified was the 41-kDa ERK-1, which is tyrosine phosphorylated within seconds after fMLF stimulation. Torres *et al.* (1993) confirmed this finding and reported the identification of two tyrosine phosphorylated proteins with apparent molecular weights of 40- and 42-kDa that were recognized by anti-MAP kinase antibodies. fMLF-stimulated MAP kinases were able to phosphorylate the substrates myelin basic protein and T-669, a peptide derived from the EGF receptor with Thr-669. The tyrosine kinase inhibitor genistein reduced fMLF stimulated phosphorylation of the 40- and 42-kDa proteins in a dose-dependent manner. Meanwhile, a decreased production of superoxide anion in fMLF-stimulated neutrophils was observed. These initial studies suggest a link between fMLF induction of MAP kinase activation and the stimulation of the NADPH oxidase system. However, Yu *et al.* (1995) suggest that MAPK activation can be dissociated from the oxidative burst in neutrophils and differentiated HL-60 cells. Worthen and co-workers (1994) immunoprecipitated Raf-1 activity and detected Ras activation in fMLF-stimulated neutrophils. They further demonstrated that this function of fMLF was sensitive to pertussis toxin treatment of the cells, but was not dependent on PKC activity. Thus, fMLF stimulation of MAP kinase activity in neutrophils appears to involve $G_{i\alpha}$-mediated receptor regulation of the Ras/Raf/MAP kinase pathway. In addition to fMLF, C5a and IL-8 have also been shown to stimulate this kinase pathway (Buhl *et al.*, 1995; Knall *et al.*, 1996).

A number of laboratories have demonstrated the activation of the phosphatidylinositol 3-kinase (PI3K) in fMLF-stimulated neutrophils. Unlike the activation of PI3K by receptor tyrosine kinases (RTK), fMLF-induced PI3K activation does not involve tyrosine phosphorylation of the protein (Vlahos and Matter, 1992). This is consistent with the finding that a newly cloned PI3K isotype, p110γ, can be activated by the α and $\beta\gamma$ subunits of G proteins without interaction with the p85 subunits of the PI3K (Stoyanov *et al.*, 1995). The neutrophil PI3K activation can be blocked by the inhibitors wortmannin and LY294002, resulting in the inhibition of fMLF-stimulated oxidant production (Okada *et al.*, 1994; Vlahos *et al.*, 1995; Ding *et al.*, 1995). However, fMLF-induced calcium flux, CD11b-dependent adhesion, and actin polymerization were not affected by the inhibitors (Vlahos *et al.*, 1995), suggesting the selective involvement of PI3K in some, but not all, neutrophil functions. More recently, it was shown that fMLF also activates the lyn tyrosine kinase, resulting in the phosphorylation of the Shc adaptor protein which contains the SH2 and SH3 domains (Ptasznik *et al.*, 1995). This finding suggests a potentially extensive overlap between the signaling pathways stimulated by chemoattractants and growth factors.

III. Molecular Characterization of the Structure of Chemoattractant Receptors

A. Biochemical Characterization and Molecular Cloning

1. Receptors for Classical Chemoattractants

Study of the classical chemoattractants began in the 1970s, when a variety of ligands were recognized as chemoattractants for phagocytes. These include the anaphylatoxin C5a and C3a, polypeptides that arise from the cleavage of the complement proteins (Shin *et al.*, 1968; Hugli and Müller-Eberhard, 1978); the N-formylated peptides derived from bacterial cells as well as mitochondrially encoded proteins (Schiffmann *et al.*, 1975a,b; Carp, 1982; Marasco *et al.*, 1984); the platelet-activating factor (1-O-alkyl-2-acetyl-*sn*-glycero-3-phosphocholine), which is a lipid mediator released from platelets, neutrophils, monocytes, macrophages, and mast cells (Benveniste *et al.*, 1972; Hanahan, 1986; Prescott *et al.*, 1990); and the leukotriene B_4, which belongs to a group of compounds derived from arachidonic acid (Samuelson *et al.,* 1987). A series of studies established the presence of functionally distinct high-affinity binding sites for ^{125}I-labeled C5a (Chenoweth *et al.,* 1978) and *N*-formyl-Nle-Leu-Phe-Nle-[^{125}I]Tyr-Lys (Niedel *et al.,* 1979) as well as [^{3}H]PAF (O'Flaherty *et al.,* 1986) and [^{3}H]LTB_4 (Goldman and Goetzl , 1982). These binding sites are found on membrane fractions isolated from human PMN phagocytes and display dissociation constants (K_d) of ~1 n*M*. A variety of cross-linking approaches, involving either radioligands derivatized with photoactivatable groups or radioligands together with homo- or heterobifunctional reagents, allowed the identification of a single molecular species in neutrophils for FPR, C5aR, and the LTB_4 receptor. A polypeptide that migrated as a broad band on SDS-PAGE, with an apparent molecular mass between 55 and 70 kDa typical of glycosylated protein, was first identified as the FPR by Niedel *et al.* (1980). Cross-linking of ^{125}I-labeled C5a identified a major species with an apparent mass at 52 kDa, indicating that the C5a-binding unit has a molecular mass of 42–43 kDa (Johnson and Chenoweth, 1987). Finally, Goldman *et al.* (1991) described the photoaffinity labeling of a compound at ~60 kDa that may represent the receptor for LTB_4. However, despite the progress in the characterization of binding sites for the classical chemoattractants, purification and sequencing of the receptor proteins remained unsuccessful.

A major progress toward the understanding of neutrophil activation by chemoattractant receptors was achieved by cloning of the cDNAs encoding these classical chemoattractant receptors. All the aforementioned receptors, with the exception of the LTB_4 receptor, have been cloned by the use of exogenous expression or homology hybridization strategies.

a. Human N-formyl Peptide Receptors and Structurally Related Receptors
Using a strategy relying on the ability of functional receptor to confer high-affinity ligand binding in COS-7 cells, two human cDNAs encoding a 350 amino acid protein were first isolated by Boulay and co-workers (1990a,b) from a cDNA library prepared from dibutyryl cyclic AMP (Bt2cAMP)-differentiated HL-60 cells. The two isolated cDNAs differ in the organization of their 5′ and 3′ sequences as well as by two nucleotides in the coding sequence, but both encode functional proteins that belong to the G protein-coupled receptor family. Further studies by others indicated that the human FPR is encoded by a single copy gene of ~6 kb with a genomic organization similar to that of the β_1- and β_2-adrenergic receptors in that the coding sequence is contained in a single exon (Perez *et al.,* 1992a; Murphy *et al.,* 1993; Haviland *et al.,* 1993). The 5′-untranslated region contains two exons separated by Alu sequences. Two mRNAs are produced by alternative splicing of exon 2 in differentiated HL-60 cells and normal blood monocytes (Murphy *et al.,* 1993). The 3′-untranslated sequence contains a third Alu sequence downstream of the polyadenylation site, thereby indicating that

the different cDNA clones originally isolated may be derived by alternative polyadenylation (Haviland *et al.*, 1993). Although cAMP regulates FPR gene expression in HL-60 cells in a time- and concentration-dependent manner, no cAMP responsive element has been found in the 5′-untranslated region (Perez *et al.*, 1992a). Sequence analysis of cDNA clones isolated from different sources revealed amino acid differences that do not alter the pharmacological profile (Boulay *et al.*, 1990a; Perez *et al.*, 1992a), suggesting that there are allelic forms of FPR and a polymorphism of the FPR gene.

Two genes encoding FPR homologs have been isolated by low-stringency cross-hybridization with the human FPR cDNA probe. These genes, designated *FPRL1* and *FPRL2,* encode proteins that are highly homologous to the human FPR. A cDNA of *FPRL1* was cloned from HL-60 cells cDNA libraries. The gene product is referred to as FPR2 (for it binds fMLF with low affinity; Ye *et al.*, 1992), FPR-like 1 (FPRL1; Murphy *et al.*, 1992), and FPR-homolog 1 (FPRH1; Bao *et al.*, 1992). It shares 69% sequence identity with the human FPR (Boulay *et al.*, 1990a,b). The sequence of these two proteins are particularly similar in the transmembrane domains and in the intracellular loops. Despite the high level of sequence homology, the gene product of *FPRL1* only binds fMLF with a low affinity (K_d = 430 n*M* with ^{3}H-labeled fMLF; Quehenberger *et al.*, 1993). This is in contrast to the rabbit counterpart of human FPR, which has slightly higher degree of sequence homology (78%) but binds fMLF with high affinity (Ye *et al.*, 1993). At micromolar concentrations, fMLF induced calcium mobilization in FPRLI-transfected L cells (Ye *et al.*, 1992) and in injected *Xenopus* oocytes expressing the *FPRL1* protein (Durstin *et al.*, 1994). This effect of fMLF could be blocked by pretreatment of the cells with pertussis toxin, indicating functional coupling of the receptor with a G_i or G_o-like protein (Quehenberger *et al.*, 1993). In an effort to identify the natural ligand for the *FPRL1* gene product, *N*-formyl peptides of various lengths and compositions as well as nonformylated peptides have been tested (R. Ye, 1997 unpublished data). None have been shown to potently activate this receptor.

Recently Fiore and Serhan reported that transfected Chinese hamster ovary (CHO) cells expressing the *FPRL1* protein displayed specific and high-affinity binding to lipoxin A_4 (Fiore *et al.*, 1994; Fiore and Serhan, 1995). Furthermore, they observed lipoxin A_4-stimulated GTPase activity in the transfected cells. These findings suggest that *FPRL1* gene encodes a functional receptor for lipoxin A_4, which is a lipoxygenase-derived eicosanoid. Lipoxin A_4-induced signaling is apparently different from signaling by fMLF. While in PMN, fMLF is a potent agonist for CD11/18 upregulation, LXA_4 does not increase the surface expression of CD11b. Addition of LXA_4 was found to result in a 30–50% inhibitory effect of the fMLF-stimulated CD11b upregulation (Fiore and Serhan, 1995). The diffferential signaling observed with LXA_4 is intriguing since FPR and FPRL1 share an extremely high degree of amino acid identity in their cytoplasmic domain and are likely to transduce signals through the same pool of pertussis toxin-sensitive G protein (Quehenberger *et al.,* 1993). Although LXA_4 has been shown to stimulate calcium mobilization in monocytes (Romano *et al.,* 1996), several laboratories were not able to obtain Lipoxin A_4-stimulated calcium mobilization in injected oocytes or transfected mammalian cells that responded to micromolar concentrations of fMLF with calcium mobilization (P. Murphy, personal communication; F. Boulay, R. Ye, unpublished data). Furthermore, LXA_4 was found to be unable to induce phosphorylation of FRPL1 expressed in cell lines in which FPR is rapidly phosphorylated in response to fMLF (F. Boulay, unpublished data). Whether there are additional ligands for this receptor remains to be investigated.

A second gene, *FPRL2,* was originally cloned from a genomic DNA library (Bao *et al.,* 1992). It encodes a protein with 56% sequence identity to the human FPR and 83% sequence identity to the *FPRL1* gene product. It was subsequently shown that the *FPRL2* gene is indeed expressed in monocytes, but not in neutrophils (Durstin *et al.,* 1994). This is different from the expression pattern of the *FPRL1* gene, which is found in neutrophils as well as in monocytes (Durstin *et al.,* 1994), and its expression is induced during myeloid differentiation of the HL-60 cells (Ye *et al.,* 1992). Expression of the *FPRL2* gene product in *Xenopus* oocytes did not result in any functional responses to fMLF (Durstin *et al.,* 1994).

b. Human C5a Receptor Elucidation of the amino acid sequence of the C5a receptor (C5aR) was independently achieved by two groups using different strategies. Making the prediction that the C5aR shares homologies with rhodopsin and the β-adrenergic receptors, Gerard and Gerard (1991) probed a cDNA library from differentiated U937 lymphoma cells with a degenerate oligonucleotides. Subsequent expression of candidate cDNAs in COS-7 allowed the identification of a cDNA that confers high-affinity binding to C5a (Gerard and Gerard, 1991). At the same time, Boulay and coworkers (1991) isolated a cDNA clone from a library prepared from Bt2cAMP-differentiated HL-60 by an expression cloning strategy similar to that used for the cloning of FPR. In contrast to FPR, a single transcript of 2.4 kb was detected in differentiated myeloid cell lines. The human C5aR is encoded by a single copy gene that contains a large intron (~9 kb) separating the ATG translation initiation site (exon 1) and the rest of the receptor coding sequence (exon 2) (Gerard *et al.,* 1993). The genomic sequence flanking the 5′-untranslated sequence was reported to possess a weak promoter activity when transfected in myeloid-derived rat basophilic leukemia RBL-1 cells, but not in SK-N-SH human neuroblastoma cells. Upstream to the promoter region, a silencing element(s) was identified which may regulate C5aR gene expression (Gerard *et al.,* 1993). Interestingly, the gene for C5aR is localized closely with that for the FPR, FPRL1, and FPRL2 on a 200-kb fragment in chromosome 19q13.3 (Bao *et al.*, 1992; Murphy *et al.*, 1992; Gerard *et al.*, 1993; Alvarez *et al.*, 1994).

The cloned receptor, when transiently expressed in COS-7 cells, bound C5a with an affinity similar to that observed in neutrophils and differentiated HL-60 cells. The deduced amino acid sequence demonstrated the relatedness of C5aR with other members of the GPCR family. The overall protein sequence identity with the FPR is 34%, with the greatest sequence similarity in the hydrophobic transmembrane segments. Subsequently, the rat, mouse, dog, and bovine C5a receptors were also characterized, revealing a striking divergence (only ~30% amino acid identity) from one species to the next in the putative hydrophilic extracellular regions. In contrast, the putative intracellular hydrophilic sequences as well as the hydrophobic transmembrane domains share a higher degree of sequence identity (70 and 78%, respectively) (Gerard *et al.*, 1992; Perret *et al.*, 1992). However, despite the marked sequence divergence, all these receptors bind human C5a with high affinity. This pattern of interspecies divergence is quite unusual in the receptor family and all the more surprising if one considers that the putative extracellular loops may establish secondary contact point for the interaction with the ligand. Inside a given species, no polymorphism has been reported, suggesting a strong selective pressure for the maintenance of a conserved structure of C5aR. In this respect, it is worth noting that most mutant C5a receptors generated *in vitro* are not functionally expressed in transfected cells (Kolakowski *et al.*, 1995).

Using the human FPR cDNA as a probe, Roglić *et al.* (1996) isolated a clone (AZ3B) from a differentiated HL-60 cDNA library that encodes a putative G protein-coupled receptor with 482 amino acids. The receptor is homologous (up to 37% identical sequence) to the human C5aR, FPR, and the two FPR-like receptors. The AZ3B protein is unique in that it contains a large extracellular loop between transmembrane domain (TMD) 4 and TMD 5. Hydropathy plot analysis reveals a loop structure of ~172 amino acids, which is the largest extracellular loop seen among all the GPCRs identified to date. The localization of this loop on the cell surface was confirmed by flow cytometry analysis of differentiated HL-60 cells as well as cells transfected to express the AZ3B protein, using antisera against fusion proteins containing a stretch to the loop sequence (Roglić *et al.*, 1996). This receptor has been subequently identified as the human C3a receptor by two independent studies. Crass *et al.* (1996) used an expression cloning approach to obtain the cDNA for the C3aR from cAMP-differentiated U937 cells, whereas Ames *et al.* (1996) used a partial cDNA sequence as a probe to isolate the full-length clone from a neutrophil cDNA library. Direct binding analysis revealed a K_d of 0.3 n*M* in transfected cells expressing the C3aR (Ames *et al.*, 1996). An intriguing finding from these studies is the tissue distribution pattern of the C3aR. The receptor message was detected not only in myeloid cells, but also in several lymphoid tissues and many regions of the brain (Roglić *et al.*, 1996; Ames *et al.*, 1996; Crass *et al.*, 1996). In addition, C3aR was immunologically detected in umbilical vein endothelial cells (Roglić *et al.*, 1996). These new observations suggest a potential role of the complement fragment in immune regulation and vascular biological functions.

Similarly, C5aR and FPR expression is traditionally thought to be restricted to cells of myeloid lineage, but several studies indicate that they are also present in nonmyeloid cells. C5a can bind to and activate endothelial cells (Foreman *et al.*, 1994), and cultured human umbilical vein endothelial cells are able to uptake and release formyl peptides (Rotrosen *et al.*, 1987). Moreover, Haviland and co-workers (1995) have shown that the human hepatoma-derived cell line HepG2 expresses high-affinity binding sites for ^{125}I-labeled C5a (K_d = 1 nM, B_{max} = 2.8 × 10^4 receptors/cell) and for a ^{125}I-labeled fMLF analog (K_d = 2.5 nM, B_{max} = 6 × 10^3 receptors/cell) (McCoy *et al.*, 1995). In *in vivo* studies, C5aR expression has been demonstrated by *in situ* hybridization and immunocytochemistry. In addition to the expression of C5aR in liver, mice treated with LPS showed an dramatic increase in C5aR mRNA in spleen, lung, heart, kidney, and intestine. Immunostaining analyses revealed that bronchial and alveolar epithelial cells, as well as smooth muscle and endothelial cells, also express C5aR (Haviland *et al.*, 1995). Interestingly, mRNAs and protein expression of C5aR, IL-8R, and FPR were reported in human astrocytes and microglia as well as in the astrocytoma cell line HSC2 (Gasque *et al.*, 1995; Lacy *et al.*, 1995). Dendritic cells, a heterogeneous system of professional antigen-presenting cells involved in the initiation of immune responses,were found to migrate in response to N-formyl peptides, C5a, but not IL-8 (Sozzani *et al.*, 1995). Thus, these observations suggest that these chemotactic factors and their cognate receptors may play an important role in modulating the inflammatory and immune responses in both the central nervous system and peripheral tissues.

c. PAF Receptor The phospholipid PAF (1-O-alkyl-2-acetyl-*sn*-glycero-3-phosphocholine) is one of the most potent phospholipid agonists. Pharmacological studies with [^{3}H]PAF and structurally different PAF antagonists have provided most of the information on the molecular properties of the PAF receptor protein. However, despite intense efforts to purify the receptor, depicting the molecular architecture of PAF receptor was not successful until Honda and co-workers (1991) isolated the guinea pig PAF receptor cDNA by expression in the oocytes from *Xenopus laevis* and electrophysiological detection of PAF-induced responses. The human PAF receptor cDNA was subsequently isolated from leukocyte cDNA libraries by others (Nakamura *et al.*, 1991; Ye *et al.*, 1991; Kunz *et al.*, 1992). Both the guinea pig and the human cDNAs encode a 342 amino acid protein exhibiting significant homologies with other members of the G protein-coupled receptor family. Overall amino acid identity between the two receptors is 83%, with a higher homology in the putative transmembrane domains. While the guinea pig receptor contains two putative N-glycosylation sites, the human PAF receptor, unlike most chemoattractant receptors, has no sites for N-glycosylation. Cells transfected with PAFR cDNA acquired the ability to bind with high affinity a radiolabeled PAF antagonist, [^{3}H]WEB 2086, and to respond to subnanomolar PAF concentrations with inositol 1,4,5-trisphosphate production and calcium mobilization that could be inhibited by PAF antagonists (Nakamura *et al.*, 1991; Ye *et al.*, 1991).

Analysis of somatic cell hybrids unequivocally suggests that human PAFR exists as a single gene located on chromosome 1 (Seyfried *et al.*, 1992). Two 5′-noncoding exons, each with distinct transcription initiation sites, are alternatively spliced to a common splice acceptor site on a third exon that contains the entire coding sequence. This particular gene organization with two promoters yields two different transcripts with distinct tissue distribution pattern. Transcript 1 (containing exon 1) is preferentially found in peripheral leukocytes, the differentiated eosinophilic cell line EoL-1, and brain, whereas transcripts 1 and 2 were both detected in heart, lung, spleen, and kidney (Mutoh *et al.*, 1993; Sugimoto *et al.*, 1992). It has been reported that the expression of PAF receptor transcript 1 can be regulated through NF-κB (Mutoh *et al.*, 1994), whereas PAF itself stimulates NF-κB activation (Kravchenko *et al.*, 1995). Thus, PAF may positively regulate the expression of its own receptor (Mutoh *et al.*, 1994).

2. *Chemokine Receptors*

Since the mid-1980s, a new class of structurally related peptides termed chemokines has emerged that chemoattract and activate a variety of cell types. This growing family of chemoattractants has been divided into two subfamilies according to the position of the first two cysteine residues, which are either separated by one amino acid residue (CXC or α chemokines) or are adjacent (CC or β chemokines). The well-studied human CXC chemokines are interleukin 8 (IL-8), GROα, β, γ, NAP-2, ENA-78, platelet factor 4 (PF4), and interferon-γ-inducible protein 10 (IP-10) that act preferentially on neutrophils, whereas the major CC chemokines include monocyte chemotactic proteins (MCP-1, MCP-2, and MCP-3), macrophage inflammatory proteins (MIP-1α and MIP-1β), I-309, and RANTES that act on monocytes, basophil and eosinophil granulocytes, and T lymphocytes. Detailed reviews on their structures, chemical properties, cellular sources, biochemistry, and biological activities have been published (Oppenheim *et al.*, 1991; Baggiolini *et al.*, 1994; Murphy, 1994). This review focuses on selected representative chemokines and their cognate receptors, i.e., IL-8, which is the best known member of the CXC chemokine subfamily, and MCP-1 and MIP-1α/RANTES in the CC chemokine subfamily.

a. Receptors for CXC Chemokines Competitive radioligand-binding studies with ^{125}I-labeled human IL-8, NAP-2, and GROα led to the identification of high-affinity binding sites on a variety of cell types. None of the tested chemokines were displaced by unrelated classical chemoattractants such as fMet-Leu-Phe, C5a, LTB_4, and PAF. However, there was no strict selectivity for related chemokines within a subfamily. The existence of shared receptors for chemokines was inferred from the analysis of the binding data and cross-desensitization studies of human neutrophils (Schnitzel *et al.*, 1991). One receptor binds all three ligands with high affinity ($K_d = 0.1–0.4$ nM) whereas another binds IL-8 with high affinity and NAP-2 and GROα with low affinity ($K_d > 100$ nM) (Moser *et al.*, 1991). However, evidence for a distinct high-affinity receptor for GROα in human melanoma cell line Hs294T has been presented (Horuk *et al.*, 1993a). The sharing of receptors by IL-8, NAP-2, and GROα in human neutrophils was corroborated by cross-desensitization experiments. As shown by intracellular Ca^{2+} measurement, stimulation of neutrophils with IL-8 resulted in a marked desensitization toward a subsequent challenge with NAP-2 and GROα. Consistent with the existence of low-affinity receptors for NAP-2 and GROα, these two chemokines cross-desensitized each other, but responses to IL-8 were moderately attenuated when cells were prestimulated with NAP-2 and GROα, presumably because IL-8 still interacts with a high-affinity receptor that binds NAP-2 and GROα with low affinity (Moser *et al.*, 1991). Further studies revealed that other members of the family, GROβ, GROγ (Geiser *et al.*, 1993), and ENA-78 (Walz *et al.*, 1991), behave similarly to NAP-2 and GROα in desensitization experiments and presumably share receptors with IL-8 in neutrophils.

The concept of "shared receptors" was further supported by affinity cross-linking experiments with ^{125}I-labeled IL-8, NAP-2, or GROα which revealed the presence of multiple IL-8-sensitive species with molecular masses ranging from 44 and 70 kDa in neutrophil membranes (Grob *et al.*, 1990; Moser *et al.*, 1991). Cross-linking could be suppressed by all three unlabeled chemokines. Treatment of neutrophil membranes with digitonin resulted in the preferential solubilization of a 44-kDa receptor species in an active form that bound NAP-2 and GROα with low affinity and IL-8 with high affinity (Schumacher *et al.*, 1992). The receptor heterogeneity observed in neutrophils was not observed in U937 cells, where affinity cross-linking with iodinated IL-8 resulted in the labeling of a single molecular species with an apparent molecular mass of 69 kDa (Horuk *et al.*, 1993a).

Two distinct human IL-8 receptors were cloned whose pharmacological profiles were consistent with the previous observations when expressed exogenously. The first cDNA, encoding a 350 amino acid protein (IL-8RA, or CXCR1 according to the new nomenclature) with high affinity for ^{125}I-labeled IL-8, was isolated from a neutrophil cDNA library by an expression cloning strategy (Holmes *et al.*, 1991). A second cDNA coding for a 360 amino acid receptor (IL-8RB, or CXCR2) was identified by probing at low stringency a cDNA library from Bt2cAMP-differentiated HL-60 cells with an oligonucleotide probe specific for the sequence of F3R, the rabbit counterpart of human IL-8RA (Murphy and Tiffany, 1991). F3R had been cloned from a rabbit neutrophil cDNA library and was originally reported to be the rabbit counterpart of the human FPR based on calcium mobilization assays in *X. laevis* oocytes (Thomas *et al.*, 1990). However, the pharmacological profile of the encoded protein was that of the IL-8 receptor after expression in mammalian cells (Thomas *et al.*, 1991; Lee *et al.*, 1992b). The genomic organizations of the two human IL-8 receptors have been characterized, and it was found that the genes are clustered on a 150-kb fragment on chromosome 2q35 (Alvarez *et al.*, 1994; reviewed in Murphy, 1994).

The two human IL-8 receptors share 77% amino acid identity. The sequence differences cluster in the putative amino-terminal segments, the hydrophilic extracellular loop e2, the transmembrane domain IV, and the carboxyl-terminal segments. Although IL-8RB was originally reported to be a "low-affinity" IL-8 receptor on the basis of ^{125}I-labeled IL-8 binding to oocytes expressing the cloned receptor, it was subsequently determined that both receptors exhibit high-affinity binding for IL-8 (K_d = 2 nM) when expressed in the same mammalian cells (Lee *et al.*, 1992a). However, there was a marked difference in the affinity for GROα. While IL-8RB binds IL-8 and GROα with high affinity (K_d = 2 nM), IL-8RA binds GROα with low affinity (K_d = 450 nM) (Lee *et al*,. 1992a; Cerretti *et al.*, 1993; Gayle *et al.*, 1993). Because both transcripts are present in human neutrophils (Lee *et al.*, 1992a), it is likely that the complex pharmacological profile observed by Moser *et al.* (1991) is derived from the expression of these two receptors in neutrophils. An approximately equal ratio of both receptors in human neutrophils was unequivocally established by flow cytometry using monoclonal antibodies specific for each receptor (Chuntharapai *et al.*, 1994b).

While initial studies with IL-8, NAP-2, and MGSA/GROα suggest preferential activation of neutrophils with these CXC chemokines, recent cloning of CXCR3 and CXCR4 demonstrates a different pattern of interaction between CXC chemokines and their target cells. CXCR3 was cloned from a tetanus toxoid-specific CD4$^+$ T cell cDNA library by a PCR-generated probe (Loetscher *et al.*, 1996). The receptor has 368 amino acids and shares 40–41% sequence identity with the IL-8 receptors CXCR1 and CXCR2. It is 34–37% identical in sequence with the 5 known CC chemokine receptors. CXCR3 expressed in transfected cell lines responded to the interferon-γ-inducible CXC chemokines IP10 and Mig (monokine induced by interferon-γ) with calcium mobilization and chemotaxis, indicating that it is an IP-10/Mig receptor. Determination of the binding kinetics with these two chemokines, however, was hampered by the presence of a high-level nonspecific binding due to the cationic nature of the chemokines. Therefore, no direct binding data was available at this time. Calcium mobilization results indicate that the receptor was able to respond to as low as 1 nM of the chemokines, and that IP-10 and Mig cross-desensitized each other. The receptor does not interact with several other known CXC and CC chemokines (Loetscher *et al.,* 1996). An interesting finding is that CXCR3 is expressed in IL-2-activated T cells and NK cells, but not in resting T lymphocytes, B lymphocytes, monocytes, or granulocytes. This highly restricted distribution pattern suggests that CXCR3 is involved in the selective recruitment of activated T lymphocytes, indicating a potential involvement of the receptor in delayed-typed hypersensitivity, viral infection and certain types of tumors.

CXCR4 was originally isolated in several laboratories as an orphan G protein-coupled receptor, most frequently referred to as LESTR (Loetscher *et al.,* 1994) but also variously named as the human homolog of the bovine NPY Y3 receptor, pBE1.3 and HM89 (Herzog *et al.,* 1993; Federsppiel *et al.,* 1993; Nomura *et al.,* 1993). The receptor, with 352 amino acids, is highly homologous (92% identical sequence) in sequence to the cloned bovine NPY Y3 receptor (Rimland *et al.,* 1991). Unlike the bovine receptor, the human homolog displays no detectable binding to neuropeptide Y (Herzog *et al.,* 1993; Loetscher *et al.,* 1994). Upon sequence alignment, it was found that the human NPY receptor homolog shares ~36% identical sequence with the two IL-8 receptors. In particular, the DRYLAIVHA sequence immediately following the third transmembrane domains of the IL-8 receptors are conserved entirely in the human NPY receptor homolog. Short stretches of sequences found in the second and the six transmembrane domains of the IL-8 receptors are also conserved in the human receptor. Loetscher and coworkers expressed the receptor in CHO cells and examined the binding of the receptor with various leukocyte chemokines. They found no binding of the transfected receptor to IL-8, GROα, NAP-2, PF4, IP-10, MCP-1, MCP-3, MIP-1α, I-309, RANTES, and several other ligands (Loetscher *et al.,* 1994).

Despite the initial negative results, identification of the functions of this receptor took a dramatic turn when Berger and colleagues found that the HIV-1 entry cofactor fusin is identical in sequence to the 3-year-old orphan receptor (Feng *et al.,* 1996). Fusin mediates the entry of T cell-tropic isolates of HIV-1 into $CD4^+$ host cells (Feng *et al.,* 1996), a process requiring physical association of the viral gp120 protein, CD4, and fusin (Lapham *et al.,* 1996). In less than 4 months after the original publication of the fusin results, two groups reported the identification of stromal cell-derived factor-1 (SDF-1) as an agonist for LESTR/fusin (Bleul *et al.,* 1996a; Oberlin *et al.,* 1996). These studies also demonstrated inhibition of fusin-mediated HIV-1 entry by SDF-1. SDF-1 is a CXC chemokine originally cloned by Tashiro *et al.* (1993) and independently by Nagasawa *et al.,* (1994) as a pre-B-cell growth-stimulating factor (PBSF). Targeted deletion of the gene for this CXC chemokine led to cardiac ventricular septal defect and perinatal death of the resultant mice (Nagasawa *et al.,* 1996). Meanwhile, Bleul *et al.* (1996b) studied chemotactic activities in the culture media of a murine bone marrow stroma cell line MS-5 and found that the purified protein factor was identical to SDF-1. When tested in leukocytes, SDF-1 attracted lymphocytes and monocytes but not neutrophils (Bleul *et al.*, 1996b). This finding is intriguing since previous study indicated the presence of large amount of CXC4 message in neutrophils (Loetscher *et al.*, 1994). Thus, CXCR4 provides another example for a CXC chemokine to preferentially interact with leukocytes other than neutrophils. It is prospose that SDF-1 may serve a role in immune surveillance and basal extravasation of selected leukocytes. Since SDF-1 appears to be constitutively expressed in a large number of tissues, its function in inflammation has yet to be determined.

b. Receptors for CC Chemokines Receptors with high affinity for MCP-1, MIP-1α, MIP-1β, and RANTES have been identified in human monocytes by direct binding studies with iodinated human chemokines. A high-affinity receptor for MCP-1 was first identified on human monocytes (Yoshimura and Leonard, 1990; Valente *et al.*, 1991) and subsequently on a human monocytic leukemia cell line THP-1 (K_d = 2 nM and B_{max} = 2000 sites/cell) (Van Riper *et al.*, 1993). No significant binding to either neutrophils or lymphocytes was observed. Steady-state binding experiments revealed approximately 3000 high-affinity binding sites/cell for MIP-1α ($K_d \leq 1$ nM) on human monocytes and monocytic THP-1 cells (Wang *et al.*, 1993b). Finally, two independent studies revealed high-affinity receptors for RANTES on THP-1, a myeloid cell type that responded to RANTES in chemotaxis and Ca^{2+} mobilization assays. Depending on the methodology used, i.e., whole cells or membranes, the analysis of binding isotherms revealed high-affinity receptors ranging from 700 to 5000 per cell and K_d values for RANTES approximately 1 nM (Van Riper *et al.*, 1993; Wang *et al.*, 1993b).

Competition binding and cross-desensitization studies revealed a complex pattern of interactions between these chemokines and the binding entities. MIP-1α and MIP-1β compete equally well for binding to monocytes, whereas MCP-1 partially displaced human MIP-1α and β binding on monocytes. Conversely, MIP-1α and β partially inhibited the binding of radioactive MCP-1 (Wang *et al.*, 1993b). Likewise, MIP-1α and β desensitized with each others in terms of monocyte chemotactic response, whereas both were only partially desensitized by MCP-1. The Ca^{2+} mobilization response of human monocyte to MCP-1 was shown to be cross-desensitized by MCP-3, but not by MCP-2, two CC chemokines that share 71 and 62% sequence similarity with MCP-1, respectively (Sozzani *et al.*, 1994). MIP-1α and MCP-1 were found to compete for RANTES binding to monocytes with a K_d of 1.6 and 6 nM, respectively. The Ca^{2+} mobilization and chemotactic responses of THP-1 to RANTES were also markedly inhibited by preincubation with MCP-1 or MIP-1α, but no cross-desensitization was observed when the chemokines were added in a reverse order (Wang *et al.*, 1993a). These studies suggest the existence of at least three subtypes of CC chemokine receptors: (1) A shared receptor for MIP-1α and MIP -1β, (2) a shared receptor for MCP-1 and MCP-3, and (3) a shared receptor that recognizes RANTES with low affinity and MCP-1 and MIP-1α with high affinity.

The cloning of several CC-chemokine receptors has partially clarified the complex relationship among these receptors and the different chemokines. The first CC-chemokine receptor cDNA was cloned from human leukocyte cDNA libraries by two groups (Neote *et al.*, 1993; Gao *et al.*, 1993). The open reading frame encodes a 355 amino acid receptor, known as CC CKR1 (which stands for CC Chemokine Receptor 1, now named CCR1), that binds MIP-1α and RANTES. Analysis of the displaceable binding isotherms of ^{125}I-labeled MIP-1α with homologous and heterologous unlabeled chemokines after the transfection of CC CKR1 in HEK 293 cells revealed a broad range of ligand specificity for CC chemokine. The dissociation constants (K_d) for MIP-1α, MCP-1, MIP-1β, and RANTES are approximately 6, 120, 230, and 460 n*M*, respectively (Neote *et al.*, 1993). However, the binding affinity values did not parallel the signaling efficacy as shown by calcium mobilization assays. Although MIP-1β and MCP-1 have a better affinity than RANTES for CC CKR1, they are poor agonists to transmit signal through the cloned receptor ($EC_{50} \geq 250$ n*M*) as compared to RANTES ($EC_{50} = 50$ n*M*) (Neote *et al.*, 1993; Gao *et al.*, 1993). Similar results were obtained with the murine counterpart of human CC CKR1 (Gao and Murphy, 1995). These results suggest that MIP-1β and MCP-1 behave as partial agonists or inverse agonists for CC CKR1. MCP-3 has been reported to induce calcium mobilization in HEK293 stably expressing CC CKR1 with a potency ranging between that of MIP-1α and RANTES (Combadiere *et al.*, 1995b). Thus, CC CKR1 appears to be a shared receptor that potently responds to MIP-1α, MCP-3, and RANTES.

Subsequently, Charo and co-workers (1994) isolated two cDNAs that encode two MCP-1-specific receptors with alternatively spliced carboxyl terminal tails. These receptors are named CC CKR2A (374 amino acids) and CC CKR2B (CCR2B, 356 amino acids). Both conferred to injected *Xenopus* oocytes a robust mobilization of intracellular calcium ($EC_{50} \approx$ 1 nM) in response to MCP-1 but not to other chemokines, despite a relatedness to CC CKR1 (51% amino acid identity). Competition binding studies with ^{125}I-labeled chemokines indicate that only MCP-1 and MCP-3 compete with each other for binding on HEK293 cells transfected with CC CKR2B. Both chemokines are equipotent agonists for calcium mobilization (Combadiere *et al.*, 1995b). CC CKR2 presents with CC CKR1 a marked divergence in the amino terminal domain. This divergence may be involved in the chemokine selectivity as it seems to be the case for the two IL-8 receptors. There is, however, a striking identity between CC CKR2 and CC CKR1 in the sequence IFFIILLTIDRYLAIVHAVFAL(K/R)ARTVTFGV at the end of the third transmembrane domain and at the beginning of the second intracellular loop. These two regions have been implicated in G protein activation (see Section IV). This sequence (and its variation) is a hallmark that identifies the CC-chemokine receptors (CCRs) thus far cloned. The alternative splicing of the C-terminal tail, is however, uncommon in the chemoattractant receptor subfamily whose genes are usually intronless for the coding sequences. Divergence at the carboxyl-terminal tail may have an important consequence on the signaling properties in that the carboxyl-terminal tail is a region that is involved in both G protein coupling and regulation of receptor activity.

A human CC chemokine receptor with a restricted eosinophil expression pattern was isolated by Combadiere *et al.* (1995). Meanwhile, the murine homolog was independently cloned by Post *et al.* (1995). This receptor, named CC CKR3 or CCR3, was also identified and cloned by several groups in their efforts to study the receptor for eotaxin (Daugherty *et al.*, 1996; Ponath *et al.*, 1996; Gao *et al.*, 1996). CCR3 is closely related to CCR1 and CCR2B, with 63 and 51% sequence identity, respectively. Stably transfected cell lines expressing CCR3 bind to eotaxin, MCP-3, and RANTES, with K_ds of 0.1, 2.7, and 3.1 n*M*, respectively (Daugherty *et al.*, 1996). In a number of functional assays, eotaxin was identified to be the most potent agonist for CCR3 (Ponath *et al.*, 1996; Daugherty *et al.*, 1996; Kitaura *et al.*, 1996; also see correction for Combadiere *et al.*, 1995, published in *J. Biol. Chem.* 270, p. 30235). Eotaxin was originally isolated as a chemotactic factor that induced eosinophil accumulation in guinea-pig lung (Griffiths-Johnson *et al.*, 1993). It was subsequently identified as a CC chemokine with increased expression in allergen-challenged guinea-pig lungs (Jose *et al.*, 1994a, 1994b; Rothenberg *et al.*, 1995a). Additional studies with the murine and human eotaxin confirmed that eotaxin is a potent chemotactic factor for eosinophils, particularly in allergen-stimulated lungs (Rothenberg *et al.*, 1995b; Garcia-Zepeda *et al.*, 1996; Ponath *et al.*, 1996). Thus, CCR3 can be an important model for the study of eosinophilia as well as a potential target for therapeutic intervention. CCR3 has recently been shown to be a cofactor for the entry of certain dual-tropic HIV-1 isolates (Choe *et al.*, 1996; Doranz *et al.*, 1996).

A fourth CC chemokine receptor, CC CKR4 or CCR4, was cloned from the immature human basophilic cell line KU-812 (Power *et al.*, 1995). It is 47% identical in sequence to CCR2B and confers to injected *Xenopus* oocytes the capability of mobilizing calcium in response to MIP-1α, RANTES, and MCP-1, but not to MCP-2, MIP-1β, and the CXC chemokine IL-8. The murine homolog of CCR4 was recently identified (Hoogewerf *et al.*, 1996). Equilibrium competition binding assays were performed in transfected HL-60 cells expressing the human and murine CCR4, resulting in IC_{50} values of 14.5 ± 9 n*M* and 10.1 ± 3 n*M*, respectively, for iodinated MIP-1α. Similar binding assays with iodinated RANTES revealed IC_{50} values of 9.3 ± 3 n*M* and 5.7 ± 2.6 n*M* for the human and murine receptors, respectively. The murine CCR4 is expressed in the thymus and several T cell lines as detected by Northern blot analysis, similar to the human CCR4 (Hoogewerf *et al.*, 1996).

The most recently cloned CC chemokine receptor is CC CKR5 or CCR5 (Samson *et al.*, 1996; Raport *et al.*, 1996; also see Combadiere *et al.*, 1995, and published correction in *J. Biol. Chem.* 270, p. 30235). CCR5 contains 352 amino acids and appears to respond to MIP-1α, MIP-1β, and RANTES when expressed in CHO-K1 and HEK293 cells. The receptor shares 71% sequence identity with CCR2B, and the genes for these two receptors are only 17.5 kb apart on human chromosome 3p21 (Samson *et al.*, 1996; Raport *et al.*, 1996). The message for CCR5 has been detected in the KG-1A promyeloblastic cell line and in $CD4^+$ T cells. Shortly after its original cloning, CCR5 was found to be a major chemokine receptor cofactor that mediates the entry of primary (macrophage-tropic) isolates of HIV-1 (Dragic *et al.*, 1996; Alkhatib *et al.*, 1996; Deng *et al.*, 1996; Choe *et al.*, 1996; Doranz *et al.*, 1996). This function apparently requires the interaction of the HIV-1 envelope protein with a receptor extracellular domain. A deletion of 32 basepairs in the gene for CCR5 has been found at a frequency of about 0.092–0.10 in the Caucasian population. This deletion is responsible for a shift of the reading frame, resulting in a much shortened receptor that cannot mediate fusion of the macrophage-tropic and dual-tropic isolates of HIV-1 (Liu *et al.*, 1996; Samson *et al.*, 1996; Dean *et al.*, 1996). Using a chimeric receptor approach, it was recently found that the N-terminal 20 amino acids harbor a determinant for macrophage-tropic envelope protein fusion (Rucker *et al.*, 1996). No signaling events have been identified in association with chemokine receptor-mediated HIV-1 entry.

B. Receptor Structure

The deduced three-dimensional model currently available for the chemoattractant receptors is a compact structure characterized by seven domains highly enriched in hydrophobic residues. These domains contain distinctive sequence patterns and are thought to form a bundle of transmembrane segments, joined by hydrophilic loops on the extracellular and cytoplasmic sides of the receptors. The transmembrane domains form the agonist-binding pocket, at least in the case of small nonpeptide ligands, and are believed to transmit conformational changes to the cytoplasmic face of receptors. The conserved amino acid patterns in transmembrane domains are likely to provide a structure necessary for G protein interaction and activation.

A variety of biophysical measurements indicate that the transmembrane segments are α-helices of 20–25 amino acids, roughly perpendicular to the plane of the membrane, as demonstrated in rhodopsin (Chabre, 1985). It has been widely assumed that G protein-coupled receptors have the same transmembrane organization as bacteriorhodopsin, a light-driven proton pump of *Halobacterium halobium*, whose seven-helix pattern was determined by high-resolution electron cryo-microscopy (Henderson *et al.,* 1990). Grotzinger and co-workers (1991) have proposed a computer-generated model for the C5a receptor making the assumption that the seven hydrophobic segments are membrane-spanning helices of known direction, arranged roughly as in the bacteriorhodopsin structure. However, modeling of G protein-coupled receptors using bacteriorhodopsin as a template may not be justified because, despite a similar profile of hydropathy, bacteriorhodopsin is not functionally coupled to G proteins and its sequence exhibits none of the amino acid patterns common to the G protein-coupled receptors.

A probable arrangement of the seven helices in the receptors has been proposed by Baldwin (1993) on the basis of a detailed alignment of 204 sequences representative of G protein-coupled receptors. Although the percentage of amino acid identity between distantly related members of the family is as low as 20%, the 204 sequences, including those for FPR and its homologs, C5aR, PAFR, IL-8RA, and IL-8RB, are convincingly aligned within the seven hydrophobic domains from motifs of residues that are characteristic of each of the transmembrane segments. Because the lengths of the interhelical loops are relatively short, as seen in most chemoattractant receptors, each helix must be positioned in the membrane next to its neighbors in the sequence. The suggested arrangement gives a more closely packed structure at the intracellular face, where the interactions with G proteins occur; whereas the extracellular face, which is in contact with the ligand, is a more open structure. Interestingly, the detailed transmembrane helix packing proposed by Baldwin fits relatively well with the projection map of bovine rhodopsin, which was determined by electron crystallography of two-dimensional crystals to a resolution of 9 Å (Schertler *et al.,* 1993). Four well-resolved peaks of density have been interpreted as transmembrane helices oriented nearly perpendicular to the membrane, whereas an arc-shaped feature is likely to be the remaining helices in a tilted orientation. Although the general arrangement of helices is similar in rhodopsin and bacteriorhodopsin, the structure of rhodopsin seen in this map is clearly different from that of bacteriorhodopsin. The detailed relative positions of amino acid motifs, particularly helices, are presently not known and await projection maps with higher resolution.

The structure of the different hydrophilic loops remains unknown. Knowledge about the folding of these structures is, however, particularly important in understanding how large peptidic ligands interact with the extracellular surface and how G proteins interact with the intracellular surface of receptors. A structural constraint is probably imposed to extracellular loops e1 and e2 by the presence of a disulfide bridge formed between a cysteine residue a few amino acids from the beginning of helix III and a second cysteine residue, which varies in position from one receptor to the next, in loop e2 between helix IV and helix V (Fig 2). The importance of this disulfide bridge has been established for rhodopsin (Karnik and Khor-

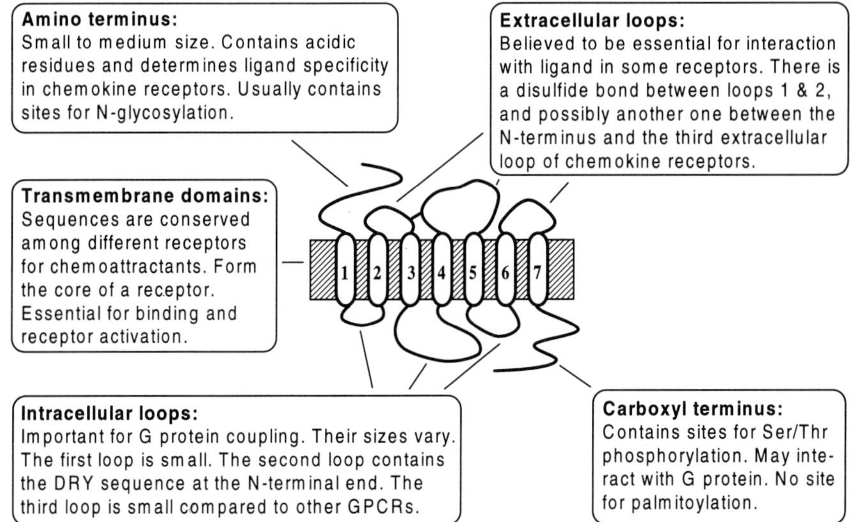

FIGURE 2 Transmembrane disposition of a prototype leukocyte chemoattractant receptor. The structure of the receptor is depicted as cylinders, numbered 1–7 for the seven transmembrane domains (TMD), and lines, representing extracellular and intracellular loops that connect the TMDs as well as the amino and carboxyl termini. The hatched area marks the membrane bilayer. The features of each receptor component are described briefly in the boxed text.

ana, 1990; Karnik *et al.*, 1988), for muscarinic receptors (Kurtenbach *et al.*, 1990) and for the β_2-adrenergic receptor (Dohlman *et al.*, 1990). Because both cysteine residues are invariant in the superfamily, the disulfide bridge is believed to occur in the majority of receptors. Its role is probably to stabilize an active conformation of receptors.

Although there are no primary structural features common to all chemoattractant receptors that allows their classification in a subfamily apart from other classes of peptide ligand receptors, the chemoattractant receptors have nevertheless a number of remarkable peculiarities: (1) they are similar in size containing, mostly 350–370 amino acids; (2) the third intracellular loop is one of the shortest in the GPCR superfamily and is enriched in positively charged residues; this loop may form a cationic amphiphilic α helix; and (3) the carboxyl-terminal domains, with the exception of PAFR, do not contain a cysteine residue generally conserved in many other members of the GPCR superfamily. This residue, which is palmitoylated and bound at the membrane surface in rhodopsin and the β_2-adrenergic receptor, appears to facilitate the formation of a short, fourth intracellular loop (Ovchinnikov *et al.*, 1988; O'Dowd *et al.*, 1989). The functional role of palmitoylation is, however, unclear. Although a human β_2-adrenergic receptor lacking this palmitoylated cysteine residue is constitutively phosphorylated and uncoupled from the G_s protein in the absence of activation (Moffett et al.,

1993), the lack of palmitoylation of the α_{2a}-adrenergic receptor does not perturb receptor–G_i protein coupling (Kennedy and Limbird, 1993). This variance may result from the fact that the latter is coupled to G_i rather than to G_s.

IV. Pharmacological and Biochemical Properties of Chemoattractant Receptors

A. Ligand–Receptor Interactions

1. Ligand Structure and Function

a. N-formylated Peptides The interest in formyl peptides, as chemoattractants and activators of leukocytes, started in 1975 when Schiffmann and co-workers reported that oligopeptides elaborated by *Escherichia coli* cultures chemoattract and activate the microbicidal respiratory burst of mammalian phagocytes *in vitro*. The peptides were found to be di- and tri-N-formylated methionyl peptides (Schiffmann *et al.*, 1975a,b). Subsequently, the structural requirement for optimal ligand binding and cellular activation was studied by systematic analyses of a series of synthetic peptides (Showell *et al.*, 1976; Freer *et al.*, 1980, 1982). The smallest active structure that emerged as the prototypic chemotactic peptide is the tripeptide N-formyl-Met-Leu-Phe-OH (fMLF).

A model for the interactions of fMLF with its receptor has been proposed by Freer *et al.* (1982). The structural requirements for optimal biological activity of the tripeptide are: (1) the N terminus of the first amino acid has to be blocked by a formyl group that may form a hydrogen bound to a residue in the receptor; acetylated and nonacetylated tripeptides have little, if any, biological activity (see below); (2) position 1 can be indifferently occupied by methionine or norleucine; (3) position 2 accommodates either valine or isoleucine, but the presence of a glycine residue dramatically reduces the biological activity; thus, the length of the aliphatic side chain may be important for interactions with hydrophobic areas; and (4) position 3 has a strict requirement for a phenylalanine residue. Studies with longer synthetic peptides containing the bioactive module f-Met/Nle-Leu-Phe-OH have indicated that positions 4 and 5 can be occupied by various substituents. The tetrapeptide f-Met-Leu-Phe-Lys-OH (Freer *et al.*, 1980) and the hexapeptide f-Nle-Leu-Phe-Nle-Tyr-Lys-OH (Niedel *et al.*, 1979) are as active as the parent tripeptide. Moreover, the lysine residue could be derivatized with bulky hydrophobic photoactivable residues (Niedel *et al.*, 1980; Schmitt *et al.*, 1983; Allen *et al.*, 1986; Boulay *et al.*, 1990a) or fluorescent moieties (Sklar *et al.*, 1984) without loss of specificity and bioactivity.

Replacing the formyl group with a t-butyloxycarbonyl (tBOC) often results in a peptide with antagonist properties (Freer *et al.*, 1980).

Cyclosporine H, a completely unrelated peptide, proved to be a potent antagonist for N-formyl peptide-mediated responses in neutrophils (Wenzel-Seifert and Seifert, 1993). The binding of [^{3}H]fMLF and the functional responses triggered by *N*-formylated peptides can be antagonized by the poorly selective N-t-butoxycarbonyl-Phe-Leu-Phe-Leu-Phe-OH peptide (tBoc-FLFLF) with a K_i value in the range of 0.1–0.2 μM and more selectively with cyclosporine H (CsH) with a K_i value of 0.1 μM (Wenzel-Seifert and Seifert, 1993).

Several N-formylated peptide chemoattractants, including f-Met-Leu-Phe-OH, have been purified from natural sources. The prototype *N*-formylated tripeptide, fMLF, is the major neutrophil chemotactic factor produced by *E. coli* (Marasco *et al.*, 1984). *N*-formylated peptides corresponding to the amino terminus of the murine mitochondrially encoded NADP dehydrogenase subunit 1 were found to trigger the chemotactic receptor (Shawar *et al.*, 1995). Thus, these two observations provide support for the current notion that the biologically relevant ligands for FPR are N-formylated peptides secreted by bacteria at sites of infection or by mitochondria released from damaged tissues. However, the biological role of the FPR may not be restricted to host defense in the light of several observations. First, it has been demonstrated that a peptide can be a potent agonist of FPR in the absence of a *N*-formyl group (Gao *et al.*, 1994). In fact, the synthetic pentapeptide Met-Nle-Leu-Phe-Phe-OH, either N-formylated or N-acetylated, is at least 10-fold more potent than the parent prototype, fMLF, in evoking a transient alteration of Ca^{2+} concentration in human neutrophils. Moreover, the unacylated form, H-MNleLFF, is also a good activator of neutrophil functions but is 100-fold less active than the acylated counterpart. Amino-terminal, urea-substituted and carbamate-modified peptides have also been shown to be potent agonists for the FPR (Higgins *et al.*, 1996; Derian *et al.*, 1996). Modification of the side chains of these amino-terminal substituted peptides can convert an agonist to an antagonist, further supporting the notion that the bioactivity of chemotactic peptides is not entirely determined by the formyl group at the amino terminus. Second, the cellular distribution of FPR is not restricted to neutrophils and monocytes as previously thought. Expression of FPR has been demonstrated in hepatocytes, dendritic cells, and astrocytes (Gasque *et al.*, 1995; Lacy *et al.*, 1995; Sozzani *et al.*, 1995). Third, several human and mouse FPR homologs have been identified that exhibit no ability to bind *N*-formylated peptides. The mouse equivalent of FPR shares 76% sequence identity with the human FPR but displays 200-fold less potency to fMLF (Gao and Murphy, 1993). These data support the idea that FPR may have wider functions than host defense against bacterial infection and that an as yet unidentified endogenous ligand may trigger the activation of FPR and its congeners.

b. C5a and C3a Anaphylatoxin Activation of the complement protein C3-C5 generates three anaphylatoxins: C3a, C4a, and C5a. The latter is the most potent with the broadest spectrum of activity. The biology of the C5a anaphylatoxin as well as its structure and function has been addressed by Gerard and Gerard (1994). Therefore, only the most salient features of this anaphylatoxin will be summarized here. Similar to fMLF, C5a is chemotactic for all the cells of myeloid lineage (granulocytes, monocytes, and macrophages) as well as dendritic cells and astrocytes at concentrations in the subnanomolar range; it elicits the activation of the NADPH oxidase and proteolytic enzyme release at higher nanomolar concentrations. The robust bioactivity of C5a contrasts with that of other classical chemoattractants such as LTB_4 and PAF, which are good chemoattractants for neutrophils but poor activators of the NADPH oxidase.

The C5a anaphylatoxin is 74 amino acids in length and is highly cationic at physiological pH. Human C5a contains seven cysteine residues which form three intrachain disulfide bonds (Mollison *et al.*, 1989). The binding of C5a is substantially inhibited by mutation at Lys_{68}, Leu_{72}, and Arg_{74} (Mollison *et al.*, 1989). The biological activity depends mostly on the carboxyl-terminal arginyl residue. Cleavage of Arg74 by serum carboxypeptidase yields C5a-desArg_{74} with its bioactivity decreased by three orders of magnitude in terms of the spasmogenic response of ileal tissue from guinea pig. The chemotactic activity on neutrophils is, however, still significant and effective in the high nanomolar range. Deletion of the last five residues (MQLGR-OH) yields a truncated molecule (C5a 1–69) that lacks bioactivity, even though it binds to the cellular receptor with an affinity in the micromolar range (Chenoweth and Hugli, 1980). These studies provided the first evidence that C5a establishes interactions with its receptor complex secondary contact that are not related to activation and signal transduction. The carboxyl-terminal pentapeptide alone or in association with the truncated fragment (1–69) fails to activate neutrophil chemotaxis. However, it was further established that the carboxyl-terminal octapeptide (HKDM-QLGR-OH) was the minimal structure that retained a weak, albeit significant, chemotactic and spasmogenic potential. A series of studies aimed at optimizing the bioactivity of the octapeptide indicated that replacement of the amino-terminal histidine by phenylalanine/tryptophan increased the activity of the peptide approximately 10-fold in terms of spasmogenicity and the capacity to induce IL-6 synthesis (reviewed in Gerard and Gerard, 1994). Siciliano and co-workers (1994) have reported a more potent synthetic peptide (Tyr-Ser-Phe-Lys-Ala-Cha-Cha-Leu-DPhe-Arg, with Cha = cyclohexylalanine), which displays a relatively high affinity ($K_d \approx 10$ nM) for C5aR in direct binding experiments, and behaves as a full agonist. The concept of secondary contact points was confirmed by combining two-dimensional (NMR) studies and site-directed mutagenesis (Mollison *et al.*, 1989). In addition to the carboxyl-terminal region, residues critical for establishing interactions with the receptor might include the amino-terminal

Ala_{26}, Lys_{19} and/or Lys_{20}, and Arg_{40}-Ile_{41} (Bubeck *et al.*, 1994; Mollison *et al.*, 1989).

As the carboxyl-terminal domain mimicks C5a in its ability to activate the receptor, it was expected that antagonists would arise from modifications of peptide analogs. Indeed, several peptides have emerged as antagonists (Kaneko *et al.*, 1995; Konteatis *et al.*, 1994), but in most cases they retained strong agonist properties (DeMartino *et al.*, 1994; Drapeau *et al.*, 1993; reviewed in Gerard and Gerard, 1994).

Similar to C5a, the carboxyl-terminal portion of C3a appears to be important for receptor binding and biologic function. C3 is a 77-residue peptide anaphylatoxin derived from the amino-terminal end of the α chain of C3. Removal of the C-terminal arginine by carboxypeptidase B abolishes tissue contractile activity (Bokisch and Muller-Eberhard, 1970). Accordingly, a synthetic 21-residue peptide, C3a 57–77, displays biological activities equivalent to that of the natural molecule (Lu *et al.*, 1984). This peptide may have a helical conformation necessary for its function. C-terminal-derived peptides of as short as five amino acids have been shown to be biologically active (Unson *et al.*, 1984). Novel synthetic peptides have been designed based on the C-terminal sequence that display several folds higher potency than the natural C3a (Ember *et al.*, 1991). With the cloning of the C3a receptor (Roglić *et al.*, 1996; Crass *et al.*, 1996; Ames *et al.*, 1996), it is now possible to study the direct interaction of the C-terminal domain of C3a with its receptor at the molecular level.

c. CXC and CC Chemokines The CXC and CC chemokines represent a new class of proinflammatory mediators that have the ability to recruit and activate multiple lineages of myeloid cells and lymphocytes. They are structurally and functionally related polypeptides of 8–10 kDa with four cysteine residues at highly conserved positions. In the CXC chemokine family the first two cysteine residues located in the amino-terminal region are separated by a single amino acid (C-X-C motif), whereas in the CC chemokine family these cysteine residues are adjacent (C-C motif). The remaining two cysteine residues are at conserved positions.

The best representatives of each family are undoubtedly IL-8 and MIP-1β in that their quaternary structure has been completely determined. The IL-8 structure has been solved by both NMR spectroscopy (Clore *et al.*, 1990) and X-ray crystallography (Baldwin *et al.*, 1991). Its quaternary structure is a noncovalent homodimer composed of two antiparallel COOH-terminal α helices lying on top of a six-stranded β sheet. The monomeric structure in solution consists of a disordered *N*-terminal sequence, a loop region, three antiparallel β strands, and a carboxyl-terminal region folded in α helix. Comparisons of the NMR and crystal structure have revealed that the *N*-terminal region is well ordered in the crystal structure as a result of a charge interaction between Glu_4 of one subunit and Lys_{23} of the other, whereas in solution this region is not restrained by ionic interaction (Clore and Gronenborn, 1991). The structures of PF4 and MGSA/GROα, two other members of the a chemokine family, have been determined as a tetramer and a dimer, respectively (Kim *et al.*, 1994; Zhang *et al.*, 1994). Both have a monomeric structure very similar to that of IL-8.

The three-dimensional structure of the CC chemokine MIP-1β, as determined by solution multidimensional NMR, is a symmetric homodimer (Lodi *et al.*, 1994). The structure of the MIP-1β monomer is also similar to that of the related α chemokine IL-8, with a COOH-terminal α helix lying on top of a triple-stranded β sheet. The Cα backbone of 59 residues in secondary structural regions can be superimposed to that of IL-8 with a 1.6-Å root-mean square deviation. However, the quaternary structure of the two chemokines is entirely different, with a dimer interface involving a completely different set of residues. In contrast to the IL-8 dimer, which is globular, the MIP-1β homodimer is elongated and cylindrical.

Thus, chemokines appear to have a strong propensity to reversibly assemble into a dimer or tetramer depending on the experimental conditions, i.e., concentration, pH, and ionic strength. However, the necessity of dimerization or oligomerization for the expression of a biological activity is unlikely despite several lines of evidence indicating that the IL-8 dimer is a structure that does bind to the receptor. First, the native IL-8 has been cross-linked as a dimer when bound to IL-8RB (Schnitzel *et al.*, 1994). Second, chemically synthesized disulfide-linked dimers of IL-8 are functional, albeit with a lower potency than native IL-8 (Clark-Lewis *et al.*, 1995). Under physiological conditions, i.e., at low concentrations, dimers or higher states of oligomerization dissociate into monomers, suggesting that the monomer is the physiologically active structure (reviewed in Clark-Lewis *et al.*, 1995). The analysis of an IL-8 mutant that has lost its ability to dimerize has provided strong support to this hypothesis. Using a synthetic IL-8 analog with the amide nitrogen of Leu_{25} methylated to selectively block the formation of hydrogen bonds between monomers and thereby prevent dimerization, Clark-Lewis and co-workers have clearly established that the IL-8 monomer *per se* is functionally active (Rajarathnam *et al.*, 1994). These findings have two major implications with respect to chemokine structure–activity relationships and chemokine–receptor interactions. First, because covalent dimers do bind receptor, the dimer interface region is unlikely to play a role in receptor activation. Additionally, because the monomeric IL-8 analog proved to be as active as native IL-8, the structure–functional studies can be directly interpreted on the basis of the monomeric structure.

Studies using alanine scanning mutagenesis of IL-8 (Hébert *et al.*, 1991) and chemically synthesized N-terminal truncated analogs (Clark-Lewis *et al.*, 1991) have revealed that the N-terminal sequence Glu_4-Leu_5-Arg_6 (ELR) is essential for IL-8 binding and neutrophil activation. The single mutation of Arg_6 to Ala or Lys results in a 1000-fold reduction in the affinity of IL-

8 for its receptors (Hébert *et al.,* 1991). Interestingly, truncated forms of IL-8 can be engineered into a potent IL-8 receptor antagonists by substituting residues in the ELR motif (see Section VI).

The importance of the ELR motif in the expression of neutrophil-activating properties is emphasized by the fact that it is common to all α chemokines that display binding to and activation of neutrophils, whereas IP-10 and PF4 that both fail to activate and recruit neutrophils lack this motif (Baggiolini *et al.,* 1994). Studies with hybrid molecules between IL-8 or NAP-2 and PF4 have further demonstrated the critical importance of the N-terminal region for high-level neutrophil activities. PF4 can be converted into a high-affinity chemokine for the IL-8 receptor by replacing the N-terminal region before the first cysteine residue with the homologous sequence of either IL-8 (Clark-Lewis *et al.,* 1993) or NAP-2 (Yan *et al.,* 1994). However, introduction of the ELR triad into IP-10 is not sufficient to confer neutrophil-activating properties to the IP-10 hybrid (Clark-Lewis *et al.,* 1993). This, along with the fact that the amino terminal truncated IL-8 molecules are potent antagonists, strongly suggests that in addition to the residues in this region, additional structural determinants are required for receptor binding. A series of additional hybrid molecules between IL-8 and IP-10 have been analyzed and informative data were generated to pinpoint these critical residues. Although the region with residues 10–22 could generally tolerate single conservative substitutions, secondary binding and/or conformational determinants were localized within residues 10–15 and 17–22 as determined by a series of hybrid constructs (Clark-Lewis *et al.,* 1994). The critical role of the 10–15 sequence is further supported by the observation that the low-affinity rabbit IL-8 can be converted into a high-affinity molecule for human IL-8RA by replacement of His_{13} and Thr_{15} with Tyr_{13} and Lys_{15} of human IL-8 (Schraufstatter *et al.,* 1995). The turn region 30–35 may also play an important role because the inactive hybrid ELR-IP-10 can be converted to a fully active molecule by replacing Ser_{31}-Gln_{32} with the Gly_{31}-Pro_{32} sequence of IL-8 (Clark-Lewis *et al.,* 1994).

2. *Receptor Structure–Function Relationships*

The understanding of the structural basis by which agonist binding induces receptor activation may aid in the rational design of antagonist molecules. For G protein-coupled receptors that bind small nonpeptidic ligands, such as positively charged biogenic amines, the sites of interaction appear to involve discrete amino acid residues within the pocket formed by the transmembrane domains (Savarese and Fraser, 1992). In the case of chemoattractants, particularly C5a and the chemokines, the size and the complexity of the activating ligand render the identification of the ligand-binding domain far more complicated. Studies on ligand structure–activity relationships for both C5a and IL-8 have already indicated that in addition to an activating domain, multiple interaction sites are required for a potent activation.

a. Role of the Extracellular Domains in Receptor–Ligand Interaction Although the amino-terminal region is highly divergent from one receptor to the next, a high occurrence of negatively charged residues emerges as a feature common to C5aR and chemokine receptors. In at least two cases, C5aR and IL-8R, the amino-terminal regions appear to play a key role in ligand binding. Replacement of the amino-terminal domain of human IL-8RB by its counterpart from the rabbit IL-8RA yields a hybrid molecule (rIL-8RA/hIL-8RB) that displayed the properties of the human and rabbit IL-8RA, i.e., high-affinity binding for ^{125}I-labeled IL-8 that could be weakly competed by unlabeled MGSA/GROα and NAP-2 (LaRosa *et al.*, 1992; Gayle *et al.*, 1993). This suggests that the amino-terminal domain of IL-8RB represents one of the determinants for MGSA/GROα and NAP-2 selectivity. Ahuja *et al.* (1996) suggested that a region comprising helix IV and the second extracellular loop (e2) contains additional determinants for MGSA/GROα and NAP-2 selectivity. Conflicting results were reported when the reciprocal chimeric molecule was tested, i.e., replacement of the amino terminus of rabbit IL-8RA by that of human IL-8RB (hIL-8RB/rIL-8RA). LaRosa *et al.* (1992) reported high-affinity binding for ^{125}I-labeled IL-8 that was efficiently competed by MGSA/GROα and NAP-2, whereas Gayle *et al.* (1993) were unable to demonstrate specific ^{125}I-labeled IL-8 binding with the same chimera. This latter observation has been corroborated by Ahuja *et al.* (1996), who could not demonstrate specific ^{125}I-labeled IL-8 binding to a similar chimera (hIL-8RB/hIL-8RA), despite the fact that IL-8 was its most potent agonist (EC_{50} = 10 n*M*) in terms of Ca^{2+} mobilization. In contrast, ^{125}I-labeled MGSA/GROα and ^{125}I-labeled NAP-2 bound to this chimera with a high affinity reminiscent of the MGSA/GROα and NAP-2 binding to IL-8RB. Moreover, they were both efficiently competed by unlabeled IL-8, indicating that IL-8 did bind to the chimera. To explain the discrepancy between the efficient calcium mobilization by IL-8 and the lack of specific binding of ^{125}I-labeled IL-8 to the chimeric molecule, Ahuja *et al.* (1996) suggested that the determinants for high-affinity binding of ^{125}I-labeled IL-8 may differ from those responsible for high agonist potency and that the amino-terminal region of IL-8RB contains determinants for high-affinity ^{125}I-labeled IL-8 binding. The latter conclusion is in agreement with the previous observation that the mouse IL-8 receptor, which exhibits low-affinity binding for human IL-8, could be converted to a high-affinity receptor for ^{125}I-labeled IL-8 if its amino-terminal region was replaced by its counterpart in rabbit IL-8RA (Suzuki *et al.*, 1994). Regarding the former conclusion, one has to consider two alternative possibilities that might explain the lack of specific ^{125}I-labeled IL-8 binding to the chimera: (1) during the course of binding at 4°C, the receptor may be rapidly shifted to the R* conformation for which ^{125}I-labeled IL-8 has a poor affinity; consequently, it will be impossible to demonstrate specific binding, whereas high agonist potency will be detected. (2) Iodination *per se* may alter the structure of ^{125}I-labeled IL-8 in such a way that it does not bind to the chimera. The damage created to the molecule of IL-8 may vary with the level of iodine incorporated and with the methodology used to iodinate the chemokine. This latter hypothesis might explain the conflicting results observed by the different groups.

All of the acidic amino acids present in the ligand-accessible surface of IL-8RA were systematically mutated to pinpoint the positions of the residues that might establish charge interactions with IL-8 (Hébert *et al.*, 1993). In the N-terminal domain, only Asp_{11} proved to be important for interaction with the receptor. Surprisingly, although its replacement with alanine had a deleterious effect on IL-8 binding, it can be substituted with another charged residue, such as Glu or Lys. The ability of Lys_{11} to confer high-affinity binding suggests that a new and favorable interaction with IL-8 has been created. From these studies it is tempting to conclude that IL-8 contacts directly with Asp_{11} or Lys_{11} in the mutant receptor. However, in the absence of structural information on the ligand–receptor complex, one cannot exclude the possibility that Asp_{11} (or Lys_{11}) establishes an ionic interaction with a charged residue in another hydrophilic extracellular loop of the receptor to form a receptacle on which IL-8 can lie.

A systematic conversion to alanine of each residue present in the putative extracellular domains was used in an attempt to identify residues mediating IL-8 binding and signal transduction (Hébert *et al.*, 1993; Leong *et al.*, 1994). In most cases, the alanine substitutions yielded receptors that bind IL-8 and transduce signal as efficiently as the wild-type receptor. Approximately 20% of the mutations cause a decrease in the binding affinity without affecting the ability of the receptors to generate calcium flux upon stimulation. The role of these amino acid residues may be to influence the overall tertiary structure of the receptor rather than to provide contact interactions with IL-8. Of all the residues present in the putative extracellular domains, only five residues proved to be essential for both IL-8 binding and signal transduction. All of them were charged residues, including Arg_{199} and Arg_{203} in the second extracellular loop e2, as well as Asp_{265}, Glu_{275}, and Arg_{280} in the third extracellular loop e3. A direct interaction of these residues with IL-8 is hypothesized but not formally established. By looking at the compensatory effects of mutations in the critical domains of IL-8 one should be able to establish whether or not these residues are involved in specific interactions with IL-8.

In the case of the C5a receptor, the contribution of the amino-terminal domain to the binding of C5a has been highlighted by several groups using different strategies. Antiserum raised to the peptide 9–29 and monoclonal antibody directed to the hexapeptide (D_{15}DKDTLD_{21}) of C5aR antagonize the binding of the C5a anaphylatoxin without activating the receptor. Conversely, the occupation of the receptor by C5a prevents the binding of the antibodies, suggesting that the binding of C5a masks the antigenic epitope (Morgan *et al.*, 1993; Oppermann *et al.*, 1993). The critical role of the amino-terminal domain of C5aR was subsequently demonstrated by a series of studies involving a strategy of amino acid deletion in the amino-terminal domain (DeMartino *et al.*, 1994) and amino-terminal sequence swapping between C5aR and FPR (Mery and Boulay, 1994). A mutant with residues 2–22 deleted displayed a 600-fold reduction in the binding affinity for C5a, whereas truncation of residues 2–31 yielded a receptor with a 45,000-fold reduction in affinity. However, both truncated mutants bind the C5a carboxyl-terminal peptide analog (Y-F-K-P-dCha-Cha-dR) as efficiently as the wild-type receptor (DeMartino *et al.*, 1994). Replacement of the first 8 residues of the amino-terminal domain of C5aR by the corresponding region in FPR has no effect on the binding of C5a. In contrast, if the first 13 amino acids are replaced with the first 12 amino acids of FPR, no detectable binding is observed. As the two replacement mutants diverge by only four residues (Asp-Tyr-Gly-His), it is possible that this four amino acid region is involved in the binding of C5a or that they influence the structure of the binding sites (Mery and Boulay, 1994). As the amino-terminal domain of C5aR contains seven aspartic acid residues, of which five are conserved in human, dog, and mouse C5aR (Gerard and Gerard, 1994), it was expected that charge alterations would affect the binding of C5a. Indeed, replacement of the aspartate residues by alanine at positions 10, 15, 16, 18, and 21 did reduce the affinity for C5a by approximately two orders of magnitude (DeMartino *et al.*, 1994). Substitution of asparagine for the aspartate residues at positions 10, 15, and 16 yielded a receptor with no ability to bind C5a, whereas substitution at position 10 or 27 and at positions 21 and 27 had no effect on the binding affinity as compared with the wild-type receptor. However, Scatchard analysis revealed a puzzling discrepancy between an apparent high level of surface expression, similar to that of the wild-type receptor, and a weak capacity to bind C5a with high affinity (<10%) (Mery and Boulay, 1993, 1994). This suggests that many of the mutant receptors, although efficiently expressed on the cell surface, might be misfolded and unable to bind C5a. In fact, although it is clear from the truncation mutants that the amino terminus provides much of binding energy for full-length C5a, none of the experiments formally demonstrate that the aspartic residues are directly interacting with C5a via a salt bridge.

In the case of FPR, domain replacement with the corresponding region of C5aR and substitution or insertion of hydrophilic sequences were used to address the importance of the amino-terminal domain and extracellular loops in N-formyl peptide binding. Replacement of the first extracellular loop by its counterpart from C5aR completely abolishes the binding of ^{125}I-labeled formyl peptide (Perez *et al.*, 1993). This loop has also been shown to be important for ligand binding by a synthetic peptide approach (Radel *et al.,* 1991). Alanine scanning mutagenesis of this region (His_{90} to Lys_{99}) has revealed that His_{90}, Phe_{96}, and Cys_{98} are essential for ligand binding. However, the role of Cys_{98} is probably structural since it is most likely involved in a disulfide bond with Cys_{176}. One cannot exclude that the role of His_{90} and Phe_{96} is also structural. Their substitution with alanine may change the overall conformation of the binding site and consequently abolish the binding of the *N*-formyl peptide. Replacement of the amino-terminal region by the corresponding sequence in C5aR was reported to decrease the binding affinity by 15-fold (Perez *et al.,* 1993) and the surface expression by 50%, whereas replacement of residues 2–9 by the FLAG sequence (Asp-Tyr-Lys-Asp-Asp-Asp-Asp-Lys) results in a dramatic reduction in the level of expression and a 7-fold decrease in binding affinity (Perez *et al.,* 1994). However, these results are in striking contrast with other domain-swapping studies demonstrating that the replacement of the amino-terminal domain by that from C5aR or FPR2 (FPRL1) does not significantly alter the affinity or the level of cell surface expression (Mery and Boulay, 1994; Quehenberger *et al.,* 1993). These latter observations are consistent with a previous study indicating that proteolytic removal of the amino terminus does not alter the binding affinity (Malech *et al.,* 1985). It is likely that the insertion of the hydrophilic FLAG sequence in the amino-terminal domain alters the folding process and the transport of the FPR to the plasma membrane.

b. Role of Transmembrane Core in Receptor–Ligand Interaction As the C5a C-terminal hexapeptide analog (Y-F-K-P-dCha-Cha-dR) activates with the same efficiency cells transfected with either the truncated mutant (Δ2-22) or the wild-type receptor, the activation domain is not expected to involve the amino-terminal region (DeMartino *et al.,* 1994). Indeed, a receptor that is proteolytically cleaved in the first extracellular loop by a metalloproteinase from the spider *Plectreurys tristes* is still activated by a potent carboxyl-terminal peptide analog (Y-F-K-A-Cha-Cha-L-dF-R; known as C-009) but not by the full-length C5a (Siciliano *et al.,* 1994). On the basis of these studies, Springer and co-workers have proposed a two-site model for C5a binding. The first site possibly involves the amino-terminal region, whereas the second interaction site is located in the transmembrane hydrophobic core and is more specifically implicated in the activation of the receptor (Siciliano *et al.,* 1994). However, the first site may not be restricted to the amino terminus and may also involve multiple contacts with other extracellular domains. High-affinity binding of full-length C5a apparently results from a cooperativity between extracellular and transmembrane core-binding interactions. Interestingly, the 4,6-diaminoquinoline (L-584,020), which competitively blocks C5a binding (Lanza *et al.,* 1992), has little, if any, effect on the binding of C-009, suggesting that this antagonist interacts with the extracellular interaction site.

Two studies have identified the amino acid residues that may interact with the carboxyl-terminal end of C5a. The carboxyl-terminal peptide contains two charged residues, Lys_{68} and Arg_{74}, which could act as counterions with negatively charged residues in the transmembrane domain. Mutation of Glu_{199} to Gln, near the extracellular end of transmembrane domain (TMD) 5, reduces by 5- to 10-fold the binding affinity and the EC_{50} for secretory responses in transfected rat basophilic leukemia cells (RBL-2H3). The use of peptides modeled on the structure of the sequence 67–74 of C5a has suggested that Lys_{68} in C5a may form a salt bridge with Glu_{199} (Monk *et al.*, 1995). The critical role of Arg_{206} for ligand recognition and receptor activation by the carboxyl-terminal hexapeptide analogs has been recognized by DeMartino *et al.* (1995). Although substitution of Ala for Arg_{206} had little effect on the recognition of C5a and the hexapeptide analogs that terminate with an arginine, it abolishes activation by hexapeptides but not that by C5a. The removal of the carboxyl-terminal guanido side chain of the hexapeptide reduces the affinity by about 100-fold, and the amidation of the carboxylic end group reduces the affinity for the wild type but not for the mutant. Based on these observations, a model for activation has been hypothesized in which the free carboxylate of the carboxyl-terminal arginine of the hexapeptide neutralizes the electrostatic repulsion between the two guanidino groups. However, the activation pathway used by C5a may not be as strongly controlled by the guanidino group of Arg_{206} because C5a can induce the activation of the R206A mutant. It has been shown that the replacement of Arg_{206} by a glutamine results in a partial loss of high-affinity binding capacity despite a normal expression level on the cell surface. Based on the observation that the number of high-affinity binding sites is upregulated by coexpression of $G_{i\alpha 2}$ and downregulated by GTPγS in the Gln_{206} C5aR mutant, it has been suggested that Arg_{206} may determine the intracellular G protein coupling (Raffetseder *et al.*, 1996).

Attempts to map the ligand binding site of FPR have been made by a chimeric approach, in which the domains of FPR were sequentially replaced by the counterpart from FPR2 (FPRL1) or vice versa (Quehenberger *et al.*, 1993; Gao and Murphy, 1993). The strategy relies on the observation that FPR2 (FPRL1), even though it is 69% identical to FPR, is unable to bind the formylpeptide ligand fMLF. Comparison of the structural and functional differences of the FPR-FPR2 chimeras has allowed the identification of domains that may be essential for binding of fMLF. The first and third extracellular loops (e1 and e3) with their adjacent transmembrane domains appear to be essential for high-affinity binding (Quehenberger *et al.*, 1993; Gao and Murphy, 1993). However, residues that specifically interact with fMLF have not been determined thus far. Preliminary results indicate that introduction into a low-affinity FPR-FPR2 chimeric receptor the positively charged residues Arg_{84} and Lys_{85} from the FPR was able to restore the binding and signaling capabilities to nearly the levels of the wild-type FPR

(O. Quehenberger and R. D. Ye, unpublished data). The same was observed when amino acids at positions 89 and 90 were restored to the wild-type FPR sequence.

B. Coupling of G Proteins to Chemoattractant Receptors

1. G Protein-Coupling Domain

The intracellular face of G protein-coupled receptors contains important determinants for G protein interactions. Studies aimed at defining the contact sites responsible for G protein-receptor coupling have been pursued with a variety of approaches, including the construction of chimeric receptors, site-directed mutagenesis, and the addition of synthetic receptor mimetic peptides to block and map the putative sites of interaction (reviewed in Savarese and Fraser, 1992). Combination of the different approaches has provided important clues about the participation of the different intracellular domains in the interactions with the G protein partner.

The second intracellular loop (i2), the carboxyl end of the third intracellular loop (i3), and the proximal end of the carboxyl-terminal domain of G protein-coupled receptors appear to be involved in G protein interaction. The i3 loop, which is most variable in length, is required for G protein activation and is thought to confer selectivity for G protein recognition (Lechleiter *et al.,* 1990). Receptors from which such conclusions have been drawn have large third intracellular loops that range from 50 to 240 amino acids, part of which can be deleted without major effect on the receptor function. In the case of the M3 muscarinic acetylcholine receptor, as few as 22 out of 239 amino acids of the i3 loop are sufficient for signaling provided that the critical charges at both ends of the loop are preserved (Kunkel and Peralta, 1993). Mutagenesis of residues in the carboxyl-end of loop i3 in several types of receptors has led to receptors that constitutively interact and activate different G proteins (Cotecchia *et al.,* 1990; Parma *et al.,* 1993; Ren *et al.,* 1993). The importance of the i2 loop was pointed out by Khorana and co-workers with rhodopsin mutants that fail to activate transducin. The ERY motif (DRY/F is found in most other receptors; except that a DRC motif is present in FPR isotypes and a NRF pattern is found in the PAF receptor) was shown to be essential for transducin binding, whereas other regions of i2 were rather critical for both transducin activation and release from rhodopsin (Franke *et al.,* 1990). The failure of a mutant with a charge reversal to couple with transducin suggests that the charged pair E/DR, which has been proposed to form the cytoplasmic border of helix III, either directly interacts with the G protein or helps other cytoplasmic sites to form the G protein-binding domain. Because the arginine residue of the DRY motif is the only residue that is invariably conserved in the entire family, it has been proposed that this amino acid may function as a switch that is "on" when the arginine side chain is exposed to the cytosol where it can interact with the G protein (Oliveira *et al.*, 1994). The shift may be caused by the release of structural constraints as a result of agonist binding or point mutations in particular regions.

Several studies have examined the role of the putative intracellular regions and cytoplasmic tail of FPR that might be involved in G_i protein binding. Ye and co-workers have studied the role of the i3 loop by the systematic substitution of charged and polar residues with uncharged or oppositely charged ones (Prossnitz *et al.*, 1993). Although some of the generated mutant receptors, in particular those with mutations at the transmembrane boundary, appear to have altered structures, none of the mutants are critically affected in G protein coupling as inferred from Ca^{2+} mobilization assays. These results suggest that the putative i3 loop (T_{226}KIHKQGLIKSSRPLRVLS$_{244}$) is not critical for FPR–G protein interaction. This conclusion is supported by additional studies employing receptor-mimetic peptides to block and map putative interaction domains. A competition assay based on the velocity sedimentation sucrose gradient in the presence of octyl glucoside was used to measure the amount of FPR complexed with G_{i2} as a function of receptor-mimetic peptide concentration (Bommakanti *et al.*, 1992, 1994). According to these studies, the most hydrophilic part of the putative i3 loop is not involved in contact with G_{i2} (Bommakanti *et al.*, 1995). However, peptides corresponding to the flanking amino- and carboxyl-terminal regions of loop i3 display a significant inhibitory activity (Bommakanti *et al.*, 1995). Interestingly, these peptides contain hydrophobic sequences corresponding to the carboxyl-terminal half of TMD 5 and the beginning of TMD 6 according to the model of transmembrane topology proposed by Baldwin (1993).

The inhibitory activity of peptides that mimic the loops i1 and i2 as well as various domains of the carboxyl-terminal tail was similarly examined. Although several studies on other receptors have suggested no role for the first intracellular loop of rhodopsin (König *et al.*, 1989) and β-adrenergic receptor (Münch *et al.*, 1991), Bommakanti *et al.* (1995) found that a peptide corresponding to loop i1 is one of the most active peptides for disrupting the interaction between FPR and G_i. Supporting evidence for a role of loop i1 in signal transduction has been provided by a study indicating that replacement of the i1 loop by its counterpart in C5aR results in a chimeric receptor that is constitutively activated (Amatruda *et al.*, 1995). The peptide corresponding to the entire predicted second cytoplasmic loop i2 (D_{122}RCVCVLHPVWTQNHRTVSLAKK$_{144}$) was the most active, with an IC_{50} value of about 20 μM, whereas a peptide corresponding to the middle region of i2 (C_{126}VLHPVWTQNHRTVS$_{140}$) was about 15-fold less effective (Schreiber *et al.*, 1994).

Likewise, peptides corresponding to various regions of the carboxyl-terminal tail were unequally effective. The sequence R_{322}ALTEDSTQTSD-

TAT_{336} has the best blocking activity and appears to be the major structural determinant for the carboxyl-terminal tail to interact with G_i (Bommakanti *et al.*, 1993, 1995; Schreiber et al., 1994). The critical role of the N-terminal part of the carboxyl tail in G protein coupling has been highlighted in a recent study (Prossnitz *et al.*, 1995b). Replacement of the triad Arg_{309}-Glu-Arg by Gly_{309}-Ala-Gly at the N-terminal end of the cytoplasmic tail results in a mutant receptor that displays a 50-fold reduction in the affinity for G_i protein. Supportive evidence for an important role of the carboxyl-terminal region of chemoattractant receptors in G protein coupling has been further provided by a study with IL-8RB (Ben-Baruch *et al.*, 1995a). Deletion of amino acids 317–355 of IL-8RB leads to a receptor that still binds IL-8 with the same affinity as the wild-type receptor but is unable to convey functional signals, whereas the deletion of the sequence beyond residue 325 has no deleterious effect on G protein coupling. This suggests that the amino acid sequence 317–324 is involved in signaling. An effect on the folding of the intracellular surface of the receptor is, however, not excluded. Some punctual mutations in the equivalent region of the C5aR result in receptors that are misfolded and retained in intracellular compartments (F. Boulay, unpublished data).

In light of these studies, it is clear that the FPR–G_i interaction most likely involves multiple contact sites with loop i1, the boundaries of loops i2 and i3, and restricted regions in the carboxyl-terminal tail as well as in transmembrane segments. The fact that some putative hydrophobic transmembrane regions are effective in blocking FPR–G_i interactions whereas most of the hydrophilic midregions of the putative cytoplasmic loops i2 and i3 are ineffective suggests that part of the G protein might be inserted as a wedge between the transmembrane domains. In this regard, some of the conserved motifs at the cytoplasmic boundaries of TMD 3 to TMD 6 may contact the G protein and impose the selectivity for a particular class of G proteins. Given the structural similarities between the different chemoattractant receptors, the conclusions drawn from the studies with FPR and IL-8R are likely to be valid for other members of this subfamily.

2. G Proteins Coupled to Chemoattractant Receptors

A series of studies initiated in the mid-1980s revealed that the biochemical and functional responses of leukocytes to the classical chemoattractants fMLF, C5a, PAF, and LTB_4, as well as the chemokine IL-8, are largely inhibited by pretreatment of cells with pertussis toxin (PTX), a toxin that inactivates the G_i class but not the G_q class ($G_{\alpha q}$, $G_{\alpha 11}$, G_z, and $G_{\alpha 16}$) (Bokoch and Gilman, 1984; Sha'afi and Molski, 1988; Thelen *et al.*, 1988; Snyderman and Uhing, 1992). However, a small PTX-resistant component has been reported for fMLF, LTB_4, and PAF in neutrophils (Verghese *et al.*, 1987) and for C5a in the monocytic cell line THP-1 (Amatruda *et al.*, 1993), suggesting the participation of other classes of G proteins. A large body of evidence indicates that the neutrophil functions activated by fMLF, C5a, and LTB_4 require the physical coupling of the agonist-occupied receptor with a common pool of G_{i2} (Gierschik *et al.*, 1989; Offermans *et al.*, 1990; Rollins *et al.*, 1991; Erbeck et al, 1993) and possibly G_{i3} (Wennogle *et al.*, 1994). These two G proteins are the main PTX-sensitive G proteins found in HL-60 myeloid cells (Murphy *et al.*, 1987). Neither G_{i1} nor G_o could be detected by Western blot analyses in this cell line (Goldsmith *et al.*, 1988). The mechanism by which G_{i2} is able to mediate PI-PLC activation in myeloid cells remained unclear until Gierschick and co-workers (Camps *et al.*, 1992a,b) established that the G protein $\beta\gamma$ subunit is involved in the activation of PI-$PLC_{\beta 2}$, which is the major PI-PLC isoform expressed in myeloid cells (Park *et al.*, 1992).

The pattern of G proteins activated in response to chemoattractants is dependent on the background in which chemoattractant receptors are expressed. In contrast to PAF-stimulated neutrophil responses, PAFR signaling is not blocked by PTX in platelets (Hwang, 1988) or in COS-7 cells transiently transfected with the neutrophil PAFR (Amatruda *et al.*, 1993). In COS-7 cells, the transfected PAFR is able to couple to endogenous G proteins and activates PI-PLC in a PTX-resistant manner most likely through $G_q/_{11}$ (Amatruda *et al.*, 1993). The result with PAF is in marked contrast with other chemoattractants that fail to stimulate inositol formation in COS-7 cells. This deficiency may be attributable to the fact that COS-7 cells express PI-$PLC_{\beta 1}$ but not the myeloid cell-specific PI-$PLC_{\beta 2}$ isotype, which is the major target for the $\beta\gamma$ subunit (Camps *et al.*, 1992a,b; Katz *et al.*, 1992). However, a PTX-dependent signaling pathway has been reconstituted in COS-7 cells by coexpression of IL-8RA or IL-8RB with PI-$PLC_{\beta 2}$, $G_{\alpha i2/3}$, $G_{\beta 1}$, and $G_{\gamma 2}$ (Wu *et al.*, 1993). Because $G_{\alpha i2}$ is unable to directly activate the endogenous PI-PLC or transfected PI-$PLC_{\beta 2}$, the IL-8-dependent formation of inositol phosphate most likely results from the release of $\beta\gamma$, which in turn activates PI-$PLC_{\beta 2}$. A supportive evidence for such a mechanism of PI-$PLC_{\beta 2}$ activation is provided by the observation that coexpression of $PLC_{\beta 2}$ and $\beta\gamma$ along with a dominant negative $G_{i2\alpha}$, one that is unable to bind GTP but with the capacity to complex $\beta\gamma$, results in a marked decrease of inositol phosphate release (Slepak *et al.*, 1995).

A PTX-resistant signaling can be reconstituted in COS-7 and HEK 293 cells without the need of exogenous PI-$PLC_{\beta 2}$ provided that the chemoattractant receptors FPR, C5aR, and IL-8R are cotransfected with $G_{\alpha 16}$ (Amatruda *et al.*, 1993, 1995; Wu *et al.*, 1993). $G_{\alpha 16}$ is a developmentally regulated PTX-insensitive G protein α subunit of the G_q class whose expression is restricted to a subset of hematopoietic cells in the early stage of differentiation (Amatruda *et al.*, 1991). The ability of $G_{\alpha 16}$ to couple to chemoattractant receptors contrasts with the inability of $G_{\alpha q}$ and $G_{\alpha 11}$ to reconstitute PI-$PLC_{\beta 1}$ and $PLC_{\beta 2}$ activation (Amatruda *et al.*, 1993; Buhl *et al.*, 1993; Wu *et al.*, 1993). This may result from the fact that $G_{\alpha 16}$ is a rather promiscuous

G protein that can couple to a large variety of receptors (Offermans and Simon, 1995; Wu *et al.*, 1995). Although there is no doubt that chemoattractant receptors can couple to $G_{\alpha 16}$, the restricted pattern of expression of $G_{\alpha 16}$ makes its role in neutrophil activation questionable: (1) The changes in the course of differentiation; $G_{\alpha 16}$ mRNA and protein are not detectable after terminal differentiation of HL-60 and U-937 cells to the granulocyte phenotype (Amatruda *et al.*, 1991; Vanek *et al.*, 1994). (2) The classical chemoattractant receptors are only expressed when cells are differentiated. It is presently unclear whether $G_{\alpha 16}$ and chemoattractant receptors are expressed during a short "temporal window" in the course of differentiation. However, one cannot exclude that $G_{\alpha 16}$ may play a role in monocyte activation since the protein is present in mature monocytes. $G_{\alpha 16}$ coupling may be restricted to the classical chemoattractant receptors and the α chemokine receptors, as shown by the observation that CCR1 and CCR2 are not able to couple to this G protein in transfected COS-7 cells (Kuang *et al.*, 1996).

Thus, all chemoattractant receptors appear to be coupled efficiently to G_{i2} and G_{i3} in myeloid cells, and some may also couple to $G_{\alpha 16}$ in heterologous expression systems. In addition, cotransfection experiments in HEK 293 indicate that FPR and C5aR can also couple to G_{i1}, G_o, and G_z, a PTX-resistant G protein (Tsu *et al.*, 1995). However, G_z can only replace G_i in mediating the inhibition of cAMP accumulation and cannot substitute for G_i in the stimulation of PLC (Shum *et al.*, 1995; Tsu *et al.*, 1995).

C. Phosphorylation and Desensitization of Chemoattractant Receptors

The cellular responses to chemoattractants can be rapidly attenuated and cells become refractory to further stimulation with the same agonist. This loss of cellular responsiveness to agonist, termed homologous desensitization, is common to many hormonal and neurotransmitter signaling systems (Dohlman *et al.*, 1991). One mechanism for homologous desensitization is phosphorylation of the agonist-occupied state of receptors by specific receptor kinases (reviewed in Inglese *et al.*, 1993). Indeed, the carboxyl terminus of chemoattractant receptors contain serine and threonine residues that may be phosphorylated by various kinases (Fig. 3). In addition,

```
FPR     QDFRERLIHALPASLER-ALTEDSTQTSDTA-TN--STLPSAEVELQAK
C5aR    QGFQGRLRKSLP-SLLRNVLTEESVVR-ESK-SFTRSTVDTMAQKTQAV
IL8RA   QNFRHGFLKILAM---HGLVSKEF-LARHRVTSYTSSSVNV-SSNL
IL8RB   QKFRHGLLKILAI---HGLISKDSLPK-DSRPSFVGSSSGHTSTTL
                     •      •^^•    ^•  • • ••  • ••
```

FIGURE 3 Alignment of the carboxyl terminal sequences from four chemoattractant receptors. Sequences from the carboxyl termini of FPR, C5aR, IL-8RA and IL-8RB B are aligned manually. The serine and threonine residues conserved in more than one receptors are marked with filled circles, and negatively charged residues that may constitute part of the recognition site for G protein-coupled receptor kinases are indicated by carets.

agonist-occupied receptors are rapidly internalized, resulting in a net decrease in the number of receptors on the cell surface. A second phenomenon, termed heterologous desensitization, refers to a process of inactivation whereby a receptor is desensitized in response to the activation of another receptor. Heterologous desensitization may result from the phosphorylation of the receptor without ligand occupation and/or the modifications of downstream components distal from the receptor by second messenger-activated kinases, such as protein kinase C (PKC) or cAMP-dependent protein kinase A (Hausdorff *et al.*, 1990; Dohlman *et al.*, 1991).

Despite a wealth of evidence indicating that chemoattractant receptors are rapidly desensitized following agonist exposure, little is known about the underlying mechanisms that govern this process. Immunoprecipitation studies have provided evidence that FPR, C5aR, PAFR, and the two IL-8 receptors are rapidly phosphorylated upon agonist binding in differentiated HL-60 cells (Tardif *et al.*, 1993), stably transfected RBL-2H3 cells (Ali *et al.*, 1993; Tomhave *et al.*, 1994; Richardson *et al.*, 1995a), and 3ASubE nonhematopoietic cells (Mueller *et al.*, 1994, 1995). Furthermore, phorbol 12-myristate 13-acetate (PMA), a potent activator of PKC, induced the phosphorylation of C5aR, IL-8R, and PAFR, but not of FPR. Both PMA- and agonist-mediated phosphorylations have been correlated with an inhibition of agonist-mediated GTPγS binding to and GTPase activity in membranes prepared from agonist-treated cells (Ali *et al.*, 1993; Tomhave *et al.*, 1994; Richardson *et al.*, 1995a). Mutation of the potential phosphorylation sites in the cytoplasmic tail of PAFR results in receptors that produce a sustained elevation of inositol 1,4,5-trisphosphate (Takano *et al.*, 1994). Altogether these results support the notion that phosphorylation is an essential step in the balance of cellular activation. However, the precise mechanism by which the receptor–G protein interaction is impaired is still unclear. In the case of FPR, the interaction between the G_i protein and receptor can be reconstituted with the same efficiency whether receptors were solubilized from desensitized or from unstimulated cells (Klotz and Jesaitis, 1994). This suggests that the physical interaction of FPR with its G protein partner is not affected by desensitization of this receptor system in human neutrophils. Instead, Jesaitis and co-workers have proposed that desensitization may result from both a rapid association of an agonist-occupied receptor with cytoskeletal elements (Jesaitis *et al.*, 1993) and a lateral segregation of FPR and G proteins into different plasma membrane domains (Jesaitis *et al.*, 1988; Johansson *et al.*, 1993). Alternatively, by analogy with the β-adrenergic receptor (Hausdorff *et al.*, 1990), one cannot exclude that the impairment of chemoattractant receptor–G protein interaction involves an inhibitory factor which belongs to the arrestin family of regulatory proteins that specifically bind the phosphorylated form of the receptor.

In terms of Ca^{2+} mobilization, all three peptide chemoattractants desensitize one another with the following rank order of potency: fMLF > C5a >

IL-8. Moreover, all peptide chemoattractants desensitize responses to lipid chemoattractants such as LTB_4 and PAF, but neither lipids nor ATPγS was able to desensitize the Ca^{2+}-mobilizing response to peptides (Tomhave *et al.*, 1994). This has led Snyderman and co-workers to the description of a third form of desensitization referred to as cross-desensitization. However, the mechanism by which receptor cross-desensitization is orchestrated appears to be complex and most likely occurs at several levels. Thus, although C5a and IL-8 cross-desensitize the Ca^{2+}-mobilizing responses to fMLF, they are unable to induce the phosphorylation of FPR and do not alter fMLF-stimulated GTPγS binding to leukocyte membranes. This indicates that cross-desensitization of Ca^{2+}-mobilizing responses can occur independently of receptor phosphorylation by a mechanism that most likely involves the alteration of effectors distal from the receptor. In contrast, pretreatment of leukocytes or stably cotransfected RBL-2H3 cells by fMLF causes an inhibition of C5a- and IL-8-stimulated GTPγS binding to membrane (Tomhave *et al.*, 1994; Richardson *et al.*, 1995b). However, conflicting results exist in the literature as to whether the mechanism of inhibition involved receptor phosphorylation. Although Richardson and co-workers (1995b) were able to demonstrate fMLF-induced phosphorylation of C5aR and IL-8R in co-transfected RBL-2H3 cells, Tardif *et al.* (1993) were unable to demonstrate fMLF-induced phosphorylation of C5aR in differentiated HL-60 cells. This discrepancy is presently not understood, but protein kinase C isoforms with different substrate specificity may be activated in HL-60 and RBL-2H3 cells. Alternatively, the absence of cross-phosphorylation in HL-60 cells may indicate the existence of a variant cell clone.

The kinases involved in the phosphorylation of different chemoattractant receptors may vary from one receptor to the next. On the basis of phosphorylation studies with a fusion protein containing the Ser/Thr-rich carboxyl terminus of FPR, it has been suggested that FPR is phosphorylated in a sequential manner on serine and threonine residues by a neutrophil cytosolic kinase (Prossnitz *et al.*, 1995a). The fusion protein could be phosphorylated efficiently by the G protein-coupled receptor kinase, GRK2, which is most abundant in leukocytes and may be translocated from cytosolic fraction to the membrane fraction upon chemoattractant stimulation. Both second messenger-activated kinases and G protein-coupled receptor kinase(s) seem to be involved in the phosphorylation of C5aR, PAFR, and IL-8R. However, the contribution of the former type of kinases in the phosphorylation process appears to be limited upon agonist stimulation. Although phosphorylation of C5aR is promoted by PMA in HL-60 cells, C5aR is fully phosphorylated upon agonist binding when signal transduction is disrupted by pertussis toxin treatment, indicating a modest contribution of second messenger-activated kinases in the process (Giannini and Boulay, 1995). Additional support to this conclusion is provided by the observation that C5aR does not transduce a signal in COS-7 cells and yet it is hyperphosphorylated in the presence of an agonist. Moreover, staurosporine totally blocks PMA-induced phosphorylation but only partially inhibits C5a-mediated phosphorylation. This implies the participation of a dominant kinase that most likely belongs to the G protein-coupled receptor kinase family (reviewed in Inglese *et al.*, 1993). Phosphorylation sites have been identified on serine residues of the carboxyl-terminal tail whether cells are stimulated with C5a or PMA (Giannini *et al.*, 1995). Sites that are phosphorylated in the presence of PMA appear to overlap with those phosphorylated in the presence of an agonist. In the presence of C5a, C5aR is phosphorylated with a maximal stoichiometry of 6 mol of PO_4/mol of receptor at Ser_{314}, Ser_{317}, Ser_{327}, Ser_{332}, Ser_{334}, and Ser_{338}. The key phosphorylation sites are located at positions 332, 334, and 338 as a simultaneous replacement by alanine residues results in a dramatic reduction of basal as well as C5a- and PMA-mediated phosphorylation (Giannini *et al.*, 1995). The capacity of this mutant to produce inositol 1,4,5-trisphosphate is increased as compared to the wild-type receptor (Naik *et al.*, 1997). Similar to C5aR, the phosphorylation of IL-8RA is promoted by PMA. Although staurosporine completely blocks PMA-induced phosphorylation, it only partially inhibits IL-8-mediated phosphorylation. Mutagenesis studies indicate that the phosphorylation of IL-8RA mainly occurs in the carboxyl-terminal tail in three clusters of Ser/Thr residues (Fig 3). Disruption of the second cluster, Thr-Ser-Ser-Ser, by alanine replacement yields a mutant receptor that shows a four-fold increase in IL-8-induced PI hydrolysis (Richardson *et al.*, 1995b). The effect of phosphorylation of the carboxyl terminus in receptor function has also been reported for the PAF receptor (Ali *et al.*, 1994; Takano *et al.*, 1994).

V. Chemoattractant Receptor Homologs

Since the cloning of the N-formyl peptide receptor cDNA in 1990, a large number of chemoattractant receptors and their homologs have been identified. Two factors contribute to the surge of the number of cloned receptors. One is the increasing awareness of the presence of new chemoattractant receptors, and the necessity of and interest in finding these receptors by molecular cloning. At present, there is a mismatch between the large (and still growing) number of characterized chemoattractants, including chemokines, and a relatively small number of the cloned receptors. Pharmacological studies indicate that many of these chemoattractants interact with binding sites having different properties from those of cloned receptors. The other factor is the rapid development and broad application of new cloning technologies. The finding that many chemokine receptors contain the DRYLAIVHA sequence led to the design and use of degenerate oligonucleotides to isolate new receptor cDNAs by polymerase chain reaction (PCR) (Neote *et al.*, 1993). The PCR-based method is replacing the conventional low-stringency hybridization method and has contributed to the cloning of several CCRs. The use of cDNA subtraction and differential display technologies has further facilitated the identification of novel receptor cDNAs.

Many cloned chemoattractant receptor homologs remain orphan receptors, i.e., receptors without known physiological ligands. The tissue distribution pattern of these receptors, as well as their binding profile with characterized chemoattractants, is summarized in Table I. It is hoped that sequence comparison will give hints for the identification of possible ligands for these receptors. The properties of some of these receptors are discussed next.

1. Viral Homologs of Chemoattractant Receptors

In 1990, Chee and co-workers reported the identification of three predicted open reading frames (ORF) within the genome of the human cytomegalovirus (HCMV) that encode putative proteins homologous to the sequence of mammalian G protein-coupled receptors. Two of the three ORF, US27 and US28, are arranged in tandem in the genome and are likely to be the result of gene duplication. The third, UL33, is 173 bp apart from US27 and US28. The three ORF encode proteins of 390 (UL33), 362 (US27), and 323 (US28) amino acids, respectively. Alignment of the sequences of these ORF with subsequently cloned G protein-coupled chemokine receptors revealed global and regional homology of approximately 36 and 50% to the human IL-8 receptors and CC CKR1. Neote and co-workers (1993) demonstrated that the protein product of US28, which is most homologous to CC CKR1, could bind MIP-1α, MCP-1, MIP-1β, and RANTES. It, however, did not interact with the CXC chemokines such as IL-8. This finding was confirmed by Gao and Murphy (1994), indicating that the ORF of US28 indeed encodes a promiscuous receptor for the CC chemokines.

The herpesvirus saimiri was also found to contain a gene (ECRF3) that encodes a GPCR-like protein (Nicholas *et al.,* 1992). The ECRF3 product contains 321 amino acids. The sequence homology between the ECRF3 product and the chemokine receptors is not significantly higher than that for other GPCRs, with the exception that the amino terminus of the ECRF3 product contains a stretch of residues that aligns well with those found in similar regions of the IL-8 receptors and CCR1. This observation led to the investigation by Ahuja and Murphy (1993), who found that the ECRF3 protein is a functional receptor for the CXC chemokines in the rank order of GROα/MGSA > MAP-2 > IL-8. The ECRF3, when expressed in *Xenopus* oocytes, mediated ligand-specific calcium mobilization only to the previously described CXC chemokines but not to several CC chemokines tested, including MIP-1α/β, MCP-1, and RANTES. Thus, the ligand-binding profile for the ECRF3 protein is most similar, but not identical, to that of the IL-8 receptor B (IL-8 > GROα = NAP-2). The differences in the hierarchy of potency to various CXC chemokines are possibly due to the fact that these

TABLE I Chemoattractant Receptors and Homologs: Ligands and Tissue Distribution[a]

Name of receptor	*Accession no.*[b]	*Ligand/Function*	*Tissue distribution*[c]
N-formyl peptide receptor (FPR)	M60626	*N*-formyl (or non-formyl) peptides	N, M, HepG2, astrocyte
Lipoxin A_4R (FPR2/FPRL1)	B42009/P25089	Lipoxin A_4; fMet-Leu-Phe (low affinity)	N, M, HL-60
FPRL2	L14061/P25090		M. lung
C5a receptor (C5aR)	M62505	C5a	N, M, Eo, HepG2, astrocyte, Ba, Ma
C3aR (AZ3B)	U28488/Z73157	C3a	N, M, En, brain, Heart, lung, placenta
PAF receptor (PAFR)	M80436	Platelet-activating factor/AGEPC	N, M, Eo, Placenta, Fb, lung
CXCR1 (IL-8RA)	M68932/P25025	IL-8	N, M, T (NK)
CXCR2 (IL-8RB)	M73969/U03905	IL-8, GRO, NAP-2, ENA-78	N, M, melanoma cells, T (NK)
CXCR3	X95876	IP-10, Mig	Activated T cells
CXCR4 (LESTR/Fusin)	M99293/L01639	SDF-1/PBSF	N, M, PBL, HL-60
CCR1 (CC CKR1)	L09230/L10918	MIP-1α, RANTES, MCP-3	M, N, T, THP-1, U937
CCR2A,2B (CC CKR2A,2B)	U03882/U03905	MCP-1, MCP-3, MCP-4	M, Ba, MonoMac6, THP-1
CCR3 (CC CKR3/ 88-2b)	U28694	Eotaxin, RANTES, MCP-2, MCP-3, MCP-4	Eo, Ba
CCR4 (CC CKR4)	X85740	MIP-1α, RANTES, MCP-1	Ba, T
CCR5 (CC CKR5)	X91492	MIP-1α, MIP-1β, RANTES	M, T (CD4-positive), KG-1A
HCMV-US27	P09703		Human cytomegalovirus
HCMV-US28	P09704/P32952	MIP-1α, MIP-1β, MCP-1, RANTES	Human cytomegalovirus
HCMV-UL33 (AD169)	X17403		Human cytomegalovirus
HVS-ECRF3	Q01035	IL-8, NAP-2, GROα	Herpesvirus saimir
K2R	L21931		Swinepoxvirus
Q2/3L	S78201		Capripoxvirus (KS-1)

Duffy antigen receptor	U01839	IL-8, NAP-2, GROα, RANTES, MCP-1	E, kidney, brain
Burkitt's lymphoma R1 (BRL1)	X68149/P32302	Important for B-cell homing in mice[d]	Burkitt's lymphoma
MDR15 orphan receptor	X68829		B, M
EBV infected cell receptor (EBI1)	L08176		B
EBV infected cell receptor (EBI2)	L08177		U937, HL-60
R2 orphan receptor	U33448		Unknown; isolated as genomic clone
R12 orphan receptor	U33447		Unknown; isolated as genomic clone
R20 orphan receptor/APJ	U03642/P35414		Lymph node, brain, placenta, kidney
CMKBRL1/V28	U28934/U20350	MCP-3 (low affinity)	Leukocytes, spleen, brain
GPR5 orphan receptor	L36149		Unknown; isolated as genomic clone
GPR9 orphan receptor	U32674		Unknown; isolated as genomic clone
GPR-CY4 orphan receptor	U45984		Unpublished
GPR-CY6 orphan receptor	U45983		Unpublished

[a] This table and is divided into four sections (from the top): classical chemoattractant receptors and their homolog; chemokine receptors; viral homologs of chemokine receptors; and other chemoattractant receptor homologus.

[b] Accession numbers are for GenBank/EMBL and SWISSPROT databases.

[c] B, B lymphocyte; Ba, basophil; E, erythrocyte; En, endothelial cell; Eo, eosinophil; Fb, fibroblast; M, monocyte; Ma, mast cell; N, neutrophil; T, T lymphocyte; PBL, peripheral blood lymphocytes.

[d] Förster *et al.*, 1996

studies were conducted in injected oocytes rather than in mammalian cells (Ahuja and Murphy, 1993).

There may be more viral chemoattractant receptor homologs, as evidenced by the identification of these in capripoxvirus and swinepoxvirus (Cao *et al.,* 1995; Massung *et al.,* 1993). The physiological functions of these viral chemokine receptors are not understood at present. The viruses apparently acquired the chemokine genes from their respective hosts, a process termed molecular piracy (Ahuja *et al.,* 1994). It remains to be determined whether these chemokine receptor homologs are expressed in the infected cells and to what extent the expression of these chemokine receptor homologs benefits the viruses.

2. *Duffy Antigen Receptor for Chemokines (DARC)*

The Duffy antigen was originally identified as an erythrocyte-binding protein for the malarial parasite *Plasmodium vivax*. Duffy antigen-negative individuals, mostly of African origin, are resistant to invasion by *P. vivax*. The function of the Duffy antigen to bind chemokines was first discovered by Darbonne and co-workers (1991), who investigated the cause of contaminating erythrocytes on the binding of IL-8 to leukocyte cell preparations. It was subsequently found that the Duffy antigen also serves as binding sites for MGSA/GROα, NAP-2, MCP-1, and RANTES (Neote *et al.,* 1993; Horuk *et al.,* 1993b). Chaudhuri and co-workers (1993) reported the cloning of the cDNA for the Duffy antigen from a human bone marrow cDNA library. The cDNA encodes a protein of 338 amino acids that is highly hydrophobic. The predicted protein has a molecular mass of ~35 kDa, shares 26% overall sequence identity with the human IL-8RB, and contains several proline and cysteine residues in the transmembrane and extracellular domains, respectively, that are conserved among leukocyte chemokine receptors. These amino acids may provide the structural basis for the binding of multiple chemokines. Horuk and co-workers (1996) conducted a detailed study of the structure and function relationship of the Duffy antigens from mouse. The mouse homolog of the Duffy antigen binds human MGSA/GROα with a higher affinity than that for the human IL-8. Using monoclonal antibodies against the Duffy antigen and chimeric DARC/IL-8RB receptor constructs, a binding site for chemokines has been localized to the amino-terminal extracellular domain (Horuk *et al.,* 1996). Despite the capability of binding multiple chemokines, the Duffy antigen has not been shown to couple to G proteins or to transduce signals generated by ligand–receptor interaction. The DRYLAIVHA sequence, commonly seen at the end of the third transmembrane domain of chemokine receptors, is not conserved in this receptor. It may explain the absence of G protein coupling since this stretch of sequence is believed to be involved in the interaction of G protein-coupled chemoattractant receptors with the G_i proteins.

The physiological and pathological functions of the Duffy antigen as a chemokine receptor are not clear at present. This promiscuous receptor for chemokine is expressed early in erythropoiesis and its messenger RNA is detectable in bone marrow, fetal liver, spleen, and kidney, as well as in brain and the K562 erythroleukemia cells. It has been found in Purkinje cells in the cerebellum and in T cells of the CD45RA phenotype (Horuk *et al.*, 1996). The Duffy antigen is structurally conserved across species from birds to humans (Horuk, 1994). One possible role of the Duffy antigen is to negatively regulate the levels of chemokines in the circulation. However, there has not been a report of higher chemokine levels or a proinflammatory tendency in Duffy-negative individuals. Thus, until a clear role of this protein in chemokine binding is identified, the primary function of the Duffy antigen remains that associated with the invasion of *P. vivax*.

3. Lymphocyte-Derived Chemokine Receptor Homologs

While searching for genes potentially involved in the tumorogenesis of Burkitt's lymphoma (BL), Lipp and colleagues cloned a GPCR homolog from a subtractive cDNA library of the BL64 cell line (Dobner *et al.*, 1992). The cDNA encodes a peptide of 372 amino acids and is named BRL1. BLR1 is most homologous to the IL-8 receptor (35% sequence identity with IL-8RA and 37% with IL-8RB). The most conserved sequences are located in the transmembrane domains and include the DRYLAIVHA sequence in the second intracellular loop. Several acidic residues and a proline are found in the identical positions of BLR1 when aligned with the IL-8 receptors. Despite this sequence homology, no IL-8 binding to BL64- and BLR1-transfected COS-7 cells was detected (Dobner *et al.*, 1992). There has not been a report of BLR1 binding to other chemoattractants.

The expression pattern of BLR1 has been studied with human and murine BLR1 probes (Kaiser *et al.*, 1993). In human cells, BLR1 expression is independent of EBV infection, but is B cell specific and is associated with cell differentiation (Dobner *et al.*, 1992). Treatment with cycloheximide induced the expression of the BLR1 transcript in some cells. The mouse BLR1 has been cloned by two groups (Kaiser *et al.*, 1993; Kouba *et al.*, 1993), one of which obtained the cDNA by homologous hybridization with a rat cDNA probe that encodes a similar receptor named NLR (Kouba *et al.*, 1993). In mice, the BLR1 message is detected in secondary lymphatic organs and to a lesser extent in the brain and fetal liver (Kaiser *et al.*, 1993). SCID mice with severely impaired B-cell development have much less expression of the BLR1 message in the spleen. Using a monoclonal Ab against the receptor, it was found that in addition to the B cells, a subset of T cells also express BLR1 (Forster *et al.*, 1994). These T cells have the phenotype of CD45R0-positive, IL-2R-negative, high levels of CD44 and low levels of L-selectin. BRL1 was detected in the majority of $CD4^+$ cells originating from secondary lymphatic tissue, but was not seen in cord blood-derived T cells, indicating that BLR1 is a marker for memory T cells. The cell surface expression of BLR1 was downregulated by stimulating the B and T cells with anti-CD40 and anti-CD3 mAb, respectively.

A variant of BLR1 cDNA has been isolated from a monocyte cDNA library (Barella *et al.*, 1995). This cDNA encodes a protein of 327 amino acids that lacks the amino-terminal 45 residues found in the original BLR1. This variation is believed to be the result of alternative RNA splicing. Alternative splicing at the 5′ end of the RNA may result in receptors with different amino termini and hence a distinct ligand-binding profile. This possibility remains to be tested as the ligand for BLR1 has not been identified to date.

In 1993, Kieff and co-workers cloned two GPCRs from Epstein–Barr virus (EBV)-infected Burkitt's lymphoma cells (Birkenback *et al.*, 1993). One of the proteins, EBI 1, is homologous to the chemokine receptors IL-8R (40% sequence identity overall to either IL-8RA or IL-8RB). The other protein, EBI 2, is most homologous to the thrombin receptor. The natural ligand for these receptors is unknown. EBI 1 is a 377 residue peptide expressed in human spleen and tonsil tissues and in the T-cell line HSB-2. The message for EBI 1 is not detected in promyelocytic and monocytic cell lines such as HL-60 and U937. A more recently isolated cDNA from activated lymphocytes, which was named BLR2, turned out to be identical to EBI 1 (Burgstahler *et al.*, 1995). In addition to the observation that the EBI 1 message is detected in all EBV-positive B-cell lines surveyed, it was also reported that mitogen and anti-CD3 stimulate the expression of EBI 1 in peripheral blood lymphocytes. Further experiments are necessary to examine whether EBI 1 is involved in viral pathogenesis and in the migration of activated lymphocytes.

4. Chemokine Receptor Homolog CMKBRL1/V28

CMKBRL1 is encoded by a isolated cDNA clone from a human eosinophilic leukemia library (Combadiere *et al.*, 1995c). CMKBRL1 contains 355 amino acids and shares approximately 40% sequence identity with the cloned α chemokine receptor IL-8Rα and the α chemokine receptor MIP-1αR (CC CKR1). The protein is most homologous in its transmembrane domains with these two cloned receptors, and the DRYLAIV sequence at the end of the third transmembrane domain is found in CMKBRL1. The amino terminus of CMKBRL1, which contains 29 residues, displays no significant sequence homology with several already characterized chemokine receptors, suggesting that the biological ligand for CMKBRL1 may be quite different from the presently cloned chemokines because the amino terminus of a chemokine receptor is in general a determinant for ligand specificity. Interestingly, CMKBRL1 is highly homologous to a previously cloned rat receptor RBS11 (83% sequence identity), which is also an orphan GPCR

(Harrison *et al.*, 1994). Of the 16 chemokines and nonchemokine chemoattractants tested, none induced calcium mobilization in transfected cells expressing CMKBRL1 (Combadiere *et al.*, 1995c). Northern blot analysis indicated that the message is expressed in neutrophils, monocytes, and in the brain, as well as in solid tissues, including the placenta, lung, liver, and skeletal muscle. It is likely that CMKBRL1 encodes a GPCR that serves a broad range of functions in these tissues.

The V28 cDNA was independently isolated from a human peripheral blood leukocyte DNA library (Raport *et al.*, 1995) and was identical in sequence to CMKBRL1. Tissue distribution studies with Northern blots indicate the expression of V28 transcript in brain and skeletal muscles, but not in detectable levels in placenta, lung, and liver. Exogenously expressed V28 in a human cell line showed that the receptor interacts with low affinity to the CC chemokine MCP-3 (Raport *et al.*, 1996).

The collection of chemoattractant receptor homologs shown in Table I is by no means complete, as several of these receptors expressed in T cells are not included due to the high level sequence homology to tachykinin receptors rather than to leukocyte chemoattractant receptors. Furthermore, novel receptor cDNAs continue to be identified, at an increasingly fast pace, to match the equally rapid expansion of the family of chemoattractants. With the development of large-scale, high throughput ligand-screening technologies, it is anticipated that the ligands for many orphan GPCRs will be identified soon. However, a full understanding of the biological functions of chemoattractant receptor homologs is likely to be a task for many years.

VI. Potential Therapeutic Interventions for Chemoattractant Receptor Activation

Chemoattractants have been implicated in a large number of inflammatory diseases. These range from acute inflammation involving activated neutrophils, such as adult respiratory distress syndrome, to chronic conditions involving mononuclear cells, such as allergic asthma, psoriasis, atopic dermatitis, and arthritis. The important functions that chemoattractant receptors play during inflammatory cell activation suggest that they are targets for therapeutic modulation. Because leukocyte activation by chemoattractants involves agonist binding, functional coupling of the agonist-occupied receptor to G proteins, and activation of the effectors, any intervention at one or more of these steps is likely to disrupt the activation of the cells by a given chemoattractant. Based on this assumption, current efforts are focused on the development of receptor antagonists, blocking antibodies against the receptors or the agonists, and agents that can selectively inhibit one or more signaling pathways. A few examples are given in the following sections.

A. Receptor Antagonists

The development of specific chemoattractant receptor antagonists started long before the molecular cloning of these receptors. It is best exemplified with the identification of PAF receptor antagonists. Various compounds have been chemically synthesized since the early 1980s (reviewed in Hwang, 1990). This traditional drug screening approach has been remarkably successful, yielding antagonists that display affinities for the PAF receptor higher than PAF itself (Herbert, 1992). It is not uncommon that the most potent PAF antagonists have little structural resemblance to PAF, whereas PAF derivatives often display partial agonist activities (Hwang, 1990). In *in vitro* studies with isolated blood cells and cultured cell lines, most PAF antagonists are able to inhibit PAF-induced cellular functions, including chemotaxis, calcium mobilization, transcription activation, and platelet aggregation. However, clinical trials of several PAF antagonists have showed only measured success in human subjects. Discovery of the juxtacrine mechanism (Zimmerman *et al.*, 1993) suggests that the tight cell–cell association may prevent PAF antagonists from reaching sufficiently high concentrations at the site of action. Thus, the effective use of these potent PAF antagonists requires further characterization of the basic mechanisms of PAF action. Antagonists for other cloned chemoattractant receptors have been developed. The tBOC-Phe-Leu-Phe-Leu-Phe is an FPR antagonist with a K_i value in the range of 0.1–0.2 μM. More potent antagonists for FPR have been developed that display IC_{50} values in the submicromolar concentrations, making them useful for diagnostic and possibly therapeutic purposes (Higgins *et al.*, 1996; Derian *et al.*, 1996). Substituted 4,6-diaminoquinolines have been found to be inhibitors for C5aR, with IC_{50} values between 3.3 and 12 μg/ml (Lanza *et al.*, 1992).

The development of chemokine receptor antagonists has been a relatively recent endeavor, hence there has not been a sizable collection of potent receptor antagonists. One of the approaches is based on structural information that suggests the importance of the amino-terminal residues of the CXC chemokines, such as the Glu-Leu-Arg at positions 4–6 of IL-8, in agonist binding and activities (Clark-Lewis *et al.*, 1991). It was predicted that modification of the agonists in this region might produce chemokine analogs with antagonist properties. Two of these modified ligands, (F1-5)R-IL-8 and (F1-3)AAR-IL-8, displayed half-maximal inhibitory effects on receptor binding and exocytosis at 300 n*M* (Moser *et al.*, 1993). More recently, this approach has been used for the CC chemokine MCP-1, resulting in amino terminal truncated analogs that are not significantly active but are able to desensitize MCP-1-induced functions (Gong and Clark-Lewis, 1995). The IC_{50} for these MCP-1 analogs can reach 20 n*M*, whereas the dissociation constant for the MCP-1 receptors is as low as 8.3 n*M*. Zhang and Rollins (1995) independently demonstrated that an amino-terminal deletion variant of MCP-1 (7ND) inhibited MCP-1-induced chemotaxis. This study indicated that MCP-1 forms dimers at physiological concentrations and that the dimer is the active form of MCP-1. Thus, it is suggested that the dominant negative inhibitory effect of 7ND is the consequence of heterodimer formation between the nonfunctional 7ND and the wild-type MCP-1. These findings suggest a novel mechanism for the antagonism by chemokine analogs. However, the general applicability of this approach remains to be investigated, as previous studies indicated that the monomer, rather than the dimer, is a functional form of IL-8 (Rajarathnam *et al.,* 1994). Conversely, the addition of residues at the amino terminus can result in molecules with antagonist properties. Extension with a single methionine at the amino terminus has been found to be sufficient to switch RANTES to a selective antagonist (Proudfoot *et al.,* 1996). The same chemokine, when truncated with the first eight residues at the N-terminus, became a less specific antagonist capable of binding to multiple chemokine receptors (Gong *et al.,* 1996). The N-terminmal truncated RANTES (9–68) has been shown to inhibit the entry of macrophage-tropic HIV into human monocytes (Arenzana-Seisdedos *et al.,* 1996). Recently, synthetic non-peptide antagonists for chemokine receptors began to emerge. The compound SKF83589 prevents IL-8 and GROα/MGSA binding to the IL-8RB with an IC_{50} value of 0.5 μM. The compound SB225002 inhibited GROα/MGSA and IL-8-induced chemotaxis with an IC_{50} of 20 and 50 n*M*, respectively. None of these antagonists display an inhibitory effect for IL-8RA (J.R. White, personal communication).

B. Blocking Antibodies

Antibodies against the amino termini and other regions of several chemoattractant receptors have been shown to block the binding of chemoattractants and their functions. Both the polyclonal (Morgan *et al.,* 1993) and the monoclonal (Oppermann *et al.,* 1993) antibodies against the human C5a receptor have been shown to partially inhibit the function of this receptor. The blocking effect is conveyed by inhibition of one of the two steps of C5a binding, the initial contact of the agonist with the amino terminus of the receptor (see Section IV,A), likely by steric hindrance due to the size of the blocking IgG. Antibodies specific for the type A and type B IL-8 receptors have also been developed and have been shown to neutralize the functions of these receptors (Chuntharapai *et al.,* 1994a; Hammond *et al.,* 1995). The use of these antibodies has led to the finding that the type A IL-8 receptor predominantly mediates chemotaxis (Hammond *et al.,* 1995). In addition, monoclonal antibodies against DARC have been prepared (Horuk *et al.,* 1996). One of the antibodies was mapped to the amino terminus of the receptor and was shown to inhibit chemokine binding to DARC expressed in K562 cells. More recently, an anti-peptide antibody against the amino-terminal sequence of fusin (LESTR) was shown to block HIV-1 entry mediated by the orphan receptor (Feng *et al.*, 1996).

C. Inhibitors for Chemoattractant-Induced Signal Transduction

Although there are a large number of available inhibitors that disrupt various intracellular signaling pathways, few have been shown to be specific for chemoattractant receptor-mediated signaling. This is due to the fact that chemoattractants induce many of the signaling events that are similar or identical to those induced by other GPCRs and receptors of other types. Depending on the development of special delivery systems, agents known for their inhibitory properties on leukocyte functions may eventually prove to be useful tools for therapy. These can be classified as (1) cytoskeleton-disrupting agents for the inhibition of chemotaxis; (2) natural and synthetic inhibitors for kinases that are involved in NADPH oxidase activation; (3) antisense oligonucleotides that disrupt the interaction between the receptors and G proteins, and between G protein subunits; (4) dominant negative signaling components and other engineered scavenger molecules that can block one or more steps of the signaling pathways; and (5) inhibitors for transcription activation that may reduce the expression of key leukocyte proteins necessary for chemoattractant signaling.

Inflammation serves the dual functions of host defense and tissue damage. Therefore the control of chemoattractant receptor-mediated inflammatory cell activation must be quantitative and requires the consideration of temporal and spatial factors. It is further complicated by the presence of a large number of chemoattractants and the promiscuity or shared binding properties with some members of the chemoattractant receptor family. It is difficult to identify a single antagonist for all chemoattractant receptors. The development of effective therapeutic means, therefore, requires a multipronged approach and demands a better understanding of the mechanisms with which chemoattractant receptors activate cells.

VII. Summary and Future Perspectives

Recent advances in the molecular cloning of chemoattractant receptors have generated enormous amounts of information regarding the structure–function relationships of these receptors. It is now clear that chemoattractant receptors, as a subgroup of the GPCR superfamily, have their own unique pharmacological and biochemical properties. There is no doubt that many of these receptors can be targets for therapeutic intervention. In the near future, research in this field is likely to address several issues that are currently unresolved. First, the discovery of a large number of chemoattractants indicates the presence of as yet unidentified cell surface receptors. A combination of phamacological analysis and molecular cloning approach is necessary to identify these receptors. Second, the rapid increase in the number of orphan receptors requires the development of more powerful screening methods for the identification of the biological ligands for these receptors. Third, leukocyte chemoattractant receptors have been shown to mediate other important cellular functions and biological processes, such as virus entry and gene transcription. The discovery that some chemokine receptors serve as cofactors for HIV-1 fusion will certainly stimulate new research efforts to understand the underlying mechanisms. The functions of chemoattractant receptors in nonleukocytic cells are essentially unknown at present, but will be undoubtedly identified in the future. Last but not least, chemoattractant receptor-mediated signaling mechanisms will continue to be analyzed in greater detail. Understanding of the signaling mechanisms is essential to the development of new strategies for the control of inflammatory cell activation, which can be mediated by a plethora of cell surface receptors capable of responding to numerous inflammatory stimuli.

Acknowledgements

The authors would like to thank Charley Cochrane for encouragement, Eric Prossnitz and Darren Browning for helpful discussions, and Lilia Lomibao for assistance in reference organization. We are indebted to the many investigators who made their data available prior to publication.

REFERENCES

Ahuja, S. K., and Murphy, P. M. (1993). Molecular piracy of mammalian interleukin-8 receptor type B by herpesvirus saimiri. *J. Biol. Chem.* **268**, 20691–20694.

Ahuja, S. K., Gao, J.-L., and Murphy, P. M. (1994). Chemokine receptors and molecular mimicry. *Immunol. Today* **15**, 281–287.

Ahuja, S. K., Lee, J. C., and Murphy, P. M. (1996). CXC chemokines bind to unique sets of selectivity determinants that can function independently and are broadly distributed on multiple domains of human interleukin-8 receptor B. *J. Biol. Chem.* **271**, 225–232.

Ali, H., Richardson, R. M., Tomhave, E. D., Didsbury, J. R., and Snyderman, R. (1993). Differences in phosphorylation of formulpeptide and C5a chemoattractant receptors correlated with differences in densensitization. *J. Biol. Chem.* **268**, 24247–24254.

Ali, H., Richardson, R. M., Tomhave, E. D., DuBose, R. A., Haribabu, B., and Snyderman, R. (1994). Regulation of stably transfected platelet activating factor receptor in RBL-2H3 cells. Role of multiple G proteins and receptor phosphorylation. *J. Biol. Chem.* **269**, 24557–24563.

Alkhatib, G., Combadiere, C., Broder, C. C., Feng, Y., Kennedy, P. E., Murphy, P. M., and Berger, E. A. (1996). CC CKR5: A RANTES, MIP-1-alpha, MIP-1-beta receptor as a fusion cofactor for macrophage-tropic HIV-1. *Science* **272,** 1955–1958.

Allen, R. A., Tolley, J. O., and Jesaitis, A. J. (1986). Preparation and properties of an improved photoaffinity ligand for the N-formylpeptide receptor. *Biochim. Biophy. Acta* **882,** 271–280.

Allen, R. A., Jesaitis, A. J., and Cochrane, C. G. (1990). N-formyl peptide receptor structure-function relationships. *Cell. Mol. Mech. Inflammation* **1,** 83–112.

Alvarez, V., Coto, E., Setien, F., and Lopez-Larrea, C. (1994). A physical map of two clusters containing the genes for six proinflammatory receptors. *Immunogenetics* **40,** 100–103.

Amatruda, T. T., Steele, D. A., Slepak, V. Z., and Simon, M. I. (1991). Gα16, a G protein a subunit specifically expressed in hematopoietic cells. *Proc. Natl. Acad. Sci. U.S.A.* **88,** 5587–5591.

Amatruda, T. T., Gerard, N. P., Gerard, C., and Simon, M. I. (1993). Specific interactions of chemoattractant factor receptors with G-proteins. *J. Biol. Chem.* **268,** 10139–10144.

Amatruda, T. T., Dragas-Graonic, S., Holmes, R., and Perez, H. D. (1995). Signal transduction by the formyl petide receptor. *J. Biol. Chem.* **270,** 28010–28013.

Ames, R. S., Li, Y., Sarau, H. M., Nuthulaganti, P., Foley, J. J., Ellis, C., Zeng, Z., Su, K., Jurewicz, A. J., Hertzberg, R. P., Bergsma, D. J., and Kumar, C. (1996). Molecular cloning and characterization of the human anaphylatoxin C3a receptor. *J. Biol. Chem.* **271,** 20231–20234.

Arenzana-Seisdedos, F., Virelizier, J.-L., Rousset, D., Clark-Lewis, I., Loetscher, P., Moser, B., and Baggiolini, M. (1996). HIV blocked by chemokine antagonist. *Nature* **383,** 400.

Bacon, K. B., Premack, B. A., Gardner, P., and Schall, T. J. (1995). Activation of dual T cell signaling pathways by the chemokine RANTES. *Science* **269,** 1727–1729.

Baggiolini, M., Dewald, B., and Moser, B. (1994). Interleukin-8 and related chemotactic cytokines—CXC and CC chemokines. *Adv. Immunol.* **55,** 97–179.

Baldwin, E. T., Weber, I. T., St. Charles, R., Xuan, J.-C., Appella, E., Yamada, M., Matsushima, K., Edwards, B. F. P., Clore, G. M., Gronenborn, A. M., and Włodawer, A. (1991). Crystal structure of interleukin 8: Symbiosis of NMR and crystallography. *Proc. Natl. Acad. Sci. U.S.A.* **88,** 502–506.

Baldwin, J. M. (1993). The probable arrangement of the helices in G protein-coupled receptors. *EMBO J.* **12,** 1693–1703.

Bao, L., Gerard, N. P., Eddy, R., Jr., Shows, T. B., and Gerard, C. (1992). Mapping of genes for the human C5a receptor (C5AR), human FMLP receptor (FPR), and two FMLP receptor homologue orphan receptors (FPRH1, FPRH2) to chromosome 19. *Genomics* **13,** 437–440.

Barella, L., Loetscher, M., Tobler, A., Baggiolini, M., and Moser, B. (1995). Sequence variation of a novel heptahelical leukocyte receptor through alternative transcript formation. *Biochem. J.* **309,** 773–779.

Ben-Baruch, A., Bengali, K. M., Biragyn, A., Johnston, J. J., Wang, J. M., Kim, J., Chuntharapai, A., Michiel, D. F., Oppenheim, J. J., and Kelvin, D. J. (1995a). Interleukin-8 receptor β. The role of the carboxyl terminus in signal transduction. *J. Biol. Chem.* **270,** 9121–9128.

Ben-Baruch, A., Michiel, D. F., and Oppenheim, J. J. (1995b). Signal and receptors involved in recruitment of inflammatory cells. *J. Biol. Chem.* **270,** 11703–11706.

Benveniste, J., Henson, P. M., and Cochrane, C. G. (1972). Leukocyte-dependent histamine release from rabbit platelets: The role of IgE, basophils and a platelets-activating factor. *J. Exp. Med.* **136,** 1356–1367.

Berson, J. F., Long, D., Doranz, B. J., Rucker, J., Jirik, F. R., and Doms, R. W. (1996). A seven transmembrane domain receptor involved in fusion and entry of T-cell tropic human immunodeficiency virus type-1 strains. *J. Virol.* **70,** 6280–6295.

Billah, M. M. (1993). Phospholipase D and cell signaling. *Curr. Opin. Immunol.* **5,** 114–123.

Birkenback, M., Josefsen, K., Yalamanchili, R., Lenoir, G., and Kieff, E. (1993). Epstein-Barr virus-induced genes: First lymphocyte-specific G protein-coupled peptide receptors. *J. Virol.* **67**, 2209–2220.

Blank, J. L., Brattain, K. A., and Exton, J. H. (1992). Activation of cytosolic phosphoinositide phospholipase C by G-protein $\beta\gamma$ subunits. *J. Biol Chem.* **267**, 23069–23075.

Bleul, C. C., Farzan, M., Choe, H., Parolin, C., Clark-Lewis, I., Sodroski, J., and Springer, T. A. (1996a). The lymphocyte chemoattractant SDF-1 is a ligand for LESTR/fusin and blocks HIV-1 entry. *Nature* **382,** 829–833.

Bleul, C. C., Fuhlbrigge, R. C., Casasnovas, J. M., Aiuti, A., and Springer, T. A. (1996b) A highly efficacious lymphocyte chemoattractant, stromal cell-derived factor 1 (SDF-1). *J. Exp. Med.* **184,** 1101–1109.

Bokisch, V. A., and Muller-Eberhard, H. J. (1970). Anaphylatoxin inactivator of human plasma: its isolation and characterization as a carboxypeptidase. *J. Clin. Invest.* **49,** 2429–2436.

Bokoch, G. M., and Der, C. J. (1993) Emerging concepts in the Ras super-family of GTP-binding proteins. *FASEB J.* **7,** 750–759.

Bokoch, G. M., and Gilman, A.G. (1984). Inhibition of receptor-mediated release of arachidonic acid by pertussis toxin. *Cell* (*Cambridge, Mass.*) **39,** 301–309.

Bommakanti, R. K., Bokoch, G. M., Tolley, J. O., Schreiber, R. E., Siemsen, D. W., Klotz, K. N., and Jesaitis, A. J. (1992). Reconstitution of a physical complex between the N-formyl chemotactic peptide receptor and G protein. Inhibition by pertussis toxin-catalyzed ADP ribosylation. *J. Biol. Chem.* **267,** 7576–7581.

Bommakanti, R. K., Klotz, K. N., Dratz, E. A., and Jesaitis, A. J. (1993). A carboxyl-terminal tail peptide of neutrophil chemotactic receptor disrupts its physical complex with G protein. *J. Leukocyte Biol.* **54,** 572–577.

Bommakanti, R. K., Dratz, E. A., Siemsen, D. W., and Jesaitis, A. J. (1994). Characterization of complex formation between Gi_2 and octyl glucoside solubilized neutrophil N-formyl peptide chemoattractant receptor by sedimentation velocity. *Biochim. Biophys. Acta* **1209,** 69–76.

Bommakanti, R. K., Dratz, E. A., Siemsen, D. W., and Jesaitis, A. J. (1995). Extensive contact between Gi_2 and N-formyl peptide receptor of human neutrophils: Mapping of binding sites using receptor-mimetic peptides. *Biochemistry* **34,** 6720–6728.

Boulay, F., Tardif, M., Brouchon, L., and Vignais, P. (1990a). Synthesis and use of a novel N-formyl peptide derivative to isolate a human N-formyl peptide receptor cDNA. *Biochem. Biophys. Res. Commun.* **168,** 1103–1109.

Boulay, F., Tardif, M., Brouchon, L., and Vignais, P. (1990b). The human N-formylpeptide receptor. Characterization of two cDNA isolates and evidence for a new subfamily of G-protein-coupled receptors. *Biochemistry* **29,** 11123–11133.

Boulay, F., Mery, L., Tardif, M., Brouchon, L., and Vignais, P. (1991). Expression cloning of a receptor for C5a anaphylatoxin on differentiated HL-60 cells. *Biochemistry* **30,** 2993–2999.

Boyden, S. E. J. (1962). The chemotactic effects of mixtures of antibody and antigen on polymorphonuclear leukocytes. *J. Exp. Med.* **115,** 453–466.

Bubeck, P., Grotzinger, J., Winkler, M., Kohl, J., Wollmer, A., Klos, A., and Bautsch, W. (1994). Site-specific mutagenesis of residues in the human C5a anaphylatoxin which are involved in possible interaction with the C5a receptor. *Eur. J. Biochem.* **219,** 897–904.

Buhl, A. M., Eisfelder, B. J., Worthen, G. S., Johnson, G. L., and Russell, M. (1993). Selective coupling of the human anaphylatoxin C5a receptor and alpha 16 in human kidney 293 cells. *FEBS Lett.* **323,** 132–134.

Buhl, A. M., Osawa, S., and, Johnson, G. L. (1995). Mitogen-activated protein kinase activation requires two signal inputs from the human anaphylatoxin C5a receptor. *J. Biol. Chem.* **270,** 19828–19832.

Burgstahler, R., Kempkes, B., Steube, K., and Lipp, M. (1995). Expression of the chemokine receptor BLR2/EBI1 is specifically transactivated by Epstein-Barr virus nuclear antigen 2. *Biochem. Biophys. Res. Commun.* **215,** 737–743.

Camps, M., Carozzi, A., Schnabel, P., Scheer, A., Parker, P. J., and Gierschik, P. (1992a). Isozyme-selective stimulation of phospholipase C-$\beta 2$ by G protein $\beta\gamma$-subunits. *Nature (London)* **360,** 684–689.

Camps, M., Hou, C., Sidiropoulos, D., Stock, J. B., Jakobs, K. H., and Gierschik, P. (1992b). Stimulation of phospholipase C by guanine-nucleotide binding protein $\beta\gamma$-subunits. *Eur. J. Biochem.* **206,** 821–823.

Cao, J. X., Gershon, P. D., and Black, D. N. (1995). Sequence analysis of HindIII Q2 fragment of Capripoxvirus reveals a putative gene encoding a G-protein-coupled chemokine receptor homologue. *Virology* **209,** 207–712.

Carp, H. (1982). Mitochondrial N-formylmethionylprotein as chemoattractants for neutrophils. *J. Exp. Med.* **155,** 264–275.

Cassatella, M. A., Bazzoni, F., Ceska, M., Ferro, I., Baggiolini, M., and Berton, G. (1992). IL-8 production by human polymorphonuclear leukocytes: The chemoattractant formyl-methionyl-leucyl-phenylalanine induces the gene expression and release of IL-8 through a pertussis toxin-sensitive pathway. *J. Immunol.* **148,** 3216–3220.

Cerretti, D. P., Kozlosky, C. J., Vanden-Bos, T., Nelson, N., Gearing, D. P., and Beckmann, M. P. (1993). Molecular characterization of receptors for human interleukin-8, GRO/melanoma growth-stimulatory activity and neutrophil activating peptide-2. *Mol. Immunol.* **30,** 359–367.

Chabre, M. (1985). Trigger and amplification mechanisms in visual phototransduction. *Annu. Rev. Biophys. Chem.* **14,** 331–360.

Charo, I. F., Myers, S. J., Herman, A., Franci, C., Connolly, A. J., and Coughlin, S. R. (1994). Molecular cloning and functional expression of two monocyte chemoattractant protein 1 receptors reveals alternative splicing of the carboxyl-terminal tails. *Proc. Natl. Acad. Sci. U.S.A.* **91,** 2752–2756.

Chaudhuri, A., Polyakova, J., Zbrzezna, V., Williams, K., Gulati, S., and Pogo, A. O. (1993). Cloning of glycoprotein D cDNA, which encodes the major subunit of the Duffy blood group system and the receptor for the Plasmodium vivax malaria parasite. *Proc. Natl. Acad. Sci. U.S.A.* **90,** 10793–10797.

Chee, M. S., Satchwell, S. C., Preddie, E., Weston, K. M., and Barrell, B. G. (1990). Human cytomegalovirus encodes three G protein-coupled receptor homologues. *Nature (London)* **344,** 774–777.

Chenoweth, D. E., and Hugli, T. E. (1980). Human C5a and C5a analogs as probes of the neutrophil C5a receptor. *Mol. Immunol.* **17,** 151–161.

Chenoweth, D. E., Goodman, M. G., and Hugli, T. E. (1978). Demonstration of specific C5a receptors on intact human polymorphonuclear leukocytes. *Proc. Natl. Acad. Sci. U.S.A.* **75,** 3943–3947.

Choe, H., Farzan, M., Sun, Y., Sullivan, N., Rollins, B., Ponath, P. D., Wu, L., Mackay, C. R., laRosa, G., Newman, W., Gerard, N., Gerard, C., and Sodroski, J. (1996). The beta-chemokine receptors CCR3 and CCR5 facilitate infection by primary HIV-1 isolates. *Cell* **85,** 1135–1148.

Chuntharapai A., Lee, J., Burnier, J., Wood, W. I., Hebert, C., and Kim, K. J. (1994a). Neutralizing monoclonal antibodies to human IL-8 receptor A map to the NH_2-terminal region of the receptor. *J. Immunol.* **152,** 1783–1789.

Chuntharapai, A., Lee, J., Hebert, C. A., and Kim, K. J. (1994b). Monoclonal antibodies detect different distribution patterns of IL-8 receptor A and IL-8 receptor B on human peripheral blood leukocytes. *J. Immunol.* **153,** 5682–5688.

Clark-Lewis, I., Dewald, B., Geiser, T., Moser, B., and Baggiolini, M. (1993). Platelet factor 4 binds interleukin 8 receptors and activates neutrophils when its N terminus is modified with Glu-Leu-Arg. *Proc. Natl. Acad. Sci. U.S.A.* **90,** 3574–3577.

Clark-Lewis, I., Dewald, B., Loetscher, M., Moser, B., and Baggiolini, M. (1994). Structural requirements for interleukin-8 function identified by design of analogs and CXC chemokine hybrids. *J. Biol. Chem.* **269,** 16075–16081.

Clark-Lewis, I., Kim, K. S., Rajarathnam, K., Gong, J. H., Dewald, B., Moser, B., Baggiolini, M., and Sykes, B. D. (1995). Structure-activity relationships of chemokines. *J. Leukocyte Biol.* **57**, 703–711.

Clark-Lewis, I., Schumacher, C., Baggiolini, M., and Moser, B. (1991). Structure-activity relationships of interleukin-8 determined using chemically synthetized analogs. *J. Biol. Chem.* **266**, 23128–23134.

Clore, G. M., and Gronenborn, A. M. (1991). Comparison of the solution nuclear magnetic resonance and crystal structures of interleukin-8. Possible implications for the mechanism of receptor binding. *J. Mol. Biol.* **217**, 611–620.

Clore, G. M., Appella, E., Yamada, M., Matsushima, K., and Gronenborn, A. M. (1990). Three-dimensional structure of interleukin 8 in solution. *Biochemistry* **29**, 1689–1696.

Cocchi, F., DeVico, A. L., Garzino-Demo, A., Arya, S. K., Gallo, R. C., and Lusso, P. (1995). Identification of RANTES, MIP-1α, and MIP-1β as the major HIV-suppressive factors produced by CD8$^+$ T cells. *Science* **270**, 1811–1815.

Cockcroft, S. (1992). G protein regulated phospholipases C, D and A_2 mediated signalling in neutrophils. *Biochim. Biophys. Acta* **1113**, 135–160.

Combadiere, C., Ahuja, S. K., and Murphy, P. M. (1995a). Cloning and functional expression of a human eosinophil CC chemokine receptor. *J. Biol. Chem.* **270**, 16491–16494 (correction published in *J. Biol. Chem.* **270**, 30235).

Combadiere, C., Ahuja, S. K., Van Damme, J., Tiffany, H. L., Gao, J.-L., and Murphy, P. M. (1995b). Monocyte chemoattractant protein-3 is a functional ligand for CC chemokine receptors 1 and 2B. *J. Biol. Chem.* **270**, 29671–29675.

Combadiere, C., Ahuja, S. K., and Murphy, P. M. (1995c). Cloning, chromosomal localization, and RNA expression of a human beta chemokine receptor-like gene. *DNA Cell Biol.* **14**, 673–680.

Cotecchia, S., Exum, S., Caron, M. G., and Lefkowitz, R. J. (1990). Regions of the α1-adrenergic receptor involved in coupling to phosphatidylinositol hydrolysis and enhanced sensitivity of biological function. *Proc. Natl. Acad. Sci. U.S.A.* **87**, 2896–2900.

Crass, T., Raffetseder, U., Martin, U., Grove, M., Klos, A., Kohl, J., and Bautsch, W. (1996). Expression cloning of the human C3a anaphylatoxin receptor (C3aR) from differentiated U-937 cells. *Eur. J. Immunol.* **26**, 1944–1950.

Cundell, D. R., Gerard, N. P., Gerard, C., Idanpaan-Heikkila, I., and Tuomanen, E. I. (1995). Streptococcus pneumoniae anchor to activated human cells by the receptor for platelet-activating factor. *Nature (London)* **377**, 435–438.

Darbonne, W. C., Rice, G. C., Mohler, M. A., Apple, T., Hebert, C. A., Valente, A. J., and Baker, J. B. (1991). Red blood cells are a sink for interleukin 8, a leukocyte chemotaxin. *J. Clin. Invest.* **88**, 1362–1369.

Daugherty, B. L., Siciliano, S. J., DeMartino, J. A., Malkowitz, L., Sirotina, A., and Springer, M. S. (1996). Cloning, expression, and characterization of the human eosinophil eotaxin receptor. *J. Exp. Med.* **183**, 2349–2354.

Dean, M., Carrington, M., Winkler, C., Huttley, G. A., Smith, M. W., Allikmets, R., Goedert, J. J., Buchbinder, S. P., Vittinghoff, E., Gomperts, E., Donfield, S., Vlahov, D., Kaslow, R., Saah, A., Rinaldo, C., Detels, R., *et al.* (1996). Genetic restriction of HIV-1 infection and progression to AIDS by a deletion allele of the CKR5 structural gene. *Science* **273**, 1856–1862.

DeMartino, J. A., Konteatis, Z. D., Siciliano, S. J., Van Riper, G., Underwood, D. J., Fischer, P. A., and Springer, M. S. (1995). Arginine 206 of the C5a receptor is critical for ligand recognition and receptor activation by C-terminal hexapeptide analogs. *J. Biol. Chem.* **270**, 15966–15969.

DeMartino, J. A., Van Riper, G., Siciliano, S. J., Molineaux, C. J., Konteatis, Z. D., Rosen, H., and Springer, M. S. (1994). The amino terminus of the human C5a receptor is required for high affinity C5a binding and for receptor activation by C5a but not C5a analogs. *J. Biol. Chem.* **269**, 14446–14450.

Deng, H., Liu, R., Ellmeier, W., Choe, S., Unutmaz, D., Burkhart, M., Di Marzio, P., Marmon, S., Sutton, R. E., Hill, C. M., Davis, C. B., Peiper, S. C., Schall, T. J., Littman, D. R., and Landau, N. R. (1996). Identification of the major co-receptor for primary isolates of HIV-1. *Nature (London)* **381**, 661–666.

Derian, C. K., Solomon, H. F., Higgins, J. D., Beblavy, M. J., Santulli, R. J., Bridger, G. J., Pike, M. C., Kroon, D. J., and Fischman, A. J. (1996). Selective inhibition of N-formylpeptide-induced neutrophil activation by carbamate-modified peptide analogues. *Biochemistry* **35**, 1265–1269.

Ding, J., Vlahos, C. J., Liu, R., Brown, R. F., and Badwey, J. A. (1995). Antagonists of phosphatidylinositol 3-kinase block activation of several novel protein kinases in neutrophils. *J. Biol. Chem.* **270**, 11684–11691.

Dobner, T., Wolf, I., Emrich, T., and Lipp, M. (1992). Differentiation-specific expression of a novel G protein-coupled receptor from Burkitt's lymphoma. *Eur. J. Immunol.* **22**, 2795–2799.

Dohlman, H. G., Caron, M. G., DeBlasi, A., Frielle, T., and Lefkowitz, R. J. (1990). Role of extracellular disulfide-bonded cysteines in the ligand binding function of the β2-adrenergic receptor. *Biochemistry* **29**, 2335–2342.

Dohlman, H. G., Thorner, J., Caron, M., and Lefkowitz, R. J. (1991). Model systems for the study of seven-transmembrane-segment receptors. *Annu. Rev. Biochem.* **60**, 653–688.

Doranz, B. J., Rucker, J., Yi, Y., Smyth, R. J., Samson, M., Peiper, S. C., Parmentier, M., Collman, R. G., and Doms, R. W. (1996). A dual-tropic primary HIV-1 isolate that uses fusin and the beta-chemokine receptors CKR-5, CKR-3, and CKR-2b as fusion cofactors. *Cell* **85**, 1149–1158.

Dragic, T., Litwin, V., Allaway, G. P., Martin, S. R., Huang, Y., Nagashima, K. A., Cayanan, C., Maddon, P. J., Koup, R. A., Moore, J. P., and Paxton, W. A. (1996). HIV-1 entry into $CD4^+$ cells is mediated by the chemokine receptor C-C CKR-5. *Nature (London)* **381**, 667–673.

Drapeau, G., Brochu, S., Godin, D., Levesque, L., Rioux, F., and Marceau, F. (1993). Synthetic C5a receptor agonists. Pharmacology, metabolism and *in vivo* cardiovascular and hematologic effects. *Biochem. Pharmacol.* **45**, 1289–1299.

Durstin, M., Gao, J.-L., Tiffany, H. L., McDermott, D., and Murphy, P. M. (1994). Differential expression of members of the N-formylpeptide receptor gene cluster in human phagocytes. *Biochem. Biophys. Res. Commun.* **201**, 174–179.

Erbeck, K., Klein, J. B., and McLeish, K. R. (1993). Differential uncoupling of chemoattractant receptors from G proteins in retinoic acid-differentiated HL-60 granulocytes. *J. Immunol.* **150**, 1913–1921.

Federsppiel, B., Melhado, I. G., Duncan, A. M. V., Delaney, A., Schappert, K., Clark-Lewis, I., and Jirik, F. R. (1993). Molecular cloning of the cDNA and chromosomal localization of the gene for a putative seven-transmembrane segment (7-TMS) receptor isolated from human spleen. *Genomics* **16**, 707–712.

Feng, Y., Broder, C. C., Kennedy, P. E., and Berger, E. A. (1996). HIV-1 entry cofactor: Functional cDNA cloning of a seven-transmembrane, G protein-coupled receptor. *Science* **272**, 872–877.

Fiore, S., and Serhan, C. N. (1995). Lipoxin A_4 receptor activation is distinct from that of the formyl peptide receptor in myeloid cells: Inhibition of CD11/18 expression by lipoxin A4-lipoxin A_4 receptor interaction. *Biochemistry* **34**, 16678–16686.

Fiore, S., Maddox, J. F., Perez, H. D., and Serhan, C. N. (1994). Identification of a human cDNA encoding a functional high affinity lipoxin A4 receptor. *J. Exp. Med.* **180**, 253–260.

Foreman, K. E., Vaporciyan, A. A., Bonish, B. K., Jones, M. L., Johnson, K. J., Glovsky, M. M., Eddy, S. M., and Ward, P. A. (1994). C5a-induced expression of P-selectin in endothelial cells. *J. Clin. Invest.* **94**, 1147–1155.

Förster, R., Emrich, T., Kremmer, E., and Lipp, M. (1994). Expression of the G-protein-coupled receptor BLR1 defines mature, recirculating B cells and a subset of T-helper memory cells. *Blood* **84**, 830–840.

Förster, R., Mattis, A. E., Kremmer, E., Wolf, E., Brem, G., and Lipp, M. (1996). A putative chemokine receptor, BLR1, directs B cell migration to defined lymphoid organs and specific anatomic compartments of the spleen. *Cell* **87**, 1037–1047.

Franke, R. R., König, B., Sakmar, T. P., Khorana, H. G., and Hofman, K. P. (1990). Rhodopsin mutants that bind but fail to activate transducin. *Science* **250**, 123–125.

Freer, R. J., Day, A. R., Muthukumaraswamy, N., Pinon, D., Wu, A., Showell, H. J., and Becker, E. L. (1982). Formyl peptide chemoattractants: A model of the receptor on rabbit neutrophils. *Biochemistry* **21**, 257–263.

Freer, R. J., Day, A. R., Radding, J. A., Schiffmann, E., Aswanikumar, S., Showell, H. J., and Becker, E. L. (1980). Further studies on the structural requirements for synthetic peptide chemoattractants. *Biochemistry* **19**, 2404–2410.

Gao, J. L., Becker, E. L., Freer, R. J., Muthukumaraswamy, N., and Murphy, P. M. (1994). A high potency nonformylated peptide agonist for the phagocyte N-formylpeptide chemotactic receptor. *J. Exp. Med.* **180**, 2191–2197.

Gao, J. L., Kuhns, D. B., Tiffany, H. L., McDermott, D., Li, X., Francke, U., and Murphy, P. M. (1993). Structure and functional expression of the human macrophage inflammatory protein 1 alpha/RANTES receptor. *J. Exp. Med.* **177**, 1421–1427.

Gao, J. L., and Murphy, P. M. (1993). Species and subtype variants of the N-formyl peptide chemotactic receptor reveal multiple important functional domains. *J. Biol. Chem.* **268**, 25395–25401.

Gao, J. L., and Murphy, P. M. (1994). Human cytomegalovirus open reading frame US28 encodes a functional beta chemokine receptor. *J. Biol. Chem.* **269**, 28539–28542.

Gao, J. L., and Murphy, P. M. (1995). Cloning and differential tissue-specific expression of three mouse beta chemokine receptor-like genes, including the gene for a functional macrophage inflammatory protein-1 alpha receptor. *J. Biol. Chem.* **270**, 17494–17501.

Gao, J. L., Sen, I., Kitaura, M., Yoshie, O., Rothengerg, M. E., Murphy, P. M., and Luster, A. D. (1996). Identification of a mouse eosinophil receptor for the CC chemokine eotaxin. *Biochem. Biophys. Res. Commun.* **223**, 679–684.

Garcia-Zepeda, E. A., Rothenberg, M. E., Ownbey, R. T., Celestin, J., Leder, P., and Luster, A. D. (1996). Human eotaxin is a specific chemoattractant for eosinophil cells and provides a new mechanism to explain tissue eosinophilia. *Nat. Med.* **2**, 449–456.

Gasque, P., Chan, P., Fontaine, M., Ischenko, A., Lamacz, M., Götze, O., and Morgan, B. P. (1995). Identification and characterization of the complement C5a anaphylatoxin receptor on human astrocytes. *J. Immunol.* **155**, 4882–4889.

Gayle, R., III, Sleath, P. R., Srinivason, S., Birks, C. W., Weerawarna, K. S., Cerretti, D. P., Kozlosky, C. J., Nelson, N., Vanden Bos, T., and Beckmann, M. P. (1993). Importance of the amino terminus of the interleukin-8 receptor in ligand interactions. *J. Biol. Chem.* **268**, 7283–7289.

Geiser, T., Dewald, B., Ehrengruber, M. U., Clark-Lewis, I., and Baggiolini, M. (1993). The interleukin-8-related chemotactic cytokines GROα, GROβ, and GROγ activate human neutrophil and basophil leukocytes. *J. Biol. Chem.* **268**, 15419–15424.

Gerard, C., Bao, L., Orozco, O., Pearson, M., Kunz, D., and Gerard, N. P. (1992). Structural diversity in the extracellular faces of peptidergic G-protein-coupled receptors. Molecular cloning of the mouse C5a anaphylatoxin receptor. *J. Immunol.* **149**, 2600–26006.

Gerard, C., and Gerard, N. P. (1994). C5A anaphylatoxin and its seven transmembrane-segment receptor. *Annu. Rev. Immunol.* **12**, 775–808.

Gerard, N. P., Bao, L., Xiao-Ping, H., Eddy, R., Jr., Shows, T. B., and Gerard, C. (1993). Human chemotaxis receptor genes cluster at 19q13.3-13.4. Characterization of the human C5a receptor gene. *Biochemistry* **32**, 1243–1250.

Gerard, N. P., and Gerard, C. (1991). The chemotactic receptor for human C5a anaphylatoxin. *Nature (London)* **349**, 614–617.

Giannini, E., and Boulay, F. (1995). Phosphorylation, dephosphorylation, and recycling of the C5a receptor in differentiated HL60 cells. *J. Immunol.* **154**, 4055–4064.

Giannini, E., Brouchon, L., and Boulay, F. (1995). Identification of the major phosphorylation sites in human C5a anaphylatoxin receceptor in vivo. *J. Biol. Chem.* **270,** 19166–19172.

Gierschik, P., Sidoropoulos, D., and Jakobs, K. H. (1989). Two distinct G_i-proteins mediate formyl peptide receptor signal transduction in human leukemia (HL-60) cells. *J. Biol. Chem.* **264,** 21470–21473.

Goldman, D. W., Gifford, L. A., Young, R. N., Marotti, T., Cheung, M. K. L., and Goetzl, E. J. (1991). Affinity labeling of the membrane protein-binding component of human polymorphonuclear leukocyte receptors for leukotriene B_4. *J. Immunol.* **146,** 2671–2677.

Goldman, D. W., and Goetzl, E. J. (1982). Specific binding of leukotriene B_4 to receptors on human polymorphonuclear leukocytes. *J. Immunol.* **129,** 1600–1603.

Goldsmith, P., Rossiter, K., Carter, A., Simonds, W., Unson, C. G., Vinitsky, R., and Spiegel, A. M. (1988). Identification of the GTP-binding protein encoded by Gi_3 complementary DNA. *J. Biol. Chem.* **263,** 6476–6479.

Gong, J.-H., and Clark-Lewis, I. (1995). Antagonists of monocyte chemoattractant protein 1 identified by modification of functionally critical NH_2-terminal residues. *J. Exp. Med.* **181,** 631–640.

Gong, J.-H., Uguccioni, M., Dewald, B., Baggiolini, M., and Clark-Lewis, I. (1996). RANTES and MCP-3 antagonists bind multiple chemokine receptors. *J. Biol. Chem.* **271,** 10521–10527.

Goodman, M. G., Chenoweth, D. E., and Weigle, W. O. (1982). Induction of interleukin 1 secretion and enhancement of humoral immunity by binding of human C5a to macrophage surface C5a receptors. *J. Exp. Med.* **1156,** 912–917.

Griffiths-Hohnson, D. A., Collins, P. D., Rossi, A. G., Jose, P. J., and Williams, T. J. (1993). The chemokine, eotaxin, activates guinea-pig eosinophils *in vitro* and causes their accumulation into the lung in vivo. *Biochem. Biophys. Res. Commun.* **197,** 1167–1172.

Grinstein, S., and Furuya, W. (1992). Chemoattractant-induced tyrosine phosphorylation and activation of microtubule-associated protein kinase in human neutrophils. *J. Biol. Chem.* **267,** 18122–18125.

Grob, P. M., David, E., Warren, T. C., DeLeon, R. P., Farina, P. R., and Homon, C. A. (1990). Characterization of a receptor for human monocyte-derived neutrophil chemotactic factor/interleukin-8. *J. Biol. Chem.* **265,** 8311–8316.

Grotzinger, J., Engels, M., Jacoby, E., Wollmer, A., and Strassburger, W. (1991). A model for the C5a receptor and for its interaction with the ligand. *Protein Eng.* **4,** 767–771.

Hall, A. (1992). Ras-related GTPases and the cystoskeleton. *Mol. Biol. Cell* **3,** 475–479.

Hammond, M. E. W., Lapointe, G. R., Feucht, P. H., Hilt, S., Gallegos, C. A., Gordon, C. A., Giedlin, M. A., Mullenbach, G., and Tekamp-Olson, P. (1995). IL-8 induces neutrophil chemotaxis predominantly via type I IL-8 receptors. *J. Immunol.* **155,** 1328–1433.

Hanahan, D. J. (1986). Platelet-activating factor: A biologically active phosphoglyceride. *Annu. Rev. Biochem.* **55,** 483–509.

Harrison, J. K., Barber, C. M., and Lynch, K. R. (1994). cDNA cloning of a G-protein-coupled receptor expressed in rat spinal cord and brain related to chemokine receptors. *Neurosci. Lett.* **169,** 85–89.

Hausdorff, W. P., Caron, M. G., and Lefkowitz, R. J. (1990). Turning off the signal: Desensitization of β-adrenergic receptor function. *FASEB J.* **4,** 2881–2889.

Haviland, D. L., Borel, A. C., Fleischer, D. T., Haviland, J. C., and Wetsel, R. A. (1993). Structure, 5′-flanking sequence, and chromosome location of the human N-formyl peptide receptor gene. A single-copy gene comprised of two exons on chromosome 19q.13.3 that yields two distinct transcripts by alternative polyadenylation. *Biochemistry* **32,** 4168–4174.

Haviland, D. L., McCoy, R. L., Whitehead, W. T., Akama, H., Molmenti, E. P., Brown, A., Haviland, J. C., Parks, W. C., Perlmutter, D. H., and Wetsel, R. A. (1995). Cellular expression of the C5a anaphylatoxin receptor (C5aR): Demonstration of C5aR on nonmyeloid cells of the liver and lung. *J. Immunol.* **154,** 1861–1869.

Hébert, C. A., Chuntharapai, A., Smith, M., Colby, T., Kim, J., and Horuk, R. (1993). Partial functional mapping of the human interleukin-8 type A receptor. *J. Biol. Chem.* **268,** 18549–18553.

Hébert, C. A., Vitangcol, R. V., and Baker, J. B. (1991). Scanning mutagenesis of interleukin-8 identifies a cluster of residues required for receptor binding. *J. Biol. Chem.* **266,** 18989–18994.

Henderson, R., Baldwin, J. M., Ceska, T. A., Zemlin, F., Beckmann, E., and Downing, K. H. (1990). Model for the structure of bacteriorhodopsine based on high-resolution electron cryo-microscopy. *J. Mol. Biol.* **213,** 899–929.

Herbert, J.-M. (1992). Characterization of specific binding sites of 3H-labelled platelet-activating factor ([^{3}H]PAF) and a new antagonist, [^{3}H]SR 27417, on guinea-pig tracheal epithelial cells. *Biochem. J.* **284,** 201–206.

Herzog, H., Hort, Y. J., Shine, J., and Selbie, L. A. (1993). Molecular cloning, characterization, and localization of the human homolog to the reported bovine NPY Y3 receptor: Lack of NPY binding and activation. *DNA Cell Biol.* **12,** 465–471.

Higgins, J. D., III., Bridger, G. J., Derian, C. K., Beblavy, M. J., Hernandez, P. E., Gaul, F. E., Abrams, M. J., Pike, M. C., and Solomon, H. F. (1996). N-terminus urea-substituted chemotactic peptides: New potent agonists and antagonists toward the neutrophil fMLF receptor. *J. Med. Chem.* **39,** 1013–1017.

Holmes, W. E., Lee, J., Kuang, W. J., Rice, G. C., and Wood, W. I. (1991). Structure and functional expression of a human interleukin-8 receptor. *Science* **253,** 1278–1280.

Honda, Z., Nakamura, M., Miki, I., Minami, M., Watanabe, T., Seyama, Y., Okado, H., Toh, H., Ito, K., Miyamoto, T., and Shimizu, T. (1991). Cloning by functional expression of platelet-activating factor receptor from guinea-pig lung. *Nature (London)* **349,** 342–346.

Höpken, U. E., Lu, B., Gerard, N. P., and Gerard, C. (1996). The C5a chemoattractant receptor mediates mucosal defence to infection. *Nature* **383,** 86–89.

Hoogewerf, A., Black D., Proudfoot, A. E., Wells, T. N., and Power, C. A. (1996). Molecular cloning of murine CC CKR-4 and high affinity binding of chemokines to murine and human CC CKR-4. *Biochem. Biophys. Res. Commun.* **218,** 337–343.

Horuk, R. (1994). The interleukin-8-receptor family: From chemokines to malaria. *Immunol. Today* **15,** 169–174.

Horuk, R., Yansura, D. G., Reilly, D., Spencer, S., Bourell, J., Henzel, W., Rice, G., and Unemori, E. (1993a). Purification, receptor binding analysis, and biological characterization of human melanoma growth stimulating activity (MGSA). *J. Biol. Chem.* **268,** 541–546.

Horuk, R., Chitnis, C. E., Darbonne, W. C., Colby, T. J., Rybicki, A., Hadley, T. J., and Miller, L. H. (1993b). A receptor for the malarial parasite Plasmodium vivax: The erythrocyte chemokine receptor. *Science* **261,** 1182–1184.

Horuk, R., Martin, A., Hesselgesser, J., Hadley, T., Lu, Z.-H., Wang, Z.-X., and Peiper, S. C. (1996). The Duffy antigen receptor for chemokines: structural analysis and expression in the brain. *J. Leukocyte Biol.* **59,** 29–38.

Hugli, T. E., and Müller-Eberhard, H. J. (1978). Anaphylatoxins C3a and C5a. *Adv. Immunol.* **26,** 1–53.

Hwang, S.-B. (1988). Identification of a second putative receptor of platelet-activating factor from human polymorphonuclear leukocytes. *J. Biol. Chem.* **263,** 3225–3233.

Hwang, S.-B. (1990). Specific receptors of platelet-activating factor, receptor heterogeneity, and signal transduction mechanisms. *J. Lipid Mediators* **2,** 123–158.

Inglese, J., Freedman, N. J., Koch, W. J., and Lelkowitz, R. J. (1993). Structure and mechanism of the G protein-coupled receptor kinase. *J. Biol. Chem.* **268,** 23735–23738.

Jesaitis, A. J., Bokoch, G. M., Tolley, J. O., and Allen, R. A. (1988). Lateral segregation of neutrophil chemotactic receptors into actin-and fodrin-rich plasma membrane microdomains depleted in guanyl nucleotide regulatory proteins. *J. Cell Biol.* **107,** 921–928.

Jesaitis, A. J., Erickson, R. W., Klotz, K. N., Bommakanti, R. K., and Siemsen, D. W. (1993). Functional molecular complexes of human N-formyl chemoattractant receptors and actin. *J. Immunol.* **151,** 5653–5665.

Johansson, B., Wymann, M. P., Holmgren-Peterson, K., and Magnusson, K. E. (1993). N-formyl peptide receptors in human neutrophils display distinct membrane distribution and lateral mobility when labeled with agonist and antagonist. *J. Cell Biol.* **121,** 1281–1299.

Johnson, R. J., and Chenoweth, D. E. (1987). Synthesis of a new photoreactive C5a analog that permits identification of the ligand binding component of the granulocyte C5a receptor. *Biochem. Biophys. Res. Commun.* **148,** 1330–1337.

Jose, P. J., Griffiths-Johnson, D. A., Collins, P. D., Walsh, D. T., Moqbel, R., Totty, N. F., Truong, O., Hsuan, J. J., and Williams, T. J. (1994). Eotaxin: A potent eosinophil chemoattractant cytokine detected in a guinea pig model of allergic airways inflammation. *J. Exp. Med.* **179,** 881–887.

Jose, P. J., Adcock, I. M., Griffiths-Hohnson, D. A., Wells, T. N., Williams, T. J., and Power, C. A. (1994). Eotaxin: Cloning of an eosinophil chemoattractant cytokine and increased mRNA expression in allergen-challenged guinea-pig lungs. *Biochem. Biophys. Res. Commun.* **205,** 788–794.

Kaiser, E., Forster, R., Wolf, I., Ebensperger, C., Kuehl, W. M., and Lipp, M. (1993). The G protein-coupled receptor BLR1 is involved in murine B cell differentiation and is also expressed in neuronal tissues. *Eur. J. Immunol.* **23,** 2532–2539.

Kaneko, Y., Okada, N., Baranyi, L., Azuma, T., and Okada, H. (1995). Antagonist peptides against human anaphylatoxin C5a. *Immunology* **86,** 149–154.

Karnik, S. S., and Khorana, H. G. (1990). Assembly of functional rhodopsin requires a disulfide bond between cysteine residues 110 and 187. *J. Biol. Chem.* **265,** 17520–17524.

Karnik, S. S., Sakmar, T. P., Chen, H.-B., and Khorana, H. G. (1988). Cysteine residues 110 and 187 are essential for the formation of correct structure in bovine rhodopsin. *Proc. Natl. Acad. Sci. U.S.A.* **85,** 8459–8463.

Katz, A., Wu, D., and Simon, M. I. (1992). Subunits $\beta\gamma$ of heterotrimeric G protein activate $\beta 2$ isoform of phospholipase C. *Nature (London)* **360,** 686–689.

Kennedy, M. E., and Limbird, L. E. (1993). Mutations of the a2a adrenergic receptor that eliminate detectable palmitoylation do not perturb receptor G protein coupling. *J. Biol. Chem.* **268,** 8003–8011.

Kim, K.-S., Clark-Lewis, I., and Sykes, B. D. (1994). Solution structure of GRO/MGSA determined by 1H NMR spectroscopy. *J. Biol. Chem.* **269,** 32909–32915.

Kishimoto, T. K., Jutila, M. A., Berg, E. L., and Butcher, E. C. (1989). Neutrophil Mac-1 and MEL-14 adhesion proteins inversely regulated by chemotactic factors. *Science* **245,** 1238–1241.

Kitaura, M., Nakajima, T., Imai, T., Harada, S., Combadiere, C., Tiffany, H. L., Murphy, P. M., and Yoshie, O. (1996). Molecular cloning of human eotaxin, an eosinophil-selective CC chemokine, and identification of a specific eosinophil eotaxin receptor, CC chemokine receptor 3. *J. Biol. Chem.* **271,** 7725–7730.

Klotz, K. N., and Jesaitis, A. J. (1994). Physical coupling of N-formyl peptide chemoattractant receptors to G protein is unaffected by desensitization. *Biochem. Pharmacol.* **48,** 1297–1300.

Knall, C., Young, S,., Nick, J. A., Buhl, A. M., Worthen, G. S. and Johnson, G. L. (1996). Interleukin-8 regulation of the Ras/Raf/Mitogen-activated protein kinase pathway in human neutrophils. *J. Biol. Chem.* **271,** 2832–2838.

Kolakowski, L. F., Lu, B., Gerard, C., and Gerard, N. (1995). Probing the "message: address" sites for chemoattractant binding to the C5a receptor. *J. Biol. Chem.* **270,** 18077–18082.

König, B., Arendt, A., McDowell, J. H., Kahlert, M., Hargrave, P. A., and Hofmann, K. P. (1989). Three cytoplasmic loops of rhodopsin interact with transducin. *Proc. Natl. Acad. Sci. U.S.A.* **86,** 6878–6882.

Konteatis, Z. D., Siciliano, S. J., Van Riper, G., Molineaux, C. J., Pandya, S., Fischer, P., Rosen, H., Mumford, R. A., and Springer, M. S. (1994). Development of C5a receptor antagonists. Differential loss of functional responses. *J. Immunol.* **153**, 4200–4205.

Kouba, M., Vanetti, M., Wang, X., Schafer, M., and Hollt, V. (1993). Cloning of a novel putative G-protein-coupled receptor (NLR) which is exprssed in neuronal and lymphatic tissue. *FEBS Lett.* **321**, 173–178.

Kravchenko, V. V., Pan, Z., Han, J., Herbert, J. M., Ulevitch, R. J., and Ye, R. D. (1995). Platelet-activating factor induces NF-κB activation through a G protein-coupled pathway. *J. Biol. Chem.* **270**, 14928–14934.

Kuang, Y., Wu, Y., Jiang, H., and Wu, D. (1996). Selective G protein coupling by C-C chemokine receptors. *J. Biol. Chem.* **271**, 3975–3978.

Kunkel, M. T., and Peralta, E. (1993). Charged amino acids required for signal transduction by m3 muscarinic acetylcholine receptor. *EMBO J.* **12**, 3809–3815.

Kunz, D., Gerard, N. P., and Gerard, C. (1992). The human leukocyte platelet-activating factor receptor. *J. Biol. Chem.* **267**, 9101–9106.

Kurtenbach, E., Curtis, C. A. M., Pedder, E. K., Aitken, A., Harris, A. C. M., and Hulmes, E. C. (1990). Muscarinic acetylcholine receptors. *J. Biol. Chem.* **265**, 13702–13708.

Lacy, M., Jones, J., Whittemore, S. R., Haviland, D. L., Wetsel, R. A., and Barnum, S. R. (1995). Expression of the receptors for the C5a anaphylatoxin, interleukin-8 and FMLP by human astrocytes and microglia. *J. Neuroimmunol.* **61**, 71–78.

Lanza, T. J., Durette, P. L., Rollins, T., Siciliano, S., Cianciarulo, D. N., Kobayashi, S. V., Caldwell, C. G., Springer, M. S., and Hagmann, W. K. (1992). Substituted 4,6-diaminoquinolines as inhibitors of C5a receptor binding. *J. Med. Chem.* **35**, 252–258.

Lapham, C. K., Ouyang, J., Chandrasekhar, B., Nguyen, N. Y., Dimitrov, D. S., and Golding, H. (1996). Evidence for cell-surface association between fusin and the CD4-gp120 complex in human cell lines. *Science* **274**, 602–605.

LaRosa, G. J., Thomas, K. M., Kaufmann, M. E., Mark, R., White, M., Taylor, L., Gray, G., Witt, D., and Navarro, J. (1992). Amino terminus of the interleukin-8 receptor is a major determinant of receptor subtype specificity. *J. Biol. Chem.* **267**, 25402–25406.

Laudanna, C., Campbell, J. J. and Butcher, E. C. (1996). Role of Rho in chemoattractant-activated leukocyte adhesion through integrins. *Science* **271**, 981–983.

Lechleiter, J., Hellmiss, R., Duerson, K., Ennulat, D., David, N., Clapham, D., and Peralta, E. (1990). Distinct sequence elements control the specificity of G protein activation by muscarinic acetycholine receptor subtypes. *EMBO J.* **9**, 4381–4390.

Lee, J., Horuk, R., Rice, G. C., Bennett, G. L., Camerato, T., and Wood, W. I. (1992a). Characterization of two high affinity human interleukin-8 receptors. *J. Biol. Chem.* **267**, 16283–16287.

Lee, J., Kuang, W. J., Rice, G. C., and Wood, W. I. (1992b). Characterization of complementary DNA clones encoding the rabbit IL-8 receptor. *J. Immunol.* **148**, 1261–1264.

Leong, S. R., Kabakoff, R. C., and Hébert, C. A. (1994). Complete mutagenesis of the extracellular domain of interleukin-8 (IL-8) type A receptor identifies charged residues mediating IL-8 binding and signal transduction. *J. Biol. Chem.* **269**, 19343–19348.

Liu, R., Paxton, W. A., Choe, S., Ceradini, D., Martin, S. R., Horuk, R., MacDonald, M. E., Stuhlmann, H., Koup, R. A., and Landau, N. R. (1996). Homozygous defect in HIV-1 coreceptor accounts for resistance of some multiply-exposed individuals to HIV-1 infection. *Cell* **86**, 367–377.

Lodi, P. J., Garret, D. S., Kuszewski, J., Tsang, M. L.-S., Weatherbee, J. A., Leonard, W. J., Gronenborn, A. M., and Clore, G. M. (1994). High-resolution solution structure of the b chemokine hMIP-1b by multidimensional NMR. *Science* **263**, 1762–1767.

Loetscher, M., Gerber, B., Loetscher, P., Jones, S. A., Piali, L., Clark-Lewis, I., Baggiolini, M., and Moser, B. (1996). Chemokine receptor specific for IP10 and Mig: Structure, function, and expression in activated T-lymphocytes. *J. Exp. Med.* **184**, 963–969.

Loetscher, M., Geiser, T., O'Reilly, T., Zwahlen, R., Gaggiolini, M., and Moser, B. (1994). Cloning of a human seven-transmembrane domain receptor, LESTR, that is highly expressed in leukocytes. *J. Biol. Chem.* **269**, 232–237.

Lu, Z.-X., Fok, K. F., Erickson, B. W., and Hugli, T. E. (1984). Conformational analysis of COOH-terminal segments of human C3a. Evidence of ordered conformation in an active 21-residue peptide. *J. Biol. Chem.* **259**, 7367–7370.

Malech, H. L., Gardner, J. P., Heiman, D. F., and Rosenzweig, S. A. (1985). Asparagine-linked oligosaccharides on formyl peptide chemotactic receptors of human phagocytic cells. *J. Biol. Chem.* **260**, 2509–2514.

Marasco, W. A., Phan, S. H., Krutzsch, H., Showell, H. J., Feltner, D. E., Nairn, R., Becker, E. L., and Ward, P. A. (1984). Purification and identification of formyl-methionyl-leucyl-phenylalanine as the major peptide neutrophil chemotactic factor produced by *Escherichia coli*. *J. Biol. Chem.* **259**, 5430–5439.

Massung, R. F., Jayarama, V., and Moyer, R. W. (1993). DNA sequence analysis of conserved and unique regions of Swinepox virus: Identification of genetic elements supporting phenotypic observations including a novel G protein-coupled receptor homologue. *Virology* **197**, 511–528.

McCoy, R., Haviland, D. L., Molmenti, E. P., Ziambaras, T., Wetsel, R. A., and Perlmutter, D. H. (1995). N-formylpeptide and complement C5a receptors are expressed in liver cells and mediate hepatic acute phase gene regulation. *J. Exp. Med.* **182**, 207–217.

Mery, L., and Boulay, F. (1993). Evidence that the extracellular N-terminal domain of C5aR contains amino-acid residues crucial for C5a binding. *Eur. J. Haematol.* **51**, 282–287.

Mery, L., and Boulay, F. (1994). The NH2-terminal region of C5aR but not that of FPR is critical for both protein transport and ligand binding. *J. Biol. Chem.* **269**, 3457–3463.

Moffett, S., Mouillac, B., Bonin, H., and Bouvier, M. (1993). Altered phosphorylation and desensitization patterns of a human b2-adrenergic receptor lacking the palmitoylated Cys341. *EMBO J.* **12**, 349–356.

Mollison, K. W., Mandecki, W., Zuiderweg, E. R. P., Fayer, L., Fey, T. A., Krause, R. A., Conway, R. G., Miller, L., Edalji, R. P., Shallcross, M. A., Lane, B., Fox, J. L., Greer, J., and Carter, G. W. (1989). Identification of the receptor-binding residues in the inflammatory complement protein C5a by site-directed mutagenesis. *Proc. Natl. Acad. Sci. U.S.A.* **86**, 292–296.

Monk, P. N., Barker, M. D., Partridge, L. J., and Pease, J. E. (1995). Mutation of glutamate 199 of the human C5a receptor defines a binding site for ligand distinct from the receptor N-terminus. *J. Biol. Chem.* **270**, 16625–16629.

Morgan, E. L., Ember, J. A., Sanderson, S. D., Scholz, W., Buchner, R., Ye, R. D., and Hugli, T. E. (1993). Anti-C5a receptor antibodies. Characterization of neutralizing antibodies specific for a peptide, C5aR-(9-29), derived from the predicted amino-terminal sequence of the human C5a receptor. *J. Immunol.* **151**, 377–388.

Moser, B., Schumacher, C., von Tscharner, V., Clark-Lewis, I., and Baggiolini, M. (1991). Neutrophil-activating peptide 2 and gro/melanoma growth-stimulatory activity interact with neutrophil-activating peptide 1/interleukin 8 receptors on human neutrophils. *J. Biol. Chem.* **266**, 10666–10671.

Moser, B., Dewald, B., Barella, L., Schumacher, C., Baggiolini, M., and Clark-Lewis, I. (1993). Interleukin-8 antagonists generated by N-terminal modification. *J. Biol. Chem.* **268**, 7125–7128.

Mueller, S. G., Schraw, W. P., and Richmond, A. (1994). Melanoma growth stimulatory activity enhances the phosphorylation of the class II interleukin-8 receptor in non-hematopoietic cells. *J. Biol. Chem.* **269**, 1973–1980.

Mueller, S. G., Schraw, W. P., and Richmond, A. (1995). Activation of protein kinase C enhances the phosphorylation of the type B interleukin-8 receptor and stimulates its degradation in non-hematopoietic cells. *J. Biol. Chem.* **270**, 10439–10448.

Münch, G., Dees, C., Hekman, M., and Palm, D. (1991). Multisite contacts involved in coupling of the $_b$-adrenergic receptor with the stimulatory guanine-nucleotide-binding regulatory protein. *Eur. J. Biochem.* **198,** 357–364.

Murphy, P. M. (1994). The molecular biology of leukocyte chemoattractant receptors. *Annu. Rev. Immunol.* **12,** 593–633.

Murphy, P. M., and Tiffany, H. L. (1991). Cloning of complementary DNA encoding a functional human interleukin-8 receptor. *Science* **253,** 1280–1283.

Murphy, P. M., Eide, B., Goldsmith, P., Brann, M., Gierschik, P., Spiegel, A., and Malech, H. L. (1987). Detection of multiple forms of $G_{i\alpha}$ in HL60 cells. *FEBS Lett.* **221,** 81–86.

Murphy, P. M., Ozcelik, T., Kenney, R. T., Tiffany, H. L., McDermott, D., and Francke, U. (1992). A structural homologue of the N-formyl peptide receptor. Characterization and chromosome mapping of a peptide chemoattractant receptor family. *J. Biol. Chem.* **267,** 7637–7643.

Murphy, P. M., Tiffany, H. L., McDermott, D., and Ahuja, S. K. (1993). Sequence and organization of the human N-formyl peptide receptor-encoding gene. *Gene* **133,** 285–290.

Mutoh, H., Bito, H., Minami, M., Nakamura, M., Honda, Z., Izumi, T., Nakata, Y., Terano, A., and Shimizu, T. (1993). Two different promoters direct expression of two distinct forms of mRNAs of human platelet-activating factor receptor. *FEBS Lett.* **322,** 129–134.

Mutoh, H., Ishii, S., Izumi, T., Kato, S., and Shimizu, T. (1994). Platelet-activating factor (PAF) positively auto-regulates the expression of human PAF receptor transcript 1 (leukocyte-type) throught NF-kappa B. *Biochem. Biophys. Res. Commun.* **205,** 1137–1142.

Nagasawa, T., Kikutani, H., and Kishimoto, T. (1994). Molecular cloning and structure of a pre-B-cell growth stimulating factor. *Proc. Natl. Acad. Sci. USA* **91,** 2305–2309.

Nagasawa, T., Hirota, S., Tachibana, K., Takakura, N., Nishikawa, S.-I., Kitamura, Y., Yoshida, N., Kikutani, H., and Kishimoto, T. (1996). Defects of B-cell lymphopoiesis and bone-marrow myelopoiesis in mice lacking the CXC chemokine PBSF/SDF-1. *Nature* **382,** 635–638.

Naik, N., Giannini, E., and Boulay, F. (1997). Unpublished data.

Nakamura, M., Honda , Z. I., Izumi, T., Sakanaka, C., Mutoh, H., Minami, M., Bito, H., Seyama, Y., Matsumoto, T., Noma, M., and Shimizu, T. (1991). Molecular cloning and expression of platelet-activating factor receptor from human leukocytes. *J. Biol. Chem.* **266,** 20400–20405.

Neote, K., DiGregorio, D., Mak, J. Y., Horuk, R., and Schall, T. J. (1993). Molecular cloning, functional expression, and signaling characteristics of a C-C chemokine receptor. *Cell (Cambridge, Mass.)* **72,** 415–425.

Nicholas, J., Cameron, K. R., and Honess, R. W. (1992). Herpesvirus saimiri encodes homologous of G protein-coupled receptors and cyclins. *Nature (London)* **355,** 362–365.

Niedel, J., Wilkinson, S., and Cuatrecasas, P. (1979). Receptor-mediated uptake and degradation of ^{125}I-chemotactic peptide by human neutrophils. *J. Biol. Chem.* **254,** 10700–10706.

Niedel, J., Davis, J., and Cuatrecasas, P. (1980). Covalent affinity labeling of the formyl peptide chemotactic receptor. *J. Biol. Chem.* **255,** 7063–7066.

O'Dowd, B. F., Hnatowich, M., Caron, M. G., Lefkowitz, R. J., and Bouvier, M. (1989). Palmitoylation of the human b2-adrenergic receptor. *J. Biol. Chem.* **264,** 7564–7569.

Offermans, S., and Simon, M. I. (1995). G alpha 15 and G alpha 16 couple a wide variety of receptors to phospholipase C. *J. Biol. Chem.* **270,** 15175–15180.

Offermans, S., Schäfer, R., Hoffmann, B., Bombien, E., Spicher, K., Hinsch, K.-D., Schultz, G., and Rosenthal, W. (1990). Agonist-sensitive binding of a photoreactive GTP analog to a G-protein a-subunit in membranes of HL-60 cells. *FEBS Lett.* **260,** 14–18.

O'Flaherty, J. T., Surles, J. R., Redman, J., Jacobson, D., Piantadosi, C., and Wykle, R. L. (1986). Binding and metabolism of platelet-activating factor by human neutrophils. *J. Clin. Invest.* **78,** 381–388.

Okada, T., Sakuma, L., Fukui, Y., Hazeki, O., and Ui, M. (1994). Blockage of chemotactic peptide-induced stimulation of neutrophils by worthmannin as a result of selective inhibition of phosphatidylinositol 3-kinase. *J. Biol. Chem.* **269,** 3563–3567.

Oliveira, L., Paiva, A. C. M., Sander, C., and Vriend, G. (1994). A common step for signal transduction in G protein-coupled receptor. *Trends Pharmacol. Sci.* **15,** 170–172.

Oppenheim, J. J., Zachariae, C. O. C., Mukaida, N., and Matsushima, K. (1991). Properties of the novel proinflammatory supergene "intercrine" cytokine family. *Annu. Rev. Immunol.* **9,** 617–648.

Oppermann, M., Raedt, U., Hebell, T., Schmidt, B., Zimmermann, B., and Götze, O. (1993). Probing the human receptor for C5a anaphylatoxin with site-directed antibodies. *J. Immunol.* **151,** 3785–3794.

Ovchinnikov, Y. A., Abdulaev, N. G., and Bogachuk, A. S. (1988). Two adjacent cysteine residue in the C-terminal cytoplasmic fragment of bovine rhodopsin are palmitylated. *FEBS Lett.* **230,** 1–5.

Pan, Z., Kravchenko, V. V., and Ye, R. D. (1995). Platelet-activating factor stimulates transcription of the heparin-binding epidermal growth factor-like growth factor in monocytes. *J. Biol. Chem.* **270,** 7787–7790.

Park, D., Jhon, D. Y., Kriz, R., Knopf, J., and Rhee, S. G. (1992). Cloning , sequencing, expression, and Gq-independent activation of phospholipase C-β2. *J. Biol. Chem.* **267,** 16048–16055.

Parma, J., Duprez, L., Van Sande, J., Cochaux, P., Gervy, C., Mockel, J., Dumont, J., and Vassart, G. (1993). Somatic mutations in the thyrotropin receptor gene cause hyperfunctioning thyroid adenomas. *Nature (London)* **365,** 649–651.

Perez, H. D., Holmes, R., Kelly, E., McClary, J., Chou, Q., and Andrews, W. H. (1992a). Cloning of the gene coding for the human receptor for formyl peptides: Characterization of a promoter region and evidence for polymorphic expression. *Biochemistry* **31,** 11595–11599.

Perez, H. D., Holmes, R., Vilander, L. R., Adams, R. R., Manzana, W., Jolley, D., and Andrews, W. H. (1993). Formyl peptide receptor chimeras define domains involved in ligand binding. *J. Biol. Chem.* **268,** 2292–2295.

Perez, H. D., Kelly, E., and Holmes, R. (1992b). Regulation of formyl peptide receptor expression and its mRNA levels during differentiation of HL-60 cells. *J. Biol. Chem.* **267,** 358–363.

Perez, H. D., Vilander, L., Andrews, W. H., and Holmes, R. (1994). Human formyl peptide receptor ligand binding domain(s). *J. Biol. Chem.* **269,** 22485–22487.

Perret, J. J., Raspe, E., Vassart, G., and Parmentier, M. (1992). Cloning and functional expression of the canine anaphylatoxin C5a receptor. Evidence for high interspecies variability. *Biochem. J.* **288,** 911–917.

Ponath, P. D., Qin, S., Ringler, D. J., Clark-Lewis, I., Wang, J., Kassam, N., Smith, H., Shi, X., Gonzalo, J. A., Newman, W., Gutierrez-Ramos, J. C., and Mackay, C. R. (1996). Cloning of the human eosinophil chemoattractant, eotaxin. Expression, receptor binding, and functional properties suggest a mechanism for the selective recruitment of eosinophils. *J. Clin. Invest.* **97,** 604–612.

Post, T. W., Bozic, C. R., Rothenberg, M. E., Luster, A. D., Gerard, N., and Gerard, C. (1995). Molecular characterization of two murine eosinophil beta chemokine receptor. *J. Immunol.* **155,** 5299–5305.

Power, C. A., Meyer, A., Nemeth, K., Bacon, K. B., Hoogewerf, A. J., Proudfoot, A. E. I., and Wells, T. N. C. (1995). Molecular cloning and functional expression of a novel CC chemokine receptor cDNA from a human basophilic cell line. *J. Biol. Chem.* **270,** 19495–19500.

Prescott, S. M., Zimmerman, G. A., and McIntyre, T. M. (1990). Platelet-activating factor. *J. Biol. Chem.* **265,** 17381–17384.

Prossnitz, E. R., Quehenberger, O., Cochrane, C. G., and Ye, R. D. (1993). The role of the third intracellular loop of the neutrophil N-formyl peptide receptor in G protein coupling. *Biochem. J.* **294,** 581–587.

Prossnitz, E. R., Kim, C. M., Benovič, J. L., and Ye, R. D. (1995a). Phosphorylation of the N-formyl peptide receptor carboxyl terminus by the G protein-coupled receptor kinase, GRK2. *J. Biol. Chem.* **270,** 1130–1137.

Prossnitz, E. R., Schreiber, R. E., Bokoch, G. M., and Ye, R. D. (1995b). Binding of low affinity N-formyl peptide receptors to G protein. Characterization of a novel inactive receptor intermediate. *J. Biol. Chem.* **270,** 10686–10694.

Proudfoot, A. E. I., Power, C. A., Hoogewerf, A. J., Montjovent, M.-O., Borlat, F., Offord, R. E., and Wells, T. N. C. (1996). Extention of recombinant human RANTES by the retention of the initiating methionine produces a potent antagonist. *J. Biol. Chem.* **271,** 2599–2603.

Ptasznik, A., Traynor-Kaplan, A. and Bokoch, G. M. (1995). G protein-coupled chemoattractant receptors regulate lyn tyrosine kinase-Shc adapter protein signaling complexes. *J. Biol. Chem.* **270,** 19969–19973.

Quehenberger, O., Prossnitz, E. R., Cavanagh, S. L., Cochrane, C. G., and Ye, R. D. (1993). Multiple domains of the N-formyl peptide receptor are required for high-affinity ligand binding. Construction and analysis of chimeric N-formyl peptide receptors. *J. Biol. Chem.* **268,** 18167–18175.

Quinn, M. T. (1995). Low-molecular-weigh GTP-binding proteins and leukocyte signal transduction. *J. Leukocyte Biol.* **58,** 263–276.

Radel, S. J., Genco, R. J., and De Nardin, E. (1991). Localization of ligand binding regions of the human formyl peptide receptor. *Biochem. Int.* **25,** 745–753.

Raffetseder, U., Roper, D., Meryk L., Gietz, C., Klos, A., Grotzinger, J., Wollmer, A., Boulay, F., Kohl, J., and Bautsch, W. (1996). Site-directed mutagenesis of conserved charged residues in the helical region of human C5aR: Arg206 determines high-affinity binding sites of C5a receptor. *Eur. J. Biochem.* **235,** 82–90.

Rajarathnam, K., Sykes, B. D., Kay, C. M., Dewald, B., Geiser, T., Baggiolini, M., and Clark-Lewis, I. (1994). Neutrophil activation by monomeric interleukin-8. *Science* **264,** 90–92.

Raport, C. J., Schweickart, V. L., Eddy, R. L., Jr., Shows, T. B., and Gray, P. W. (1995). The orphan G-protein-coupled receptor-encoding gene V28 is closely related to genes for chemokine receptors and is expressed in lymphoid and neural tissues. *Gene* **163,** 295–299.

Raport, C. J., Gosling, J., Schweickart, V. L., Gray, P. W., and Charo, I. R. (1996b). Molecular cloning and functional characterization of a novel human CC chemokine receptor (CCR5) for RANTES, MIP-1-beta, and MIP-1-alpha. *J. Biol. Chem.* **271,** 17161–17166.

Raport, C. J., Schweickart, V. L., Chantry, D., Eddy, R. L., Jr., Shows, T. B., Godiska, R., and Gray, P. W. (1996). New members of the chemokine receptor gene family. *J. Leukocyte Biol.* **59,** 18–23.

Ren, Q., Kurose, H., Lefkowitz, R. J., and Cotecchia, S. (1993). Constitutively active mutants of a2-adrenergic receptor. *J. Biol. Chem.* **268,** 16483–16487.

Richardson, R. M., Ali, H., Tomhave, E. D., Haribabu, B., and Snyderman, R. (1995a). Cross-desensitization of chemoattractant receptors occurs at multiple levels. *J. Biol. Chem.* **270,** 27829–27833.

Richardson, R. M., DuBose, R. A., Ali, H., Tomhave, E. D., Haribabu, B., and Snyderman, R. (1995b). Regulation of human interleukin-8 receptor A: Identification of a phosphorylation site involved in modulating receptor functions. *Biochemistry* **34,** 14193–14201.

Rimland, J., Xin, W., Sweetnam, P., Saijoh, K., Nestler, E. J., and Duman, R. S. (1991). Sequence and expression of a neuropeptide Y receptor cDNA. *Mol. Pharmacol.* **40,** 869–875.

Roglić, A., Prossnitz, E. R., Cavanagh, S. L., Pan, Z., Zou, A., and Ye, R. D. (1996). cDNA cloning of a novel G protein-coupled receptor with a large extracellular loop structure. *Biochim. Biophys. Acta* **1305,** 39–43.

Rollins, T. E., Siciliano, S., Kobayashi, S., Cianciarulo, D. N., Bonilla-Argudo, V., Collier, K., and Springer, M. S. (1991). Purification of the active C5a receptor from human polymorphonuclear leukocytes as a receptor-Gi complex. *Proc. Natl. Acad. Sci. U.S.A.* **88,** 971–975.

Romano, M., Maddox, J. F., and Serhan, C. N. (1996). Activation of human monocytes and the acute monocytic leukemia cell line (THP-1) by lipoxins involves unique signaling pathways for lipoxin A_4 versus lipoxin B_4: Evidence for differential Ca^{2+} mobilization. *J. Immunol.* **157,** 2149–2154.

Rothenberg, M. E., Luster, A. D., Lilly, C. M., Drazen, J. M., and Leder, P. (1995a). Constitutive and allergen-induced expression of eotaxin mRNA in the guinea pig lung. *J. Exp. Med.* **181,** 1211–1216.

Rothenberg, M. E., Luster, A. D., and Leder, P. (1995b). Murine eotaxin: An eosinophil chemoattractant inducible in endothelial cells and in interleukin 4-induced tumor suppression. *Proc. Natl. Acad. Sci. USA* **92,** 8960–8964.

Rotrosen, D., Malech, H. L., and Gallin, J. I. (1987). Formyl peptide leukocyte chemoattractant uptake and release by cultured human umbilical vein endothelial cells. *J. Immunol.* **139,** 3034–3040.

Rucker, J., Samson, M., Doranz, B. J., Libert, F., Berson, J. F., Yi, Y., Smyth, R. J., Collman, R. G., Broder, C. C., Vassart, G., Doms, R. W., and Parmentier, M. (1996). Regions in beta-chemokine receptors CCR5 and CCR2b that determine HIV-1 cofactor specificity. *Cell* **87,** 437–446.

Samson, M., Labbe, O., Mollereau, C., Vassart, G., and Parmentier, M. (1996). Molecular cloning and functional expression of a new human CC-chemokine receptor gene. *Biochemistry* **35,** 3362–3367.

Samson, M., Libert, F., Doranz, B. J., Rucker, J., Liesnard, C., Farber, C.-M., Saragosti, S., Lapoumeroulie, C., Cognaux, J., Forceille, C., Muyldermans, G., Verhofstede, C., Burtonboy, G., Georges, M., Imai, T., Rana, S., Yi, Y., Smyth, R. J., Collman, R. G., Doms, R. W., Vassart, G., and Parmentier, M. (1996b). *Nature* **382,** 722–725.

Samuelson, B., Dahlén, S.-E., Lindgren, J. A., Rouzer, C. A., and Serhan, C. N. (1987). Leukotrienes and lipoxins: Structures, biosynthesis, and biological effects. *Science* **237,** 1171–1176.

Savarese, T., and Fraser, C. M. (1992). In vitro mutagenesis and the search for structure-function relationship among G protein-coupled receptors. *Biochem. J.* **283,** 1–19.

Schertler, G. F. X., Villa, C., and Henderson, R. (1993). Projection structure of rhodopsin. *Nature* (*London*) **362,** 770–772.

Schiffmann, E., Corcoran, B. A., and Wahl, S. (1975a). N-formylmethionyl peptides as chemoattractants for leucocytes. *Proc. Natl. Acad. Sci. U.S.A.* **72,** 1059–1062.

Schiffmann, E., Showell, H. V., Corcoran, B. A., Ward, P. A., Smith, E., and Becker, E. L. (1975b). The isolation and partial characterization of neutrophil chemotactic factors from *Escherichia coli. J. Immunol.* **114,** 1831–1837.

Schmitt, M., Painter, R. G., Jesaitis, A. J., Preissner, K., Sklar, L. A., and Cochrane, C. G. (1983). Photoaffinity labeling of the N-formyl peptide receptor binding site of intact human polymorphonuclear leukocytes. A label suitable for following the fate of the receptor-ligand complex. *J. Biol. Chem.* **258,** 649–654.

Schnitzel, W., Garbeis, B., Monschein, U., and Besemer, J. (1991). Neutrophil activating peptide-2 binds with two affinities to receptor(s) on human neutrophils. *Biochem. Biophys. Res. Commun.* **180,** 301–307.

Schnitzel, W., Monschein, U., and Besemer, J. (1994). Monomer-dimer equilibria of interleukin-8 and neutrophil-activating peptide 2. Evidence for IL-8 binding as a dimer and oligomer to IL-8 receptor B. *J. Leukocyte Biol.* **55,** 763–770.

Schraufstatter, I. U., Ma, M., Oades, Z. G., Barritt, D. S., and Cochrane, C. G. (1995). The role of Tyr13 and Lys15 of interleukin-8 in the high affinity interaction with the interleukin-8 receptor type A. *J. Biol. Chem.* **270,** 10428–10431.

Schreiber, R. E., Prossnitz, E. R., Ye, R. D., Cochrane, C. G., and Bokoch, G. M. (1994). Domains of the human neutrophil N-formyl peptide receptor involved in G protein coupling. *J. Biol. Chem.* **269,** 326–331.

Schumacher, C., Clark-Lewis, I., Baggiolini, M., and Moser, B. (1992). High- and low-affinity binding of GRO α and neutrophil-activating peptide 2 to interleukin 8 receptors on human neutrophils. *Proc. Natl. Acad. Sci. U.S.A.* **89,** 10542–10546.

Seyfried, C. E., Schweickart, V. L., Godiska, R., and Gray, P. W. (1992). The human platelet-activating factor receptor gene (PTAFR) contains no introns and maps to chromosome 1. *Genomics* **13,** 832–834.

Sha'afi, R. I., and Molski, T. F. P. (1988). Activation of the neutrophil. *Prog. Allergy* **42,** 1–64.

Shawar, S. M., Rich, R. R., and Becker, E. L. (1995). Peptides from the amino-terminus of mouse mitochondrially encoded NADH dehydrogenase subunit 1 are potent chemoattractants. *Biochem. Biophys. Res. Commun.* **211,** 812–818.

Shin, H. S., Snyderman, R., Friedman, E., Mellors, A., and Mayer, M. M. (1968). Chemotactic and anaphylatoxic fragment cleaved from the fifth component of guinea pig complement. *Science* **162,** 361–363.

Showell, H. J., Freer, R. J., Zigmond, S. H., Schiffmann, E., Aswanikumar, S., Corcoran, B., and Becker, E. L. (1976). The structure-activity relations of synthetic peptides as chemotactic factors and inducers of lysosomal enzyme secretion for neutrophils. *J. Exp. Med.* **143,** 1155–1169.

Shum, J. K., Allen, R. A., and Wong, Y. H. (1995). The human chemoattractant complement C5a receptor inhibits cyclic AMP accumulation through Gi and Gz proteins. *Biochem. Biophys. Res. Commun.* **208,** 223–229.

Siciliano, S. J., Rollins, T. E., DeMartino, J., Konteatis, Z., Malkowitz, L., Van Riper, G., Bondy, S., Rosen, H., and Springer, M. S. (1994). Two-site binding of C5a by its receptor: an alternative binding paradigm for G protein-coupled receptors. *Proc. Natl. Acad. Sci. U.S.A.* **91,** 1214–1218.

Sklar, L. A., Finney, D. A., Oades, Z. G., Jesaitis, A. J., Painter, R. G., and Cochrane, C. G. (1984). The dynamics of ligand-receptor interactions. *J. Biol. Chem.* **259,** 5661–5669.

Slepak, V. Z., Katz, A., and Simon, M. I. (1995). Functional analysis of a dominant negative mutant of G alpha i_2. *J. Biol. Chem.* **270,** 4037–4041.

Snyderman, R., and Uhing, R. J. (1992). Phagocytic cells: Stimulus-response coupling mechanisms. *In* "Inflammation: Basic Principles and Clinical Correlates" (J. I. Gallin, I. M. Goldstein, and R. Snyderman, eds.), 2nd ed., pp. 421–439. Raven Press, New York.

Sozzani, S., Sallusto, F., Luini, W., Zhou, D., Piemonti, L., Allavena, P., Van Damme, J., Valitutti, S., Lanzavecchia, A., and Mantovani, A. (1995). Migration of dendritic cells in response to formyl peptides, C5a, and a distinct set of chemokines. *J. Immunol.* **155,** 3292–3295.

Sozzani, S., Zhou, D., Locati, M., Rieppi, M., Proost, P., Magazin, M., Vita, N., Van Damme, J., and Mantovani, A. (1994). Receptors and transduction pathways for monocyte chemotactic protein-2 and monocyte chemotactic protein-3. Similarities and differences with MCP-1. *J. Immunol.* **152,** 3615–3622.

Stoyanov, B., Volinia, S., Hanck, T., Rubio, I., Loubtchenkov, M, Malek, D., Stoyanova, S., Vanhaesebroeck, B., Dhand, R., Nurnberg, B., Gierschik, P., Seedorf, K., Hsuan, J. J., Waterfield, M. D., and Wetzker, R. (1995). Cloning and characterization of a G protein-activated human phosphoinositide-3 kinase. *Science* **269,** 690–693.

Sugimoto, T., Tsuchimochi, H., McGregor, C. G., Mutoh, H., Shimizu, T., and Kurachi, Y. (1992). Molecular cloning and characterization of the platelet-activating factor receptor gene expressed in the human heart. *Biochem. Biophys. Res. Commun.* **189,** 617–624.

Suzuki, H., Prado, G. N., Wilkinson, N., and Navarro, J. (1994). The N terminus of interleukin-8 (IL-8) receptor confers high affinity binding to human IL-8. *J. Biol. Chem.* **269,** 18263–18266.

Takano, T., Honda, Z.-I., Sakanaka, C., Izumi, T., Kameyama, K., Haga, K., Haga, T., Kurokawa, K., and Shimizu, T. (1994). Role of cytoplasmic tail phosphorylation sites of platelet-activating factor receptor in agonist-induced desensitization. *J. Biol. Chem.* **269**, 22453–22458.

Tardif, M., Mery, L., Brouchon, L., and Boulay, F. (1993). Agonist-dependent phosphorylation of N-formylpeptide and activation peptide from the fifth component of C (C5a) chemoattractant receptors in differentiated HL60 cells. *J. Immunol.* **150**, 3534–3545.

Tashiro, K., Tada, H., Heilker, R., Shirozu, M., Nakano, T., and Honjo, T. (1993). Signal sequence trap: A cloning strategy for secreted proteins and type I membrane proteins. *Science* **261**, 600–603.

Thelen, M., Peveri, P., Kernen, P., von Tscharner, V., Walz, A., and Baggiolini, M. (1988). Mechanism of neutrophil activation by NAF, a novel monocyte-derived peptide agonist. *FASEB J.* **2**, 2702–2706.

Thelen, M., and Wirthmueller, U. (1994). Phospholipases and protein kinases during phagocyte activation. *Curr. Opin. Immunol.* **6**, 106–112.

Thomas, K. M., Pyun, H. Y., and Navarro, J. (1990). Molecular cloning of the f-Met-Leu-Phe receptor from neutrophils. *J. Biol. Chem.* **265**, 20061–20064.

Thomas, K. M., Taylor, L., and Navarro, J. (1991). The interleukin-8 receptor is encoded by a neutrophil-specific cDNA clone, F3R. *J. Biol. Chem.* **266**, 14839–14841.

Tomhave, E. D., Richardson, R. M., Didsbury, J. R., Menard, L., Snyderman, R., and Ali, H. (1994). Cross-desensitization of receptors for peptide chemoattractants. *J. Immunol.* **153**, 3267–3275.

Torres, M., Hall, F. L. and O'Neill, K. (1993). Stimulation of human neutrophils with fMLP induces tyrosine phosporylation and activation of two distinct mitogen-activated protein kinases. *J. Immunol.* **150**, 1563–1578.

Tsu, R. C., Lai, H. W. L., R. A., A., and Wong, Y. H. (1995). Differential coupling of the formyl peptide receptor to adenylate cyclase and phospholipase C by the pertussis toxin-insensitive G_z protein. *Biochem. J.* **309**, 331–339.

Unson, C. G., Erickson, B. W., and Hugli, T. E. (1984). Active site of C3a anaphylatoxin: Contributions of the lopophilic and orienting residues. *Biochemistry* **23**, 585–589.

Valente, A. J., Rozek, M. M., Schwartz, C. J., and Graves, D. T. (1991). Characterization of monocyte chemotactic protein-1 binding to human monocytes. *Biochem. Biophys. Res. Commun.* **176**, 309–314.

Vanek, M., Hawkins, L. D., and Gusovsky, F. (1994). Coupling of the C5a receptor to Gi in U-937 cells and in cells transfected with C5a receptor cDNA. *Mol. Pharmacol.* **46**, 832–839.

Van Riper, G., Siciliano, S., Fischer, P. A., Meurer, R., Springer, M. S., and Rosen, H. (1993). Characterization and species distribution of high affinity GTP-coupled receptor for human rantes and monocyte chemoattractant protein 1. *J. Exp. Med.* **177**, 851–856.

Verghese, M. W., Charles, L., Jakoi, L., Dillon, S. B., and Snyderman, R. (1987). Role of a guanine nucleotide regulatory protein in the activation of phospholipase C by different chemoattractants. *J. Immunol.* **138**, 4374–4380.

Vlahos, C. J. and Matter, W. F. (1992). Signal transduction in neutrophil activation phosphatidylinositol 3-kinease is stimulated without tyrosine phosporylation. *FEBS Lett.* **309**, 242–248.

Vlahos, C. J., Matter, W. F., Brown, R. F., Traynor-Kaplan, A. E., Heyworth, P. G., Prossnitz, E. R., Ye, R. D., Marder, P., Schelm, J. A., Rothfuss, K. J., Serlin, B. S., and Simpson, P. J. (1995). Investigation of neutrophil signal transduction using a specific inhibitor of phosphatidylinositol 3-kinase. *J. Immunol.* **154**, 2413–2422.

Walz, A., Burgener, R., Car, B., Baggiolini, M., Kunkel, S. L., and Strieter, R. M. (1991). Structure and neutrophil-activating properties of a novel inflammatory peptide (ENA-78) with homology to interleukin 8. *J. Exp. Med.* **174**, 1355–1362.

Wang, J. M., McVicar, D. W., Oppenheim, J. J., and Kelvin, D. J. (1993a). Identification of RANTES receptors on human monocytic cells: Competition for binding and desensitization by homologous chemotactic cytokines. *J. Exp. Med.* **177**, 699–705.

Wang, J. M., Sherry, B., Fivash, M. J., Kelvin, D. J., and Oppenheim, J. J. (1993b). Human recombinant macrophage inflammatory protein-1 alpha and -beta and monocyte chemotactic and activating factor utilize common and unique receptors on human monocytes. *J. Immunol.* **150**, 3022–3029.

Wennogle, L. P., Conder, L., Winter, C., Braunwalder, A., Vlattas, S., Kramer, R., Cioffi, C., and Hu, S. I. (1994). Stabilization of C5a receptor-G-protein interactions through ligand binding. *J. Cell. Biochem.* **55**, 380–388.

Wenzel-Seifert, K., and Seifert, R. (1993). Cyclosporin H is a potent and selective formylpeptide receptor antagonist. *J. Immunol.* **150**, 4591–4599.

Weyrich, A. S., McIntyre, T. M., McEver, R. P., Prescott, S. M., and Zimmerman, G. A. (1995). Monocyte tethering by P-selectin regulates monocyte chemotactic protein-1 and tumor necrosis factor-α secretion. *J. Clin. Invest.* **95**, 2297–2303.

Worthen, G. S., Avdi, N., Buhl, A. M., Suzuki, N., and Johnson, G. L. (1994). FMLP activates Rac and Raf in human neutrophils. *J. Clin. Invest.* **94**, 815–823.

Wu, D., LaRosa, G. J., and Simon, M. I. (1993). G protein-coupled signal transduction pathways for interleukin-8. *Science* **261**, 101–103.

Wu, D., Jiang, H., and Simon, M. I. (1995). Different a1-adrenergic receptor sequences required for different Gasubunits of G_q class of G proteins. *J. Biol. Chem.* **270**, 9828–9832.

Yan, Z., Zhang, J., Holt, J. C., Stewart, G. J., Niewiarowski, S., and Poncz, M. (1994). Structural requirements of platelet chemokines for neutrophil activation. *Blood* **84**, 2329–2339.

Ye, R. D., Prossnitz, E. R., Zou, A., and Cochrane, C. G. (1991). Characterization of a human cDNA that encodes a functional receptor for platelet activating factor. *Biochem. Biophys. Res. Commun.* **180**, 105–111.

Ye, R. D., Cavanagh, S. L., Quehenberger, O., Prossnitz, E. R., and Cochrane, C. G. (1992). Isolation of a cDNA that encodes a novel granulocyte N-formyl peptide receptor. *Biochem. Biophys. Res. Commun.* **184**, 582–589.

Ye, R. D., Quehenberger, O., Thomas, K. M., Navarro, J., Cavanagh, S. L., Prossnitz, E. R., and Cochrane, C. G. (1993). The rabbit neutrophil N-formyl peptide receptor. cDNA cloning, expression, and structure/function implications. *J. Immunol.* **150**, 1383–13894.

Ye, R. D., Pan, Z., Kravchenko, V., Browning, D. D., and Prossnitz, E. R. (1996). Gene transcription through activation of G protein-coupled chemoattractant receptors. *Gene Expression* **5**, 205–215.

Yoshimura, T., and Leonard, E. J. (1990). Identification of high affinity receptors for human monocyte chemoattractant protein-1 on human monocytes. *J. Immunol.* **145**, 292–297.

Yu, H., Suchard, S. J., Nairn, R., and Jove, R. (1995). Dissociation of mitogen-activated protein kinase activation from the oxidative burst in differentiated HL-60 cells and human neutrophils. *J. Biol. Chem.* **270**, 15719–15724.

Zhang, X., Chen, L., Bancroft, D. P., Lai, C. K., and Maione, T. E. (1994). Crystal structure of recombinant human platelet factor 4. *Biochemistry* **33**, 8361–8366.

Zhang, Y., and Rollins, B. J. (1995). A dominant negative inhibitor indicates that monocyte chemoattractant protein 1 functions as a dimer. *Mol. Cell. Biol.* **15**, 4851–4855.

Zimmerman, G. A., Lorant, D. E., McIntyre, T. M., and Prescott, S. M. (1993). Juxtacrine intercellular signaling: another way to do it. *Am. J. Respir. Cell Mol. Biol.* **9**, 573–577.

James T. Willerson

Department of Cardiovascular Research
Texas Heart Institute
Division of Cardiology, Department of Internal Medicine
The University of Texas Health Science Center at Houston
Houston, Texas 77030

Pharmacologic Approaches to Reperfusion Injury

I. Introduction

Various pharmacologic and mechanical approaches have been developed and used successfully to reduce mortality from cardiovascular disease and acute myocardial infarction. Early intervention after the onset of ischemia is important in preventing myocardial cell death and in restoring cellular functions to the myocardial tissues that have been altered by the ischemic process. In clinical studies, early reperfusion of the myocardium has been shown to reduce infarct size and mortality after acute coronary artery occlusion (Guerci *et al.*, 1987; Flaherty *et al.*, 1982).

Techniques used to restore blood flow to the myocardium, however, including thrombolytic therapy, percutaneous transluminal coronary angioplasty (PTCA), and cardiac surgery, may lead to damage to the myocardium beyond that generated by the ischemic process alone. Reperfusion of the

Advances in Pharmacology, Volume 39

1054-3589/97/$25.00

previously ischemic myocardium is often followed by detrimental morphologic and functional changes in the affected coronary arteries and myocardial tissues, which ultimately results in tissue damage known as *reperfusion injury*. In a biochemical sense, reperfusion injury has been described as a complex interaction between substances that accumulate during ischemia and those that are delivered as a result of reperfusion (Park *et al.*, 1992). The degree of injury is dependent on the extent of collateral blood flow and duration of ischemia, as well as the influx of neutrophils and the generation of free radicals during reperfusion, which exacerbate the injury. The injury, known as "reperfusion injury," occurs as a consequence of the reintroduction of oxygen to the previously ischemic tissue by pharmacologic or mechanical means of reperfusion. In some studies, damage to the coronary vascular endothelium has been noted to occur within 2.5 to 5 min after the initiation of reperfusion (Tsao *et al.*, 1990). In others, endothelial injury has been noted after 1 hr (Blann *et al.*, 1993). It appears that a considerable amount of time passes, however, before myocyte necrosis, or irreversible injury, occurs as a result of reperfusion of injury (Tsao *et al.*, 1990; Lefer *et al.*, 1991).

Although reperfusion causes injury to the myocardium, paradoxically perfusion must be reestablished for the ischemic myocardium to recover. Optimally, blood flow should be restored within at least 2 to 4 hr after an acute ischemic event. However, the longer the period of ischemia, the greater the number of myocytes that become irreversibly damaged as a consequence of a wave front of necrosis that progresses from the endocardium to the epicardium.

A variety of mechanisms are responsible for reperfusion injury: the generation of oxygen free radicals, loss of antioxidant enzymes, neutrophil-initiated damage, calcium abnormalities, loss of normal adenosine triphosphate concentration, vascular endothelial and myocyte edema, and hemorrhage (Hudson, 1994). These mechanisms of injury are manifested in various ways, including the development of arrhythmias, contractile dysfunction or myocardial "stunning," ultrastructural damage, and defects in intracellular biochemical homeostasis (Fig. 1) (Karmazyn, 1991; Kloner, 1993).

Because of the complex, deleterious effects of reperfusion, developing treatment approaches to lessen or prevent injury to the myocardium is challenging. The goal of current research is to go beyond the palliative treatments available for management of the coronary heart disease patient—to attack directly the pathogenic determinants of reperfusion injury (Janero, 1995).

Ongoing studies include the evaluation of antioxidants and free radical scavengers, membrane stabilizers, calcium antagonists, endogenous agents, protease inhibitors, and nucleoside transport inhibition agents. This review includes current theories regarding the mechanisms behind reperfusion in-

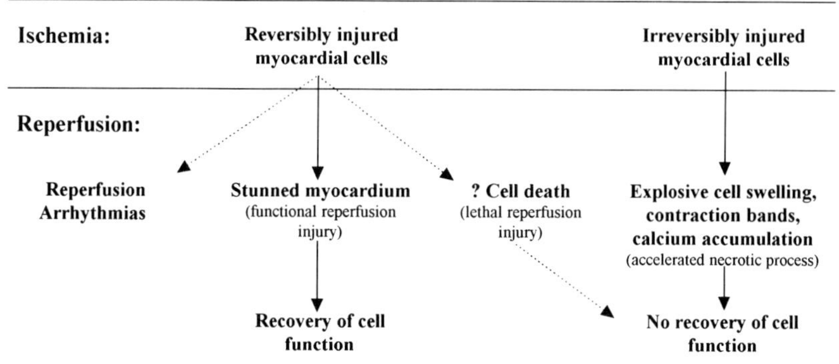

FIGURE 1 Schematic diagram of possible outcomes of ischemia and reperfusion. At the end of a period of ischemia, myocardial cells are injured either reversibly or irreversibly. Reperfusion of reversibly injured myocardial cells results in the salvage of ischemic tissue but also in reperfusion arrhythmias during the first few minutes of reperfusion, and stunned myocardium, which may represent a functional component of reperfusion injury. Still controversial is whether a certain population of cells that were reversibly injured at the end of a period of ischemia die because of reperfusion itself (lethal reperfusion injury). Myocardial cells that are irreversibly injured at the end of a period of ischemia often demonstrate an acceleration of the necrotic process when exposed to reperfusion, including massive swelling, contraction band necrosis, and accumulation of intracellular calcium. Adapted from Kloner (1993). See also Kloner *et al.* (1974b), Whalen *et al.* (1974), Willerson *et al.* (1975), Hearse (1977), and Fishbein (1990).

jury and the pharmacologic approaches used in the treatment of this difficult problem.

II. Oxygen Free Radicals

Oxygen free radicals are believed to play a major role in postischemic injury. This concept has been debated extensively by both experimental and clinical investigators, as discussed by Werns (1994). Oxygen free radicals may be involved in all types of reperfusion injury, including arrhythmias, microvascular injury, myocardial stunning, and lethal reperfusion injury.

A free radical is a molecule with an unpaired electron that renders the molecule unstable, highly reactive, and cytotoxic. PTCA induces an ischemic reperfusion injury by producing toxic oxygen-derived free radicals and other metabolites, such as the superoxide anion (O_2^-), hydrogen peroxide (H_2O_2), and the hydroxyl radical (OH°) (Braunwald and Kloner, 1985; Nayler and Elz, 1986; Flaherty and Weisfeldt, 1988).

Oxygen radical production appears to peak within the first minutes of reperfusion, but continues at a lower level for hours (Bolli *et al.*, 1988). Small concentrations of oxygen free radicals are present in normal oxidative metabolism, but are controlled by the body's defense mechanisms, such as the enzymes superoxide dismutase, catalase, and glutathione peroxidase. During acute ischemic events, however, the defense mechansims against oxygen toxicity are altered. At the time of reflow, there is a decrease in cellular levels of superoxide dismutase and an increase in oxygen free radicals. The sudden burst of oxygen free radicals that emerge at reflow overwhelm the natural superoxide dismutase defense system and cause cell and tissue death or lethal reperfusion injury (Coombs *et al.*, 1992; Kloner, 1993).

A. Sources of Oxygen Free Radicals

Several theories abound as to the source of oxygen free radicals during reperfusion injury (Korthuis and Granger, 1993). The primary source appears to be the xanthine oxidase pathway (Fig. 2).

B. Neutrophil Activation

Neutrophil activation is believed to play a critical role in the inflammatory reaction occurring in oxygen-deprived tissue (Lucchesi and Mullane, 1986; Engler and Covell, 1987; Opie, 1989; Kloner *et al.*, 1989; Entman *et al.*, 1992; Youker *et al.*, 1992, 1993; Dore *et al.*, 1995; Kukielka *et al.*, 1995; Lefer, 1995a; Silver *et al.*, 1995). When activated, the neutrophils produce large quantities of superoxide radicals. Neutrophil attachment in

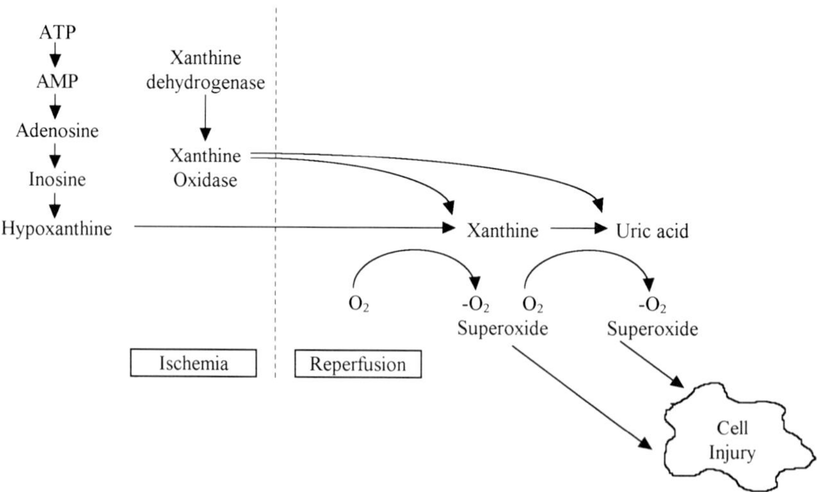

FIGURE 2 Free radical production by the xanthine oxidase pathway. During ischemia, ATP is degraded to adenosine, inosine, and hypoxanthine. The enzyme xanthine dehydrogenase is converted to xanthine oxidase. At the moment of reperfusion, oxygen combines with hypoxanthine in the presence of xanthine oxidase and produces uric acid and the superoxide radical. AMP, adenosine monophosphate; ATP, adenosine triphosphate. Adapted from Coombs *et al.* (1992).

ischemic areas may contribute to the development of cellular edema and subsequent cell necrosis, and in capillary plugging, contributing to the subsequent *no-reflow phenomenon* (Wiggers, 1954; Willerson *et al.*, 1975; Kloner *et al.*, 1974a, 1983; Hashimoto *et al.*, 1991).

The no-reflow phenomenon is a reduction in perfusion despite restoration of flow in the conductance artery. The no-reflow phenomenon is believed to be caused by leukocyte trapping and plugging of reperfused vessels and, in some circumstances, possibly by compression or obstruction of intramyocardial arteries by edematous endothelial and perivascular cells. It is also possible that the local accumulation of platelet-derived mediators, such as thromboxane A_2, serotonin, and/or platelet activating factor; the local generation of thrombin; or the endothelial release of the potent vasocontrictor endothelin also play a role in increasing coronary vascular resistance in the reperfused vessel, thereby reducing myocardial perfusion.

Inflammation in oxygen-deprived tissue is characterized by phagocytic cells that include neutrophils and macrophages. During reperfusion of the ischemic myocardium, circulating neutrophils come into contact with vascular endothelium by a process known as "tethering." This process is mediated by three lectin-like carbohydrate-binding molecules called selectins: *P-selectin* is localized on endothelial cells and platelets, *L-selectin* on neutrophils (leukocytes), and *E-selectin* on endothelium. The function of selectins is to mediate the binding of leukocytes to the vascular endothelium. It has been proposed that the cascade of inflammatory events involved in neutrophil-mediated reperfusion injury may be altered by the use of monoclonal antibodies (MAbs) directed specifically toward these selectins and their associated ligands (Dore *et al.*, 1993a,b; Buerke *et al.*, 1994; Lefer, 1995a; Silver *et al.*, 1995) (Table I).

Earlier experimental studies exploring the role of neutrophils in reperfusion injury focused on neutrophil depletion before induction of regional ischemia (Romson *et al.*, 1983; Mullane *et al.*, 1984) or pharmacological suppression of neutrophil activation as a means of limiting infarct size (Simpson *et al.*, 1987, 1988; Bednar *et al.*, 1985; Nicolini *et al.*, 1991).

III. Selectin Blockers

Lefer (1995a) and colleagues (Lefer *et al.*, 1991, 1994) have been instrumental in delineating the role of selectins in reperfusion injury and in determining the efficacy of MAbs directed against certain selectins. In a feline model, DREG-200 (a MAb developed at Stanford University against L-selectin) was given as a single intravenous dose before the onset of reperfusion. DREG-200 did not specifically bind to feline neutrophils, but did cause their margination or removal from the circulation (Ma *et al.*, 1993). Further studies in left anterior descending coronary artery rings from the same

TABLE I Adhesion Molecules Involved in Neutrophil–Coronary Endothelial Cell Interactions[a]

Type	*Location*	*Expression*	*Time course*	*Ligand*[c]
Selectins				
P	Platelets, endothelium	Stimulated: thrombin, histamine, H_2O_2	10–20 min	SLe^x on PMN, SLe^a on PMN
E	Endothelium	Stimulated: cytokines, lipopolysaccharide	4–6 hr	SLe^x on PMN, SLe^a on PMN
L	Leukocytes	Constitutive	Shed on activation	SLe^x on PMN
Immunoglobins				
ICAM-1[b]	Endothelium, monocytes, lymphocytes	Constitutive, low concentrations	Constitutive, increases slowly over 6–12 hr	CD11a/CD18, CD11b/CD18
β2 Integrins				
CD11a/CD18	Neutrophils	Stimulated by chemotactic stimuli	Activated in minutes	ICAM-1, ICAM-2
CD11b/CD18	Neutrophils	Stimulated by chemotactic stimuli	Activated in minutes	ICAM-1

[a] From Lefer (1995a).

[b] Intercellular adhesion molecule 1.

[c] PMN, polymorphonuclear leukocyte; SLe^x and SLe^a, cell surface; (PMN) oligosaccharides (Sialyl Lewis).

animals supported the hypothesis that an MAb directed against the L-selectin adhesion molecule prevented neutrophil accumulation and endothelial dysfunction and reduced myocardial necrosis. Other studies by this research team (Weyrich *et al.,* 1993) using the MAb PB1.3 against P-selectin in the feline model of ischemia–reperfusion showed a similar degree of cardioprotection.

All three selectins (P, L, and E) interact with a common ligand, sialyl Lewis^x, a tetrasaccharide containing both sialic acid and fucose. Oligosaccharide analogs of sialyl Lewis^x can be used to block the entire family of selectin adhesion molecules; nonsialylated or nonfucosylated analogs can be used as control agents (Lefer, 1995a). An active sialyl Lewis^x oligosaccharide analog, CY-1503, has been developed by Cytel Corporation (San Diego, CA).

In the feline model, use of this active analog reduced infarct size by approximately 75% relative to the nonactive analog and a saline solution-treated control (Lefer 1995a). Similar results have been shown in a canine model of coronary occlusion plus reperfusion (Lefer *et al.,* 1994). Other investigators (Buerke *et al.,* 1994) examined the effects of sialyl Lewis^x on neutrophil–endothelial interactions in a feline model of ischemia–reperfusion. Cardioprotection was confirmed by significantly lower plasma creatine kinase activities in sialyl Lewis^x-treated cats than in control animals. These students indicate that sialyl Lewis^x may be important in neutrophil accumulation, endothelial dysfunction, and myocardial injury in myocardial ischemia and reperfusion.

Silver and associates (1995) assessed the efficacy of CY-1503 as an adjunct to thrombolytic therapy using recombinant tissue-type plasminogen activator (rTPA) in a canine model. By blocking neutrophil interaction with E- and P-selectin, CY-1503 may limit the recruitment of neutrophils to myocardial tissue after ischemia–reperfusion and subsequently reduce myocardial infarct size. Animals that received the selectin blocker in this study had a significant reduction (69%) in infarct size when expressed as a percentage of the area at risk, as well as a marked reduction in myeloperoxidase activity compared with the placebo group. No difference was shown between the treated animals and the control group in the occurrence of reperfusion arrhythmias. This study also underscored the role of the neutrophil as a potent mediator of reperfusion injury.

IV. Antioxidant Therapy

Studies with antioxidants have focused on the potential of these agents to lessen postischemic myocardial injury and to increase the beneficial effects of acute interventional recanalization (Janero, 1994; 1995). Antioxidants have been divided into two broad classes: small molecule and enzymatic.

Small-molecule antioxidants are derived from natural sources, such as vitamins, as well as synthetic sources (Table II). Synthetic molecules are designed as antioxidants or as proprietary drugs whose primary pharmacologic action is independent of their antioxidant activity.

Mickle and Weisel (1993) have proposed that vitamin E—the major lipid soluble, chain-breaking antioxidant in the heart—and its analogs may offer protection from reperfusion injury.

Blann and colleagues (1993) examined the roles of lipid peroxides and the antioxidant enzyme glutathione peroxidase in oxygen free radical damage to the endothelium after PTCA. They took samples of plasma at various time intervals in 16 patients undergoing PTCA. They measured levels of von Willebrand factor (vWf, a marker of damage), thiobarbituric acid reactive substances (TBARS, an indirect measure of the activity of free radicals in

TABLE II Naturally Occurring Substances with Anti-ischemic Cardioprotective Potential as Antioxidants[a]

Substance	*Action*	*Reference*
Adenosine	Inhibits granulocyte oxidant production	Thiel and Bardenheuer (1992)
Ascorbic acid (vitamin C)	Radical scavenging, tocopherol regeneration	Lee *et al.* (1992)
Bilirubin	Radical scavenging	Wu *et al.* (1991)
Catalase	H_2O_2 scavenging	Triana *et al.* (1991)
Coenzyme Q_{10} (ubiquinone)	Redox-active electron carrier	Greenberg and Frishman (1990)
Creatine phosphate	Radical scavenging	Zucchi *et al.* (1989)
Desferrioxamine	Iron chelation	Katoh *et al.* (1993)
Fatty acid-binding protein	Radical scavenging	Srimani *et al.* (1990)
Fructose-1,6-bisphosphate	Metal chelation (?)	Lazzarino *et al.* (1992)
Low-molecular-weight mercaptans	Radical scavenging, glutathione cycle	Menasche *et al.* (1992)
Monocarboxylic α-ketoacids	H_2O_2 scavenging	Janero *et al.* (1993)
Myoinositol hexaphosphate	Metal chelation (?)	Rao *et al.* (1991)
Nitric oxide, L-arginine	Radical scavenging	Weyrich *et al.* (1992)
Propionyl carnitine	Metabolic substrate, metal chelation	Reznick *et al.* (1992)
Selenium	Selenoenzyme cofactor	Peters and Koehler (1989)
Superoxide dismutase	$O_2^{\cdot -}$ scavenging	Konya *et al.* (1992)
α-Tocopherol (vitamin E)	Chain-breaking antiperoxidant	Janero (1991)
Uric acid	Radical scavenging	Becker *et al.* (1989)

[a] From Janero (1995).

peroxidizing lipoproteins), and the antioxidant glutathione peroxidase. They observed an early peak in free radical activity associated with PTCA, causing endothelial injury 1 hr after inflation. This indicated the likelihood of reduced ability of gluathione peroxidase to scavenge oxygen-free radicals.

Initial studies with oxygen-free radical scavengers and reperfusion showed enhanced salvage of myocardium (Jolly *et al.*, 1984; Forman *et al.*, 1988). Subsequent studies in the conscious dog from several laboratories showed no effect of the radical scavengers on infarct size after reperfusion (Nejima *et al.*, 1989; Patel *et al.*, 1990; Downey, 1990). Bolli (1991) published a review of at least 44 published articles describing the effect of antioxidants on infarct size in models of ischemia following reperfusion. About half of those reported a reduction of infarct size whereas half did not. Thus, some researchers claim that no convincing evidence exists to show that antioxidant therapy can reduce infarct size after ischemia followed by reperfusion or that cell death is a manifestation of reperfusion injury (Jeroudi *et al.*, 1994).

A. Antioxidant Therapy in Myocardial Stunning

If ischemic heart muscle is reperfused before irreversible injury occurs, contractility may remain impaired for a prolonged period of hours to days, a phenomenon known as *myocardial stunning*. In experimental studies, considerable evidence supports an oxygen free, radical-mediated mechanism for myocardial stunning (Hess and Kukreja, 1995; Matheis *et al.*, 1992; Naseem *et al.*, 1995).

It is generally agreed, based on experimental evidence of oxidative stress and stunning, that antioxidant intervention made just prior to reperfusion may help restore postischemic cardiac contractile function. Janero (1995) has listed the clinical settings to which these experimental data may be extrapolated—common conditions wherein heart muscle may require days to months for functional recovery following transient ischemia. These include unstable or variant angina, exercise-induced ischemia, percutaneous transluminal coronary angioplasty, open-heart surgery with cardiac arrest, and cardiac transplantation.

Myers and co-workers (1985) and Jeroudi and co-workers (1990, 1994) from the same research group have conducted a considerable number of experiments in open-chest anesthetized dogs to determine whether administration of two antioxidant enzymes, superoxide dismutase and catalase, has a significant effect on myocardial stunning after reperfusion. In their studies, when both enzymes were combined, myocardial contractility was significantly greater than in control animals or in dogs receiving either agent alone, suggesting that both superoxide anion (O_2^-) and hydrogen peroxide (H_2O_2) contribute to myocardial stunning. Another research group used superoxide dismutase and catalase in canine studies, with similar beneficial effects on contractile function (Przyklenk and Kloner, 1986).

In other observations on a conscious dog model, Triana *et al.* (1991) and Sekili *et al.* (1991) found that the administration of several antioxidant agents, such as superoxide dismutase, catalase, *N*-(2-mercaptopropionyl)-glycine (MPG), and deferoxamine, produced a significant and sustained enhancement of the recovery of ventricular function. These experiments helped prove that the oxygen radical hypothesis is applicable to the conscious state and is therefore not influenced by nonphysiologic conditions, such as anesthesia and surgical trauma.

Based on results seen in animal studies with the antioxidant allopurinol (Werns *et al.*, 1986; Grum *et al.*, 1987; Bando *et al.*, 1988; Vinten-Johansen *et al.*, 1988), several small clinical studies have been undertaken to observe the drug's cardioprotective effects during cardiac surgery (Fabiani *et al.*, 1993; Gimpel *et al.*, 1995; Emerit *et al.*, 1995). One such study conducted by a group of French surgeons was based on the hypothesis that free radicals generated by ischemia and reperfusion in surgery can produce clastogenic factor (CF), which results in chromosomal aberration (Emerit *et al.*, 1995). *In vitro* studies in their laboratory in 1988 (Emerit *et al.*, 1988) revealed the presence of DNA-damaging material in the coronary sinus blood after reperfusion of hearts subjected to coronary bypass grafting. Clastogenic factors had been similarly observed in a variety of conditions accompanied by increased oxygen-radical production. The cellular origin of CFs was indicated by the fact that their formation was demonstrable *only* in the presence of cells, but not after exposure of cell-free medium or plasma to oxygen radicals. In the clinical study, 14 patients were divided into two groups: in one group, allopurinol was added to the cardioplegic solution during surgery; in the other group, it was not. Blood samples were used to study the patients' chromosomes after surgery. A significant difference was shown between the postischemic values in the two groups, indicating the effectiveness of allopurinol to reduce clastogenic activity in this setting. However, further clinical trials are needed to determine the efficacy of allopurinol and other antioxidants in the prevention of postoperative myocardial stunning.

B. Antioxidant Therapy for Arrhythmias

Several mechanisms may contribute to the development of arrhythmias during reperfusion, including the local release of catecholamines, ionic shifts, and free-radical injury (Coombs *et al.*, 1992). Early studies indicated that antioxidants could be used successfully to reduce the incidence of reperfusion arrhythmias (Manning and Hearse, 1984; Bernier *et al.*, 1986).

The importance of free radicals in the pathogenesis of reperfusion arrhythmias has been seriously questioned (Opie, 1989; Fox, 1992; Werns,

1994). In the European Myocardial Infarction Project (EMIP), for example, patients randomized to prehospital thrombolysis had a higher incidence of ventricular fibrillation and cardiac arrest (Fox, 1992; White, 1992; EMIP-FR Pilot Study Group, 1993). Thus, reperfusion arrhythmias may be associated with early reperfusion (<4 hr after onset of symptoms). Werns (1994) suggests that adjunctive therapy with prehospital thrombolysis may suppress reperfusion arrhythmias.

C. Calcium Antagonists

Oxygen free radicals also have the capacity to cause sarcoplasmic reticulum dysfunction or membrane damage. When membrane permeability increases, an influx of calcium into the myocytes may also contribute to cellular injury. Ambrosio and colleagues (1992) proposed that calcium antagonists may lessen several mechanisms of reperfusion injury, including neutrophil activation, oxygen radical generation via xanthine oxidase activity, membrane lipid peroxidation, calcium overload, and severity of (indirect) ischemic damage. This theory has been evaluated in a number of experimental studies, using calcium antagonists such as verapamil, nifedipine, and diltiazem (Reimer *et al.,* 1977; Yellon *et al.,* 1983; Lo *et al.,* 1985; Przyklenk and Kloner, 1988; Przyklenk *et al.,* 1989a; Taylor *et al.,* 1990).

In a study by Ambrosio's research team (Villari *et al.,* 1991), a calcium channel antagonist was combined with an oxygen radical scavenger in the treatment of anesthetized rabbits subjected to coronary artery occlusion followed by reperfusion. In one arm of the study, infarct size was significantly reduced by the administration of the calcium antagonist gallopamil during ischemia. Gallopamil administration significantly reduced the rate-pressure product (a major determinant of oxygen demand) during ischemia. These results agreed with other studies indicating that calcium channel blockers can decrease the severity of ischemic injury and reduce myocardial cell necrosis (Ambrosio *et al.,* 1992).

In the clinical setting of cardiac surgery, calcium antagonists have been shown to enhance the recovery of systolic and diastolic function of the stunned myocardium when administered before reperfusion (Mazer, 1993).

One theory regarding reperfusion injury is based on the idea that a less severe degree of ischemia might reduce the development of reperfusion injury. Calcium antagonists may work by indirectly reducing oxygen radical damage after reflow, while allowing extension of the time window of reperfusion therapy by thrombolysis.

V. Endogenous Agents

The heart's ability to protect itself during ischemia and reperfusion is impaired by a reduction in the endogenous oxygen radical scavengers. Other endogenous agents, namely adenosine and nitric oxide, are produced during ischemia, reperfusion, or both. As shown in surgical and nonsurgical models of ischemia and reperfusion, both exert cardioprotective actions by inhibiting endothelial–neutrophil interactions (Vinten-Johansen *et al.*, 1995) and both agents share similar physiologic effects in the myocardium (Table III).

A. Adenosine

The exact mechanisms underlying the cardioprotective effects of adenosine are not fully understood. Adenosine has been shown to protect the myocardium during both ischemia and reperfusion, covering both periods during which myocardial injury may be sustained during a cardiac operation. Importantly, adenosine directly inhibits the production of superoxide radicals by neutrophils (endothelium independent action), as well as neutrophil adherence and subsequent damage to the endothelium (Nakanishi *et al.*, 1994). In the nonischemic heart, adenosine works by interacting with specific membrane proteins, referred to as adenosine A_1 and A_2 receptors. Adenosine A_1 receptors, located primarily on cardiac myocytes, mediate the agent's negative chronotropic/dromotropic and antiadrenergic effects. Adenosine A_2 receptors, located predominantly on endothelial cells, mediate its effects on coronary blood flow (Lasley and Mentzer, 1995).

The A_1 adenosine receptor antagonists 1,3-dipropyl-8-cyclopentylxanthine (DPCPX) and xanthine amine congener (XAC) have been shown to be effective for prevention and early treatment of ischemia–reperfusion injury of the lung (Neely and Keith, 1995). Based on the hypothesis that adenosine receptor antagonists are protective against reperfusion injury in

TABLE III Physiologic Actions of Adenosine and Nitric Oxide[a]

Action[b]	*Adenosine*	*Nitric oxide*
Endogenous	Yes	Yes
Endothelium	Yes	Yes
Myocyte	Yes	Yes
Vasodilatory	Yes	Yes
Inhibits PMN	Yes	Yes
Reduces infarct	Yes	Yes
Reperfusion	Yes	Yes
Compartmental	Yes	?
cAMP	Yes	No
cGMP	No	Yes
Receptor-mediated	Yes	No

[a] From Vinten-Johansen *et al.* (1995).
[b] cAMP, adenosine monophosphate; cGMP, cyclic guanosine monophosphate; PMN, neutrophils.

the heart, DiPierro and co-workers (1995) conducted a study using an *in vivo* feline heart regional infarct model. They administered the selective A_1 adenosine receptor antagonists bamiphylline (BAM) (10 mg/kg/hr) or XAC (0.1 mg/kg/hr) as a continuous intravenous infusion for 60 min, prior to 1 hr of ischemia followed by 2 hr of reperfusion. Both BAM and XAC reduced infarct size from 54.7 ± 3.0% (controls, $n = 6$) to 34.9 ± 3.6% (BAM, $n = 5$, $P = 0.002$) or 23.4 ± 6.6% (XAC, $n = 4$, $P = 0.002$).

Adenosine has also been shown to reduce postischemic myocardial stunning (Lasley and Mentzer, 1995). Kitakaze and co-workers (1990, 1991) evaluated the potential protective effect of adenosine in experiments conducted in a canine model. Contractile function was assessed by measuring fractional shortening during 3 hr of reperfusion following 15 min of occlusion of the left anterior descending coronary artery. Administration of adenosine decreased the severity of myocardial stunning, whereas 8-phenyltheophylline increased it. N^6-Cyclohexyladenosine and 5′-*N*-ethyl-carboxamidoadenosine synergistically improved myocardial stunning, thereby suggesting that stimulation of both adenosine A_1 and A_2 receptors attenuates stunning.

In further studies, Kitakaze *et al.* (1993) evaluated whether the release of noradrenaline during ischemia could be beneficial in modulating the severity of reperfusion injury. After injecting prazosin or methoxamine in the canine model, they assessed regional myocardial contractility. They concluded that moderate α_1-adrenoceptor activation reduces the severity of myocardial stunning by increasing adenosine production.

The adenosine A_1 receptor mechanism appears to be contingent on the accumulation of adenosine in the interstitial fluid that bathes the cardiac myocytes. According to Randhawa and associates (1996), few *in vivo* studies have directly tested this hypothesis because of the rapid metabolism of adenosine and potential systemic hemodynamic side effects. Randhawa's group undertook a study to determine whether exogenous adenosine, administered *before* ischemia, could attenuate postischemic myocardial dysfunction. Regional myocardial stunning was induced by 15 min of coronary artery occlusion and 90 min of reperfusion in an open-chest canine preparation. Regional ventricular function was assessed by measuring systolic wall thickening. In these studies, adenosine treatment during the early reperfusion period failed to attenuate stunning; however, pretreatment with adenosine attenuated stunning. Preischemic adenosine administration increased coronary flow six- to sevenfold without altering regional function, mean arterial pressure, or left ventricular end-diastolic pressure. These results indicate that adenosine should be administered (the adenosine A_1 receptor activated) before the onset of, or during, ischemia to attenuate postischemic ventricular dysfunction. Because of its rapid metabolism and systemic effects, adenosine administered intravenously may not be practical for protecting the ischemic myocardium. However, Randhawa's study and human studies (Cox *et al.*,

1989; Biaggioni *et al.*, 1991) suggest that the intracoronary administration of adenosine is well tolerated and may be cardioprotective in the clinical settings of angioplasty and cardiac surgery.

Randhawa and associates (1996) believe that the apparent positive inotropic effect of adenosine in the stunned heart is related to increased coronary blood flow, inasmuch as it dissipated with the same time course as adenosine-induced hyperemia when infusion was terminated. This effect could be related to the hyperemia-induced increase in wall thickness or could be caused by an increase in oxygen delivery.

B. Nitric Oxide

Nitric oxide, which is derived from the vascular endothelium and other cells of the cardiovascular system, is important in the physiological regulation of blood flow and may have pathophysiological functions in cardiovascular disease (Dusting and MacDonald, 1995). Originally called endothelium-derived relaxing factor (EDRF), nitric oxide is generated during the conversion of L-arginine to citrulline by the highly substrate-specific NO synthase (Vinten-Johansen *et al.*, 1995; Lefer, 1995a) (Fig. 3).

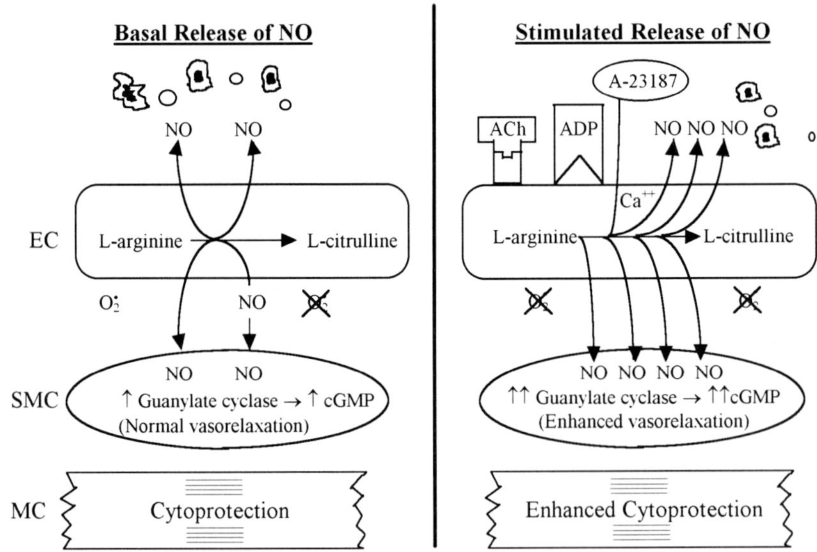

FIGURE 3 (Left) Basal and (right) agonist-stimulated release of nitric oxide (NO) during conversion of L-arginine to L-citrulline by NO synthase in endothelial cells (EC). The NO released to the abluminal side produces relaxation in the vascular smooth muscle cell (SMC). Neutralization of superoxide anions ($O_2^{\bullet}$) by a biradical coupling reaction may be part of the cytoprotective properties to the myocyte (MC). ACh, acetylcholine; ADP, adenosine diphosphate; A-23187, calcium ionophore; CA^{2+}, ionized calcium; cGMP, cyclic guanosine monophosphate. Adapted from Lefer *et al.* (1991). See also Lefer (1995a).

In reperfusion injury, nitric oxide is believed to have cytoprotective properties (Lefer, 1995b). Whereas adenosine has cardioprotective benefits during both ischemia and reperfusion, nitric oxide exerts cardioprotection mainly during reperfusion. Excess nitric oxide can be detrimental, however. Nitric oxide is also involved in neurogenic control of the microcirculation through autonomic efferent nerves, and it contributes to vasodilatation and inflammation associated with the activation of sensory nerves (Dusting, 1995). Excess nitric oxide produced by inducible nitric oxide synthase compromises circulatory function during ischemia and reperfusion injury, as well as in septic shock and transplant rejection, and contributes to the development of hypotension. Reversal of the nitric oxide effect with agents such as angiotensin-converting enzyme (ACE) inhibitors may be protective in such situations.

Seccombe and Schaff (1995) have explored the hypothesis that injury to the coronary endothelium may contribute to the pathophysiology of global (and regional) cardiac ischemia and reperfusion. During ischemia and reperfusion, there is injury to a component in the receptor/G-protein complex linking receptor–stimulus coupling to the activation of nitric oxide synthase. Oxygen radicals may contribute to the injury. Investigations have shown that oxygen radicals impair the receptor/G-protein complex specific to the nitric oxide signal transduction pathway, rather than causing global receptor/G-protein dysfunction. Further elucidation of the nitric oxide pathway and its connection in endothelial injury is needed.

Lefer (1995c) has noted that nitric oxide release by the coronary vasculature is impaired within 5 min after reperfusion of ischemic myocardium and results in a profound loss of vascular homeostasis. Therapeutic strategies, then, should be aimed at preservation or replenishment of nitric oxide concentrations in the coronary vasculature for future treatment of reperfusion injury.

VI. Angiotensin-Converting Enzyme Inhibitors

Angiotensin-converting enzyme inhibitors have long been used therapeutically in the management of hypertension and congestive heart failure. Clinical trials have shown their potential role in limiting myocardial reperfusion injury as well. The pharmacological effects of ACE inhibitors and the mechanism of cardioprotection they provide at the cellular level are not well known, however. The sulfydryl group (SH)-containing ACE inhibitor captopril has been used in most studies (Juggi *et al.*, 1993). A cardioprotective effect has also been shown in non-SH-containing ACE inhibitors, such as ramipril and enalapril (Juggi *et al.*, 1993). Captopril and zofenopril, administered either before occlusion (Westlin and Mullane, 1988) or upon reperfusion (Westlin and Mullane, 1988; Przyklenk *et al.*, 1989b), have been shown to attenuate myocardial stunning. Multicenter, clinical trials are needed to establish a definitive role for these agents in limiting reperfusion injury.

VII. Cardiac Preconditioning

One area that holds promise in the pharmacologic approach to reperfusion injury is that of cardiac preconditioning, a phenomenon whereby brief exposure to ischemia renders the heart more tolerant of a subsequent sustained ischemic insult. Preconditioning may be particularly useful in cardiopulmonary bypass surgery and in cardiac transplantation (Meldrum *et al.*, 1993).

In cardiac surgery, reperfusion injury may be avoided by infusing hyperosmotic solutions at moderate pressures and by incorporating oxygen radical scavengers or inhibitors to reduce membrane lipid peroxidation, myocellular and microcirculatory damage (Vinten-Johansen and Nakanishi, 1993).

VIII. Conclusion

For more than a decade, the concept of reperfusion injury has been known to investigators and clinicians. The growing technologies of molecular biology, immunology, cell biology, and biochemistry have contributed to the understanding and treatment of this complex problem. Much of the pharmacological research in this field is still in the early, experimental phases. As greater knowledge of the pathogenic factors associated with reperfusion injury is achieved, the development of better, more effective target-specific and event-specific approaches to myocardial protection will be possible.

Acknowledgment

The author acknowledges the expert technical assistance provided by Rebecca Teaff at the Texas Heart Institute in the preparation of this manuscript.

References

Ambrosio, G., Villari, B., and Chiariello, M. (1992). Calcium antagonists and experimental myocardial ischemic reperfusion. *J. Cardiovasc. Pharmacol.* **20**, Suppl. 7, S26–S29.

Bando, K., Tago, M., and Teramoto, S. (1988). Prevention of free radical induced myocardial injury by allopurinol. *J. Thorac. Surg.* **95**, 465–473.

Becker, B. F., Reinholz, N., Ozcelik, T., Leipert, B., and Gerlach, E. (1989). Uric acid as radical scavenger and antioxidant in the heart. *Pfluegers Arch.* **415**, 127–135.

Bednar, M., Smith, B., Pinto, A., and Mullane, K. (1985). Nafazatrom-induced salvage of ischemic myocardium in anesthetized dogs is mediated through inhibition of neutrophil function. *Circ. Res.* **57**, 131–141.

Berneir, M., Hearse, D., and Manning, A. (1986). Ability of 6 anti-free radical interventions to reduce reperfusion-induced arrhythmias caused by addition of a free radical generating system. *J. Mol. Cell. Cardiol.* **18**, 100.

Biaggioni, I., Killian, T. J., Mosqueda-Garcia, R., and Robertson, R. M. (1991). Adenosine increases sympathetic nerve traffic in humans. *Circulation* **83**, 1668–1675.

Blann, A., Midgley, H., Burrows, G., Maxwell, S., Utting, S., Davies, M., Waite, M., and McCollum, C. (1993). Free radicals, antioxidants, and endothelial cell damage after percutaneous transluminal coronary angioplasty. *Coronary Artery Dis.* **4**, 905–910.

Bolli, R. (1991). Oxygen-derived free radicals and myocardial reperfusion injury: An overview. *Cardiovasc. Drugs Ther.* **5**, Suppl. 2, 249–268.

Bolli, R., Patel, B. S., Jeroudi, M. D., Lai, E. K., and McCay, P. B. (1988). Demonstration of free radical generation in "stunned" myocardium of intact dogs with the use of the spin trap alpha-phenyl N-tert-Butyl nitrone. *J. Clin. Invest.* **82**, 476–485.

Braunwald, E., and Kloner, R. A. (1985). Myocardial reperfusion: A double edged sword? *J. Clin. Invest.* **76**, 1713–1719.

Buerke, M., Weyrich, A. S., Zheng, Z., Gaeta, F. C., Forrest, M. J., and Lefer, A. M. (1994). Sialyl Lewis^x-containing oligosaccharide attenuates myocardial reperfusion injury in cats. *J. Clin. Invest.* **3**, 1140–1148.

Coombs, V. J., Black, L., and Townsend, S. N. (1992). Myocardial reperfusion injury: The critical challenge. *Crit. Care Nurs. Clin. North Am.* **4**, 339–346.

Cox, D. A., Vita, J. A., Treasure, C. B., Fish, R. D., Selwyn, A. P., and Ganz, P. (1989). Reflex increase in blood pressure during the intracoronary administration of adenosine in man. *J. Clin. Invest.* **84**, 592–596.

DiPierro, F. V., Neely, C. F., Kong, M., and Gardner, T. J. (1995). A_1 Adenosine receptor antagonists reduce ischemia/reperfusion injury in a feline heart regional infarct model. *Circulation* **92**, I–513 (Abstr. No. 2446).

Dore, M., Hawkins, H. K., Entman, M. L., and Smith, C. W. (1993a). Production of a monoclonal antibody against canine GMP-140 (P-selectin) and studies of its vascular distribution in canine tissues. *Vet. Pathol.* **30**, 213–222.

Dore, M., Korthuis, R. J., Granger, D. N., Entman, M. L., and Smith, C. W. (1993b). P-selectin mediates spontaneous leukocyte rolling in vivo. *Blood* **82**, 1308–1316.

Dore, M., Simon, S. I., Hughes, B. J., Entman, M. L., and Smith, C. W. (1995). P-selectin- and CD18-mediated recruitment of canine neutrophils under conditions of shear stress. *Vet. Pathol.* **32**, 258–268.

Downey, J. M. (1990). Free radicals and their involvement during long-term myocardial ischemia and reperfusion. *Annu. Rev. Physiol.* **52**, 487–504.

Dusting, G. J. (1995). Nitric oxide in cardiovascular disorders. *J. Vasc. Res.* **32**, 143–161.

Dusting, G. J., and MacDonald, P. S. (1995). Endogenous nitric oxide in cardiovascular disease and transplantation. *Ann. Med.* **27**, 395–406.

Emerit, I., Fabiani, J.-N., Ponzio, O., Murday, A., Lunel, F., and Carpentier, A. (1988). Clastogenic factor in ischemia-reperfusion injury during open-heart surgery; protective effect of allopurinol. *Ann. Thorac. Surg.* **46**, 619–624.

Emerit, I., Faviani, J.-N., Ponzio, O., Murday, A., Lunel, F., and Carpentier, A. (1995). Clastogenic factor in ischemia-reperfusion injury during open-heart surgery: Protective effect of allopurinol. *Ann. Thorac. Surg.* **60**, 736–737.

EMIP-FR Pilot Study Group (1993). Free radicals, reperfusion and myocardial infarction therapy: European Myocardial Infarction Project—Free Radicals Pilot Study. *Eur. Heart J.* **14**, Suppl. G, 48–51.

Engler, R., and Covell, J. (1987). Granulocytes cause reperfusion ventricular dysfunction after 15-minute ischemia in the dog. *Circ. Res.* **61**, 20–28.

Entman, M. L., Youker, K., Shoji, T., Kukielka, G., Shappell, S. B., Taylor, A. A., and Smith, C. W. (1992). Neutrophil-induced oxidative injury of cardiac myocytes. A compartmented system requiring CD11b/CD18-ICAM-1 adherence. *J. Clin. Invest.* **90,** 1335–1345.

Fabiani, J. N., Farah, B., Vuilleminot, A., Lecompte, T., Emerit, I., Chardigny, C., and Carpentier, A. (1993). Chromosomal aberrations and neutrophil activation induced by reperfusion in the ischaemic human heart. *Eur. Heart J.* **14 (Suppl G),** 12–17.

Fishbein, M. C. (1990). Reperfusion injury. *Clin. Cardiol.* **13,** 213–217.

Flaherty, J., and Weisfeldt, M. (1988). Reperfusion injury. *Free Radical Biol. Med.* **5,** 409.

Flaherty, J. T., Weisfeldt, M. D., Bulkley, B. H., Gardner, T. J., Gott, V. L., and Jacobus, W. E. (1982). Mechanisms of ischemic myocardial cell damage assessed by phorphorus 31 nuclear magnetic resonance. *Circulation* **65,** 561–571.

Forman, M. B., Puett, D. W., Cates, C. U., McCroskey, D. E., Beckman, J. K., Greene, H. L., and Virmani, R. (1988). Glutathione redox pathway and reperfusion injury: Effect of N-acetylcysteine on infarct size and ventricular function. *Circulation* **78,** 202–213 [comment in *Circulation* **80,** 712–713 (1989)].

Fox, K. A. A. (1992). Reperfusion injury: Laboratory phenomenon or clinical reality? *Cardiovasc. Res.* **26,** 656–659.

Gimpel, J. A., Lahpor, J. R., van der Molen, A.-J., Damen, J., and Hitchcock, J. F. (1995). Reduction of reperfusion injury of human myocardium by allopurinol: A clinical study. *Free Radical Biol. Med.* **19,** 251–255.

Greenberg, S., and Frishman, W. H. (1990). Coenzyme A_{10}: A new drug for cardiovascular disease. *J. Clin. Pharmacol.* **30,** 596–608.

Grum, C. M., Ketai, L. H., Meyers, C. L., and Schlafer, M. (1987). Purine reflux after cardiac ischemia: Relevance to allopurinol cardioprotection. *Am. J. Physiol.* **252,** H368–H373.

Guerci, A. D., Gerstenblith, G., Brinker, J. A., Chandra, N. C., Gottlieb, S. O., Bahr, R. D., Weiss, J. L., Shapiro, E. P., Flaherty, J. T., and Bush, D. W. (1987). A randomized trial of intravenous tissue plasminogen activator for acute myocardial infarction with subsequent randomization to elective coronary angioplasty. *N. Engl. J. Med.* **317,** 1613–1618.

Hashimoto, K., Pearson, P. J., Schaff, H. V., and Cartier, R. (1991). Endothelial cell dysfunction after ischemic arrest and reperfusion. A possible mechanism of myocardial injury during reflow. *J. Thorac. Cardiovasc. Surg.* **102,** 688–694.

Hearse, D. J. (1977). Reperfusion of the ischemic myocardium. *J. Mol. Cell. Cardiol.* **9,** 605–616.

Hess, M. L., and Kukreja, R. C. (1995). Free radicals, calcium homeostasis, heat shock proteins, and myocardial stunning. *Ann. Thorac. Surg.* **60,** 760–766.

Hudson, K. F. (1994). A phenomenon of paradox: myocardial reperfusion injury. *Heart Lung* **23,** 384–393.

Janero, D. R. (1991). Therapeutic potential of vitamin E against myocardial ischemic-reperfusion injury. *Free Radical Biol. Med.* **10,** 315.

Janero, D. R. (1994). Myocardial ischemia-reperfusion injury and the cardioprotective potential of natural antioxidants. *In* "Natural Antioxidants in Human Health and Disease" (B. Frei, ed.), p. 411. Academic press, San Diego, CA.

Janero, D. R. (1995). Ischemic heart disease and antioxidants: Mechanistic aspects of oxidative injury and its prevention. *Crit. Rev. Food Sci. Nut.* **35,** 65–81.

Janero, D. R., Hreniuk, D., and Sharif, H. M. (1993). Hydrogen peroxide-induced oxidative stress to the mammalian heart-muscle cell (cardiomyocyte): Nonperoxidative purine and pyrimidine nucleotide depletion. *J. Cell. Physiol.* **155,** 494.

Jeroudi, M. O., Triana, F. J., Patel, B. S., and Bolli, R. (1990). Effect of superoxide dismutase and catalase, given separately, on myocardial "stunning." *Am. J. Physiol.* **259,** H889–H901.

Jeroudi, M. O., Hartley, C. J., and Bolli, R. (1994). Myocardial reperfusion injury: Role of oxygen radicals with potential therapy with antioxidants. *Am. J. Cardiol.* **73,** 2B–7B.

Jolly, S. R., Kane, W. J., Bailie, M. D., Abrams, G. D., and Lucchesi, B. R. (1984). Canine myocardial reperfusion injury: Its reduction by the combined administration of superoxide dismutase and catalase. *Circ. Res.* **54,** 277–285.

Juggi, J. S., Koenig-Berard, E., and Van Gilst, W. H. (1993). Cardioprotection by angiotensin-converting enzyme (ACE) inhibitors. [Review]. *Can. J. Cardiol.* **9**, 336–352.

Karmazyn, M. (1991). The 1990 Merck Forsst Award. Ischemic and reperfusion injury in the heart. Cellular mechansims and pharmacological interventions. *Can. J. Physiol. Pharmacol.* **69**, 719–730.

Katoh, S., Toyama, J., Kodama, I., Akita, T., and Abe, T. (1993). Deferoxamine, an iron chelator, reduces myocardial injury and free radical generation in isolated neonatal rabbit hearts subjected to global ischemia-reperfusion. *J. Mol. Cell. Cardiol.* **24**, 1267–1275.

Kitakaze, M., Takashima, S., and Sato, H. (1990). Stimulation of adenosine A_1 and A_2 receptors prevents myocardial stunning. *Circulation* **82**, III-37 (abstr.).

Kitakaze, M., Hori, M., Sato, H., Iwakura, K., Gotoh, K., Inoue, M., Kitabatake, A., and Kamada, T. (1991). Beneficial effects of $alpha_1$ adrenoceptor activity on myocardial stunning in dogs. *Circ. Res.* **68**, 1322–1339.

Kitakaze, M., Hori, M., and Kamada, T. (1993). Role of adenosine and its interaction with alpha adrenoceptor activity in ischaemic and reperfusion injury of the myocardium. *Cardiovasc. Res.* **27**, 18–27.

Kloner, R. A. (1993). Does reperfusion injury exist in humans? *J. Am. Coll. Cardiol.* **21**, 537–545.

Kloner, R. A., Ganote, C. E., and Jennings, R. B. (1974a). The "no-reflow" phenomenon after temporary coronary occlusion in the dog. *J. Clin. Invest.* **54**, 1496–1508.

Kloner, R. A., Ganote, C. E., Whalen, D., and Jennings, R. B. (1974b). Effect of a transient period of ischemia on myocardial cells. II. Fine structure during the first few minutes of reflow. *Am. J. Pathol.* **74**, 399–422.

Kloner, R. A., Ellis, S. G., Lange, R., and Braunwald, E. (1983). Studies of experimental coronary artery reperfusion: Effects on infarct size, myocardial function, biochemistry, ultrastructure and microvascular damage. *Circulation* **68**, Suppl. 1, 8–15.

Kloner, R. A., Przyklenk, K., and Whittaker, P. (1989). Deleterious effects of oxygen radicals in ischemia/reperfusion: resolved and unresolved issues. *Circulation* **80**, 1115–1127.

Konya, L., Kekesi, V., Juhasz-Nagy, S., and Feher, J. (1992). The effect of superoxide dismutase in the myocardium during reperfusion in the dog. *Free Radical Biol. Med.* **13**, 527.

Korthuis, R. J., and Granger, D. N. (1993). Reactive oxygen metabolites, neutrophils, and the pathogenesis of ischemic-tissue/reperfusion. *Clin. Cardiol.* **16**(4), Suppl. 1, I19–I26.

Kukielka, G. L., Smith, C. W., Manning, A. M., Youker, K. A., Michael, L. H., and Entman, M. L. (1995). Induction of interleukin-6 synthesis in the myocardium. Potential role in postreperfusion inflammatory injury. *Circulation* **92**, 1866–1875.

Lasley, R. D., and Mentzer, R. M., Jr. (1995). Protective effects of adenosine in the reversibly injured heart. *Ann. Thorac. Surg.* **60**, 843–846.

Lazzarino, G., Tavazzi, B., DiPierro, D., and Giardina, B. (1992). Ischemia and reperfusion: Effect of fructose-1,6-biphosphate. *Free Radical Res. Commun.* **16**, 325–329.

Lee, K. C., Horan, P. J., Canniff, P. C., Silver, P. J., and Ezrin, A. M. (1992). Myocardial salvage by Trolox and ascorbic acid, but not ascorbic acid alone, in anesthetized dogs and rabbits. *Drug Dev. Res.* **27**, 345.

Lefer, A. M. (1995a). Role of selectins in myocardial ischemia-reperfusion injury. *Ann. Thorac. Surg.* **60**, 773–777.

Lefer, A. M. (1995b). Attenuation of myocardial ischemia-reperfusion injury with nitric acid replacement therapy. *Ann. Thorac. Surg.* **60**, 847–851.

Lefer, A. M. (1995c). Myocardial protective actions of nitric oxide donors after myocardial ischemia and reperfusion. *New Horizons* **3**, 105–112.

Lefer, A. M., Tsao, P. S., Lefer, D. J., and Ma, X. (1991). Role of endothelial dysfunction in the pathogenesis of reperfusion injury after myocardial ischemia. *FASEB J.* **5**, 2029–2034.

Lefer, D. J., Flynn, D. M., Phillips, L., Ratcliffe, M., and Buja, A. J. (1994). A novel sialyl $Lewis^x$ analog attenuates neutrophil accumulation and myocardial necrosis after ischemia and reperfusion. *Circulation* **90**, 2390–2401.

Lo, H.-M., Kloner, R. A., and Braunwald, E. (1985). Effect of intracoronary verapamil on infarct size in the ischemic reperfused canine heart: Critical importance of the timing of treatment. *Am. J. Cardiol.* **56**, 672–677.

Lucchesi, B., and Mullane, K. (1986). Leukocytes and ischemia-induced myocardial injury. *Annu. Rev. Pharmacol. Toxicol.* **26**, 201–224.

Ma, X., Weyrich, A. S., Lefer, D. J., Buerke, M., Albertine, K. H., Kishimoto, T. K., and Lefer, A. M. (1993). Monoclonal antibody to L-selectin attenuates neutrophil accumulation and protects ischemic reperfused cat myocardium. *Circulation* **88**, 649–658.

Manning, A., and Hearse, D. (1984). Reperfusion-induced arrhythmias: Mechanisms and prevention. *J. Mol. Cell. Cardiol.* **16**, 497–518.

Matheis, G., Sherman, M. P., Buckberg, G. D., Haybron, D. M., Young, H. H., and Ignarro, L. J. (1992). Role of L-argninine-nitric oxide pathway in myocardial reoxygenation injury. *Am. J. Physiol.* **262**, H616–H620.

Mazer, C. D. (1993). Calcium and stunned myocardium. *J. Cardiac Surg.* **8(2 Suppl),** 329–331.

Meldrum, D. R., Mitchell, M. B., Banerjee, A., and Harken, A. H. (1993). Cardiac preconditioning. Induction of endogenous tolerance to ischemia-reperfusion injury. *Arch. Surg. (Chicago)* **128**, 1208–1211.

Menasche, P., Grousset, C., Gauduel, Y., Mouas, C., and Piwnica, A. (1992). Maintenance of the myocardial thiol pool by *N*-acetylcysteine. An effective means of improving cardioplegic protection. *J. Thorac. Cardiovasc. Surg.* **103**, 936.

Mickle, D. A., and Weisel, R. D. (1993). Future directions of vitamin E and its analogues in minimizing myocardial ischemia–reperfusion injury. *Can. J. Cardiol.* **9**, 89–93 [see comment in *Can. J. Cardiol.* **9**, 29–31 (1993)].

Mullane, K., Read, N., Salmon, J., and Moncada, S. (1984). Role of leukocytes in acute myocardial infarction in anesthetized dogs: Relationship to myocardial salvage by anti-inflammatory drugs. *J. Pharmacol. Exp. Ther.* **228**, 510–522.

Myers, M. L., Bolli, R., Lekich, R. F., Hartley, C. J., and Roberts, R. (1985). Enhancements of recovery of mycoardial function by oxygen free-radical scavengers after reversible regional ischemia. *Circulation* **72**, 915–921.

Nakanishi, K., Zhao, Z.-Q., Vinten-Johansen, J. H., Lewis, J. C., McGee, D. S., and Hammon, J. W., Jr. (1994). Coronary artery endothelial dysfunction after ischemia, blood cardioplegia, and reperfusion. *Ann. Thorac. Surg.* **58**, 191–199.

Naseem, S. A., Kontos, M. C., Rao, P. S., Jesse, R. L., Hess, M. L., and Kukreja, R. C. (1995). Sustained inhibition of nitric oxide by N^G-nitro-L-arginine improves myocardial function following ischemia/reperfusion in isolated rat heart. *J. Mol. Cell. Cardiol.* **27**, 419–426.

Nayler, W. G., and Elz, J. S. (1986). Reperfusion injury: Laboratory artifact or clinical dilemma? *Circulation* **74**, 215–221.

Neely, C. F., and Keith, I. M. (1995). A_1 adenosine receptor antagonists block ischemia-reperfusion injury of the lung. *Am. J. Physiol.* **268**, L1036–L1046.

Nejima, J., Knight, D. R., Fallon, J. T., Uemura, N., Manders, W. T., Canfield, D. R., Cohen, M. V., and Vatner, S. F. (1989). Superoxide dismutase reduces reperfusion arrhythmias but fails to salvage regional myocardial function or myocardium at risk in conscious dogs. *Circulation* **79**, 143–153.

Nicolini, F., Mehta, J., Nichols, W. I. Luostarinen, R., and Saldeen, T. (1991). Leukocyte elastase inhibition and t-PA-induced coronary artery thrombolysis in dogs: Beneficial effects on myocardial histology. *Am. Heart J.* **122**, 1245–1251.

Opie, L. H. (1989). Reperfusion injury and its pharmacologic modification. *Circulation* **80**, 1049–1062.

Park, J. W., Braum, P., Mertens, S., and Heinrich, K. W. (1992). Ischemic reperfusion injury and restenosis after coronary angioplasty. *Ann. N.Y. Acad. Sci.* **669**, 215–236.

Patel, B. S., Jeroudi, M. O., O'Neill, P. G., Roberts, R., and Bolli, R. (1990). Effect of human recombinant superoxide dismutase on canine myocardial infarction. *Am. J. Physiol.* **258** (2 Pt 2), H369–H380.

Peters, H. J., and Koehler, H. (1989). Selenium and lipid peroxidation in human and experimental cardiovascular disease. *In* "CRC Handbook of Free Radicals and Antioxidants in Biomedicine." (J. Miguel, A. T. Quintanilha, and H. Weber, eds.), Vol. 2, p. 237. CRC Press, Boca Raton, FL.

Przyklenk, K., and Kloner, R. A. (1986). Superoxide dismutase plus catalase improve contractile function in the canine model of the stunned myocardium. *Circ. Res.* **58,** 148–156.

Przyklenk, K., and Kloner, R. A. (1988). Effect of verapamil on postischemic "stunned" myocardium: Importance of timing of treatment. *J. Am. Coll. Cardiol.* **11,** 614–623.

Przyklenk, K., Ghafari, B. G., Eitzman, D. T., and Kloner, R. A. (1989a). Nifedipine administered after reperfusion ablasts systolic contractile dysfunction of postischemic "stunned" myocardium. *J. Am. Coll. Cardiol.* **13,** 1176–1183.

Przyklenk, K., Whittaker, P., and Kloner, R. A. (1989b). Zofenopril, a newly developed sulfhydryl-containing converting enzyme inhibitor, enhances contractile function of "stunned" myocardium. *In* "Current Advances in Ace Inhibition" (G. A. MacGregor and P. S. Sever, eds.), p. 279. Churchill-Livingstone, Edinburgh.

Rao, P. S., Lui, X. K., Das, D. K., Weinstein, G. S., and Tyras, D. H. (1991). Protection of ischemic heart from reperfusion injury by myo-inositol hexaphosphate, a natural antioxidant. *Ann. Thorac. Surg.* **52,** 908–912.

Randhawa, M. P., Lasley, R. D., and Mentzer, R. M., Jr. (1996). Salutary effects of exogenous adenosine administration on *in vivo* myocardial stunning. *J. Thorac. Cardiovasc. Surg.* **112,** 202–204.

Reimer, K. A., Lowe, J. E., and Jennings, R. B. (1977). Effect of calcium antagonist verapamil on necrosis following temporary coronary occlusion in dogs. *Circulation* **55,** 581–590.

Reznick, A. Z., Kagan, V. E., Ramsey, R., Tsuchiya, M., Khwaja, S., Servinova, E. A., and Packer, L. (1992). Antiradical effects in L-propionyl carnitine protection of the heart against ischemia-reperfusion injury: The possible role of iron chelation. *Arch. Biochem. Biophys.* **296,** 394–401.

Romson, J., Hook, B., Kunel, S., Abrams, G., Schork, M., and Lucchesi, B. (1983). Reduction of the extent of ischemia myocardial injury by neutrophil depletion in the dog. *Circulation* **67,** 1016–1023.

Seccombe, J. F., and Schaff, H. V. (1995). Coronary artery endothelial function after myocardial ischemia and reperfusion (review). *Ann. Thorac. Surg.* **60,** 778–788.

Sekili, S., Li, X. Y., Zughayb, M., Sun, J. Z., and Bolli, R. (1991). Evidence for a major pathogenetic role of hydroxyl radical in myocardial "stunning" in the conscious dog. *Circulation* **84,** Suppl. 2, II-656.

Silver, M. J., Sutton, J. M., Hook, S., Lee, P., Malycky, J. L., Phillips, L., Ellis, S. G., Topol, E. J., and Nicolini, F. A. (1995). Adjunctive selectin blockade successfully reduces infarct size beyond thrombolysis in the electrolytic canine coronary artery model. *Circulation* **92,** 492–499.

Simpson, P., Mitsos, S., Ventura, A., Gallagher, K., Fantone, J., and Lucchesi, B. (1987). Prostacyclin protects ischemic reperfusion myocardium in the dog by inhibition of neutrophil activation. *Am. Heart J.* **113,** 129–137.

Simpson, P., Mickelson, J., Fantone, J., Gallagher, K., and Lucchesi, B. (1988). Reduction of experimental myocardial infarct size with prostaglandin E_1-inhibition of neutrophil migration and activation. *J. Pharmacol. Exp. Ther.* **244,** 619–624.

Srimani, B. N., Engelman, R. M., Jones, R., and Das, D. K. (1990). Protective role of intracoronary fatty acid binding protein in ischemic and reperfused myocardium. *Circ. Res.* **66,** 1535–1543.

Taylor, A. E., Golino, P., Eckels, R., Pastor, P., Buja, L. J., and Willerson, J. T. (1990). Differential enhancement of postischemic segmental systolic thickening by diltiazem. *J. Am. Coll. Cardiol.* **15,** 737–747.

Thiel, M., and Bardenheuer, H. (1992). Regulation of oxygen radical production of human polymorphonuclear leukocytes by adenosine: The role of calcium. *Pfluegers Arch.* **420,** 522.

Triana, J. F., Li, X.-Y., Jamaluddin, U., Thronby, J. I., and Bolli, R. (1991). Postischemic myocardial "stunning": Identification of major differences between the open-chest and the conscious dog and evaluation of the oxygen radical hypothesis in the conscious dog. *Circ. Res.* **69,** 731–747.

Tsao, P. S., Aoki, N., Lefer, D. J., Johnson, G., III, and Lefer, A. M. (1990). Time course of endothelial dysfunction and myocardial injury during myocardial ischemia and reperfusion in the cat. *Circulation* **82,** 1402–1412.

Villari, B., Ambrosio, G., Golino, P. Ragni, M., and Chiariello, M. (1991). Reduction of severity of ischemia decreases reperfusion injury in rabbit hearts. *Eur. Heart J.* **12**(2), 136 (abstr.).

Vinten-Johansen, J., and Nakanishi, K. (1993). Postcardioplegia acute cardiac dysfunction and reperfusion injury. *J. Cardiothorac. Vasc. Aneth.* 7(4), Suppl. 2, 6–18.

Vinten-Johansen, J., Chiantella, V., Faust, K. B., Jonston, W. E., McCain, B., Hartman, M., Mills, S. A., Hester, T. O., and Cordell, A. R. (1988). Myocardial protection with blood cardioplegia in ischemically injured heart: Reduction of reoxigenation injury with allopurinol. *Am. Thorac. Surg.* **45,** 319–326.

Vinten-Johansen, J., Zhao, Z.-Q., and Sato, H. (1995). Reduction in surgical ischemia-reperfusion injury with adenosine and nitric oxide therapy. *Ann. Thorac. Surg.* **60,** 852–857.

Werns, S. (1994). Free radical scavengers and leukocyte inhibitors. *In* "Textbook of Interventional Cardiology" (E. J. Topol, ed.), Vol. 2, pp. 137–160. Saunders, Philadelphia.

Werns, S. W., Shea, M. J., Mitsos, S. E., Dysko, R. C., Fantone, J C., Schort, M. A., Abrams, G. D., and Lucchesi, B. R. (1986). Reduction of the size of infarction by allopurinol in the ischemic reperfused heart. *Lab. Invest.* **73,** 518–524.

Westlin, W., and Mullane, K. (1988). Does captopril attentuate reperfusion induced myocardial dysfunction by scavenging free radicals? *Circulation* **77,** Suppl. 1, 30–39.

Weyrich, A. S., Ma, X., and Lefer, A. M. (1992). The role of L-arginine in ameliorating reperfusion injury after myocardial ischemia in the cat. *Circulation* **86,** 279.

Weyrich, A. S., Ma, X., Lefer, D. J., Albertine, K. H., and Lefer, A. M. (1993). In vivo neutralization of P-selectin protects feline heart and endothelium in myocardial ischemia and reperfusion injury. *J. Clin. Invest.* **91,** 2620–2629.

Whalen, D. A., Hamilton, D. G., Ganote, C. E., and Jennings, R. B. (1974). Effect of a transient period of ischemia on myocardial cells. I. Effects on cell volume regulation. *Am. J. Pathol.* **74,** 381–398.

White, H. D. (1992). Reperfusion injury—a reply to Keith Fox. *Cardiovasc. Res.* **26,** 660–661.

Wiggers, C. J. (1954). The interplay of coronary vascular resistance and myocardial compression in regulating coronary flow. *Circ. Res.* **2,** 217–279.

Willerson, J. T., Watson, J. T., Hutton, I., Templeton, G. H., and Fixler, D. E. (1975). Reduced myocardial reflow and increased coronary vascular resistance following prolonged myocardial ischemia in the dog. *Circ. Res.* **36,** 771–781.

Wu, T. W., Wu, J., Li, R. K., Mickle, D., and Carey, D. (1991). Albumin-bound bilirubins protect human ventricular myocytes against oxyradical damage. *Biochem. Cell Biol.* **639,** 683–688.

Yellon, D. M., Hearse, D. J., Maxwell, M. P., Chambers, D. E., and Downery, J. M. (1983). Sustained limitation of myocardial necrosis 24 hours after coronary artery occlusion: Verapamil infusion in dogs with small myocardial infarcts. *Am. J. Cardiol.* **51,** 1409–1414.

Youker, K. A., Smith, C. W., Anderson, D. C., Miller, D., Michael, L. H., Rossen, R. D., and Entman, M. L. (1992). Neutrophil adherence to isolated adult cardiac myocytes. Induction by cardiac lymph collected during ischemia and reperfusion. *J. Clin. Invest.* **89,** 602–609.

Youker, K. A., Hawkins, H. K., Kukielka, G. L., Perrard, J. L., Michael, L. H., Ballantyne, C. M., Smith, C W., and Entman, M. L. (1993). Molecular evidence for a border zone vulnerable to inflammatory reperfusion injury. *Trans. Assoc. Am. Physicians* **106,** 145–154.

Zucchi, R., Poddighe, R, Limbruno, U., Mariani, M., Ronca-Testoni, S., and Ronca, G. (1989). Protection of isolated rat heart from oxidative stress by exogenous creatine phosphate. *J. Mol. Cell. Cardiol.* **21,** 67–73.

Joan A. Keiser
Andrew C. G. Uprichard
Cardiovascular Therapeutics
Parke-Davis Pharmaceutical Research
Warner Lambert Company
Ann Arbor, Michigan 48105

Restenosis: Is There a Pharmacologic Fix in the Pipeline?

I. Introduction

Originally introduced in 1975 as a treatment option for refractory, stable, single-vessel angina pectoris (Gruentzig *et al.*, 1979), percutaneous transluminal coronary angioplasty (PTCA) has now become a widely accepted treatment for a variety of presentations of occlusive coronary artery disease. It has been reported that as many as 400,000 procedures are performed annually in the United States (Franklin and Faxon, 1993), with more than 700,000 interventions worldwide. The most common device used clinically continues to be the balloon angioplasty catheter; although a number of other tools have been introduced, including directional and rotational atherectomy devices, excimer lasers, and stents (Margolis *et al.*, 1991; Serruys *et al.*, 1991; Simpson *et al.*, 1991; Wong *et al.*, 1993). Although all of these procedures share excellent early patency rates, a major long-

Advances in Pharmacology, Volume 39

1054-3589/97/$25.00

term complication common to all is a chronic renarrowing of the coronary artery, reported to occur in up to 50% of patients (Hillegass *et al.*, 1994). This phenomenon of restenosis (Fig. 1) usually presents with recurrence of clinical symptoms some 3 to 6 months after the initial procedure and frequently requires further intervention. Indeed, such is the cost of repeat coronary angiography and angioplasty (or bypass surgery) in affected patients that an intervention capable of reducing the rate of restenosis by 25% would save the U.S. economy $400 million annually (Topol *et al.*, 1993a). An equally stark reminder of the extent of the problem is evident when one considers the amount of time and effort that have been devoted to finding a treatment for restenosis, for the one common thread connecting all our experience to date has been a singular lack of success. Despite many exciting scientific approaches and a number of promising preclinical experiments, enthusiasm has time and again been tempered by the latest in the series of negative clinical trials. Yet there is reason to believe that there may be light at the end of the tunnel. As more is discovered about the basic pathophysiological mechanisms underlying the restenotic process in humans, so we have witnessed the development of more clinically relevant models and novel strategies for delivering targeted therapeutic interventions for what is currently a major public health burden.

This review details the molecular, cellular, and structural mechanisms thought to be involved in restenosis; summarizes current research strategies; and discusses developments which may impact clinical therapies in the future. Where references are cited, efforts have been made to restrict these, as much as possible, to recent literature.

II. Pathophysiology: Insights from Clinical and Animal Studies

The mechanisms responsible for restenosis in humans remain the subject of intense debate, although it is accepted that a cascade of events is precipitated in the vessel wall following balloon injury (Clowes *et al.*, 1983a,b; Karas *et al.*, 1991; Muller *et al.*, 1992; Casscells, 1992). As a direct result of the invasive procedure, the endothelium of the blood vessel wall is disrupted, exposing the underlying smooth muscle cells and connective tissue. This thrombogenic surface can precipitate rapid clot formation and bring about abrupt closure of the treated vessel. The incidence of such immediate (24–48 hr) postangioplasty failures, however, has been markedly reduced by the use of a variety of anticoagulant and antithrombotic therapies. Thus the use of routine anticoagulation with aspirin and heparin in routine balloon angioplasty has resulted in an expected early closure rate of 4–8% (Holmes *et al.*, 1995).

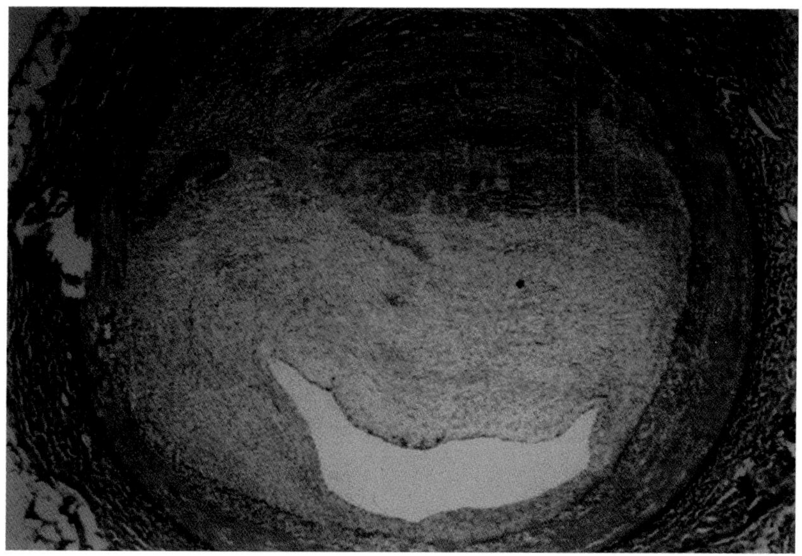

FIGURE 1 Cross section of human restenotic coronary artery. The medial wall, bordered by the internal and external elastic laminae, is stained red. Both an atherosclerotic lesion (blue) and a subsequent proliferative lesion (light blue/white) are apparent inside the internal elastic laminae.

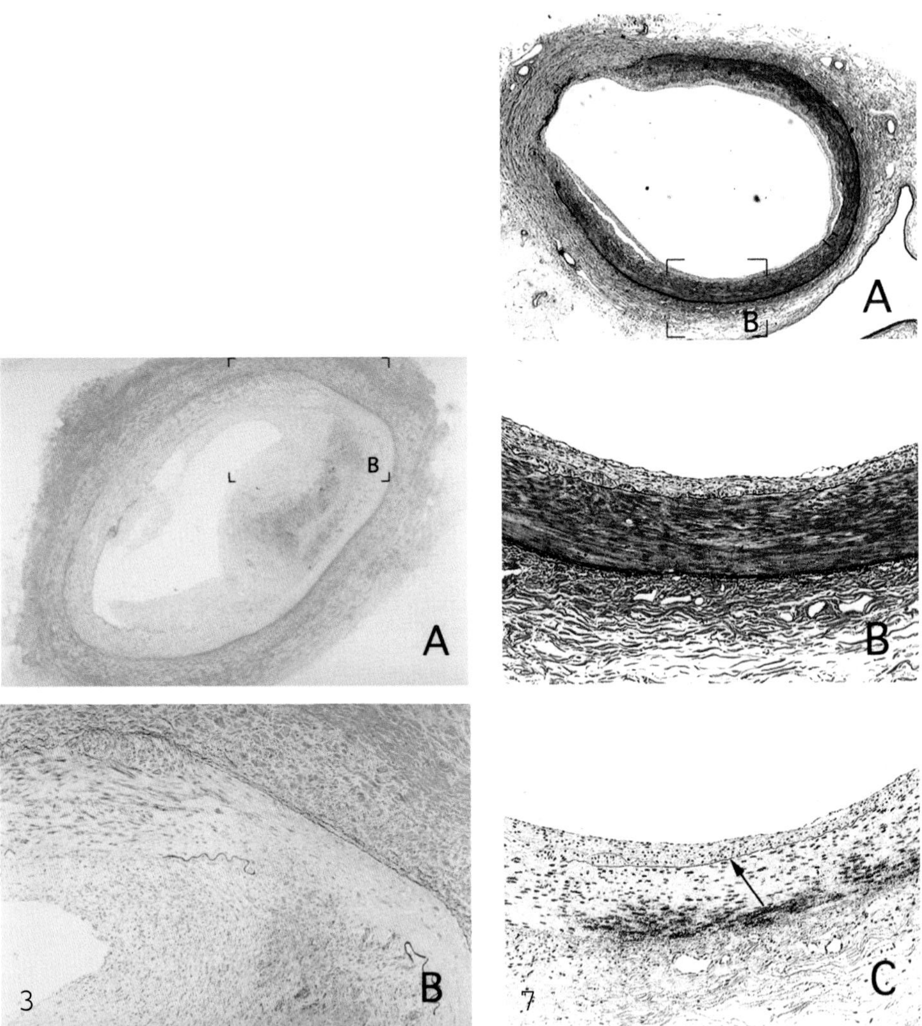

FIGURE 3 Cross section of a ballon-injured iliofemoral artery from a cynomolgus monkey 2 weeks postinjury. (A) The full cross section; (B) an enlarged view of the region noted on A. Note the disruption of the internal elastic laminae and eccentric nature of the lesion.

FIGURE 7 Immunostaining for Lp(a) in a monkey iliofemoral artery following balloon injury. (A) Cross section of a balloon-injured monkey iliofemoral artery with a trichrome stain; (B) x10 magnification of A; (C) serial section adjacent to the section in B immunostained (reddish-brown) for Lp(a) which is apparent at the medial/adventitial border. The arrow indicates the internal elastic laminae.

Damage is not only an inevitable consequence of the angioplasty, but may be essential for the procedure to be successful. In balloon angioplasty, for example, it is important that the atherosclerotic plaque is not only stretched but cracked in order to achieve any initial gain (Faxon, 1993). In animal models, researchers have developed "injury scales" to be used as variables in determining the effects of experimental interventions (Schneider *et al.,* 1993), and it is clear that the more vigorous the injury, the more robust the response (Indolfi *et al.,* 1995). However, it is not clear whether the extent of injury in humans is correlated with the incidence of subsequent restenosis. Although atherectomy devices may not result in the degree of stretching associated with balloon angioplasty, these catheters carry the risk of cutting deep into the medial smooth muscle layers, risking dissection or even aneurysm formation, both likely contributing factors in the increased risk of early complications compared with balloon angioplasty (Topol *et al.,* 1993b). To date, the reported rate of restenosis associated with atherectomy devices has not been less than that seen with balloon angioplasty, and results of a recent clinical trial have raised questions over the safety of the former procedure (Elliott *et al.,* 1995).

In response to the denuding of the endothelium, a cascade of events occur (Fig. 2). Platelets, fibrin, and other cells adhere to the thrombotic

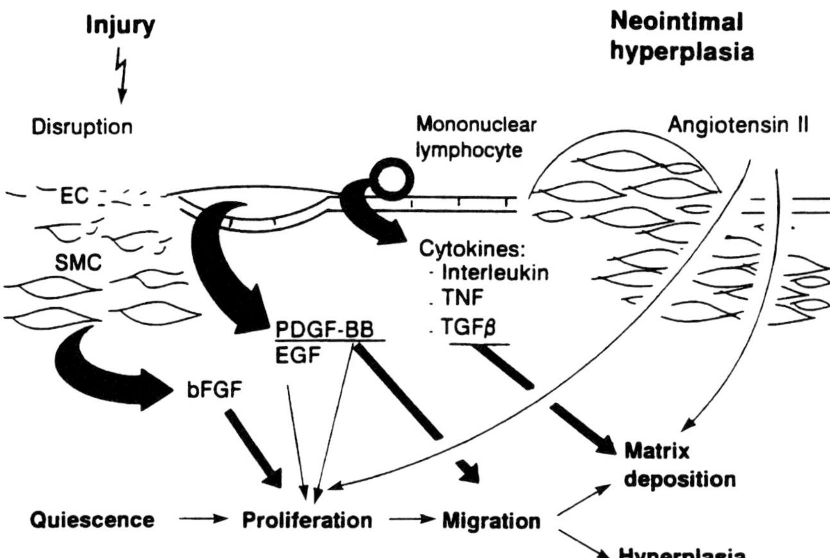

FIGURE 2 Proposed mechanisms involved in the arterial response to injury. Stimulation of smooth muscle cells by several growth factors and formation of connective tissue contributing to neointimal growth. Reprinted with permission from Herrman, J. P. R., Hermans, W. R. M., Vos, J., and Serruys, P. W., (1993). Pharmacological approaches to the prevention of restenosis following angioplasty. Drugs 46, 18–52. Copyright by Adis International Ltd., 1993.

surface of the vessel wall. Lymphocytes and monocytes are recruited to the lesion in response to the release of a number of growth factors and cytokines. These include platelet-derived growth factor (PDGF), epidermal growth factor (EGF), transforming growth factor β (TGF-β), insulin-like growth factor (IGF-1), interleukins, and potentially other vasoactive agents such as angiotensin and endothelin. It is thought that these agents, acting locally at the site of vessel injury, induce migration and proliferation of smooth muscle cells in the lesion (Casscells, 1992). Cells from rapidly expanding intima in animal models do not exhibit a typical contractile phenotype and may be responsible for the secretion of the large amounts of extracellular matrix (Majesky *et al.*, 1992). Although there are no sequential pathological studies in humans to confirm these cellular events, the final result is one of a thickened neointima, containing smooth muscle cells, fibroblasts, and a large extracellular matrix component extending into the lumen of the vessel and compromising myocardial blood flow.

Another element of the restenotic process that has commanded increasing attention in the recent literature is that of vascular remodeling, or changes in vessel diameter unrelated to proliferation (Kuntz and Baim, 1993; Glagov, 1994). Studies with intracoronary ultrasound have demonstrated a compensatory enlargement of the vessel itself, presumably an adaptive response, which may accommodate the increased neointimal area (Luo *et al.*, 1994). Ironically, therefore, it would be in those patients where remodeling is prevented, or inadequate, that restenosis is a problem. That remodeling may be particularly important in humans is suggested by a study that demonstrated similar neointimal areas in patients with and without symptoms of restenosis after angioplasty: the two groups were distinguished only by the degree of vascular remodeling (and, accordingly, lumen diameter) (Luo *et al.*, 1994). The remodeling hypothesis would also explain the enigma resulting from rates of cellular proliferation in human atherectomy specimens, which are lower than that calculated from animal models (O'Brien *et al.*, 1993).

In an attempt to explain some of the questions generated from clinical studies, a number of animal models have been developed, including balloon injury in rats, rabbits, pigs, and monkeys (Moore, 1979; Clowes *et al.*, 1983a,b; Faxon *et al.*, 1984; Steele *et al.*, 1985; Vesselinovitch, 1988; Carter *et al.*, 1994; Ryan *et al.*, 1996, Geary *et al.*, 1996). A murine model of wire-induced injury has been introduced to study the response to injury in transgenic mice (Lindner *et al.*, 1993). Balloon catheter-induced injury in the rat carotid artery is the model most often described and discussed (Clowes *et al.*, 1983a,b, 1986; Clowes and Schwartz, 1985). This injurious procedure results in the reproducible formation of a histologically distinct neointima within 10 to 14 days of injury and describes four distinct waves involving smooth muscle cell proliferation and migration as well as matrix deposition. There is no pre-existing intima in the rat carotid artery; thus migration of cells from the underlying media is a prerequisite for lesion formation. Using a variety of labeling techniques, the proliferation of smooth muscle cells can be readily confirmed in the media at 2–4 days postinjury and in the intima with a peak at approximately 7 days. Active neointimal formation subsides at 14–28 days postinjury in this model, resulting in a smooth muscle and matrix-rich lesion which persists indefinitely. Apoptosis, programmed cell death, has been reported in a rat aortic balloon injury model (Bochaton-Piallat *et al.,* 1995); however, to elucidate a role of apoptosis in the remodeling of lesions will require further study.

Balloon injury in normal rabbit, pig, and monkey vessels also induces the formation of a neointima which grows rapidly and appears to stabilize within the first few weeks after injury (Schwartz *et al.,* 1990; Faxon *et al.,* 1984; Sarembock *et al.,* 1989; Vesselinovitch, 1988; Carter *et al.,* 1994; Ryan *et al.,* 1996). An example of an iliofemoral artery from a cynomolgus monkey injured by balloon angioplasty is shown in Fig. 3 and illustrates the typical neointimal formation, disruption of the internal elastic lamina (high-power view, Fig. 3B), and persistence of thrombosis. Overt cracking and disruption of the internal elastic lamina are commonly seen in pig and primate models; these points of disruption appear to serve as niduses for proliferation in the vessel wall, resulting in eccentric lesions. Although some work has been performed in pig coronary arteries (Schwartz *et al.,* 1990; Schneider *et al.,* 1993; Shi *et al.,* 1994), accessibility and experimental limitations have meant that the majority of animal data have been gathered from noncoronary beds. Because no detailed comparisons of the histologic lesions in different blood vessels exist, it is unclear if the mechanisms of restenosis in anatomically distinct vascular beds are similar. Unlike other vascular smooth muscle cells, coronary arterial cells are derived from a distinct site in the chick embryo. In addition, the diversity of smooth muscle cells has been described based on distinct phenotypic patterns of cells when grown in culture or challenged with various growth stimuli (Majesky and Schwartz, 1990). Injury to rat carotid artery has been shown to result in changes in the phenotypic pattern of smooth muscle cells in the vessel wall (Majesky *et al.,* 1992). These examples of smooth muscle cell diversity have led to speculation that the coronary vessels may have distinct regulatory responses to injury.

Animal models of vascular injury on a substrate of underlying atherosclerotic plaque are much more difficult to establish and have been employed less frequently to model restenosis. Varying degrees of cholesterol feeding in rabbits have been used to generate a model with abnormal lipid parameters; however, balloon injury in these settings often results in a neointimal lesion with a high lipid burden that is not typical of human restenosis (Culp *et al.,* 1992). Some investigators have combined an initial denuding injury in the rabbit or the pig with a cholesterol diet to induce atherosclerosis and have subsequently angioplastied these lesions with varying success (Faxon *et al.*, 1982). These studies are inherently more difficult to interpret: variability is evident in the development of the primary atherosclerotic lesion as well as in the angioplasty-induced lesion. The use of vascular imaging techniques such as angiography and intravascular ultrasound make these studies easier to perform, but confine researchers to larger animal models due to the limits of resolution of the various imaging techniques. In a rabbit double injury model, investigators have reported that injured vessels can be seen to undergo abnormal vascular remodeling and that this may be more important to the restenotic response than smooth muscle proliferation per se (Lafont *et al.*, 1995). Similarly, others have assessed angiographic indices of late lumen loss in balloon-injured atherosclerotic minipigs and concluded that arterial remodeling and intimal proliferation both contribute to the chronic loss of lumen (Post *et al.*, 1994). However, remodeling in animal models has not been universally observed (Gertz *et al.*, 1994).

In an attempt to address the role of matrix deposition in the restenotic process, investigators have begun to examine collagen gene expression in the vessel wall. One study of human autopsy material demonstrated that collagen constituted from 41 to 60% of total plaque protein (Smith, 1965). In rat balloon injury models the percentage of smooth muscle cells in the neointima drops from 41% at 2 weeks postinjury to 20% at 8 weeks postinjury (Clowes *et al.*, 1983b; Snow *et al.*, 1990). These data suggest that long-term lesion expansion may be primarily dependent on matrix deposition. Thus, although most of the animal models used to assess the efficacy of antirestenotic agents focus on smooth muscle cell proliferation and morphologic end points, researchers are beginning to gain an appreciation for the role of other vascular changes, including matrix deposition and remodeling. End points that involve an assessment of functional lumen diameter *in vivo* and more clinically relevant measures of coronary artery *restenosis* (as opposed to primary *stenosis*) in animal models will be crucial to continued progress in this field.

III. Pharmacologic Therapies

A. Antithrombotic Approaches

It is well recognized that antithrombotic treatment reduces the incidence of abrupt (24–48 hr) closure after angioplasty. Reference has already been made to the standard cocktail of aspirin and heparin with balloon angioplasty, but what remains unknown is whether antithrombotic therapy can reduce the risk of subsequent restenosis. The argument would be that nonocclusive thrombus formation would involve the recruitment and aggregation of platelets which, upon degranulation, would release various growth factors to initiate the restenosis process (Barry and Sarembock, 1994). A number of agents have accordingly been tested in experimental and clinical studies.

1. Heparins and Direct Antithrombins

Continuously administered heparin has been shown to inhibit intimal proliferation in the rat carotid artery model of balloon injury (Clowes and Karnovsky, 1977). Similar results were seen in a rabbit model of atherosclerosis and restenosis with nonanticoagulant doses (0.1–0.6 mg/kg/hr) of the heparin analog Astenose, which inhibited restenosis when administered intravenously for 28 days (Timms *et al.,* 1995). These data suggest that the efficacy of heparin in experimental models may be unrelated to its anticoagulant properties and point to data demonstrating the *in vitro* inhibition by heparin of early growth response genes (c-*fos* and c-*myc*) in rodent and bovine vascular smooth muscle cells (Pukac *et al.,* 1990). It is interesting, therefore, that clinical trials have failed to document efficacy with unfractionated heparin when given at therapeutic doses (12500 U administered subcutaneously twice a day) for 4 months after the procedure (Brack *et al.,* 1994). One possible explanation for this may relate to dosing paradigms and pharmacokinetics of the drug, as more recent animal studies have shown that intermittent administration of heparin not only does not prevent neointimal proliferation, but may actually exacerbate the injury response (Edelman and Karnovsky, 1994).

In a double-blind, placebo-controlled multicenter evaluation of the low molecular weight heparin, enoxaparin, the drug failed to prevent angiographically determined restenosis when administered for 1 month in 227 patients (231 patients received placebo) (Faxon *et al.,* 1994). The dose of enoxaparin chosen for this trial (40 mg subcutaneously once daily) was previously shown to be an effective anticoagulant therapy (Planes *et al.,* 1988).

In addition to its role as a potent platelet activator, thrombin is also known to release PDGF and plasminogen activator inhibitor. Thrombin is mitogenic for both vascular smooth muscle cells and lymphocytes *in vitro.* Thus a thrombin inhibitor would, in theory, impact several of the mechanisms implicated in restenosis. The selective thrombin inhibitor hirudin was compared with heparin for the prevention of restenosis in the 1141 patient clinical trial HELVETICA (Serruys *et al.,* 1995). Two groups of patients with unstable angina received 24 hr of hirudin intravenously followed by either hirudin or placebo subcutaneously for a further 3 days. A third group received 24 hr of heparin followed by subcutaneous placebo. Although both regimens of hirudin significantly reduced clinical events occurring within the first 96 hr, event-free survival at 7 months (the primary end point of the study) was similar across groups. Mean lumen diameters by angiography were 1.54, 1.47, and 1.56 mm for the heparin, intravenous hirudin, and intravenous/subcutaneous hirudin groups, respectively (P = NS). More recently, Topol's group compared hirudin with tick anticoagulant peptide (TAP, a factor Xa inhibitor), recombinant tissue factor pathway inhibitor (TFPI), and active-site inactivated factor VIIa in a rabbit model of atherosclerosis and angioplasty. Although no benefit was seen with TAP or hirudin treatment, the active-site inactivated VIIa and TFPI groups showed significant reductions in absolute neointimal areas compared with controls (Jang *et al.*, 1995). Taken in conjuction with the observation that tissue factor may be responsible for the prolonged procoagulant activity seen after injury (Speidel *et al.*, 1995), these data suggest that inhibition of the early initiators of the extrinsic coagulation pathway may be a more appropriate target for interventions in restenosis.

2. *Antiplatelets*

The antirestenotic effects of a monoclonal antibody Fab fragment (c7E3) directed against the platelet glycoprotein IIb/IIIa integrin were assessed by Topol and co-workers in a double-blind, placebo-controlled, dose-ranging evaluation as add on to standard therapy with heparin and aspirin in 2099 patients determined to be at "high risk" from the angioplasty procedure (EPIC Investigators, 1994; Topol *et al.*, 1994). Although the primary end point of the study was the 30-day composite incidence of major cardiac events, all patients were followed up for 6 months to evaluate the effects of intervention on restenosis. At this time point, the absolute difference in numbers of patients with either major ischemic events or need for subsequent revascularization was 8.1% (35.1% in placebo vs 27% in c7E3-treated groups, respectively, $P = 0.001$). Thus, in this hypothesis-generating exercise (the study was not designed for a restenosis end point), c7E3 significantly lowered these clinical signs of restenosis (Fig. 4). Although these data are promising, it is of note that 7E3 is not absolutely specific for the GPIIb/IIIa integrin: evidence exists for an effect on the $\alpha v\beta 3$ integrin receptor, another surface adhesion receptor which binds vitronectin and could be implicated in the restenotic process. A prospective, hypothesis-testing clinical trial with angiographic end points and assessment of luminal diameter will be needed to complement these clinical findings.

Blockade of the thromboxane pathway with sulotroban, a selective thromboxane A2 receptor blocker, failed to inhibit restenosis in a clinical trial of 752 patients when compared to aspirin therapy or placebo (Savage *et al.*, 1995). Additionally, a double-blinded clinical trial was conducted with the prostacyclin epoprostenol administered for 36 hr postangioplasty (Gershlick *et al.*, 1994). This short-term infusion of prostacyclin did not significantly reduce the rate of restenosis at 6 months after PTCA. It is of interest that these agents had previously shown positive effects in animal models (Groves *et al.*, 1979).

The purported antiplatelet agent, dipyridamole, inhibited neointimal formation in a rabbit model of injury to carotid or femoral arteries when

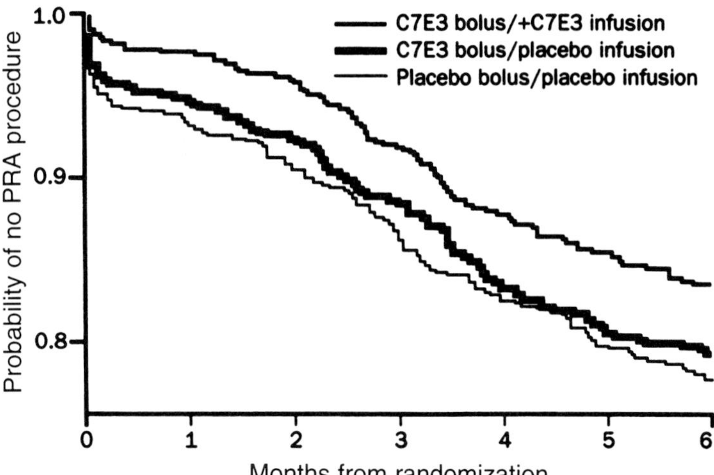

FIGURE 4 Six month EPIC results. Need for subsequent target vessel revascularization, either by coronary angioplasty of coronary bypass surgery. Repeat revascularization was significantly reduced in the c7E3 bolus + infusion group compared with placebo (p = 0.007). Reprinted with permission from Topol, E. J., Califf, R. M., Weisman, H. F., Ellis, S. G., Tcheng, J. E., Worley, S., Ivanhoe, R., George, B. S., Fintel, D., Weston, M. (1994). Randomised trial of coronary intervention with antibody against platelet IIb/IIIa integrin for reduction of clinical restenosis: results at six months. Lancet 343(8902), 881–886. Copyright by the Lancet Ltd., 1994.

administered locally to the periadventitial surface via an osmotic minipump, but was ineffective when administered systemically (Singh *et al.,* 1994). Although the locally administered doses of dipyridamole ranged from 0.6 to 600 μg/day, only the two highest doses (300 and 600 μg/day) significantly inhibited smooth muscle cell proliferation. The explanation offered by the investigators for the lack of a systemic effect was that the systemic administration of dipyridamole failed to achieve plasma drug levels that were sufficient to block smooth muscle cell replication. Earlier clinical trials using various doses and combinations of dipyridamole with other antiplatelet agents had been inconclusive (Schwartz *et al.,* 1988; Chesebro *et al.,* 1989; Okamato *et al.,* 1992).

B. Antiproliferatives

Within the developing intima of several animal models of vascular injury, smooth muscle cell proliferation has been described at rates ranging from 5 to 50% of total cells at early time points postinjury. Although we cannot be sure that the same phenomena occur clinically, the observation of a neointima after angioplasty in humans is suggestive of a proliferative process and lends weight to the pursuit of antiproliferative strategies.

I. Growth Factor Inhibitors

A number of antiproliferative strategies have targeted growth factor pathways in an attempt to prevent neointimal formation. It has been shown that application of growth factors by a variety of methods can exacerbate neointimal formation *in vivo* (see Table I).

Blockade of growth factor signaling has been attempted through a number of pathways. A synthetic analog of insulin-like growth factor-1 (IGF-1) known to inhibit receptor activation prevented neointimal formation in balloon-injured rat carotid arteries, whereas a "scrambled" control peptide was without effect (Hayry *et al.*, 1995). Similarly, studies with a cytotoxin fusion protein (DAB-389EGF) directed to the EGF receptor inhibited neointimal formation 40% (vs control) in the rat when administered systemically (Pastore *et al.*, 1995). DAB-389EGF was more efficacious (74% reduction in neointimal area) when administered locally and lacked some of the side effects (of the cytotoxin) noted with systemic administration.

Although the role of growth factors in smooth muscle cell proliferation has received considerable attention experimentally, most investigators believe that multiple growth factors are probably involved, suggesting the futility of blocking a specific growth factor. In addition, several growth factors signal through multiple receptors. Thus attention has turned to the intracellular signaling pathways believed to be common to many of the growth factors; an example is provided in Fig. 5. Tyrphostins, receptor tyrosine kinase inhibitors with some selectivity for the PDGF receptor, have been reported to inhibit neointimal formation in the rat carotid artery when administered locally (Colomb *et al.*, 1994). Trapidil (triazolopyrimidine) is also reported to inhibit PDGF-induced mitogenic activity (Ohnishi *et al.*, 1981), although the mechanism (or specificity) with which this compound blocks PDGF signaling is unclear. In the rat carotid model, trapidil inhibited PDGF-stimulated neointimal formation (Tiell *et al.*, 1983), complementing the decreased neointimal formation and increased luminal area seen in the atherosclerotic rabbit (Liu *et al.*, 1990).

TABLE I Growth Factors in Animal Models of Vascular Injury

Agent	*Animal model*	*Effect*	*Reference*
PDGF	Rat carotid artery	↑ Neointimal area, ↑ Smooth muscle migration	Jawien *et al.* (1992)
	Porcine femoral artery	↑ Neointimal area	Nabel *et al.* (1993b)
FGF	Rat carotid artery	Neointimal hyperplasia	Lindner *et al.* (1991) Edelman *et al.* (1992)
	Rabbit aorta	Transient ↑ neointimal area	Parish *et al.* (1995)
	Porcine femoral artery	↑ Neointimal area, angiogenesis	Nabel *et al.* (1993a)
TGF $\beta 1$	Porcine femoral artery	↑ extracellular matrix, intimal and medial hyperplasia	Nabel *et al.* (1993c)

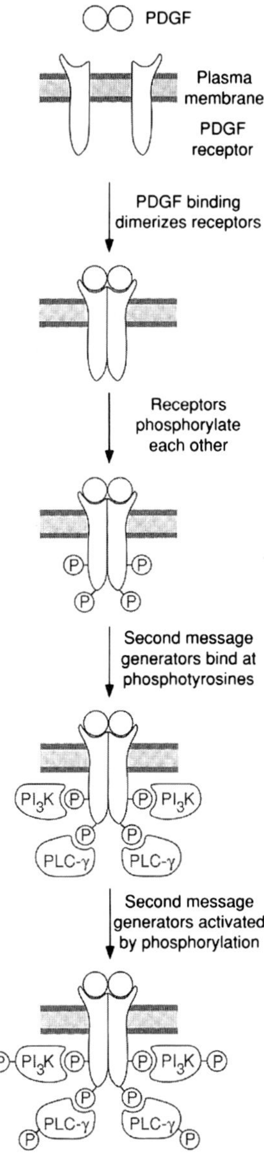

FIGURE 5 A representative growth factor signaling pathway indicating autophosphorylation of the receptor and subsequent second messenger generation. From: The Cell Cycle by Murray and Hunt. Copyright (c) 1993 by W. H. Freeman and Company. Used with permission.

Given the structural similarity between growth factor receptors, it was previously thought unlikely that compounds could be identified with selectivity for one tyrosine kinase over others (Waltenberger *et al.*, 1994). Fry *et al.* (1994), however, described a class of quinazalines with marked selectivity for the EGF receptor tyrosine kinase. It is believed that a number of companies are currently exploring specific growth factor tyrosine kinase inhibitors as potential drug targets. CGP 53716, a 2-phenylaminopyrimidine, is reported to selectively inhibit PDGF receptor tyrosine kinase activity (Buchdunger *et al.*, 1995), but no data are available on the effects of this compound in cardiovascular systems. Leflunomide is a novel isoxazole (Nair *et al.*, 1995) that has been characterized as an EGF growth factor tyrosine kinase inhibitor, although the specificity of leflunomide for a particular growth factor remains to be demonstrated. Leflunomide inhibits vascular smooth muscle cell proliferation *in vitro;* however, there are no *in vivo* studies reported to date.

Angiopeptin is a somatostatin analog that has been reported to inhibit early response oncogene expression in rabbit aorta after balloon injury (Bauters *et al.*, 1994). Studies from Foegh and co-workers (1989; Lundergan *et al.*, 1991) detailed the effects of angiopeptin in a rabbit model of transplant atherosclerosis. When administered subcutaneously at a dose of 60 μg/day for 6 weeks, angiopeptin inhibited intimal hyperplasia in the transplanted group by approximately 50% (Foegh *et al.*, 1989). Similar results were seen with the drug (20 or 50 μg/kg daily) in injured rat carotid arteries assessed 15 days postinjury, although the effects of angiopeptin were not dose related in this model (Lundergan *et al.*, 1991).

Clinical experience with angiopeptin provides an interesting story: a pilot study randomized 112 patients to receive continuous subcutaneous angiopeptin or placebo infusion for 1 day before and 4 days after angioplasty. Quantitative coronary angiography was performed at 6 months with clinical follow-up at 1 year. Results demonstrated a statistically significant ($P = 0.003$) reduction in restenosis at 6 months and a trend toward fewer clinical events at 1 year (Eriksen *et al.*, 1995). A subsequent European study of 553 patients used a similar protocol, but this time there was a significant reduction in clinical events at 12 months (36.4% vs 28.4%, $P = 0.046$), with no effect on angiographic variables (Emanuelsson *et al.*, 1995). In a parallel U.S. study of over 1200 patients, there were no beneficial effects on either end point (Faxon and Currier, 1995). This has been attributed to the twice-daily subcutaneous dosing regimen imposed on the trial by regulatory agencies.

The importance of inflammatory components in vessel wall injury is evidenced by the fact that cholesterol-containing foam cells are monocyte/macrophage in origin. The T-cell cytokine, interferon-γ, will inhibit cholesterol accumulation into foam cells. In addition, interferon-γ will inhibit smooth muscle cell proliferation directly (Hansson, 1994). Cytokine therapy with interferon-γ administered as daily injections (200,000 units) for 1 week reduced neointimal formation in balloon-injured rat carotid arteries assessed after 14 days (Castronuovo *et al.*, 1995). The investigators reported that although interferon-γ treatment had smaller lesions, the rates of vascular smooth muscle cell (VSMC) proliferation as determined by immunocytochemistry were not different. It should be noted, however, that proliferation rates are returning toward baseline levels at this time point in this model, thus making interpretation difficult.

2. *Vasoactive Agents*

Powell and co-workers first reported that angiotensin-converting enzyme (ACE) inhibitors inhibited neointimal formation in the balloon-injured rat carotid artery in 1989. This finding was heralded widely in the research community because a local tissue renin angiotensin system had been described in the vessel wall and angiotensin was known to potentiate the mitogenic activity of other growth factors *in vitro* (Rakugi *et al.*, 1994; Pratt and Dzau, 1996). Subsequently, researchers demonstrated that *in vivo* administration of angiotensin selectively enhanced smooth muscle cell proliferation in the intima compared with the media in balloon-injured rodent vessels (Daemen *et al.*, 1991), lending further credence to the possible involvement of angiotensin in restenosis. Although numerous investigators have since described the positive effects of ACE inhibitors and angiotensin receptor type 1 (AT1) antagonists in the rat carotid artery balloon injury model (Prescott *et al.*, 1991; Azuma *et al.*, 1992; Kawamura *et al.*, 1993), the effects of angiotensin blockade have been less clear cut in other animal models with negative results from rabbit, porcine, and primate vascular injury studies (Clozel *et al.*, 1991; Bilazarian *et al.*, 1992; Huber *et al.*, 1993). Unpublished data from the authors' laboratories have failed to demonstrate any beneficial effect of the selective angiotensin type 2 receptor (AT2) antagonist, PD 123319, in the rat carotid model. More recently, two well-controlled clinical trials of cilazapril failed to document any benefit in angiographic or clinical end points in more than 2000 patients postangioplasty (MERCATOR Study Group, 1992; Faxon, 1995). Enalapril (10 mg/day) also failed to prevent restenosis in a small clinical trial (Kaul *et al.*, 1994). The QUinapril Ischemic Event Trial (QUIET) should add further information in evaluating the effects of the ACE inhibitor quinapril on a number of cardiac ischemic events in a population of patients followed for 3 years after angioplasty (Texter *et al.*, 1993).

Like angiotensin a decade earlier, endothelin is currently attracting the attention of researchers because of its profound vasoconstrictor and mitogenic properties. Endothelin receptors are found on both endothelial and vascular smooth muscle cells, changes in endothelin receptor expression have been described in response to vascular injury (Azuma *et al.*, 1994), and endothelin can potentiate the mitogenic effects of growth factors such as PDGF (Kohno *et al.*, 1994; Irons *et al.*, 1996). Studies with the nonselective ET_A/ET_B) endothelin receptor antagonist SB 209670 demonstrated inhibition of neointimal formation in the balloon-injured rat carotid artery (Douglas *et al.*, 1994). When administered at 2.5 mg/kg IP twice daily for 3 days prior to injury and throughout a subsequent 14-day period, the drug blocked neointimal formation by approximately 50%. In addition, the administration of endothelin to balloon-injured rats dose dependently exacerbated the formation of neointimal lesions (Fig. 6). These same investigators have subsequently shown that blockade of ET_A receptors with the selective ET_A receptor antagonist BQ-123 does not inhibit neointimal formation in the same rat model (Douglas *et al.*, 1995) and have concluded that both ET_A and ET_B receptors must contribute to neointimal formation in the rat. Work from Moreland's laboratory indicated that the ET_A selective compound BMS-182874 (100 mg/kg PO once daily for 3 weeks beginning 1 week prior to injury) suppresses neointimal formation 34% in the rat 14 days postangioplasty (Ferrer *et al.*, 1995). Based on the current literature, the role of endothelin receptor subtypes in restenosis is unclear; additional studies in more complex models of vascular injury are urgently needed.

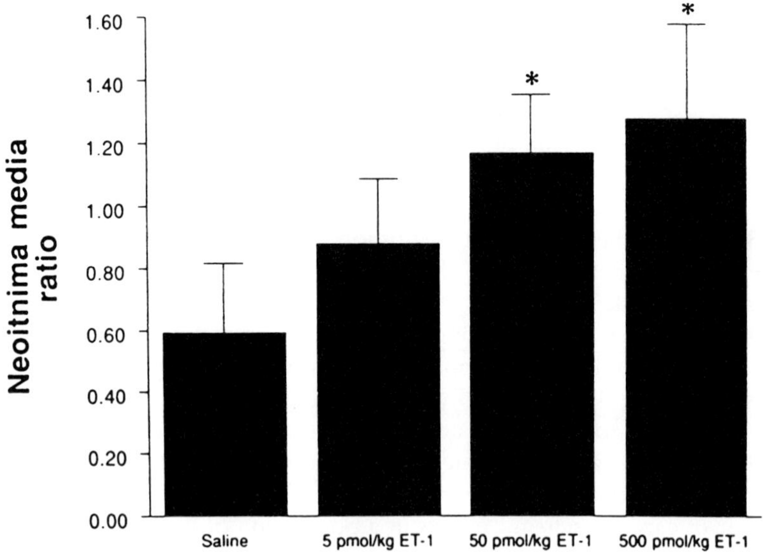

FIGURE 6 An acute thirty minute intra-arterial infusion of endothelin-1 (ET-1) dose-dependently enhances neointimal formation, expressed as the ratio of neointima to media, in rat carotid arteries examined 14 days after balloon angioplasty. ET-1 was administered at 5, 50 or 500 pmol/kg; n = 6, 8, and 7, respectively. Reprinted with permission from Douglas, S. A., Louden, C., Vickery-Clark, L. M., Storer, B. L., Hart, T., Feurstein, G. Z., Elliott, J. D., and Ohlstein, E. H. (1994). A role for endogenous endothelin-1 in neointimal formation after carotid artery balloon angioplasty: Protective effects of the novel nonpeptide endothelin receptor antagonist SB 209670. Circ Res 75(1), 190–197. Copyright by The American Heart Association, 1994.

The long-acting calcium channel blocker benedipine inhibited serum stimulated VSMC proliferation *in vitro* (Ide *et al.*, 1994a) and inhibited proliferation *in vivo* (5 mg/kg PO, BID) after 48 hr (Ide *et al.*, 1994a) or 14 days (Ide *et al.*, 1994b) in the rat carotid injury model. Although three clinical trials failed to demonstrate any benefit of various calcium antagonists (Corcos *et al.*, 1985, Whitworth *et al.*, 1986; O'Keefe *et al.*, 1991), a recent metaanalysis of five studies involving 919 patients did show a small, but statistically significant, reduction in restenosis (Hillegas *et al.*, 1994).

The role of endothelium-derived vasodilating substances in the vasculature continues to command increasing attention for many cardiovascular conditions. Previously known as endothelium-derived relaxing factor, or EDRF, nitric oxide (NO) plays a major role in mediating the control between vasodilatation and vasoconstriction in addition to its known effects on platelet adhesion and aggregation (Moncada *et al.*, 1991). In this latter capacity, NO may play a beneficial role by indirectly preventing the release of platelet-derived mitogens, but it has also been argued that disruption of the endothelium by angioplasty may destroy normal dilator responses to shear stress in the vessel and lead to a chronic constrictor/dilator imbalance and failure of the vessel wall adequately to remodel.

A novel study using chronically inhaled NO (80 ppm for 14 days) inhibited neointimal formation in rats by 43% (Lee *et al.*, 1996). In addition, the nitric oxide donor SPM-5185, when infused into rats for 7 days after balloon injury, inhibited neointimal formation by 85% compared to vehicle controls (Guo *et al.*, 1994). SPM-5185 also accelerated regeneration of the endothelium in injured vessels and restored endothelium-dependent relaxation assessed *in vitro*. Similarly, Groves and coworkers demonstrated that the nitric oxide donor molsidomine could inhibit indices of proliferation (PCNA labeling) in balloon-injured porcine carotid arteries, although the effect did not translate into any morphologic benefit (Groves *et al.*, 1995). Furthermore, the effect on proliferation was evident only in those cases where the internal elastic lamina was not ruptured by the angioplasty, prompting the authors to conclude that the inhibitory effects of NO were overwhelmed by more severe injury. Systemic hypotension and bleeding times, however, are likely to be dose-limiting and suggest that the side effect potential of exogenous NO may argue for a locally directed therapy (see later under Gene Therapy). Despite these findings a recent multicenter clinical restenosis trial with molsidomine is reported to have demonstrated significant clinical and angiographic benefit (Faxon and Currier, 1995b).

Antitumor Agents

In the 1980s a number of studies addressed the potential utility of antiproliferative agents by studying antimitogenic agents in animal models (Muller *et al.*, 1991). Of these, only colchicine appears to have been tested clinically, in the 253-patient CART (Colchicine Angioplasty Restenosis

Trial). When used at conventional doses, the drug was well tolerated, but was without effect (Grines *et al.*, 1991). Two clinical trials evaluated systemic steroids in over 1000 patients in the United States, again without benefit (Stone *et al.*, 1989; Pepine *et al.*, 1990).

More recently, the antitumor agent taxol blocked serum-stimulated VSMC migration and proliferation *in vitro* at nanomolar concentrations (Sollott *et al.*, 1995). Similarly, taxol blocked neointimal formation *in vivo* in the rat balloon injury model when assessed at 14 days postinjury. Mithramycin, a G-C specific DNA binding drug (intercalater) and cytotoxic antibiotic also known as plicamycin, is reported selectively to inhibit transcription of early response genes such as c-*myc*. In the rat carotid injury model mithramycin administered as two doses 1 hr prior to and 1 hr postinjury (150 μg/kg IP) blocked the induction of c-*myc* mRNA levels by 66% 2 hr after injury and inhibited neointimal formation by 50% when assessed 2 weeks later (Chen *et al.*, 1994).

C. Others

Lipid-Lowering Therapies

The 3-hydroxy-3-methylglutaryl coenzyme A (HMG CoA) reductase inhibitors effectively reduce plasma total and low density lipoprotein cholesterol levels (Hagemenas *et al.*, 1990; Endo, 1992). In addition, these agents have antiatherosclerotic activity in animals (Kobayashi *et al.*, 1989; Zhu *et al.*, 1992) and humans (Brown *et al.*, 1990; Illingworth, 1991; Blakenworth, 1991). Although there is no correlation between elevated serum cholesterol levels and risk of restenosis in PTCA patients (Sahni *et al.*, 1991), reductase inhibitors have also been shown to inhibit smooth muscle cell growth *in vitro* (Corsini *et al.*, 1991), a finding which has provided the rationale for their use in models of restenosis.

In a comparative study, the effects of several HMG CoA reductase inhibitors (pravastatin, lovastatin, simvastatin, and fluvastatin) on neointimal formation was determined in normocholesterolemic rabbits (Soma *et al.*, 1993). Three of the drugs significantly inhibited neointimal formation determined morphometrically and all four agents reduced proliferation assessed by index of percent proliferating cells in the vessel wall. These effects of the HMG CoA reductase inhibitors were independent of effects on plasma cholesterol concentrations.

Despite these findings, however, neither lovastatin nor pravastatin inhibited angiographic restenosis in clinical trials (Weintraub *et al.*, 1994; Onaka *et al.*, 1994; Beigel *et al.*, 1995). Although the doses of these agents used in animal models were higher than used clinically, it is unclear if the lack of clinical efficacy lies in dose alone. Clinical trials of fluvastatin are ongoing (Foley *et al.*, 1994).

Elevated levels of lipoprotein a [Lp(a)] have been implicated as a risk factor for restenosis based on retrospective clinical trials (Hearn *et al.*, 1992; Tenda *et al.*, 1993), although the literature remains controversial (Cooke *et al.*, 1994). Animal studies of Lp(a) in models of restenosis are hampered as Lp(a) is only expressed in humans, nonhuman primates, and hedgehogs. Lp(a) shares structural homology with plasminogen, and investigators have proposed that Lp(a) may indirectly potentiate smooth muscle cell proliferation by interfering with TGF-β activation as well acting directly (Grainger *et al.*, 1993). Immunocytochemical studies have shown the presence of Lp(a) in nonhuman primate lesions following balloon angioplasty (Fig. 7) (Ryan *et al.*, 1996). However, the causative role of Lp(a) remains to be proven.

A natural variant of the apolipoprotein (apo) A-1 known as ApoA-1 Milano is reported to confer significant protection against atherosclerotic disease (Soma *et al.*, 1995). Rabbits treated with a recombinant ApoA-1 Milano preparation also demonstrated significant reductions in neointimal formation in response to vascular injury if the therapy was initiated prior to injury. Although the study was conducted in 1% of cholesterol-fed rabbits, treatment had no significant effects on plasma cholesterol levels.

2. *Antioxidants*

Rao and Berk (1992) demonstrated that active oxygen species could stimulate vascular smooth muscle cell growth and proto-oncogene expression. If, in fact, inflammatory cells, recruited to the site of vascular injury, release active oxygen species, the argument would follow for a potential benefit from the use of antioxidants. The antioxidant properties of probucol have been implicated in the antiatherogenic effects of the drug (Carew *et al.*, 1987) and have been studied in models of endothelial reactivity (Nunes *et al.*, 1995). Ferns and co-workers (1992) found that probucol treatment inhibited macrophage accumulation and neointimal formation in a rabbit balloon injury model. More recently, King's group at Emory demonstrated significant improvements in intimal area and residual lumen with high-dose (2 g/day) probucol in pigs (Schneider *et al.*, 1993). Baumann and co-workers (1994) reported that probucol reduced the cellularity of intimal lesions in cholesterol-fed rabbits with prosthetic grafts, suggesting an antiproliferative effect on vascular smooth muscle cells.

Daily vitamin C and E therapy inhibited neointimal formation in a porcine model of balloon-injured coronary arteries, but neither intervention alone was effective (Nunes *et al.*, 1995). The beneficial effects of vitamins correlated with changes in the lipid redox state in the vessel wall, suggesting that the mechanism of action was based on the known antioxidant properties of these agents.

3. *Inhibitors of Cell Adhesion and Migration*

Adhesion of platelets and inflammatory cells to the injured vessel wall is believed to play an important role in the initial cascade of events occurring after balloon injury to the vessel. Balloon injury of the vessel wall disrupts endothelial cells and the cytokine milieu postinjury may promote the upregulation of a host in integrin receptors. A specific arginine–glycine–aspartic acid antagonist of the $\alpha v\beta 3$ integrin receptor GpenGRGDSPCA prevented smooth muscle cell migration *in vitro* and prevented neointimal formation in rabbits when administered locally to balloon-injured carotid arteries (Choi *et al.*, 1994). Because this compound appears to be an inhibitor of VSMC migration, these data provide more evidence to the earlier suggestion that migration is important in the development of neointima in the rabbit model.

Vascular smooth muscle cells have been shown to synthesize a complement of enzymes required for extracullar matrix digestion (Galis *et al.*, 1994); however, the role these matrix metalloproteinases play in smooth muscle cell migration and vessel wall remodeling is controversial. Interstitial collagenase (matrix metalloproteinase type 1) expression is increased in late human restenotic lesions (>4 years) and in atheromatous plaques (Nikkari *et al.*, 1996). Arterial injury in the rat carotid artery balloon model results in an induction of 88-kDa gelatinase and an increase in 68-kDa gelatinase above constitutive levels (Bendeck *et al.*, 1994), and administration of a matrix metalloproteinase inhibitor (GM-6001) reduced smooth muscle cell migration from the media into the neointima by 97%. However, two studies using different matrix metalloproteinase inhibitors failed to demonstrate reductions in neointimal formation in rat models of balloon injury (Bendeck *et al.*, 1996; Zempo *et al.*, 1996).

IV. Gene Therapy

Several molecular-based therapeutic strategies have been advanced for the control of restenosis and a number of reviews are available (Epstein *et al.*, 1994; Mazur *et al.*, 1994a; Nabel *et al.*, 1994). Antisense approaches to inhibition of proliferation have also been widely explored both in cell culture and *in vivo* with varying degrees of efficacy. Table II provides a summary of published studies and a discussion of these approaches follows.

Bennett and co-workers (1994) described the inhibitory effects of c-*myc* antisense oligonucleotides both *in vitro* and in a rat carotid artery balloon injury model. The *in vivo* experiments applied c-*myc* antisense molecules directly to the adventitial surface of the injured vessel with the use of a pluronic gel. Peak vessel wall c-*myc* expression was reduced by 75% and neointimal formation was inhibited at 14 days postinjury compared with sense c-*myc* controls. Experiments conducted in a procine model of coronary artery balloon injury also described growth inhibitory effects of c-*myc* antisense (Shi *et al.*, 1994) (Fig. 8). The porcine studies used a transcatheter approach to deliver antisense oligomers directly to the lumenal surface of the injured vessel during no-flow conditions.

TABLE II Antisense and Gene Therapy Interventions for the Prevention of Restenosis

Target/mechanism	*Animal model*	*Effect*	*Reference*
Antisense strategies			
c-*myc*	Rat carotid artery	↓ neointima	Bennett *et al.* (1994)
		No effect	Guzman *et al.* (1994a)
	Porcine coronary artery	↓ neointima	Shi *et al.* (1994)
c-*myb*	Rat carotid artery	↓ neointima	Simons *et al.* (1992)
		No effect	Guzman *et al.* (1994a)
PCNA	Rat carotid artery	No effect	Guzman *et al.* (1994a)
cdk2	Rat carotid artery	↓ neointima	Abe *et al.* (1994)
cdc2	Rat carotid artery	↓ neointima	Abe *et al.* (1994)
Gene therapy			
tk–ganciclovir	Rat carotid artery	↓ neointima	Guzman *et al.* (1994b) Ohno *et al.* (1994)
	Porcine femoral artery	↓ neointima	Ohno *et al.* (1994)
Retinoblastoma protein	Rat carotid artery	↓ neointima	Chang *et al.* (1995a)
	Porcine femoral artery	↓ neointima	Chang *et al.* (1995a)
p21	Rat carotid artery	↓ neointima	Chang *et al.* (1995b)
E2F decoy	Rat carotid artery	↓ neointima	Morishita *et al.* (1995)
ecNOS	Rat carotid artery	↓ neointima	Von Der Leyen *et al.* (1995)

Antisense oligonucleotides to cdk2 kinase and cdc2 kinase inhibited neointimal formation in a balloon-injured rat carotid artery (Morishita *et al.*, 1994a). The same study found that a combination of cdc2 and cdk2 kinase antisense oligomers was more efficacious than monotherapy targeting just one kinase. In these experiments the investigators delivered the product by means of a hemagglutinating virus of Japan (HVJ) liposome-mediated transfer. This vehicle appears to be unique in achieving a prolonged transfection efficiency in that fluorescently labeled oligoes had a sevenfold increase in vessel wall residence time compared to non-HVJ controls (Morishita *et al.*, 1994b).

Abe and co-workers (1994) also described the use of both cdc2 and cdk2 antisense oligomers to inhibit rat carotid artery balloon injury; neointimal formation was reduced approximately 50% when assessed 14 days after injury. In these experiments, Abe and co-workers (1994) delivered their antisense molecules to the injured vessel topically in a pluronic gel using a similar methodology to that described previously (Bennett *et al.*, 1994).

Although a number of experiments have detailed the efficacy of various antisense strategies in models of restenosis, not all investigators are in agreement. Guzman and co-workers (1994a) reported that antisense strategies to c-*myb*, c-*myc*, and PCNA (proliferating cell nuclear antigen) were ineffective

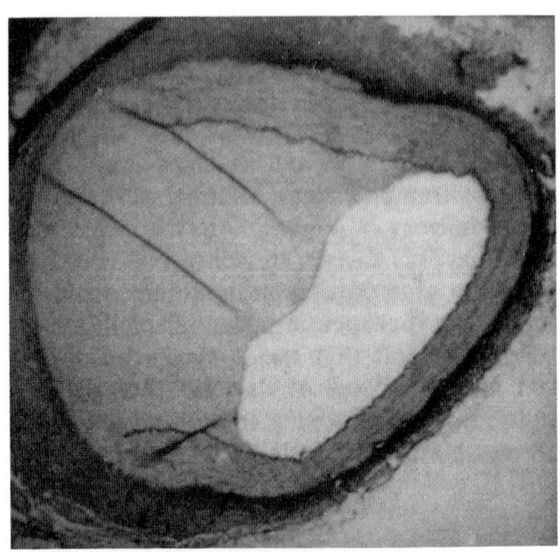

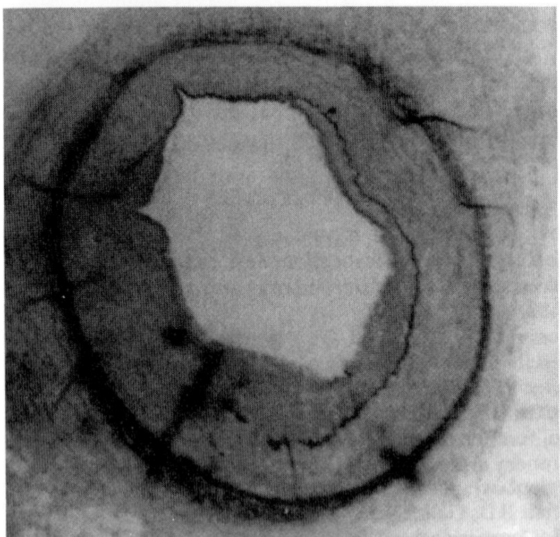

FIGURE 8 Antisense oligomers directed against c-*myc* inhibit neointimal formation in a porcine coronary artery model of balloon injury. The severity of injury was similar as evidenced by the disruption in the internal elastic laminae in both vessels; however neointimal formation was attenuated with antisense treatment. Reprinted with permission from Shi, Y., Fard, A., Galeo, A., Hutchinson, H. G., Vermani, P., Dodge, G. R., Hall, D. J., Shaheen, F., and Zalewski, A., (1994). Transcatheter delivery of c-*myc* antisense oligomers reduces neointimal formation in a porcine model of coronay artery balloon injury. Circulation 90(2), 944–951. Copyright by The American Heart Association, 1994.

at inhibiting the growth response to injury in rat carotid arteries. Others have cautioned that although antisense molecules block smooth muscle cell proliferation, the mechanism of action may not be due to specific hybridization to target DNA as previously hypothesized (Burgess *et al.*, 1995; Bennett and Schwartz, 1995).

In addition to antisense approaches, some researchers have transfected the arterial wall with genes encoding growth inhibitory molecules. Two laboratories have described adenovirus-mediated gene transfer of the herpes simplex virus thymidine kinase (tk) gene (Guzman *et al.*, 1994b; Ohno *et al.*, 1994) (Fig. 9). When exposed to the prodrug ganciclovir, cells expressing the tk gene form an agent that blocks DNA synthesis. The tk–ganciclovir strategy inhibited neointimal formation and smooth muscle cell proliferation in both balloon-injured rat carotid arteries and procine iliofemoral arteries. In a separate series of experiments, adenovirus-mediated overexpression of the cyclin/cyclin-dependent kinase inhibitor p21 *in vitro* arrested vascular smooth muscle cells in the G1 phase of the cell cycle and inhibited phosphorylation of the retinoblastoma gene product (Chang *et al.*, 1995a). Transfection of injured rat carotid arteries with the p21 gene construct also inhibited neointimal formation *in vivo*. A slightly different approach has used overexpression of a mutated form of the retinoblastoma protein, which can also arrest cell cycle progression both *in vitro* and *in vivo* (Chang *et al.*, 1995b). An additional gene therapy strategy has utilized a transcription factor decoy of the E2F-binding site to inhibit neointimal formation in the balloon-injured rat carotid artery (Morishita *et al.*, 1995).

As mentioned earlier, NO donors have been shown to inhibit neointimal formation *in vivo* (Lee *et al.*, 1996; Guo *et al.*, 1994). At Stanford, Dzau and co-workers transfected constitutive nitric oxide synthase into injured rat carotid arteries using HVJ liposome-mediated gene transfer (Von Der Leyen *et al.*, 1995). Results suggested that this enzyme, responsible for the generation of NO, inhibited neointimal formation 70% at 14 days postinjury. In addition to inhibition of neointimal formation, the authors also demonstrated that NO production was restored in injured vessels and that the impaired vascular reactivity in response to injury was normalized.

Although gene therapy has received enormous attention, a number of issues remain about the efficiency of gene transfer and techniques for local delivery. Adenoviral vectors are far more effective than earlier lipofectin formulations for delivering foreign genes into arteries *in vivo* (French *et al.*, 1994; Mazur *et al.*, 1994b), and evidence suggests that the efficiency of adenoviral transfection is not altered in the presence of atherosclerosis (French *et al.*, 1994). Other investigators have reported a 10-fold increase in the transduction rate of a reporter gene when adenoviral gene constructs were administered in the presence of a biocompatible polyol. It is thought that polyol may have maintained high pericellular vector concentrations, thereby enhancing transfection efficiency (March *et al.*, 1995). Losordo and

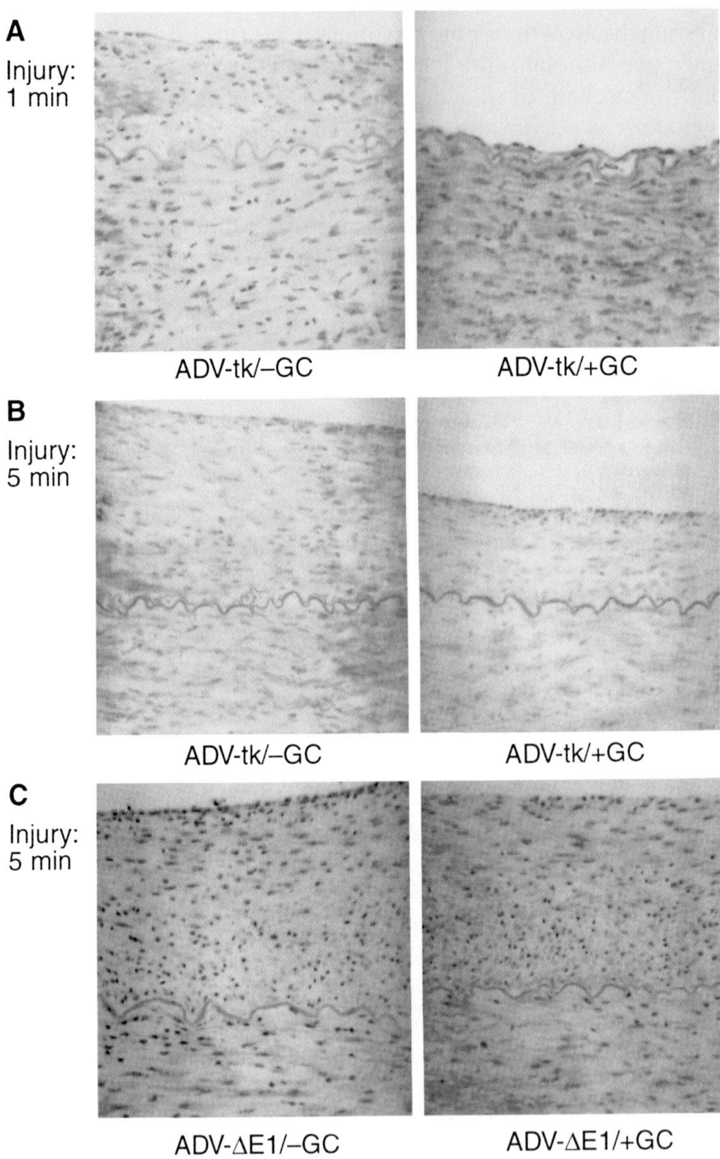

FIGURE 9 Effect of ganciclovir treatment on intimal and medial areas in porcine femoral arteries after balloon injury and infection with an adenoviral construct containing the gene encoding for thymidine kinase (ADV-tk/+GC). Vehicle treatments included the tk transfection without ganciclovir therapy (ADV-tk/-GC) or transfection with an adenoviral vector lacking E1 and containing no insert (ADVΔE1/+GC) and ganciclovir. Reprinted with permission from Ohno, T., Gordon, D., San, H., Pompili, V., Imperiale, M. J., Nabel, G. J., and Nabel, E. G., (1994). Gene therapy for vascular smooth muscle cell proliferation after arterial injury. Science 265, 781–784. Copyright by The American Association for the Advancement of Science, 1994.

co-workers (1994) have cautioned that quantification of gene transfer by histological techniques such as immunocytochemistry or *in situ* hybridization may underestimate the true magnitude of transgene expression: the authors suggest that measurements of secreted protein from the vessel wall may be more appropriate.

In summary, the gene therapy trials in animal models of vascular injury have been uniquely exciting in their positive results; however, a number of hurdles remain. Adenoviral vectors appear to be the best means of vessel wall transfection with respect to efficiency of transfection. However, inflammation associated with the administration of adenovirus to the normal vessel wall (Newman *et al.,* 1995) argues strongly against its utility in the clinic. Although HVJ liposome-mediated gene transfer has been utilized successfully by one laboratory, a wider experience with this methodology is needed to confirm the success. Clearly attention to nonviral vectors and novel means of gene delivery are needed to advance the field.

V. Nonpharmacologic Approaches

A. Irradiation/Light Therapy

Gamma radiation as a means of limiting intimal hyperplasia following balloon injury has been assessed in the rat carotid artery model (Shimotakahara and Mayberg, 1994). Radiation doses of 1.5 or 2.25 rads significantly inhibited neointimal formation when delivered by external beam 1 or 2 days after the injury. Similarly, low-dose intracoronary radiation (2 rads administered by catheter immediately prior to injury) significantly inhibited neointimal formation and reduced the percentage stenosis in porcine coronary arteries when evaluated 6 months later (Wiedermann *et al.,* 1995). Additional dose and time to treatment studies in pigs have demonstrated a radiation dose–response relationship and documented that treatment 2 days postinjury is more efficacious than immediate therapy (Waksman *et al.,* 1995b). The use of ionizing radiation in conjunction with stent implantation, whether given externally (Waksman *et al.,* 1995a) or in the form of radioactive stents (Hehrlein *et al.,* 1995), has been shown to confer additional benefit.

Photodynamic therapy, or the light-based activation of photosensitizing agents to generate cytotoxic mediators, is another technique that has been evaluated for the prevention of restenosis. 5-Aminolevulinic acid-induced protoporphyrin IX was administered to rats undergoing balloon injury; laser illumination of the carotid arteries was used for activation (Nyamekye *et al.,* 1994). Photodynamic therapy completely inhibited neointimal formation determined at either 14 or 28 days postinjury. Using a different photosensitizer, aluminum disulfonated phthalocyanine, these same authors again demonstrated efficacy in a balloon-injured rat carotid artery (Nyamekye *et al.,*

1995). However, it should be noted that both studies also described cellular depletion and damage in normal vessels, raising concerns of nonspecificity in the uptake of the photosensitizing agents and an inability to accurately restrict the laser to localized areas of the vasculature.

B. Mechanical Interventions

The prevention of restenosis has also been tackled using mechanical interventions, and data are beginning to document that intracoronary stenting can significantly reduce restenosis in clinical trials (Yellai and Schatz, 1994) (Fig. 10). The current Benestent (Belgian–Netherlands Stent Trial) Serruys *et al.,* 1994) and Stress (Stent Restenosis Study) (Fischman *et al.,* 1994) trials are generating enormous enthusiasm in the cardiovascular community. Although information from these trials is still being accumulated, restenosis rates as low as 8–10% have been suggested. In addition to their use in coronary arteries, stents have been successfully employed in hemodialysis shunt access sites, atherosclerotic renal artery stenosis, and saphenous vein graft lesions (Beathard, 1992; Dorros *et al.,* 1995; Dunlop *et al.,* 1995; Gray *et al.,* 1995; Wong *et al.,* 1995). By maintaining the anatomical lumen of the artery, it has been suggested that stents prevent acute elastic recoil and achieve a larger postprocedural luminal diameter (Carrozza *et al.,* 1994). Similar, longer-term mechanisms may account for the observed benefits of stents in restenosis by preventing chronic narrowing of the luminal diameter

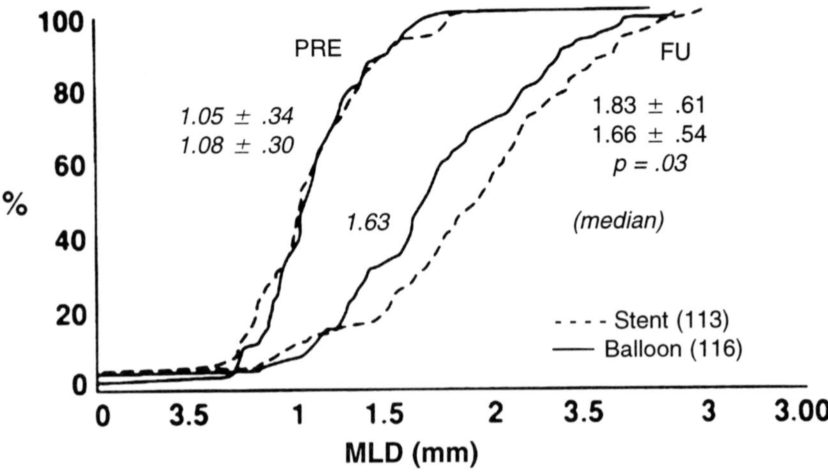

FIGURE 10 Results of the BENESTENT trial comparing minimum luminal diameter (MLD) in stent-treated vs. PTCA treated patients. The MLD in stent treated patients is 1.83 mm compared to 1.66 mm in PTCA-treated patients at 6 month follow-up. Reprinted with permission from Yellai, S. S., and Schatz, R. A., (1994). Indications and use of the Palmaz-Schatz coronary stent. Cardiol Clin 12(4), 651–663. Copyright by Harcourt Brace & Co., 1994.

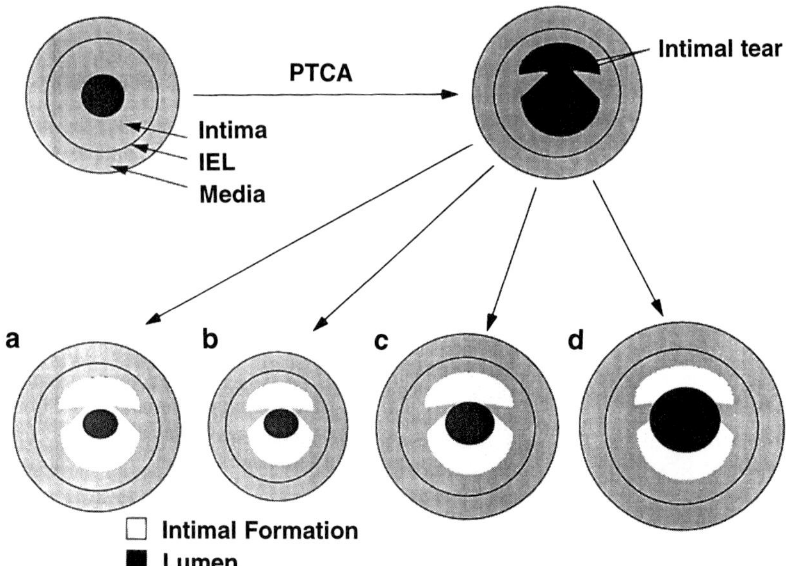

FIGURE 11 Expanded paradigm of restenosis after angioplasty. Several possible responses to balloon injury are illustrated. The classical paradigm (a) is intimal formation with no remodeling. If vascular constriction occurs (b), even minimal amounts of neointimal may result in restenosis. A moderate amount of compensatory enlargement (c) may accommodate neointima with less lumen narrowing. Augmented compensatory enlargement (d) may result in a widely patent artery despite significant intimal formation. IEL = internal elastic lamina, PTCA = percutaneous transluminal coronary angioplasty. Reprinted with permission from the American College of Cardiology (Currier and Faxon, Journal of the American College of Cardiology, 1995, 25(2), 516–520).

(Currier and Faxon, 1995) (Fig. 11). Ultrasound and angiographic data from the stent trials suggest that the mechanism by which stents "prevent" restenosis is by achieving a larger initial postprocedural lumen area (Kimura *et al.*, 1994). Interestingly, investigators have suggested that "stent restenosis" can be attributed soley to intimal proliferation (Klauss *et al.*, 1993), suggesting the combination of stents with antiproliferatives may provide an added benefit.

VI. Issues Related to Local Product Delivery

Local delivery of drugs, proteins, or genes permits a therapeutic effect at the site of action without exposing the rest of the body to the particular agent (Riessen and Isner, 1994). Although local delivery has been considered for many diseases, a confounding issue in many has been the technology for the delivery itself, as in most cases this requires an invasive process. Local delivery to the arterial wall is therefore particularly attractive in an angioplasty setting because the intravascular access has already been accomplished by virtue of the intervention. Several delivery systems have been explored clinically, including a hydrogel-coated balloon used to deliver a gene-encoding vascular endothelial cell growth factor to peripheral vessels (Isner *et al.*, 1995) and a porous balloon used to deliver tissue plasminogen activator to coronary vessels (Cumnerland *et al.*, 1994). A number of issues regarding pressure and volume are currently being explored with local-delivery catheters (Fram *et al.*, 1994; Lambert *et al.*, 1994).

In addition to specialized catheters, a variety of drug polymer composites are under evaluation as controlled release reservoirs (Levy *et al.*, 1994, 1995; March *et al.*, 1994). Labhesetwar and co-workers (1995) reported on a nanoparticle system used to deliver the antiproliferative agent U-86983 to pig coronary arteries. In this study, neointimal formation was significantly reduced in treated pigs and histologic examination demonstrated the presence of U-86983 in the vessel wall 2 weeks after injury. Local delivery of microparticles containing colchicine in an atherosclerotic rabbit model similarly showed a beneficial effect; importantly, local delivery of colchicine alone (i.e., without microparticle formulation) was ineffective in this model (Gradus-Pizlo *et al.*, 1995).

Given the success with intracoronary stenting, the use of coated stents is likely to be our first successful "local delivery" in the coronary vasculature. Clinical trials using heparin-coated stents are currently in progress.

Our understanding of some of the mechanisms involved in the pathological mechanisms involved in restenosis has resulted in some novel approaches: Crawford and co-workers (1995) loaded platelets with the prostacycline analog iloprost *ex vivo* and used the thrombogenicity of the vessel wall to deliver the drug to balloon-injured rat carotid arteries. By adhering to the thrombogenic surface and releasing iloprost, the platelets effectively acted as a local delivery system, resulting in a significant reduction in the neointimal area.

VII. Summary and Conclusions

One of the most frustrating aspects of restenosis is that it is the result of advances in medical care (there was no restenosis before the days of balloon angioplasty), yet it seems to be resistant to all that science has to offer. Still we believe there is reason to be optimistic. We are at last beginning to see some promise from clinical trials, and data being generated confirm some of the hypotheses previously generated from animal experiments. Thus the effects seen with the GP IIb/IIIa antibody 7E3 suggest that thrombosis may be as important in its long-term sequelae as it is for acute reocclusion. The jury is still out on whether antiproliferative approaches will be a therapeutic option, but local delivery paradigms using novel formulations delivered by catheter or impregnated in stents may allow the concept to be tested without the risk of systemic toxicity. Plans are also underway for gene therapy trials, although we may have to wait for better vector technology before taking these into the coronary bed. Perhaps we should move away from the "single pill" approach and accept that, like many infections, malignancies, or even heart failure, a multifaceted approach with combination therapy will provide the first glimmer of that brighter tomorrow.

References

Abe, J. I., Zhou, W., Taguchi, J. I., Takuwa, N., Miki, K., and Okazaki, H. (1994). Suppression of neointimal smooth muscle cell accumulation in vivo by antisense cdc2 and cdk2 oligonucleotides in rat carotid artery. *Biochem. Biophys. Res. Commun.* **198**(1), 16–24.

Azuma, H., Niimi, Y., and Hamasaki, H. (1992). Prevention of intimal thickening after endothelial removal by a nonpeptide angiotensin II receptor antagonist, losartan. *Br. J. Pharmacol.* **106**(3), 665–671.

Azuma, H., Hamasaki, H., and Niimi, Y. (1994). Endothelin (ET-1) plays a role in the intimal hyperplasia after endothelial removal. *Can. J. Physiol. Pharmacol.* **72**, Suppl. 1, I54.

Barry, W. L., and Sarembock, I. J. (1994). Antiplatelet and anticoagulant therapy in patients undergoing percutaneous transluminal coronary angioplasty. *Cardiol. Clin.* **12**(3), 571–535.

Baumann, D. S., Doblas, M., Schonfeld, G., Sicard, G. A., and Daugherty, A. (1994). Probucol reduces the cellularity of aortic intimal thickening at anastomotic regions adjacent to prosthetic grafts in cholesterol-fed rabbits. *Arterioscler. Thromb.* **14**, 162–167.

Bauters, C., Van Belle, E., Wernert, N., Delcayre, C., Thomas, F., Dupuis, B., Lablanche, J. M., Bertrand, M. E., and Swynghedauw, B. (1994). Angiopeptin inhibits oncogene induction in rabbit aorta after balloon denudation. *Circulation* **89**(5), 2327–2331.

Beathard, G. A. (1992). Percutaneous transvenous angioplasty in the treatment of vascular access stenosis. *Kidney Int.* **42**, 1390–1397.

Beigel, Y., Zafrir, N., Teplitzky, Y., Neuman, Y., Gavish, D., Wurzel, M., and Fainaru, M. (1995). The effect of lovastatin on early restenosis. *J. Clin. Pharmacol.* **35**(6), 599–605.

Bendeck, M. P., Zempo, N., Clowes, A. W., Galardy, R. E., and Reidy, M. A. (1994). Smooth muscle cell migration and matrix metalloproteinase expression after arterial injury in the rat. *Circ. Res.* **75**, 539–545.

Bendeck, M. P., Irvin, C., and Reidy, M. A. (1996). Inhibition of matrix metalloprteinase activity inhibits smooth muscle cell migration but not neointimal thickening after arterial injury. *Circ. Res.* **78**, 38–43.

Bennett, M. R., and Schwartz, S. M. (1995). Antisense therapy for angioplasty restenosis: Some critical considerations. *Circulation* **92**(7), 1981–1993.

Bennett, M. R., Anglin, S., McEwan, J. R., Jagoe, R., Newby, A. C., and Evan, G. I. (1994). Inhibition of vascular smooth muscle cell proliferation in vitro and in vivo by c-myc antisense oligodeoxynucleotides. *J. Clin. Invest.* **93**(2), 820–828.

Bilazarian, S. D., Currier, J. W., Tsunekazu, K., Haudenschild, C. C., and Faxon, D. P. (1992). Angiotensin II antagonism does not prevent restenosis after rabbit iliac angioplasty. *Circulation* **86**(4), I–187.

Blakenworth, D. H. (1991). Blood lipids and human atherosclerosis regression: The angiographic evidence. *Curr. Opin. Lipidol.* **2**, 2324–2329.

Bochaton-Piallat, M. L., Gabbiani, F., Redard, M., Desmouliere, A., and Gabbiani, G. (1995). Apoptosis participates in cellularity regulation during rat aortic intimal thickening. *Am. J. Pathol.* **146**(5), 1059–1064.

Brack, M., Ray, S., Chauhan, A., Fox, J., Schofield, P., and Harley, A. (1994). Subcutaneous heparin and angioplasty restenosis prevention: Results of a multicentre randomised trial evaluating unfractionated heparin. *Br. Heart J.* **71**(5), P29.

Brown, G., Albers, J. J., Fisher, L. D., Schaeffer, S. M., Lin, J. T., Kaplan, C., Zhao, X. Q., Bisson, B. D., Fitzpatrick, V. F., and Dodge, H. T. (1990). Regression of coronary artery disease as a result of intensive lipid-lowering therapy in men with high levels of apolipoprotein B. *N. Engl. J. Med.* **323**, 1289–1298.

Buchdunger, E., Zimmermann, J., Mett, H., Meyer, T., Muller, M., Regenass, U., and Lydon, N. B. (1995). Selective inhibition of the platelet-derived growth factor signal transduction pathway by a protein-tyrosine kinase inhibitor of the 2-phenylaminopyrimidine class. *Proc. Natl. Acad. Sci. U.S.A.* **92**, 2558–2562.

Burgess, T. L., Fisher, E. F., Ross, S. L., Bready, J. V., Qian, Y. X., Bayewitch, L. A., Cohen, A. M., Herrera, C. J., Hu, S. S. F., Kramer, T. B., Lott, F. D., Martin, F. H., Pierce, G. F., Simonet, L., and Farrell, C. (1995). The antiproliferative activity of c-myb and c-myc antisense oligonucleotides in smooth muscle cells is caused by a nonantisense mechanism. *Proc. Natl. Acad. Sci. U.S.A.* **92**(9), 4051–4055.

Carew, T. E., Schwenke, D. C., and Steinberg, D. (1987). Antiatherogenic effect of probucol unrelated to its hypocholesterolemic effect: Evidence that antioxidants in vivo can selectively inhibit low density lipoprotein degradation in macrophage-rich fatty streaks and slow the progression of atherosclerosis in the Watanabe heritable hyperlipidemic rabbit. *Proc. Natl. Acad. Sci. U.S.A.* **84**, 7725–7729.

Carrozza, J. P., Kuntz, K. R., Schatz, R. A., Leon, M., Goldberg, S., Savage, M., Fischman, D., Senerchia, C., Diver, D. J., and Baim, D. S. (1994). Inter-series differences in the restenosis rate of Palmaz-Schatz coronary stent placement: Differences in demographics and post-procedure lumen diameter. *Catheterization Cardiovasc. Diagn.* **31**(3), 173–178.

Carter, A. J., Laird, J. R., Farb, A., Kufs, W., Wortham, D. C., and Virmani, R. (1994). Morphologic characteristics of lesion formation and time course of smooth muscle cell proliferation in a porcine proliferative restenosis model. *J. Am. Coll. Cardiol.* **24**(5), 1398–1405.

Casscells, W. (1992). Migration of smooth muscle and endothelial cells, critical events in restenosis. *Circulation* **86**(3), 723–729.

Castronuovo, J. J., Jr., Guss, S. B., Mysh, D., Sawhney, A., Wolff, M., and Gown, A. M. (1995). Cytokine therapy for arterial restenosis: Inhibition of neointimal hyperplasia by gamma-interferon. *Cardiovasc. Surg.* **3**(5), 463–468.

Chang, M. W., Barr, E., Lu, M. M., Seltzer, J., Jiang, Y. Q., Nabel, G. J., Nabel, E. G., Parmacek, M. S., and Leiden, J. M. (1995a). Cytostatic gene therapy for vascular proliferrative disorders with a constitutively active form of the retinoblastoma gene product. *Science* **267**, 520–522.

Chang, M. W., Barr, E., Lu, M. M., Barton, K., and Leiden, J. M. (1995b). Adenovirus-mediated over-expression of the cyclin/cyclindependent kinase inhibitor, p21 inhibits vascular smooth muscle cell proliferation and neointima formation in the rat carotid artery model of balloon angioplasty. *J. Clin. Invest.* **96**(5), 2260–2268.

Chen, S. J., Chen, Y. F., Miller, D. M., Li, H., and Oparil, S. (1994). Mithramyacin inhibit myointimal proliferation after balloon injury of the rat carotid artery in vivo. *Circulation* **90**(5), 2468–2473.

Chesebro, J. H., Webster, M. W., Reeder, G. S., Mock, M. B., Grill, D. E., and Bailey, K. R. (1989). Coronary angioplasty: Antiplatelet therapy reduces acute complications but not restenosis. *Circulation* **80**, II–64.

Choi, E. T., Engel, L., Callow, A. D., Sun, S., Trachtenberg, J., Santoro, S., and Ryan, U. S. (1994). Inhibition of neointimal hyperplasia by blocking alpha-v-beta-3 integrin with a small peptide antagonist GpenGRGDSPCA. *J. Vasc. Surg.* **19**(1), 125–134.

Clowes, A. W., and Karnovsky, M. J. (1977). Suppression by heparin of smooth muscle cell proliferation in injured arteries. *Nature (London)* **265**, 625–626.

Clowes, A. W., and Schwartz, S. M. (1985). Significance of quiescent smooth muscle migration in the injured rat carotid artery. *Circ. Res.* **56,** 139–145.

Clowes, A. W., Reidy, M. A., and Clowes, M. M. (1983a). Mechanisms of stenosis after arterial injury. *Lab. Invest.* **49**(2), 208–215.

Clowes, A. W., Reidy, M. A., and Clowes, M. M. (1983b). Kinetics of cellular proliferation after arterial injury. I. Smooth muscle cell growth in the absence of endothelium. *Lab. Invest.* **49,** 327–333.

Clowes, A. W., Clowes, M. M. and Reidy, M. A. (1986). Kinetics of cellular proliferation after arterial injury. III. Endothelial and smooth muscle cell growth in chronically denuded vessels. *Lab. Invest.* **54,** 295–303.

Clozel, J. P., Hess, P., Michael, C., Schietinger, K., and Baumgartner, H. R. (1991). Inhibition of converting enzyme and neointima formation after vascular injury in rabbits and guinea pigs. *Hypertension (Dallas)* **18,** Suppl. 4, I155–I159.

Colomb, G., Fishbein, I., Banai, S., Moscovitz, D., Msihaly, D., Gertz, S. D., Gazit, A., and Levitski, A. (1994). Restenosis therapy by site-specific delivery of tyrphostins in animal models. *Pharm. Res.* **11**(S10), 610.

Cooke, T., Sheahan, R., Foley, D., Reilly, M., D'Arcy, G., Jauch, W., Gibney, M., Gearty, G., Crean, P., and Walsh, M. (1994). Lipoprotein (a) in restenosis after percutaneous transluminal coronary angioplasty and coronary artery disease. *Circulation* **89,** 1593–1598.

Corcos, T., David, P. R., Val, P. G., Renkin, J., Dangoisse, V., and Rapold, H. G. (1985). Failure of diltiazem to prevent restenosis after percutaneous transluminal coronary angioplasty. *Am. Heart J.* **109,** 926–931.

Corsini, A., Raiteri, M., Soma, M. R., Fumagalli, R., and Paoletti, R. (1991). Simvastatin but not pravastatin inhibits the proliferation of rat aorta myocytes. *Pharmacol. Res.* **23,** 173–180.

Crawford, N., Chajara, A., Pfielgler, G., El Gamal, D., Brewer, L., and Capron, L. (1995). Targeting platelets containing electro-encapsulated iloprost to balloon injured aorta in rats. *Thromb. Haemostasis* **73**(3), 535–542.

Culp, S. C., Zidar, J. P., Jackman, J. D., Phillips, H. R., Overman, A. B., and Stack, R. S. (1992). An improved rabbit model of atherosclerosis. *Circulation* **86**(4), I–188.

Cumnerland, D. C., Gunn, J., Tsikaderis, D., Arafa, S., and Ahsan, A. (1994). Initial clinical experience of local drug delivery via a porous balloon during percutaneous coronary angioplasty. *J. Am. Coll. Cardiol.* **23,** 186A.

Currier, J. W., and Faxon, D. P. (1995). Restenosis after percutaneous transluminal angioplasty: Have we been aiming at the wrong target? *J. Am. Coll. Cardiol.* **25**(2), 516–520.

Daemen, M. J. A. P., Lombardi, D. M., Bosman, F. T., and Schwartz, S. M. (1991). Angiotensin II induces smooth muscle cell proliferation in the normal and injured rat arterial wall. *Circ. Res.* **68,** 450–456.

Dorros, G., Jaff, M., Jain, A., Dufek, C., and Mathiak, L. (1995). Follow-up of primary Palmaz-Schatz stent placement for atherosclerotic renal artery stenosis. *Am. J. Cardiol.* **75**(1), 1051–1055.

Douglas, S. A., Louden, C., Vickery-Clark, L. M., Storer, B. L., Hart, T., Feurstein, G. Z., Elliott, J. D., and Ohlstein, E. H. (1994). A role for endogenous endothelin-1 in neointimal formation after carotid artery balloon angioplasty: Protective effects of the novel nonpeptide endothelin receptor antagonist SB 209670. *Circ. Res.* **75**(1), 190–197.

Douglas, S. A., Vickery-Clark, L. M., Louden, C., and Ohlstein, E. H. (1995). Selective ETA receptor antagonism with BQ-123 is insufficient to inhibit angioplasty induced neointimal formation in the rat. *Cardiovasc. Res.* **29**(5), 641–646.

Dunlop, P., Varty, K., Hartshorne, T., Bell, P. R., Bolia, A., and London, N. J. (1995). Percutaneous transluminal angioplasty of infrainguinal vein graft stenosis: Long-term outcome. *Br. J. Surg.* **82**(2), 204–206.

Edelman, E. R., and Karnovsky, M. J. (1994). Contrasting effects of the intermittant and continuous administration of heparin in experimental restenosis. *Circulation* **89**(2), 770–776.

Edelman, E. R., Nugent, M. A., Smith, L. T., and Karnovsky, M. J. (1992). Basic fibroblast growth factor enhances the coupling of intimal hyperplasia and proliferation of vasa vasorum in injured rat arteries. *J. Clin. Invest.* **89**, 465–473.

Elliott, J. M., Berdan, L. G., Holmes, D. R., Isner, J. M., King, S. B., III, Keeler, G. P., Kearney, M., Califf, R. M., and Topol, E. J., for the CAVEAT Study Investigators (1995). One-year follow-up in the coronary angioplasty versus excisional atherectomy trial (CAVEAT I). *Circulation* **91**, 2158–2166.

Emanuelsson, H., Beatt, K. J., Bagger, J. P., Balcon, R., Heikkila, J., Piessen, J., Schaeffer, M., Suryapranta, H., and Foegh, M. (1995). Long-term effects of angiopeptin treatment in coronary angioplasty. Reduction of clinical but not angiographic restenosis. *Circulation* **91**(6), 1689–1696.

Endo, A. (1992). The discovery and development of HMG-CoA reductase inhibitors. *J. Lipid Res.* **33**, 1569–1582.

EPIC Investigators (1994). Use of a monoclonal antibody directed against the platelet gylocoprotein IIb/IIIa receptor in high-risk coronary angioplasty. *N. Engl. J. Med.* **330**, 956–961.

Epstein, S. E., Speir, E., Unger, E. F., Guzman, R. J., and Finkel, T. (1994). The basis of molecular strategies for treating coronary restenosis after angioplasty. *J. Am. Coll. Cardiol.* **23**(6), 1278–1288.

Eriksen, U. H., Amtorp, O., Bagger, J. P., Emanuelsson, H., Foegh, M., Henningsen, P., Saunamaki, K., Schaeffer, M., Thayssen, P., Orskov, H., Kuntz, R. E., and Popma, J. J. (1995). Randomized double-blind Scandinavian trial of angiopeptin versus placebo for the prevention of clinical events and restenosis after coronary balloon angioplasty. *Am. Heart J.* **130**(1), 1–8.

Faxon, D. P. (1993). Mechanisms of angioplasty and pathophysiology of restenosis based on cell biology. *In* "Practical Angioplasty" (D. Faxon, ed.), pp. 5–13. Raven Press, New York.

Faxon, D. P. (1995). On behalf of the multicenter American research trial with cilazapril after angioplasty to prevent transluminal coronary obstruction and restenosis (MARCATOR) study group. Effect of high dose angiotensin-converting enzyme inhibition on restenosis: Final results of the MARCATOR study, a multicenter, double-blind, placebo-controlled trial of cilazapril. *J. Am. Coll. Cardiol.* **2**, 362–369.

Faxon, D. P., and Currier, J. W. (1995). Prevention of post-PTCA restenosis. *Ann. N.Y. Acad. Sci.* **748**, 419–427.

Faxon, D. P., Weber, V. J., Haudenschild, C., Gottsman, S. B., McGovern, W. A., and Ryan, T. J. (1982). Acute effects of transluminal angioplasty in three models of atherosclerosis. *Arteriosclerosis (Dallas)* **2**, 125–133.

Faxon, D. P., Sanborn, T. A., and Weber, V. J. (1984). Restenosis following transluminal angioplasty in experimental atherosclerosis. *Arteriosclerosis (Dallas)* **4**, 189–195.

Faxon, D. P., Spiro, T. E., Minor, S., Cote, G., Douglas, J., Gottlieb, R., Califf, R., Dorosti, K., Topol, E., Gordon, J. B., Ohmen, M., and the ERA Investigators (1994). Low molecular weight heparin in prevention of restenosis after angioplasty. *Circulation* **90**, 908–914.

Ferns, G. A. A., Forster, L., Stewart-Lee, A., Konneh, M., Nourooz-Zadeh, J., and Anggard, E. E. (1992). Probucol inhibits neointimal thickening and macrophage accumulation after balloon injury in the cholesterol-fed rabbit. *Proc. Natl. Acad. Sci. U.S.A.* **89**, 11312–11316.

Ferrer, P., Valentine, M., Jenkins-West, T., Weber, H., Goller, N. L., Durham, S. K., Molloy, C. J., and Moreland, S. (1995). Oraly active endothelin receptor antagonist BMS-182874 suppresses neointimal development in balloon-injured rat carotid arteries. *J. Cardiovasc. Pharmacol.* **26**, 908–915.

Fischman, D. L., Leon, M. L., Baim, D. S., Schatz, R. A., Savage, M. P., Penn, I., Detre, K., Veltri, L., Ricci, D., Nobuyoshi, M., Cleman, M., Heuser, R., Almond, D., Teirstein,

P. S., Fish, R. D., Colombo, A., Brinker, J., Moses, J., Shaknovich, A., Hirshfeld, J., Bailey, S., Ellis, S. G., Rake, R., and Goldberg, S. for the Stent Restenosis Investigators (1994). A randomised comparison of coronary stent placement and balloon angioplasty in the treatment of coronary artery disease. *N. Engl. J. Med.* **331**, 496–501.

Foegh, M. L., Khirabadi, B. S., Chambers, E., Amamoo, S., and Ramwell, R. W. (1989). Inhibition of coronary artery transplant atherosclerosis in rabbits with angiopeptin, an octapeptide. *Atherosclerosis (Shannon, Irel.)* **78**, 229–236.

Foley, D. P., Bonnier, H., Jackson, G., Macaya, C., Shepherd, J., and Vrolix, M. (1994). Prevention of restenosis after coronary balloon angioplasty: Rationale and design of the Fluvastatin Angioplasty Restenosis (FLARE) Trial. *Am. J. Cardiol.* **73**(14), 50D–61D.

Fram, D. B., Aretz, T., Azrin, M. A., Samady, H., Gillam, L. D., Sahatijan, R., Waters, D., and McKay, R. G. (1994). Localized intramural drug delivery during balloon angioplasty using hydrogel-coated balloons and pressure-augmented diffusion. *J. Am. Coll. Cardiol.* **23**(7), 1570–1577.

Franklin, S. M., and Faxon, D. P. (1993). Pharmacologic prevention of restenosis after coronary angioplasty: Review of randomised clinical trials. *Coronary Artery Dis.* **4** 232–242.

French, B. A., Mazur, W., Ali, N. M., Geske, R. S., Finnigan, J. P., Rodgers, G. P., Roberts, R., and Raizner, A. E. (1994). Percutaneous transluminal in vivo gene transfer by recombinant adenovirus in normal porcine coronary arteries, atherosclerotic arteries, and two models of coronary restenosis. *Circulation* **90**(5), 2402–2413.

Fry, D., Kraker, A. J., McMichael, A., Ambroso, L. A., Nelson, J. M., Leopold, W. R., Connors, R. W., and Bridges, A. J. (1994). A specific inhibitor of the epidermal growth factor receptor tyrosine kinase. *Science* **265**, 1093–1095.

Galis, Z. S., Muszynski, M., Sukhova, G. K., Simon-Morrissey, E., Unemori, E. N., Lark, M. W., Amento, E., and Libby, P. (1994). Cytokine-stimulated human vascular smooth muscle cells synthesize a complement of enzymes required for extracellular matrix digestion. *Circ. Res.* **75**, 181–189.

Geary, R. L., Williams, J. K., Golden, D., Brown, D. G., Benjamin, M. E., and Adams, M. R. (1996). Time course of cellular proliferation, intimal hyperplasia, and remodeling following angioplasty in monkeys with established atherosclerosis. *Arterioscler. Thromb. Vasc. Biol.* **16**, 34–43.

Gershlick, A. H., Spriggins, D., Davies, S. W., Syndercombe-Court, Y. D., Timmins, J., Timmis, A. D., Rothman, M. T., Layton, C., and Balcon, R. (1994). Failure of epoprostenol (prostacyclin, PGI2) to inhibit platelet aggregation and to prevent restenosis after coronary angioplasty: results of a randomised placebo controlled trial. *Br. Heart J.* **71**(1), 7–15.

Gertz, S. D., Gimple, L. W., Banai, S., Ragosta, M., Powers, E. R., Roberts, W. C., Perez, L. S., and Sarembock, I. J. (1994). Geometric remodeling is not the principal pathogenetic process in restenosis after balloon angioplasty. Evidence from correlative angiographic-histomorphometric studies of atherosclerotic arteries in rabbits. *Circulation* **90**(6), 3001–3008.

Glagov, S. (1994). Intimal hyperplasia, vascular remodeling and the restenosis problem. *Circulation* **89**(6), 2888–2891.

Gradus-Pizlo, I., Wilensky, R. L., March, K. L., Fineberg, N., Michaels, M., Sandusky, G. E., and Hathaway, D. R. (1995). Local delivery of biodegradable microparticles containing colchicine or a colchicine analog: Effects on restenosis and implications for catheter-based drug delivery. *J. Am. Coll. Cardiol.* **26**(6), 1549–1557.

Grainger, D., Kirchenlohr, H., Metcalfe, J., Weissberg, P., Wade, D., and Lawn, R. (1993). Proliferation of human smooth muscle cells promoted by lipoprotein (a). *Science* **260**, 1655–1658.

Gray, R. J., Horton, K. M., Dolmatch, B. L., Runback, J. H., Anaise, D., Aquino, A. O., Currier, C. B., Light, J. A., and Sasaki, T. M. (1995). Use of Wallstents for hemodialysis access-related venous stenosis and occlusions untreatable with balloon angioplasty. *Radiology* **195**(2), 479–484.

Grines, C. L., Rizik, D., Levine, A., Schreiber, T., Gangadharan, V., Ramos, R., Choksi, N., Gangadharan, C., and Timmis, G. C. (1991). Colchicine angioplasty restenosis trail (CART). *Circulation* **84,** II–365.

Groves, H. M., Kinlough-Rathbone, R. L., and Richardson, M. (1979). Platelet interaction with damaged rabbit aorta. *Lab. Invest.* **40,** 194–200.

Groves, P. H., Banning, A. P., Penny, W. J., Newby, A. C., Cheadle, H. A., and Lewis, M. J. (1995). The effects of exogenous nitric oxide on smooth muscle cell proliferation following porcine carotid angioplasty. *Cardiovasc. Res.* **30**(1), 87–96.

Gruentzig, A. R., King, S. B., III, Schlumpf, M., Siegenthaler, W. (1979). Nonoperative dilation of caronary-artery stenosis. *N. Engl. J. Med.* **301,** 61–73.

Guo, J. P., Milhoan, K. A., Tuan, R. S., and Lefer, A. M. (1994). Beneficial effect of SPM-5185, a cysteine-containing nitric oxide donor, in rat carotid artery intimal injury. *Circ. Res.* **75**(1), 77–84.

Guzman, L. A., Farrel, C. L., Poptic, E. J., Dicorleto, P. E., and Topol, E. J. (1994a). Despite in vivo cellular and nuclear uptake, antisense oligonucleotides do not have a significant anti-proliferative effect after vascular injury. *Circulation* **90**(4, Part 2), I-147.

Guzman, R. J., Hirschowitz, E. A., Brody, S. L., Crystal, R. G., and Epstein, S. E. (1994b). In vivo suppression of injury-induced vascular smooth muscle cell accumulation using adenovirus-mediated transfer of the herpes simplex virus thymidine kinase gene. *Proc. Natl. Acad. Sci. U.S.A.* **91**(22), 10732–10736.

Hagemenas, F. C., Pappu, A. S., and Illingsworth, D. R. (1990). The effect of simvastatin on plasma lippoproteins and cholesterol homeostasis in patients with heterozygous familial hypercholesterolemia. *Eur. J. Clin. Invest.* **20,** 150–157.

Hansson, G. K. (1994). Immunological control mechanisms in plaque formation. *Basic Res. Cardiol.* **89,** Suppl. 1, 41–46.

Hayry, P., Myllarniemi, M., Aavik, E., Alatalo, S., Aho, P., Yilmaz, S., Raisanen-Sokolowski, A., Cozzone, G., Jameson, B. A., and Baserga, R. (1995). Stabile D-peptide analog of insulin-like growth factor-1 inhibits smooth muscle cell proliferation after carotid ballooning injury in the rat. *FASEB J.* **9**(13), 1336–1344.

Hearn, J., Donohue, B., Ba'alkabi, H., Douglas, J. S., King, S. B., Lembo, N. J., Roubin, G. S., and Sgoutas, D. S. (1992). Usefulness of serum lipoprotein (a) as a predictor of restenosis after percutaneous transluminal coronary angioplasty. *Am. J. Cardiol.* **69,** 736–739.

Hehrlein, C., Gollan, C., Doenges, K., Metz, J., Riessen, R., Fehsenfeld, P., von Hodenberg, E., and Kuebler, W. (1995). Low-dose radioactive endovascular stents prevent smooth muscle cell proliferation and neointimal hyperplasia in rabbits. *Circulation* **92**(6), 1570–1575.

Herrman, J. P. R., Hermans, W. R. M., Vos, J., and Serruys, P. W. (1993). Pharmacological approaches to the prevention of restenosis following angioplasty. *Drugs* **46,** 18–52.

Hillegass, W. B., Ohman, E. M., and Califf, R. A. (1994). Restenosis: The clinical issues. *In* "Textbook of Interventional Cardiology" (E. J. Topol, ed.), pp. 415–435. Saunders, Philadelphia.

Holmes, D. R., Simpson, J. B., Berdan, L. G., Gottlieb, R. S., Leya, F., Keeler, G. P., Califf, R. M., and Topol, E. J. for the CAVEAT I Investigators (1995). Abrupt closure: The CAVEAT I experience. *J. Am. Coll. Cardiol.* **26,** 1494–1500.

Huber, K. C., Schwartz, R. S., Edwards, W. D., Camrud, A. R., Bailey, K. R., Jorgenson, M. A., and Holmes, D. R. (1993). Effects of angiotensin converting enzyme inhibition on neointimal proliferation in a porcine coronary injury model. *Am. Heart J.* **125**(3), 695–701.

Ide, S., Kondoh, M., Satoh, H., and Karasawa, A. (1994a). Anti-proliferative effects of benidipine hydrochloride in porcine cultured vascular smooth muscle cells and in rats subjected to balloon catheter-induced endothelial denudation. *Biol. Pharm. Bull.* **17**(5), 627–631.

Ide, S., Kondoh, M., Satoh, H., and Karasawa, A. (1994b). Inhibitor action of benidipine on balloon catheterization-induced intimal thickening of the carotid artery in rats. *Jpn. J. Pharmacol.* **65**(1), 89–92.

Illingworth, D. G. (1991). HMG CoA reductase inhibitors. *Curr. Opin. Lipidol.* **2,** 24–30.

Indolfi, C., Esposito, G., DiLorenzo, E., Rapacciuolo, A., Feliciello, A., Porcellini, A., Avvedimento, V. E., Condorelli, M., and Chiariello, M. (1995). Smooth muscle cell proliferation is proportional to the degree of balloon injury in a rat model of angioplasty. *Circulation* **92,** 1230–1235.

Irons, C. E., Flynn, M. A., Mok, L. L., and Reynolds, E. E. (1996). Endothelin and platelet-derived growth factor enhance arachadonic acid release and DNA synthesis in vascular smooth muscle cells. *Am. J. Physiol.* **270**(6 Pt. 1), C1642–1646.

Isner, J. M., Walsh, K., Symes, J., Piecek, A., Takeshita, S., Lowry, J., Rossow, S., Rosenfield, K., Weir, L., Brogi, E., and Schainfeld, R. (1995). Arterial gene therapy for therapeutic angiogenesis in patients with peripheral artery disease. *Circulation* **91,** 2687–2692.

Jang, Y., Guzman, L. A., Lincoff, M., Gottsauner-Wolf, M., Forudi, F., Hart, C. E., Courtman, D. W., Ezban, M., Ellis, S. G., and Topol, E. J. (1995). Influence of blockade at specific levels of the coagulation cascade on restenosis in a rabbit atherosclerotic femoral artery injury model. *Circulation* **92,** 3041–3050.

Jawien, A., Bowen-Pope, D., Lindner, V., Schwartz, S. M., and Clowes, A. W. (1992). Platelet-derived growth factor promotes smooth muscle migration and intimal thickening in a rat model of balloon angioplasty. *J. Clin. Invest.* **89,** 507–511.

Karas, S. P., Santoian, E. C., and Gravanis, M. B. (1991). Restenosis following coronary angioplasty. *Clin. Cardiol.* **14,** 791–801.

Kaul, U., Chandra, S., Bahl, V. K., Sharma, S., and Wasir, H. S. (1994). Enalapril for prevention of restenosis after coronary angioplasty. *Indian Heart J.* **45**(6), 469–473.

Kawamura, M., Terashita, Z. I., Okida, H., Imura, Y., Shino, A., Nakao, M., and Nishikawa, K. (1993). TCV-116, a novel angiotensin II receptor antagonist, prevents intimal thickening and impairment of vascular function after carotid injury in rats. *J. Pharmacol. Exp. Ther.* **266**(3), 1664–1669.

Kimura, T., Shinoda, E., Sato, Y., Yokoi, H., Tamura, T., Nakagawa, Y., Nosaka, H., and Nobuyoshi, M. (1994). Difference in acute gain (AG) and late loss (LL) relationship among three different new angioplasty devices (NAD). *Circulation* **90**(4), Part 2, I-59.

Klauss, V., Blasini, R., and Regar, E. (1993). Mechanisms of coronary in-stent restenosis: neointimal proliferation or stent compression? Serial assessment by intracoronary ultrasound. *Circulation* **88,** I-598.

Kobayashi, M., Ishida, F., Takhashi, T., Taguchi, K., Watanabe, K., Ohmura, I., and Kamei, T. (1989). Preventive effects of MK-733 (Simvastatin), an inhibitor of HMG-CoA reductase, on hypercholesterolemia and atherosclerosis induced by cholesterol feeding in rabbits. *Jpn. J. Pharmacol.* **49,** 125–133.

Kohno, M., Horio, T., Yokokawa, K., Yasunari, K., Kurihara, N., and Takeda, T. (1994). Endothelin modulates the mitogenic effect of PDGF on glomerular mesangial cells. *Am. J. Physiol.* **266,** F894–F900.

Kuntz, R. E., and Baim, D. S. (1993). Defining coronary restenosis: newer clinical and angiographic paradigms. *Circulation* **88,** 1310–1323.

Labhasetwar, V., Song, C., Humphrey, W., Shebuski, R., and Levy, R. J. (1995). Nanoparticles for site specific delivery of U-86983 in restenosis in pig coronary arteries. *Proc. Int. Symp. Control Relat. Bioact. Mater.* **22,** 182–183.

Lafont, A., Guzman, L. A., Whitlow, P. L., Goormastic, M., Cornhill, J. F., and Chilsom, G. M. (1995). Restenosis after experimental angioplasty. *Circ. Res.* **76,** 996–1002.

Lambert, C. R., Taylor, S., and Smith, T. (1994). Pressure and volume control for local drug-delivery catheters: Development of a new microprocessor-controlled system. *Coronary Artery Dis.* **5**(2), 163–167.

Lee, J. S., Adrie, C., Jacob, H. J., Roberts, J. D., Jr., Zapol, W. M., and Bloch, K. D. (1996). Chronic inhalation of nitric oxide inhibits neointimal formation after balloon-induced arterial injury. *Circ. Res.* **78,** 337–342.

Levy, R. J., Golomb, G., Trachy, J., Labhasetwar, V., Song, Muller, D., and Topol, E. (1994). Strategies for treating arterial restenosis using polymeric controlled release implants. *In* "Biotechnology and Bioactive Polymers" (C. G. Gebelein and C. E. Carraher, eds.), pp. 342. Plenum, London.

Levy, R. J., Labhasetwar, V., Song, C., Lerner, E., Chen, W., Vyavahare, N., and Qu, X. (1995). Polymeric drug delivery systems for treatment of cardiovascular calcification, arrhythmias and restenosis. *J. Controlled Release* **36**(1–2), 137–147.

Lindner, V., Lappi, D. A., Baird, A., Majack, R. A., and Reidy, M. A. (1991). Role of basic fibroblast growth factor in vascular lesion formation. *Circ. Res.* **68,** 106–113.

Lindner, V., Fingerle, J., and Reidy, M. A. (1993). Mouse model of arterial injury. *Circ. Res.* **73,** 792–796.

Liu, M. W., Roubin, G. S., Robinson, K. A., Black, A. J. R., Hearn, J. A., Siegel, R. J., and King, S. P., III (1990). Trapidil in preventing restenosis after balloon angioplasty in the atherosclerotic rabbit. *Circulation* **81,** 1089–1093.

Losordo, D. W., Pickering, J. G., Takeshita, S., Leclerc, G., Gal, D., Weir, L., Kearney, M., Jekanowski, J., and Isner, J. M. (1994). Use of the rabbit ear artery to serially assess foreign protein secretion after site-specific arterial gene transfer in vivo. *Circulation* **89**(2), 785–792.

Lundergan, C. F., Foegh, M. L., and Ramwell, P. W. (1991). Peptide inhibition of myointimal proliferation by angiopeptin, a somatostatin analogue. *J. Am. Coll. Cardiol.* **17**(6), 132B–136B.

Luo, H., Nishoka, T., Eigler, N., Tabak, S., and Siegel, R. J. (1994). Chronic vessel constriction is an important mechanism of restenosis after balloon angioplasty: An intravascular ultrasound study. *Circulation* **90**(4, Part 2), I-61.

Majesky, M. W., and Schwartz, S. M. (1990). Smooth muscle diversity in arterial wound repair. *Toxicol. Pathol.* **18**(4), 554–559.

Majesky, M. W., Giachelli, C. M., Reidy, M. A., and Schwartz, S. M. (1992). Rat carotid neointimal smooth muscle cells reexpress a developmentally regulated mRNA phenotype during repair of arterial injury. *Circ. Res.* **71**(4), 759–768.

March, K. L., Mohanraj, S., Ho, P. P. K., Wilensky, R. L., and Hathaway, D. R. (1994). Biodegradable microspheres containing a colchicine analogue inhibit DNA synthesis in vascular smooth muscle cells. *Circulation* **89**(5), 1929–1933.

March, K. L., Madison, J. E., and Trapnell, B. C. (1995). Pharmacokinetics of adenoviral-mediated gene delivery to vascular smooth muscle cells: Modulation by polyxamer 407 and implications for cardiovascular gene therapy. *Hum. Gene Ther.* **6**(1), 41–53.

Margolis, J. R., Krauthamer, D., Litvak, F., Rothbaum, D. A., and Untereker, W. J. (1991). Six month follow-up of excimer laser coronary angioplasty registry patients. *J. Am. Coll. Cardiol.* **17,** 218A.

Mazur, W., Ali, N. M., Raizner, A. E., and French, B. A. (1994a). Coronary restenosis and gene therapy. *Tex. Heart Inst. J.* **21**(1), 104–111.

Mazur, W., Ali, N. M., Grinstead, W. C., Schulz, D. G., Raizner, A. E., and French, B. A. (1994b). Lipofectin-mediated versus adenovirus-mediated gene transfer in vito and in vivo: Comparison of canine and procine modelsystems. *Coronary Artery Dis.* **5**(9), 779–786.

MERCATOR Study Group (1992). Does the angiotensin converting enzyme inhibitor cilazapril prevent restenosis after percutaneous angioplasty? Results of the MERCATOR study: A multicenter, randomized, double-blinded placebo-controlled trial. *Circulation* **86,** 100–110.

Moncada, S., Palmer, R. M. J., and Higgs, E. A. (1991). Nitric oxide: Physiology, pathophysiology and pharmacology. *Pharmacol. Rev.* **43,** 109–142.

Moore, S. (1979). Thromboatherosclerosis in normolipemic rabbits: A result of continued endothelial damage. *Lab. Invest.* **29,** 478–487.

Morishita, R., Gibbons, G. H., Ellison, K. E., Nakajima, M., Von Der Leyen, H., Zhang, L., Kaneda, Y., Ogihara, T., and Dzau, V. J. (1994a). Intimal hyperplasia after vascular injury is inhibited by antisense cdk 2 kinase oligonucleotides. *J. Clin. Invest.* **93**(4), 1458–1464.

Morishita, R., Gibbons, G. H., Kaneda, Y., Ogihara, T., and Dzau, V. J. (1994b). Pharmacokinetics of antisense oligodeoxyribonucleotides (cyclin B1 and CDC 2 kinase) in the vessel wall in vivo: Enhanced therapeutic utility for restenosis by HVJ-liposome delivery. *Gene* **149**(1), 13–19.

Morishita, R., Gibbons, G. H., Horiuchi, M., Ellison, K. E., Nakajima, M., Zhang, L., Kaneda, Y., Ogihara, T., and Dzau, V. J. (1995). A gene therapy strategy using a transcription factor decoy of E2F binding sites inhibits smooth muscle cell proliferation in vivo. *Proc. Natl. Acad. Sci. U.S.A.* **92,** 5855–5859.

Muller, D. W. M., Ellis, S. G., and Topol, E. J. (1991). Colchicine and antineoplastic therapy for the prevention of restenosis after percutaneous coronary interventions. *J. Am. Coll. Cardiol.* **17**(6), 126B–131B.

Muller, D. W. M., Ellis, S. G., and Topol, E. J. (1992). Experimental models of coronary artery restenosis. *J. Am. Coll. Cardiol.* **19**(2), 418–432.

Murray, A., and Hunt, T. (1993). "The Cell Cycle," p. 106. Freeman, New York.

Nabel, E. G., Yang, Z., Plautz, G., Frough, R., Zhan, X., Haudenschild, C. C., Maciag, T., and Nabel, G. J. (1993a). Recombinant fibroblast growth factor-1 promotes intimal hyperplasia and angiogenesis in arteries in vivo. *Nature (London)* **362,** 844–846.

Nabel, E. G., Yang, Z., Liptay, S., San, H., Gordon, D., and Haudenschild, C. C. (1993b). Recombinant platelet derived growth factor B gene expression in porcine arteries induces intimal hyperplasia in vivo. *J. Clin. Invest.* **91,** 1822–1829.

Nabel, E. G., Shum, L., Pompili, V. J., Yang, Z., San, H., Shu, H. B., Liptay, L., Gold, L., Gordon, D., Derynck, R., and Nabel, G. J. (1993c). Direct transfer of transforming growth factor β1 gene into arteries stimulates fibrocellular hyperplasia. *Proc. Natl. Acad. Sci. U.S.A.* **90,** 10759–10763.

Nabel, E. G., Pompili, V. J., Plautz, G. E., and Nabel, G. J. (1994). Gene transfer and vascular disease. *Cardiovasc. Res.* **28,** 713–719.

Nair, R. J., Cao, W., and Morris, R. E. (1995). Inhibition of smooth muscle cell proliferation in vitro by leflunomide, a new immunosuppressant, is antagonized by uridine. *Immunol. Lett.* **47,** 171–174.

Newman, K. D., Dunn, P. F., Owens, J. W., Schulick, A. H., Virmani, R., Sukhova, G., Libby, P., and Dichek, D. A. (1995). Adenovirus-mediated gene transfer into normal rabbit arteries results in prolonged vascular cell activation, inflammation, and neointimal hyperplasia. *J. Clin. Invest.* **96,** 2955–2965.

Nikkari, S. T., Geary, R. L., Hatsukami, T., Ferguson, M., Forough, R., Alpers, C. E., and Clowes, A. W. (1996). Expression of collagen, interstitial collagenase, and tissue inhibitor of metalloproteinases-1 in restenosis after carotid endarterectomy. *Am. J. Pathol.* **148**(3), 777–783.

Nunes, G. L., Sgoutas, D. S., Redden, R. A., Sigman, S. R., Gravanis, M. B., King, S. B., III, and Berk, B. C. (1995). Combination of vitamins C and E alters the response to coronary balloon injury in the pig. *Arterioscler. Thromb. Vasc. Biol.* **15**(1), 156–165.

Nyamekye, I., Anglin, S., Bown, S., Bishop, C., and McEwan, J. (1994). Inhibition of intimal hyperplasia by photodynamic therapy in the rat carotid artery model of angioplasty restenosis. *Br. Heart J.* **71** Suppl. 5, 17.

Nyamekye, I., Anglin, S., McEwan, J., Macrobert, A., Bown, S., and Bishop, C. (1995). Photodynamic therapy of normal and balloon-injured rat carotid arteries using 5-aminolevulinic acid. *Circulation* **91**(2), 417–425.

O'Brien, E. R., Alpers, E. C., Stewart, D. K., Ferguson, M., Tran, N., Gordon, D., Bensitt, E. P., Hinohara, T., Simpson, J. B., and Schwartz, S. M. (1993). Proliferation in primary and restenotic coronary atherectomy tissue. Implications for antiproliferative therapy. *Circ. Res.* **73,** 223–231.

Ohnishi, H., Yamaguchi, K., Shimada, S., Suzuki, Y., and Kumagai, A. (1981). A new approach to treatment of atherosclerosis and trapidil as an antagonist to platelet derived growth factor. *Life Sci.* **28**(14), 1641–1646.

Ohno, T., Gordon, D., San, H., Pompili, V., Imperiale, M. J., Nabel, G. J., and Nabel, E. G. (1994). Gene therapy for vascular smooth muscle cell proliferation after arterial injury. *Science* **265**, 781–784.

Okamato, S., Inden, M., Setsuda, M., Konishi, T., and Nakano, T. (1992). Effects of trapidil (triazolopyrimidine), a platelet-derived growth factor antagonist, in preventing restenosis after percutaneous transluminal coronary angioplasty. *Am. Heart J.* **123**, 1439–1444.

O'Keefe, J. H., Giorgi, L. V., Hartzler, G. O., Good, T. H., Ligon, R. W., and Webb, D. L. (1991). Effects of diltiazem on complications and restenosis after coronary angioplasty. *Am. J. Cardiol.* **67**, 373–376.

Onaka, H., Hirota, Y., Kita, Y., Tsuji, R., Ishii, K., Ishimura, T., and Kawamura, K. (1994). The effect of pravastatin on prevention of restenosis after successful percutaneous transluminal coronary angioplasty. *Jpn. Circ. J.* **58**(2), 100–106.

Parish, M. A., Grossi, E. A., Baumann, F. G., Asai, T., Rifkin, D. B., Colvin, S. B., and Galloway, A. C. (1995). Effects of a single administration of fibroblast growth factor on vascular wall reaction to injury. *Ann. Thorac. Surg.* **59**(4), 948–954.

Pastore, C. J., Isner, J. M., Bacha, P. A., Kearney, M., and Pickering, J. G. (1995). Epidermal growth factor receptor-targeted cytotoxin inhibits neointimal hyperplasia in vivo: Results of local versus systemic administration. *Circ. Res.* **77**(3), 519–529.

Pepine, C. J., Hirshfeld, J. W., Macdonald, R. G., Henderson, M. A., Bass, T. A., Goldberg, S., Savage, M. P., Vetrovec, G., Cowley, M., Taussig, A. S., Whitworth, H. B., Margolis, J. R., Hill, J. A., Bove, A. A., and Jugo, R. for the M-HEART Group (1990). A controlled trial of corticosteroids to prevent restenosis after coronary angioplasty. *Circulation* **81**, 1753–1761.

Planes, A., Vochelle, N., Mazas, C., Zucman, J., Landais, A., Pascariello, J., Weill, D., and Butel, J. (1988). Prevention of postoperative venous thrombosis: A randomized trial comparing unfractionated heparin with low molecular weight heparin in patients undergoing total hip replacement. *Thromb. Haemostasis* **60**, 407–410.

Post, M. J., Borst, C., and Kuntz, R. E. (1994). The relative importance of arterial remodeling compared with intimal hyperplasia in lumen renarrowing after balloon angioplasty. *Circulation* **89**, 2816–2821.

Powell, J. S., Clozel, J. P., Muller, R. K. M., Kuhn, H., Hefti, F., Hosang, M., and Baumgartner, H. R. (1989). Inhibitor of angiotensin-converting enzyme prevent myointimal proliferation after vascular injury. *Science* **245**, 186–188.

Pratt, R. E., and Dzau, V. J. (1996). Pharmacologic strategies to prevent restenosis. *Circulation* **93**, 848–852.

Prescott, M. F., Webb, R. L., and Reidy, M. A. (1991). Angiotensin converting enzyme inhibitor versus angiotensin II, AT1 receptor antagonist: Effects on smooth muscle cell migration and proliferation after balloon catheter injury. *Am. J. Pathol.* **139**, 1291–1296.

Pukac, L. A., Castellot, J. J., Wright, T. C., Caleb, B. L., and Karnovsky, M. J. (1990). Heparin inhibits c-fos and c-myc mRNA expression in vascular smooth muscle cells. *Cell Regul.* **1**(5), 435–443.

Rakugi, H., Wang, D. S., Dzau, V. J., and Pratt, R. E. (1994). Potential importance of tissue angiotensin-converting enzyme inhibition in preventing neointima formation. *Circulation* **90**(1), 449–455.

Rao, G. N., and Berk, B. C. (1992). Active oxygen species stimulate vascular smooth muscle cell growth and proto-oncogene expression. *Circ. Res.* **70**, 593–599.

Riessen, R., and Isner, J. M. (1994). Prospects for site-specific delivery of pharmacologic and molecular therapies. *J. Am. Coll. Cardiol.* **23**(5), 1234–1244.

Ryan, M. J., Emig, L. E., Hicks, G. W., Ramharack, R., Spahr, M. A., Kreick, J. S., Brammer, D. W., Chien, A. J., and Keiser, J. A. (1997). Vascular localization of lipoprotein(a) in a monkey model of vessel injury. *Arterioscler. Thromb. Vasc. Biol.* **17** (in press).

Sahni, R., Maniet, A. R., Voci, G., and Banka, V. S. (1991). Prevention of restenosis by lovastatin after successful coronary angioplasty. *Am. Heart J.* **121**, 1600–1608.

Sarembock, I. J., LaVeau, P. J., Sigal, S. L., Timms, I., Sussman, J., Haudenschild, C., and Ezekowitz, M. D. (1989). Influence of inflation pressure and balloon size on the development of intimal hyperplasia after balloon angioplasty. A study in the atherosclerotic rabbit. *Circulation* **80**(4), 1029–1040.

Savage, M. P., Goldberg, S., Bove, A. A., Deutsch, E., Vetrovec, G., Macdonald, R. G., Bass, T., Margolis, J. R., Whitworth, H. B., Taussig, A., Hirshfeld, J. W., Cowley, M., Hill, J. A., Marks, R. G., Fischman, D. L., Handberg, E., Herrmann, H., and Pepine, C. J. (1995). Effect of thromboxane A2 blockade on clinical outcome and restenosis after successful coronary angioplasty: Multi-Hospital Eastern Atlantic Restenosis Trial (M-HEART II). *Circulation* **92**(11), 3194–3200.

Schneider, J. E., Berk, B. C., Gravanis, M. B., Santoian, E. C., Cipolla, G. D., Tarazona, N., Lassegue, B., and King, S. B., III (1993). Probucol decreases neointimal formation in a swine model of coronary artery balloon injury. *Circulation* **88,** 628–637.

Schwartz, R. S., Bourassa, M. G., Lesperance, J., Aldridge, H. E., Kazim, F., and Salvatori, V. A. (1988). Aspirin and dipyridamole in the prevention of restenosis after percutaneous transluminal coronary angioplasty. *N. Engl. J. Med.* **318,** 1714–1719.

Schwartz, R. S., Murphy, J. G., Edwards, W. D., Camrud, A. R., Vliestra, R. E., and Holmes, D. R. (1990). Restenosis after balloon angioplasty: a practical proliferative model in porcine coronary arteries. *Circulation* **82,** 2190–2200.

Serruys, P. W., Strauss, B. H., Beatt, K. J., Bertrand, M. E., and Puel, J. (1991). Angiographic follow-up after placement of a self-expanding coronary artery stent. *N. Engl. J. Med.* **324,** 13–17.

Serruys, P. W., Jaegewre, P., Kiemeniej, F., Macaya, C., Rutsch, W., Heyndrickx, G., Emanuelsson, H., Marco, J., Legrand, V., Materne, P., Belardi, J., Sigwart, U., Colombo, A., Goy, J. J., van den Heuvel, P., Delcan, J., and Morel, M. A. for the Benestent Study Group (1994). A comparison of balloon expandable stent implantation with balloon angioplasty in patients with coronary artery disease. *N. Engl. J. Med.* **331,** 489–495.

Serruys, P. W., Herrman, J. P. R., Simon, R., Rutsch, W., Bode, C., Laarman, G. J., Van Dijk, R., Van den Bos, A. A., Umans, V. A. W. M., Fox, K. A. A., Close, P., and Deckers, J. W. (1995). A comparison of hirudin with heparin in the prevention of restenosis after coronary angioplasty. *N. Engl. J. Med.* **333**(12), 757–763.

Shi, Y., Fard, A., Galeo, A., Hutchinson, H. G., Vermani, P., Dodge, G. R., Hall, D. J., Shaheen, F., and Zalewski, A. (1994). Transcatheter delivery of c-myc antisense oligomers reduces neointimal formation in a porcine model of coronary artery balloon injury. *Circulation* **90**(2), 944–951.

Shimotakahara, S., and Mayberg, M. R. (1994). Gamma irradiation inhibits neointimal hyperplasia in rats after arterial injury. *Stroke* **25**(2), 424–428.

Simons, M., Edelman, E. R., DeKeyser, J. L., Langer, R., and Rosenberg, R. D. (1992). Antisense c-myb oligonucleotides inhibit intimal arterial smooth muscle cell accumulation in vivo. *Nature (London)* **359,** 67–70.

Simpson, J. B., Baim, D. S., Hinohara, T., Cowley, M. J., Smucker, M. L., and the US Directional Coronary Investigator Group (1991). Restenosis of de novo lesions in native coronary arteries following directional coronary atherectomy: Multicenter experience. *J. Am. Coll. Cardiol.* **17,** 346A.

Singh, J. P., Rothfuss, K. J., Wiernicki, T. R., Lacefield, W. B., Kurtz, W. L., Brown, R. F., Brune, K. A., Bailey, D., and Dube, G. P. (1994). Dipyridamole directly inhibits vascular smooth muscle cell proliferation in vitro and in vivo: Implications in the treatment of restenosis after angioplasty. *J. Am. Coll. Cardiol.* **23**(3), 665–671.

Smith, E. B. (1965). The influence of age and atherosclerosis on the chemistry of aortic intima. *J. Atheroscler. Res.* **5,** 241–248.

Snow, A. D., Bolendar, R. P., Wight, T. N., and Clowes, A. W. (1990). Heparin modulates the composition of the extracellular matrix domain surrounding arterial smooth muscle cells. *Am. J. Pathol.* **137,** 313–330.

Sollott, S. J., Cheng, L., Pauly, R. R., Jenkins, G. M., Monticone, R. E., Kuzuya, M., Froehlich, J. P., Crow, M. T., Lakatta, E. G., Rowinsky, E. K., and Kinsella, J. L. (1995). Taxol inhibits neointimal smooth muscle cell accumulation after angioplasty in the rat. *J. Clin. Invest.* **95**(4), 1869–1876.

Soma, M. R., Donetti, E., Parolini, C., Mazzini, G., Ferrari, C., Fumagalli, R., and Paoletti, R. (1993). HMG CoA reductase inhibitors: In vivo effects on carotid intimal thickening in normocholesterolemic rabbits. *Arterioscler. Thromb.* **13**, 571–578.

Soma, M. R., Donetti, E., Parolini, C., Sirtori, C. R., Fumagalli, R., and Franceschini, G. (1995). Recombinant apolipoprotein A-I-Milano dimer inhibits carotid intimal thickening induced by perivascular manipulation in rabbits. *Circ. Res.* **76**(3), 405–411.

Speidel, C. M., Eisenberg, P. R., Ruf, W., Edgington, T. S., and Abendschein, D. R. (1995). Tissue factor mediates prolonged procoagulation activity on the luminal surface on balloon-injured aortas in rabbits. *Circulation* **92**, 3323–3330.

Steele, P. M., Chesebro, J. H., and Stanson, A. W. (1985). Balloon angioplasty: Natural history of the pathophysiologic response to injury in the pig model. *Circ. Res.* **57**, 105–112.

Stone, G. W., Rutherford, B. D., and Hartzler, G. O. (1989). A randomized trial of corticoids for the prevention of restenosis in 102 patients undergoing repeat coronary angioplasty. *Catheterization Cardiovasc. Diagn.* **18**, 227–231.

Tenda, K., Salkawa, T., Maeda, T., Sato, Y., Niwa, H., Inoue, T., Yonemochi, H., Maruyama, T., Shimoyama, N., Aragaki, S., Hara, M., and Takaki, R. (1993). The relationship between serum lipoprotein (a) and restenosis after initial elective percutaneous transluminal coronary angioplasty. *Jpn. Circ. J.* **57**, 789–795.

Texter, M., Lees, R. S., Pitt, B., Dinsmore, R. E., and Uprichard, A. C. (1993). The QUinapril Ischemic Event Trial (QUIET) design and methods: Evaluation of chronic ACE inhibitor therapy after coronary artery intervention. *Cardiovasc. Drugs Ther.* 7(2), 273–282.

Tiell, M. L., Sussman, I. I., Gordon, P. B., and Sanders, R. N. (1983). Suppression of fibroblast proliferation in vitro and of neointimal hyperplasia in vivo by the traizolopyrimidine, trapidil. *Artery (Fulton, Mich.)* **12**, 33–50.

Timms, I. D., Tomaszewski, J. E., and Shiansky-Goldberg, R. D. (1995). Effects on nonanticoagulant heparin (Astenose) on restenosis after balloon angioplasty in the atherosclerotic rabbit. *J. Vasc. Interv. Radiology* **6**(3), 365–378.

Topol, E. J., Ellis, S. G., Cosgrove, D. M., Bates, E. R., Muller, D. W., Schork, N. J., Schork, M. A., and Loop, F. D. (1993a). Analysis of coronary angioplasty practice in the United States with an insurance-claims database. *Circulation* **87**, 1489–1497.

Topol, E. J., Leya, F., Pinkerton, C. A. Whitlow, P. L., Hofling, B., Simonton, C. A., Masden, R. R., Serruys, P. W., Leon, M. B., Williams, D. O., King, S. B., III, Mark, D. B., Isner, J. M., Holmer, D. R., Jr., Ellis, S. G., Lee, K. L., Keeler, G. P., Berdan, L. G., Hinohara, T., and Califf, R. M., for the CAVEAT Study Group (1993b). A comparison of direction atherectomy with coronary angioplasty in patients with coronary artery disease. *N. Engl. J. Med.* **329**(4), 221–227.

Topol, E. J., Califf, R. M., Weisman, H. F., Ellis, S. G., Tcheng, J. E., Worley, S., Ivanhoe, R., George, B. S., Fintel, D., and Weston, M. (1994). Randomised trial of coronary intervention with antibody against platelet IIb/IIIa integrin for reduction of clinical restenosis: Results at six months. *Lancet* **343**(8902), 881–886.

Vesselinovitch, D. (1988). Animal models and the study of atherosclerosis. *Arch. Pathol. Lab. Med.* **112**, 1011–1017.

Von Der Leyen, H., Gibbons, G. H., Morishita, R., Lewis, N. P., Zhang, L., Nakajima, M., Kaneda, Y., Cooke, J., and Dzau, V. J. (1995). Gene therapy inhibiting neointimal vascular lesion: In vivo transfer of endothelial cell nitric oxide synthase gene. *Proc. Natl. Acad. Sci. U.S.A.* **92**, 1137–1141.

Waksman, R., Robinson, K. A., Crocker, I. R., Gravanis, M. B., Cipolla, G. D., and King S. B., III (1995a). Endovascular low-dose irradiation inhibits neointima formation after coronary artery balloon injury in swine: A possible role for radiation therapy in restenosis prevention. *Circulation* **91**(5), 1533–1539.

Waksman, R., Robinson, K. A., Crocker, I. R., Gravanis, M. B., Palmer, S. J., Wang, C., Cipolla, G. D., and King S. B., III (1995b). Intracoronary radiation before stent implantation inhibits neointima formation in stented porcine coronary arteries. *Circulation* **92**(6), 1383–1386.

Waltenberger, J., Kovalenko, M., Boehmer, F., Gazit, A., Hombach, V., and Levitzki, A. (1994). Characterization of receptor-tyrosine-kinase-inhibitors: Selectivity as a molecular basis for the treatment of restenosis. *Eur. Heart J.* **15**, 427 (abstr.).

Weintraub, W. S., Boccuzzi, S. J., Klein, J. L., Kosinski, A. S., King, S. B., Ivanhoe, R., Cedarholm, J. C., Stillabower, M. E., Talley, J. D., and DeMaio, S. J. (1994). Lack of effect of lovastatin on restenosis after coronary angioplasty. *N. Engl. J. Med.* **331**(20), 1331–1337.

Whitworth, H. B., Roubin, G. S., Hollman, J., Meier, B., Leimgruber, P. P., and Douglas, J. S. (1986). Effect of nifedipine on recurrent stenosis after percutaneous transluminal coronary angioplasty. *J. Am. Coll. Cardiol.* **8**, 1271–1276.

Wiedermann, J. G., Marboe, C., Amols, H., Schwartz, A., and Weinberger, J. (1995). Intracoronary irradiation markedly reduces neointimal proliferation after balloon angioplasty in swine: Persistent benefit at 6-month follow-up. *J. Am. Coll. Cardiol.* **25**(6), 1451–1456.

Wong, S. C., Leon, M. B., and Popma, J. J. (1993). New device angioplasty: The impact on restenoisis. *Coronary Artery Dis.* **4**, 243–253.

Wong, S. C., Baim, D. S., Schatz, R. A., Teirstein, P. S., King, S. B., Curry, R. C., Heuser, R. R., Ellis, S. G., Cleman, M. W., and Overlie, P. (1995). Immediate and late outcomes after stent implantation in saphenous vein graft lesions: The multicenter U.S., Palmaz-Schatz stent experience. *J. Am. Coll. Cardiol.* **26**(3), 704–712.

Yellai, S. S., and Schatz, R. A. (1994). Indications and use of the Palmaz-Schatz coronary stent. *Cardiol. Clin.* **12**(4), 651–663.

Zempo, N., Koyama, N., Kenagy, R. D., Lea, H. J., and Clowes, A. W. (1996). Regulation of vascular smooth muscle cell migration and proliferation in vitro and in injured arteries by a synthetic matrix metalloproteinase inhibitor. *Arterioscler. Thromb. Vasc. Biol.* **16**, 28–33.

Zhu, B. Q., Sievers, R. E., Sun, Y. P., Isemberg, W. M., and Parmley, W. W. (1992). Effect of lovastatin on suppression and regression of atherosclerosis in lipid-fed rabbits. *J. Cardiovasc. Pharmacol.* **19**, 246–255.

James M. Brundege*
Thomas V. Dunwiddie*,†

*Department of Pharmacology
University of Colorado Health Sciences Center
Denver, Colorado 80262

†Program in Neuroscience
University of Colorado Health Sciences Center
and Veterans Administration Medical Research Service
Denver, Colorado 80262

Role of Adenosine as a Modulator of Synaptic Activity in the Central Nervous System

I. Introduction

Adenosine has long been known to exert a number of physiological effects on the nervous system. The first demonstration that adenosine is physiologically active was made by Drury and Szent-Györgyi (1929), who observed profound effects of adenosine on the heart. Since that time it has become clear that adenosine can exert multiple effects through interactions with cell surface receptors (van Calker *et al.*, 1979; Sattin and Rall, 1970). In the nervous system adenosine has been shown to alter levels of cyclic adenosine 3′,5′-monophosphate (cAMP) (Sattin and Rall, 1970), inhibit synaptic activity and neuronal excitability (Dunwiddie and Hoffer, 1980), and modulate cerebral blood flow (Berne *et al.*, 1981), and these effects have led to numerous proposed functional roles for adenosine. Due to the lack of evidence that adenosine acts as a classical

Advances in Pharmacology, Volume 39

1054-3589/97/$25.00

neurotransmitter, it has been hypothesized to act as a local hormone that modulates the activity of tissues near its site of release (Arch and Newsholme, 1978b). The realization that adenosine levels are regulated, in part, by the metabolism of ATP and other adenine nucleotides led Newby (1984) to expand on this idea by suggesting that adenosine can act as a "retaliatory metabolite" by which cells communicate their energy status to the surrounding tissues. Adenosine has been shown to be released during cerebral ischemia (Berne *et al.,* 1974), and it increases cerebral blood flow (Berne *et al.,* 1981), inhibits synaptic activity, and decreases neuronal excitability (Phillis and Wu, 1981; Dunwiddie and Hoffer, 1980; Phillis *et al.,* 1979). These observations led to the suggestion that adenosine acts as a neuroprotectant, preventing damage from ischemia and excitotoxicity (Dragunow and Faull, 1988). Over the years, the list of possible functional roles for adenosine has grown steadily to include an involvement in epilepsy (Glass *et al.,* 1996; Zhang *et al.,* 1993; Dragunow, 1988), cerebral ischemic preconditioning (Heurteaux *et al.,* 1995), regulation of sleep (Rainnie *et al.,* 1994; Haulica *et al.,* 1973), and immune reactions within the brain (Fozard *et al.,* 1996; Sajjadi *et al.,* 1996; Fiebich *et al.,* 1996; Holgate *et al.,* 1980). Despite these advances, the precise cellular mechanisms by which cells release adenosine, and what this implies about the neuromodulatory role of this compound, have remained elusive.

A great deal of evidence shows that adenosine receptors are located throughout the nervous system and that extracellular adenosine can effectively modulate neuronal activity. However, our understanding of how cells regulate extracellular adenosine levels is considerably less clear. Adenosine does not appear to be a neurotransmitter, in that there is little evidence it is stored in synaptic vesicles and released from nerve terminals in response to an action potential, yet it is present in the extracellular space of the brain and can be released from brain cells by various stimuli. Despite many detailed investigations into the effects exerted by adenosine and adenosine receptors, it is still not clear how adenosine is released, which cells are capable of releasing adenosine, or how adenosine release fits into the mosaic of chemical and electrical signals that characterize normal brain function. A detailed understanding of these phenomenon will likely provide new insights into how the brain uses adenosine as a neuromodulatory agent. This review summarizes what is known about how adenosine exerts it effects on neuronal activity, how cells form adenosine and regulate adenosine concentrations, and how cells release adenosine into the extracellular space where it can exert its modulatory actions. By integrating these different areas of research, it is hoped that a more complete picture of how the brain uses adenosine as a modulator of synaptic activity will be formed.

II. Adenosine Receptors

One of the early pieces of evidence that helped identify adenosine as a modulator of cellular activity was the identification of adenosine receptor subtypes. The first attempt to subclassify adenosine receptors was by van Calker *et al.* (1979), who observed differential effects of adenosine on cAMP formation in cultured brain cells. They divided adenosine receptors into two subtypes which they termed R_i and R_a (now known as A_1 and A_2) based on the ability of these receptors to inhibit or activate the enzyme adenylyl cyclase, respectively. Although adenosine receptors are no longer classified by their effects on adenylyl cyclase, the present classification still uses the A_1/A_2 nomenclature. Currently there are four subtypes of adenosine receptors that have been conclusively identified and cloned: A_1, A_{2a}, A_{2b}, and A_3; all of these receptors belong to the superfamily of G-protein-coupled receptors (Fredholm *et al.*, 1994; Palmer and Stiles, 1995). A_1 receptors are the most prevalent adenosine receptors in the nervous system and bind adenosine with the highest affinity. A_1 receptors are located throughout the brain, with particularly high concentrations in the hippocampus, cortex, cerebellum, and thalamus (Stehle *et al.*, 1992; Fastbom *et al.*, 1987). A_{2a} receptors are more restricted in their brain distribution and are primarily found in the striatum, nucleus accumbens, and olfactory tubercle (Stehle *et al.*, 1992), whereas A_{2b} and A_3 receptors are expressed diffusely throughout the nervous system (Stehle *et al.*, 1992). Adenosine receptors are thus found in every region of the brain and have a variety of functions (see Table 1).

A. A_1 Receptors

A_1 receptors are the most abundant adenosine receptors in the central nervous system (CNS) and have the most prominent effects on neuronal activity. A_1 receptors can alter neuronal activity by coupling to a wide variety of effector systems. As mentioned previously, A_1 receptors can inhibit the activity of adenylyl cyclase and thus the formation of cAMP. However, it has been difficult to demonstrate any clear physiological effect of adenosine that is mediated through this mechanism. In hippocampal neurons, activation of A_1 receptors causes a hyperpolarization of the cell membrane with a concomitant decrease in the membrane resistance (Dunwiddie and Fredholm, 1989; Segal, 1982). This effect has been shown to be mediated by activation of a postsynaptic potassium conductance (Thompson *et al.*, 1992; Gerber *et al.*, 1989). A_1 receptors also inhibit calcium currents in a wide variety of neurons (Umemiya and Berger, 1994; Mogul *et al.*, 1993; Dolphin *et al.*, 1986; Schubert *et al.*, 1986; MacDonald *et al.*, 1986), and all of these postsynaptic events are mediated by a pertussis toxin sensitive G-protein (Mynlieff and Beam, 1994; Zgombick *et al.*, 1989; Fredholm *et al.*,

TABLE I Adenosine Receptors

Receptor	A_1	A_{2a}	A_{2b}	A_3
G protein	$G_{i(1-3)}$	G_s	G_s	G_iG_o?
Biochemical effectors	↓ cAMP, ↑ IP3	↑ cAMP	↑ cAMP	↑ cAMP, ↑ IP3
Electrophysiological effectors	↑ K^+ channel activity ↓ Ca^{2+} channel activity	?	?	?
Electrophysiological responses	↓ neurotransmission hyperpolarizes neurons	?	?	?
Agonists	Adenosine NECA CHA[a]	Adenosine NECA CGS 21680[a]	Adenosine NECA None[a]	Adenosine NECA 2-Cl-IB-MECA[a]
Antagonists	Theophylline XAC DPCPX[a]	Theophylline XAC CSC[a] KF 17837[a]	Theophylline XAC None[a]	BW-A 522 None[a]

[a] Selective for this receptor subtype.

1989; Trussell and Jackson, 1987). Thus, adenosine can decrease neuronal excitability through actions on multiple ion conductances. The most prominent action of adenosine in the central nervous system is its ability to inhibit the release of a wide variety of neurotransmitters, including dopamine (Harms *et al.,* 1979; Michaelis *et al.,* 1979), norepinephrine (Fredholm *et al.,* 1983; Ebstein and Daly, 1982; Harms *et al.,* 1978), glutamate (Dolphin and Archer, 1983), serotonin (Feuerstein *et al.,* 1985; Harms *et al.,* 1979), and acetylcholine (Duner-Engström and Fredholm, 1988; Jackisch *et al.,* 1984). In most systems, these effects are believed to be mediated by presynaptic A_1 receptors (Scanziani *et al.,* 1992; Lupica *et al.,* 1992; Deckert and Jorgensen, 1988; Dunwiddie and Haas, 1985). Interestingly, GABAergic neurons are not sensitive to the release-inhibiting properties of A_1 receptors in the hippocampus (Thompson *et al.,* 1992; Yoon and Rothman, 1991; Lambert and Teyler, 1991; Dolphin and Archer, 1983), suggesting that the primary role of A_1 receptors in this brain region is to inhibit excitatory neurotransmission and decrease overall neuronal activity. However, adenosine has been shown to inhibit GABA release in the substantia nigra (Wu *et al.,* 1995), ventral tegmental area (Bonci and Williams, 1996; Wu *et al.,* 1995), and the thalamus (Ulrich and Huguenard, 1995). Urlich and Huguenard (1995) demonstrated that adenosine inhibited $GABA_A$ receptor-mediated inhibitory currents in the thalamus, but due to a concurrent inhibition of excitatory currents and the interconnectivity of GABAergic interneurons in this region, the net effect of adenosine was to inhibit thalamic oscillations. It thus appears that the effects of A_1 receptors are primarily inhibitory in most brain regions.

There are several possible mechanisms for the inhibition of neurotransmitter release by A_1 receptors. Three specific hypotheses that have been proposed are: (a) presynaptic A_1 receptors may activate a potassium conductance in the presynaptic terminal, thus shunting some of the action potential and decreasing voltage-dependent calcium entry; (b) A_1 receptors may couple, via a G-protein, to presynaptic calcium channels and directly inhibit calcium entry into the nerve terminal; (c) A_1 receptors may inhibit neurotransmitter release through a direct action on the release mechanisms in the presynaptic terminal. The first proposal, that adenosine inhibits transmitter release by activating a presynaptic potassium conductance, arises from the well-characterized ability of adenosine to activate a potassium conductance postsynaptically (Thompson *et al.*, 1992; Gerber *et al.*, 1989). If adenosine activates a similar potassium conductance presynaptically, this could hyperpolarize the presynaptic terminal and thus indirectly inhibit the opening of voltage-dependent calcium channels, inhibiting transmitter release. In fact, adenosine has been shown to activate an outward potassium conductance in the presynaptic terminal of the avian ciliary ganglia (Bennett and Ho, 1992) and to have a small but significant inhibitory effect on the extracellularly recorded fiber spike in the CA1 region of the hippocampus, a measure of the strength of evoked action potentials in the Schaffer collateral/commissural afferent fibers (Dunwiddie and Miller, 1993). Furthermore, in olfactory cortex, Scholfield and Steel (1989) have found that the potassium channel blockers diaminopyridine, 4-aminopyridine, and cesium could all block the adenosine-mediated inhibition of the field excitatory postsynaptic potential (fEPSP). Despite these data, most of the evidence does not support the idea that modulation of presynaptic potassium conductances is the primary mechanism by which adenosine inhibits neurotransmitter release (see later). Dunwiddie and Miller (1993) found that the inhibition of the presynaptic fiber spike was not necessary for adenosine to inhibit excitatory postsynaptic potentials and that blocking potassium channels with diaminopyridine or barium did not decrease adenosine-mediated inhibition. Fredholm (1990) has shown that 4-aminopyridine did not block the A_1 receptor-mediated inhibition of acetylcholine release in hippocampus, although it did block the inhibition of acetylcholine (ACh) release mediated by carbachol and morphine. Furthermore, several other groups have shown that treatments which block the adenosine-mediated activation of postsynaptic potassium conductances do not alter the ability of adenosine to inhibit excitatory responses (Thompson *et al.*, 1992; Birnstiel *et al.*, 1992) or transmitter release (Cass and Zahniser, 1991). Although a presynaptic activation of potassium conductances may occur in some systems, most researchers have focused their attention on other possible mechanisms for adenosine-mediated inhibition of transmitter release.

A second potential mechanism by which A_1 receptors may inhibit the release of neurotransmitters is by directly inhibiting calcium entry into the nerve terminal, thereby decreasing the probability of calcium-dependent neurotransmitter release. Much of the support for this hypothesis has come from numerous demonstrations that adenosine can inhibit calcium currents in neurons (Umemiya and Berger, 1994; Mogul *et al.*, 1993; Dolphin *et al.*, 1986; MacDonald *et al.*, 1986; Schubert *et al.*, 1986). However, these calcium currents are mediated by calcium channels on or near the cell body, and thus do not provide direct evidence that adenosine inhibits calcium entry into the presynaptic nerve terminal. Bennett and Ho (1991) recorded directly from the axon terminal of the avian ciliary ganglia and reported that adenosine hyperpolarizes the nerve terminal, presumably by activating a presynaptic potassium conductance. However, they found that adenosine still decreased the duration of the presynaptic calcium-mediated action potential when presynaptic potassium channels were blocked, suggesting a direct inhibition of calcium influx. In this same preparation, Yawo and Chuhma (1993) used calcium-fluorescent imaging and whole cell recording to measure the actions of adenosine on calcium influx into the nerve terminal and on the excitatory postsynaptic current (EPSC). They found that adenosine inhibited the ω-conotoxin-sensitive component of calcium influx into the nerve terminal, and the magnitude of this effect was sufficient to explain the reduction in the EPSC. Furthermore, Wu and Saggau (1994a) have made similar observations in the hippocampus. By selectively loading the Schaffer collateral/commissural afferent fibers of hippocampal slices with a fluorescent calcium indicator they were able to simultaneously measure the extracellular field EPSP and calcium influx into the presynaptic nerve terminals. They found that adenosine inhibited calcium influx in a manner that was able to quantitatively account for the inhibition of the field EPSP (Fig. 1) and that adenosine preferentially inhibited ω-conotoxin-sensitive calcium channels more than ω-agatoxin-sensitive channels, although other calcium channels were also affected. These data provide a strong case for the inhibition of calcium channels as the mechanism by which adenosine inhibits neurotransmitter release. However, data from other systems suggest that this is not universally true.

Despite the evidence suggesting adenosine inhibits neurotransmitter release through an action on calcium entry, substantial data suggest that adenosine inhibits release through a mechanism downstream from calcium entry. In the seminal study supporting such a mechanism, Silinsky (1984) found that adenosine could inhibit the frequency of miniature end plate potentials at the frog motor nerve in the absence of extracellular calcium and that adenosine could also inhibit acetylcholine release induced by calcium-filled liposomes and lanthanum in the absence of extracellular calcium. Furthermore, in contrast to data obtained from central neurons and avian ciliary ganglia, Silinsky and Solsona (1992) found that adenosine did not alter the N-type calcium currents responsible for transmitter release in the frog motor nerve ending. Scholz and Miller (1992) and Scanziani *et al.* (1992) have found similar results in the hippocampus, where they showed that adenosine inhibited the frequency of miniature EPSCs (mEPSCs) in the absence of extracellular calcium and when calcium channel blockers were present. Based on these data, it seems clear that adenosine is able to inhibit neurotransmitter release via a mechanism that does not depend on calcium entry from the extracellular space.

One hypothesis that could potentially explain both the calcium imaging data (Wu and Saggau, 1994a; Yawo and Chuhma, 1993) and the data suggesting that calcium entry is not necessary for inhibition of transmitter release is that adenosine could alter calcium levels within the nerve terminal by modifying the calcium buffering capacity of the cell. Hunt *et al.* (1994) attempted to address this issue by loading the calcium chelator dimethyl-bis-(aminophenoxy)ethane-tetraacetic acid (DMBAPTA) into frog motor nerve endings and comparing the effects of this chelator to those of adenosine. They concluded that the effects of adenosine were not mediated by an alteration in the calcium buffering capacity within the nerve terminal. Further evidence that the effects of adenosine are not mediated by a change in calcium homeostasis came from Capogna *et al.* (1996), who examined the ability of adenosine to decrease the frequency of mEPSCs in hippocampal slice cultures. They found that adenosine inhibited the increase in mEPSC frequency caused by gadolinium and α-latrotoxin, compounds thought to potentiate neurotransmitter release by a mechanism completely independent of either intracellular or extracellular calcium. These data thus suggest that adenosine acts on some other part of the vesicle release mechanism and does not act by altering calcium homeostasis within the nerve terminal. Although the evidence strongly supports the idea that adenosine can inhibit neurotransmitter release through a calcium-independent mechanism under some conditions, these data are difficult to reconcile with the calcium imaging data which shows that adenosine-mediated decreases in calcium influx into the nerve terminal can quantitatively account for the magnitude of the reduction in the postsynaptic response. Although it is likely that there are multiple mechanisms by which adenosine can decrease neurotransmitter release, the contribution of each toward inhibiting synaptic activity under physiological conditions is not known. It appears that the inhibition of calcium entry can account for the inhibitory effects of adenosine on synaptic activity induced by evoked action potentials, whereas a direct action on the release apparatus is needed to explain the actions of adenosine when calcium concentrations within the nerve terminal are low. It remains to be demonstrated whether this latter mechanism has any significant impact on the normal physiological activity of central mammalian neurons.

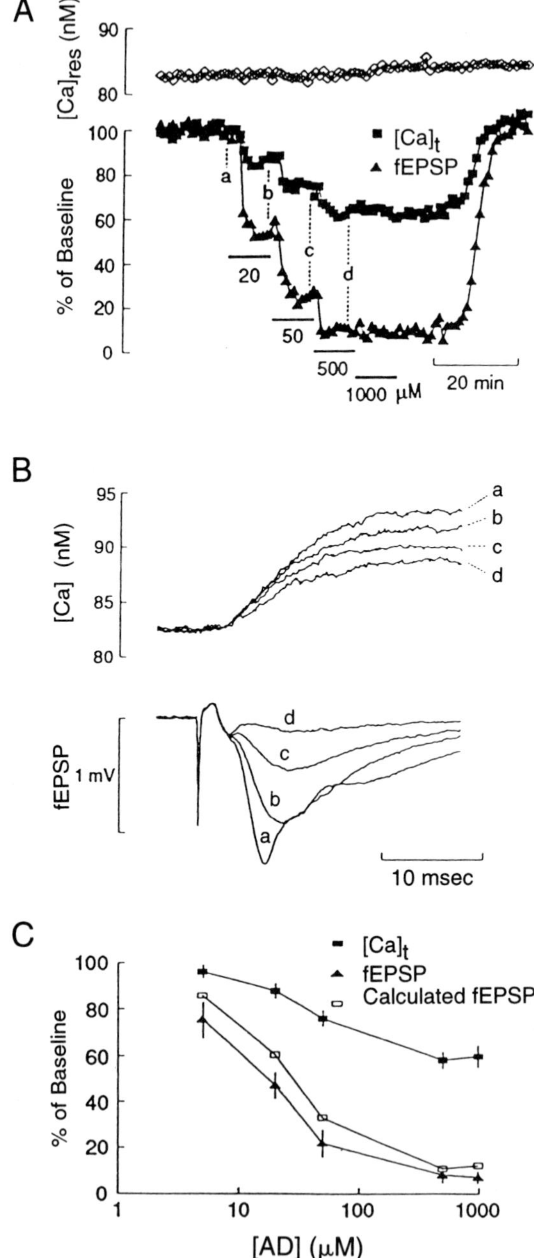

FIGURE 1 Adenosine decreases both the calcium transient ($[Ca]_t$) and the field EPSP (fEPSP) in area CA1 of hippocampus. In a hippocampal slice preparation, the Schaffer collateral/ commissural afferent fibers were selectively loaded with the fluorescent Ca^{2+} indicator fura-2 AM. Synaptic activity was evoked with a bipolar stimulating electrode, and the presynaptic $[Ca]_t$ was optically measured over an area approximately 150 μm in diameter. An extracellular

B. A_{2a} Receptors

Although A_1 receptors mediate most of the physiological effects of adenosine in the brain, A_2 receptors clearly play an important modulatory role in some brain areas. A_2 receptors exert the opposite effect on adenylyl cyclase activity as A_1 receptors, in that they stimulate adenylyl cyclase and increase cAMP formation via activation of the $G_s\alpha$ subtype of GTP-binding proteins (Parkinson and Fredholm, 1990; Li and Fredholm, 1985). A_2 receptors have been further subdivided into A_{2a} and A_{2b} subtypes, originally based on agonist binding affinity (Bruns *et al.*, 1986; Daly *et al.*, 1983), although these subtypes have now been cloned (Fredholm *et al.*, 1994; Palmer and Stiles, 1995). A_{2a} receptors bind adenosine with high affinity and are concentrated in dopamine-rich areas of the brain such as the caudate-putamen, nucleus accumbens, and olfactory tubercle (Schiffmann *et al.*, 1990; Fink *et al.*, 1994). Evidence relating the A_{2a} receptor to physiological effects has been less clear than with the A_1 receptor. In the striatum, the selective A_{2a} receptor agonist CGS 21680 has been shown to inhibit the release of acetylcholine and dopamine from tissue slices (Jin *et al.*, 1993). However, these responses could be blocked by the A_1 selective antagonist DPCPX, so the receptor type mediating this effect is uncertain. Brown *et al.*, (1990) demonstrated an adenosine receptor agonist-mediated increase in striatal acetylcholine release, and Zetterström and Fillenz (1990) showed an adenosine agonist-mediated increase in dopamine release. Both of these effects persisted in the presence of A_1 receptor antagonists, suggesting a role for A_2 receptors in these effects. However, neither study utilized A_2 selective ligands or conducted agonist potency profiles, leaving the identity of the adenosine receptor mediating these effects unclear. Ferre *et al.*, (1991) have shown that CGS 21680 can decrease the affinity of dopamine for the D_2 dopamine

---

electrode placed in the center of the fluorescent area simultaneously recorded the fEPSP. **(A)** A typical experiment showing the reduction of the $[Ca]_t$ and the fEPSP during sequential application of different concentrations of adenosine (lower panel). This reduction was not accompanied by a significant change in the resting Ca^{2+} level ($[Ca]_{res}$; upper panel). **(B)** Sampled recordings of the $[Ca]_t$ and the fEPSP taken at the times indicated in A. **(C)** Dose–response of adenosine (AD) inhibition of the amplitude of the $[Ca]_t$ and the initial slope of the fEPSP normalized to the baseline. The open squares represent the calculated slope of the fEPSP relative to the calcium transient, based on the equation $Y = X^m$, in which $m = 4$ (as determined in Wu and Saggau, 1994b) and X is taken from the mean of the measured $[Ca]_t$ at each concentration. Based on the previously determined relationship between the magnitude of the evoked calcium transient and the postsynaptic response, data show that the inhibition of calcium entry into the nerve terminals can quantitatively account for the reduction in the fEPSP. Reproduced from Wu and Saggau (1994a), with permission.

receptor in striatal membranes, suggesting an alternate manner in which A_{2a} receptors can regulate the effects of dopamine. CGS 21680 has also been shown to increase the electrically stimulated overflow of GABA from globus pallidus, an action that is opposed by dopamine D_2 receptor agonists (Mayfield *et al.,* 1993, 1996). Interestingly, this same ligand was shown to inhibit GABAergic inhibitory postsynaptic currents (IPSCs) in striatal medium spiny neurons (Mori *et al.,* 1996). Collectively, these studies suggest that the primary function of A_{2a} receptors in the CNS is to modulate the activity of dopamine and other neurotransmitters in dopamine-rich areas such as the basal ganglia.

Localization of A_{2a} receptors has been accomplished through the use of the radioligand [^{3}H]CGS 21680 (Johansson *et al.,* 1993; Wan *et al.,* 1990). These studies demonstrate that while most of the CGS 21680-binding sites are in the striatum, nucleus accumbens, and olfactory tubercle, there are lower but significant levels of binding in numerous other areas, particularly the cerebral cortex and hippocampus. Several studies have attempted to define putative A_{2a} receptor responses in these brain regions with inconsistent results. Lupica *et al.,* (1990) found no physiological responses mediated by A_{2a} receptors in the hippocampus, whereas Sebastiao and Ribeiro (1992) demonstrated an excitatory effect of CGS 21680 on population spikes in the CA1 region of the hippocampus. Furthermore, Lin and Phillis (1991) found an inhibitory effect on cortical neurons using ionophoretic application of CGS 21680 *in vivo*. One potential explanation for the differences in these results is a possible second high-affinity-binding site for CGS 21680 that does not appear to be any of the previously identified adenosine receptors (Cunha *et al.,* 1996; Johansson and Fredholm, 1995; Johansson *et al.,* 1993). At present it remains to be seen whether this putative second binding site is a new adenosine receptor, a nonadenosine receptor, or an alternate state of one of the previously identified receptors. This last possibility is intriguing considering a demonstration by Luthin and Linden (1995) that assay conditions such as temperature can alter agonist-binding profiles to the A_{2a} receptor. Which receptor mediates these non-A_1 effects in the hippocampus and cortex, and whether these responses are physiologically relevant effects of adenosine, remains to be seen.

C. A_{2b} Receptors

In contrast to the A_{2a} receptor, the function of A_{2b} receptors in the CNS has not been thoroughly investigated, primarily due to the lack of selective ligands and the diffuse distribution of these receptors. A_{2b} receptors are thought to mediate the rise in cAMP levels seen in brain slices with high concentrations of adenosine (Lupica *et al.,* 1990). A_2 receptors have been shown to potentiate P-type calcium currents in hippocampal (Mogul *et al.,*

1993) and brain stem (Umemiya and Berger, 1994) neurons, and it has been suggested that this is mediated by the A_{2b} receptor (Mogul *et al.*, 1993). A_{2b} receptors are also prominently found on glial cells, where they have been suggested to increase Ca^{2+} influx (Porter and McCarthy, 1995) and the formation of interleukin-6 (Fiebich *et al.*, 1996) as well as the formation of cAMP. Fredholm and Altiok (1994) have also shown an influence of interleukin 1β and bradykinin on the ability of A_{2b} receptors to mediate cAMP formation. Although A_{2b} receptors can mediate clear changes in messenger systems in a variety of cell types, it has proven difficult to link any significant physiological changes in neuronal activity to this receptor. Based on the apparent interaction of these receptors with inflammatory mediators, and the extremely low potency of the A_{2b} receptor for adenosine (Bruns *et al.*, 1986), it has been postulated that these receptors may mediate neuroprotective effects when extracellular adenosine levels reach exceptionally high levels (Fredholm and Altiok, 1994).

D. A_3 Receptors

The A_3 receptor is the most recently characterized adenosine receptor and its effects on central neuronal physiology are poorly understood. The A_3 receptor was not characterized by pharmacological or physiological means prior to its cloning (Zhou *et al.*, 1992; Meyerhof *et al.*, 1991). It was originally shown to be capable of inhibiting adenylyl cyclase activity when expressed in Chinese hamster ovary cells (Zhou *et al.*, 1992), although this effect has not been observed in cells naturally expressing the receptor and may have been an artifact of the expression system used. Abbracchio *et al.*, (1995) found that A_3 receptor agonists stimulated the formation of inositol phosphates in striatal and hippocampal slices, suggesting it can activate phospholipase C. Several peripheral responses to adenosine have now been attributed to the A_3 receptor, but a detailed characterization of its actions in the CNS has been difficult (Linden, 1994; Fredholm *et al.*, 1994). The first report of a possible central effect of A_3-receptor activation came from Jacobson *et al.* (1993) who showed that an ip injection of an A_3 selective agonist into mice caused locomotor depression that could not be reversed by A_1 and A_{2a} receptor antagonists. However, a peripheral site of action was not ruled out. von Lubitz *et al.* (1994b) showed that ip injection of an A_3 selective agonist into gerbils just prior to forebrain ischemia caused increased cell death and decreased survival in the animals. Chronic administration of the agonist for 10 days produced the opposite effect, decreasing neuronal cell death and increasing animal survival rates (von Lubitz *et al.*, 1994b). von Lubitz *et al.* (1994a) have also shown the opposite effect with A_1 receptor antagonists, which were found to improve survival after ischemia acutely but to worsen survival if given chronically. These data suggest that there is an interaction between the A_1 and the A_3 receptors such that they produce opposing actions in forebrain ischemia. This concept is further supported by Dunwiddie *et al.* (1997), who have shown that prior application of A_3 selective agonists can inhibit subsequent A_1 receptor-mediated responses, suggesting that A_3 receptors may produce a heterologous desensitization of A_1 receptors. Transfected A_3 receptors have been shown to desensitize after agonist exposure due to phosphorylation of the receptor (Palmer *et al.*, 1995b), and long-term agonist exposure to A_3 receptors in this system has been shown to downregulate the $G_i\alpha$-3 subunit (Palmer *et al.*, 1995a), which is a likely candidate for the $G\alpha$ subunit that interacts with A_1 receptors (Jockers *et al.*, 1994; Freissmuth *et al.*, 1991). It remains to be seen whether mechanisms such as these are responsible for the desensitization of A_1 receptors by A_3 receptor activation, and whether the deleterious effects of acute A_3 receptor activation during ischemia are related to their potential ability to alter A_1 responses. Nevertheless, the regulation of responses mediated by A_1 receptors is a potential function of A_3 receptors in the brain.

III. Intracellular Metabolism of Adenosine

Adenosine can be formed in the intracellular and extracellular spaces, and adenosine formed in both of these locations may be important in controlling the extracellular concentration of adenosine, and hence its ability to interact with adenosine receptors and modulate synaptic activity (Fig. 2). There are at least two major pathways for adenosine formation within cells: the cleavage of *S*-adenosylhomocysteine (SAH) by *S*-adenosylhomocysteine hydrolase (SAHH) and the degradation of adenine nucleotides to 5′-AMP and then to adenosine via an intracellular, cytosolic 5′-nucleotidase. Once formed, adenosine can diffuse across the cell membrane via facilitated diffusion nucleoside transporters. These transporters are bidirectional and will equilibrate the intracellular and extracellular concentrations of adenosine. Hence, adenosine flux across the membrane simply follows the concentration gradient, and changes in the intracellular concentration will affect the extracellular concentration, and vice versa. The intracellular concentration of adenosine depends not only on adenosine-forming enzymes, but also on enzymes that further metabolize adenosine. There are two major pathways of adenosine metabolism: phosphorylation to 5′-AMP via adenosine kinase and deamination to inosine via adenosine deaminase. Hence, the extracellular concentration of adenosine will ultimately depend on the rates of adenosine formation, diffusion, and degradation.

A. Adenosine Formation by S-Adenosylhomocysteine Hydrolase

S-Adenosylhomocysteine hydrolase (EC 3.3.1.1) is involved in the metabolism of *S*-adenosylhomocysteine and thus helps regulate transmethyla-

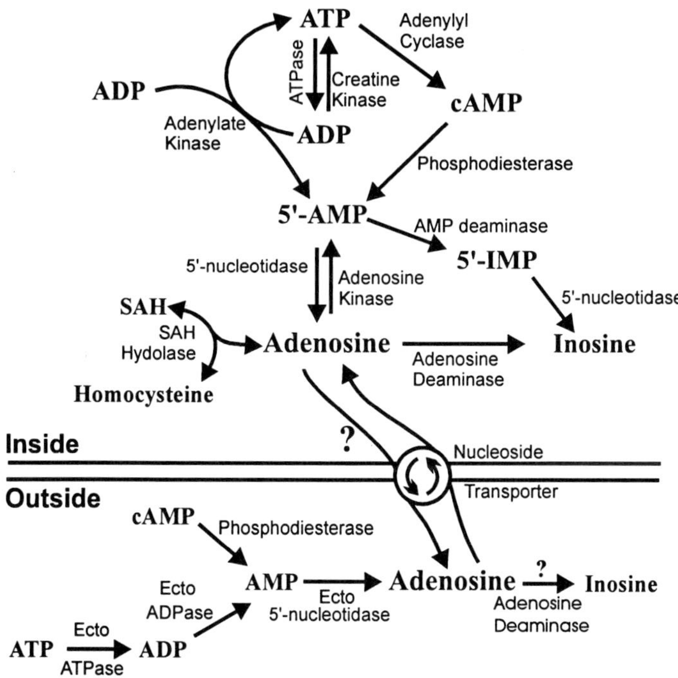

FIGURE 2 Metabolic pathways of adenosine formation and degradation both inside and outside of cells.

tion in cells. The reaction catalyzed by SAHH is reversible, so SAHH can form adenosine and homocysteine by cleavage of SAH as well as utilize adenosine during SAH synthesis (Fig. 2). SAHH is a cytoplasmic enzyme, although it may also be associated with the nucleus (Ueland, 1982), and is found in numerous brain regions (Patel and Tudball, 1986). The idea that adenosine is generated by cleavage of SAH has not received a great deal of investigation, primarily due to the assumed role of nucleotide breakdown in adenosine release during metabolic disruption and the comparatively low levels of intracellular SAH relative to ATP. However, unlike other enzymes involved in adenosine metabolism, SAHH has been shown to exist at higher levels in neurons than in glia (Ceballos *et al.,* 1994), leaving open the possibility that it is involved in adenosine release induced by synaptic stimulation or in the basal levels of adenosine present in the extracellular space. Indeed, Deussen *et al.* (1989) used the SAHH inhibitor adenosine dialdehyde to show that SAHH was responsible for approximately one-third of the basal adenosine released from the heart, but made no contribution to the much greater amount of adenosine released during hypoxia. In the hippocampus, Pak *et al.* (1994) found that adenosine dialdehyde had no effect on the ability of an adenosine kinase inhibitor to release adenosine and inhibit population spikes in the hippocampus, and Latini *et al.* (1995) saw no effect of adenosine dialdehyde on adenosine released by ischemia and electrical stimulation. These results suggest that SAHH does not play a role in most forms of evoked adenosine release in the brain, although it may play a role in determining the basal concentration of adenosine in some areas.

An interesting aspect of the SAH/adenosine metabolic pathway is that it is completely reversible. Several investigators have taken advantage of this by using exogenous homocysteine thiolactone to reduce the intracellular concentration of adenosine. The addition of homocysteine thiolactone has been shown to decrease adenosine release from neocortical (McIlwain and Poll, 1985, 1986) and hippocampal (Lloyd *et al.*, 1993) slices induced by hypoxia, electrical stimulation, and application of K^+ and glutamate. These data demonstrate that the presence of homocysteine can reduce adenosine levels through the synthesis of SAH and support an intracellular location for adenosine formation under these conditions, as SAHH is an intracellular enzyme and would be less able to utilize adenosine formed extracellularly (Lloyd *et al.*, 1993; McIlwain and Poll, 1986; Ueland, 1982). However, facilitation of adenosine uptake by increasing intracellular metabolism cannot be ruled out.

B. Adenosine Formation by Metabolism of Intracellular Nucleotides

It has long been suspected that one of the primary sources of adenosine released into the extracellular space is adenosine formed from the degradation of intracellular nucleotides. This is largely a result of the observation that almost all conditions that disrupt cellular metabolism (and thus oxidative phosphorylation) evoke the release of adenosine. It has been proposed that inhibiting cellular metabolism causes a decrease in intracellular ATP levels and a subsequent increase in ADP, AMP, and adenosine. As intracellular adenosine levels rise, it is thought that adenosine equilibrates with the extracellular space by diffusing through the cell membrane with the aid of nucleoside transporters. This model has been in generally good agreement with experimental results. Numerous studies have shown that conditions which release adenosine result in a decrease in cellular ATP (Latini *et al.*, 1995; Yoneda and Okada, 1989; Fredholm *et al.*, 1984; Lipton and Whittingham, 1982), although adenosine release does not always occur with exactly the same time course as the degradation of ATP (Latini *et al.*, 1995; Yoneda and Okada, 1989). Hence, the metabolic pathways responsible for regulating the intracellular concentration of nucleotides and nucleosides may be important in adenosine release.

Intracellular adenosine concentrations are normally extremely low and adenosine is kept in a steady state with adenine nucleotides (Fig. 2). Most of the adenine nucleotides in the intracellular space are in the form of ATP, which is estimated to be in the low millimolar concentration range. ATP is, of course, constantly being dephosphorylated to ADP by a wide variety of ATPases during most energy-requiring reactions. ADP can be rephosphorylated by creatine kinase (EC 2.7.3.2) or by oxidative phosphorylation within mitochondria. Additionally, adenylate kinase (EC 2.7.4.3) can transfer a phosphate from one ADP to another, resulting in the production of ATP and AMP. AMP can subsequently be dephosphorylated to adenosine by the action of 5′-nucleotidase (EC 3.1.3.5). Adenosine can then enter either of two metabolic pathways: rephosphorylation to AMP by adenosine kinase (EC 2.7.1.20) or deamination to inosine by adenosine deaminase (ADA; EC 3.5.4.4). Additionally, AMP can be directly deaminated by 5′-AMP deaminase to 5′-IMP, which is also a substrate for 5′-nucleotidase, resulting in inosine. It is likely that the lack of oxidative phosphorylation and/or the depletion of creatine phosphate reserves during metabolic inhibition causes an increase in the AMP pool through the actions of adenylate kinase, and subsequent dephosphorylation by 5′-nucleotidase yields high concentrations of intracellular adenosine. Hence, the energy state of the cell and the activities of 5′-nucleotidase and adenosine kinase are likely to be the dominant factors controlling intracellular (and thus extracellular) adenosine concentrations.

Despite the prevailing notion that 5′-nucleotidase must be responsible for most of the intracellular adenosine formation, relatively few studies have directly addressed this issue. It was originally thought that the predominant 5′-nucleotidase associated with the plasma membrane would fulfill this role. However, it has now been conclusively shown that the membrane-bound 5′-nucleotidase is an ecto-enzyme (Zimmermann, 1992; Pearson, 1985) that is bound to the extracellular side of the cell membrane by a glycosyl phosphatidylinositol anchor (Zimmermann, 1992). This precludes a role for this enzyme in the intracellular formation of adenosine. Attention then turned to a soluble, cytosolic, IMP-preferring form of 5′-nucleotidase that was first identified by Van den Berghe *et al.* (1977) in liver cells, and later found in leukocytes (Newby, 1980) and brain (Montero and Fes, 1982). Although Worku and Newby (1983) concluded that the IMP-preferring 5′-nucleotidase was sufficiently active in polymorphonuclear leukocytes to account for the adenosine produced during metabolic inhibition by 2-deoxyglucose, the low K_m of this enzyme for AMP is thought to preclude a role in the formation of adenosine in most tissues (Meghji *et al.*, 1988). In 1988 Truong *et al.* discovered a second cytosolic 5′-nucleotidase in rat heart for which AMP was the preferred substrate. Newby (1988) has shown that this enzyme is sufficiently active to account for the rapid adenosine production in pigeon heart induced by ischemia. Unfortunately, the AMP-preferring enzyme has not been demonstrated to exist in any tissues other than heart, so its role in adenosine production in the brain is not known. Skladanowski *et al.* (1989) have developed selective inhibitors for each of the two known cytosolic forms of 5′-nucleotidase, so future experiments need to be conducted in which the role of these enzymes in adenosine release from the brain is evaluated.

C. Degradation of Adenosine

In addition to the pathways of adenosine formation, the mechanisms of adenosine degradation are vitally important in regulating intracellular and extracellular adenosine concentrations. There are two major routes of adenosine inactivation: phosphorylation by adenosine kinase and deamination by ADA. It is important to point out that the intracellular degradation of adenosine plays a critical role in the uptake of adenosine. Uptake of adenosine occurs via nucleoside transporters that work by a facilitated diffusional mechanism and are bidirectional (Plagemann and Wohlhueter, 1984; Bender *et al.,* 1980, 1981). Hence, adenosine uptake into cells only occurs if the intracellular concentration of adenosine is kept below the extracellular concentration. Adenosine kinase activity is extremely important in maintaining this concentration gradient and in supporting the continuous uptake of adenosine (Davies and Cook, 1995; Wu *et al.,* 1984; Zimmermann *et al.,* 1979), and is therefore an important regulator of extracellular adenosine. Pak *et al.* (1994) have shown that application of the adenosine kinase inhibitor iodotubercidin to hippocampal slices can evoke the release of adenosine and the subsequent inhibition of synaptic activity. Lloyd and Fredholm (1995) have also found that iodotubercidin can potentiate the evoked release of adenosine in hippocampal slices. Both of these studies concluded that adenosine phosphorylation was the primary route of adenosine metabolism under basal conditions and was also important under stimulated conditions as was deamination by adenosine deaminase. It has been observed that the application of iodotubercidin to hippocampal slices causes an almost immediate elevation of extracellular adenosine levels, whereas the application of the nucleoside transport inhibitors dipyridamole and NBTI causes a slow, gradual increase in the extracellular adenosine concentration over the course of an hour (J. M. Brundege and T. V. Dunwiddie, unpublished observations), suggesting that intracellular adenosine formation and rephosphorylation occur continuously under basal conditions and that inhibition of adenosine kinase causes a rapid buildup of intracellular adenosine and therefore increases adenosine release. Alternatively, adenosine may be continuously released via a transporter mechanism under basal conditions, and uptake and subsequent phosphorylation occur at separate sites. In this case, inhibition of adenosine kinase would not increase the rate of release, but would selectively prevent uptake due to the collapse of the concentration gradient and therefore cause a rapid accumulation of extracellular adenosine. Transport inhibitors, however would decrease both efflux and uptake, and adenosine accumulation in the extracellular space would proceed slowly. Regardless of the mechanism involved, adenosine kinase is clearly important in regulating extracellular adenosine levels, and modulation of this enzyme could be a potential mechanism by which cells release adenosine.

In addition to metabolism by adenosine kinase, adenosine can be deaminated via ADA. Several investigators have evaluated the role of ADA in regulating adenosine levels. Under normal, basal conditions, ADA inhibitors have been found to cause a small increase in adenosine concentrations (Lloyd and Fredholm, 1995; Pak *et al.*, 1994; Ballarin *et al.*, 1991), whereas inhibition of adenosine uptake (Ballarin *et al.*, 1991) and adenosine kinase (Lloyd and Fredholm, 1995; Pak *et al.*, 1994) increase adenosine concentrations to a much larger extent. However, inhibition of ADA prior to the induction of adenosine release greatly enhanced the elevation of extracellular adenosine levels (Lloyd and Fredholm, 1995; Delaney and Geiger, 1995; Mitchell *et al.*, 1993; Lloyd *et al.*, 1993). These results suggest that ADA is not responsible for most adenosine metabolism under basal conditions, but is responsible for clearing much of the adenosine from the extracellular space when adenosine levels are elevated. This is not surprising considering the K_m for ADA is 1–2 orders of magnitude greater than the K_m for adenosine kinase (Arch and Newsholme, 1978a).

Another interesting feature of adenosine deaminase is that while predominantly a cytoplasmic enzyme, it has also been found to be associated with cell membranes (Centelles *et al.*, 1986; Franco *et al.*, 1986; Andy and Kornfeld, 1982), possibly via an interaction with a membrane-bound ADA-binding protein. Furthermore, in peripheral tissue, ADA activity has been found in the extracellular space (Hellewell and Pearson, 1983; Andy and Kornfeld, 1982) where it would be capable of directly inactivating extracellular adenosine without prior reuptake. However, ADA activity in the brain correlates with nitrobenzylthioinosine (NBTI)-binding sites (Nagy *et al.*, 1985), suggesting that much of the ADA is intracellular and requires adenosine uptake prior to metabolism. Regardless of its site of action, ADA appears to be important for clearing transiently released adenosine, leading to the proposition that ADA may be a marker for purinergic neurons or areas where adenosinergic modulation of synapses is particularly important (Nagy *et al.*, 1990). However, the localization of ADA has not been found to correlate with the localization of A_1 receptors (Geiger and Nagy, 1986), and adenosine was found to have no effect on the mesencephalic trigeminal nucleus, a target of adenosine deaminase-containing projections from the hypothalamus (Regenold *et al.*, 1988). Although these results argue against the use of ADA as a marker for purinergic neurons, there are numerous areas receiving ADA-containing projections where the role of adenosine as a neuromodulator has not been evaluated.

IV. Adenosine Levels in the Brain

As summarized earlier, it is likely that the concentration of adenosine in the extracellular space depends, in part, on the intracellular concentration of adenosine. There are, however, several mechanisms that could potentially release adenosine into the extracellular space, and the extracellular concentration of adenosine can vary depending on the physiological conditions. Normally there is a significant basal level of adenosine receptor activation, suggesting that a low, tonic level of adenosine is usually present in the extracellular space. This can be seen by the excitatory effects of adenosine receptor antagonists both *in vitro* (Dunwiddie, 1980; Dunwiddie *et al.*, 1981; Dunwiddie and Hoffer, 1980) and *in vivo* (Katims *et al.*, 1983; Snyder *et al.*, 1981). Direct measurements have been made using biochemical techniques and have yielded variable results that always suggest the presence of physiologically significant levels of adenosine. It is likely that many of these measurements overestimated the basal concentration of adenosine due to two problems: tissue damage resulting from these invasive techniques tends to increase adenosine concentrations (Fredholm *et al.*, 1984; Zetterström *et al.*, 1982) and any nucleotides present are likely to degrade into adenosine during the procedure (Pearson, 1985; Terrian *et al.*, 1989). Nevertheless, experiments have been designed to overcome these problems and have given estimates for the basal concentration of adenosine in the extracellular space that are in the nanomolar range (Dunwiddie and Diao, 1994; Ballarin *et al.*, 1991). This concentration appears to activate adenosine receptors to a modest extent, leaving open the possibility that cells might further increase the extracellular concentration in response to various stimuli.

In addition to this tonic level of adenosine, numerous other conditions cause a significant elevation of the extracellular adenosine concentration. Many of these conditions result in the inhibition of cellular metabolism. Adenosine release from brain tissue can occur in response to hypoxia (Lloyd *et al.*, 1993; Gribkoff *et al.*, 1990; Fowler, 1989; Zetterström *et al.*, 1982; Phillis *et al.*, 1987), ischemia (Pedata *et al.*, 1993; Phillis *et al.*, 1987; Berne *et al.*, 1974), electrical stimulation (Lloyd *et al.*, 1993; Schrader *et al.*, 1980; Yawo and Chuhma, 1993; Pull and McIlwain, 1972), and chemical depolarization (Hoehn and White, 1990, 1993; Shimizu *et al.*, 1970). Adenosine is also released by nonpathological nerve stimulation (Manzoni *et al.*, 1994; Mitchell *et al.*, 1993; Grover and Teyler, 1993) and by *N*-methyl-D-aspartate (NMDA) receptor activation (Chen *et al.*, 1992; Hoehn *et al.*, 1990; Hoehn and White, 1993). Although it is obvious that the brain can elevate the extracellular concentration of adenosine, the exact mechanism by which this occurs and the origins of this adenosine remain elusive.

V. Adenosine Release

Several different hypotheses have been proposed to explain the origins of extracellular adenosine. Early efforts focused on identifying purinergic neurons that use adenosine as a neurotransmitter. However, little evidence has emerged that adenosine is sequestered in nerve terminals and released in the manner of a classical neurotransmitter. Many investigators have thus shifted their attention to studying alternate ways in which adenosine can be released into or generated in the extracellular space (see Nagy *et al.*, 1990, and critiques for an excellent review of these various hypotheses). In addition to the idea that adenosine is synaptically released from purinergic nerve terminals, two major hypotheses have emerged to explain the origins of extracellular adenosine: that extracellular adenosine is formed from nucleotides released into the extracellular space and catabolized to adenosine via a series of ecto-enzymes, and that adenosine formed intracellularly is released or diffuses into the extracellular space by a nonsynaptic mechanism. These hypotheses are nonexclusive, and there is evidence that both may contribute to the effects of endogenous adenosine.

A. Extracellular Degradation of Nucleotides

Exogenously applied ATP and cAMP can elicit inhibitory responses mediated by A_1 receptors in the hippocampus as well as at peripheral synapses, presumably after their conversion to adenosine (Terrian *et al.*, 1989; Zimmermann *et al.*, 1979; Dunwiddie and Hoffer, 1980) since these nucleotides do not appear to activate adenosine receptors directly (Schwabe and Trost, 1980) (Fig. 2). The enzymes necessary to degrade extracellular nucleotides to adenosine exist in the brain (Pearson, 1985), and there is substantial evidence that ATP release and extracellular degradation to adenosine can occur in the central nervous system. Ecto-ATPase (EC 3.6.1.15), ecto-ADPase (EC 3.6.1.6), and ecto-5′-nucleotidase (EC 3.1.3.5) have all been identified in purified cholinergic synapses from the striatum (James and Richardson, 1993). Furthermore, ATP has been found to colocalize with numerous neurotransmitters in the periphery (Fredholm *et al.*, 1982; Da Prada and Pletscher, 1968) and in the CNS (Richardson *et al.*, 1987), and there is good evidence that ATP colocalized with ACh at the neuromuscular junction is released upon nerve stimulation and is subsequently degraded to adenosine in the extracellular space (Smith, 1991; Ribeiro and Sebastiao, 1987; Silinsky and Hubbard, 1973). It has proven much more difficult to demonstrate ATP colocalization with other neurotransmitters in the CNS due to the multiplicity of neurotransmitters and nerve terminals present in most brain regions. Nevertheless, several studies have demonstrated a calcium-dependent release of ATP from brain tissue (Wieraszko *et al.*, 1989; Terrian *et al.*, 1989; Potter and White, 1980; Wu and Phillis, 1978; Kuroda, 1978), suggesting that vesicular release of ATP may occur. Furthermore, Richardson *et al.* (James and Richardson, 1993; Richardson *et al.*, 1987; Richardson and Brown, 1987) have shown that ATP is colocalized with ACh in affinity-purified cholinergic nerve terminals from rat striatum, that this ATP can be released by depolarization with KCl or veratridine, and that ATP is subsequently metabolized to adenosine in the extracellular space. Although adenosine can inhibit the release of ACh from striatal synaptosomes, they found that cholinergic terminals from the cortex were not sensitive to inhibition of ACh release by adenosine and were not capable of generating high levels of adenosine from ATP due to the low activities of ecto-ADPase and ecto-5′-nucleotidase (Richardson *et al.,* 1987). This is somewhat confusing, considering that Potter and White (1980) have shown depolarization-evoked, calcium-dependent ATP release from synaptosomes from a number of different brain regions, including the cerebral cortex. However, Potter and White (1980) were studying a mixed population of synaptosomes from several types of nerve terminals, whereas Richardson *et al.* (1987) focused only on cholinergic nerve terminals. Wu and Phillis (1978) have also demonstrated that electrical stimulation directly to the motor cortex of intact rats can release ATP. In light of these data, it appears that ATP release can occur in several brain regions; however, there are numerous synapses where adenosine can modulate synaptic activity but ATP colocalization with neurotransmitters has not been demonstrated, such as glutamatergic synapses in hippocampus and cortex.

Further evidence for the formation of adenosine via release of a nucleotide comes from Hoehn and White (1990a), who conducted extensive experiments measuring adenosine outflow from cortical slice preparations. They found that the ecto-5′-nucleotidase inhibitor α,β-methylene ADP (AOPCP) decreased the basal release of adenosine, suggesting that some of the basal efflux of adenosine may be released as a nucleotide. Using the same assay, Craig and White (1993) found that NMDA-stimulated adenosine release could also be reduced by AOPCP, but adenosine release by kainate and quisqualate could not. Thus, multiple mechanisms of adenosine release appear to exist in the same preparation. Yet another mechanism of adenosine release may have been discovered by Hoehn and White (1990b), who reported that glutamate could evoke the release of adenosine from cortical synaptosomes and that the formation of adenosine was prevented by AOPCP, but there was no detectable ATP being released in their system and adenosine formation could not be blocked by a phosphodiesterase inhibitor. This led them to suggest that the synaptosomes were releasing a nucleotide other than ATP or cAMP that was metabolized to adenosine extracellularly. Interestingly, they also found that stimulation of adenosine release by glutamate was not mediated by glutamate receptors, but was rather induced by the uptake of glutamate through a sodium-dependent glutamate transporter. The relevance of these unusual results to adenosine released in other systems is not known.

Another potential source of adenosine is cAMP released into the extracellular space. Numerous receptors are positively coupled to the enzyme adenylyl cyclase and can thus stimulate the formation of cAMP (Mons and Cooper, 1995). Release of cAMP has been demonstrated from striatal slices

(Headley and O'Shaughnessy, 1986; Stoof and Kebabian, 1981), cortex cell cultures (Rosenberg *et al.*, 1994; Rosenberg and Dichter, 1989), *in vivo* spinal cord (Sweeney *et al.*, 1990, 1991), and the cortex of conscious rats (Stone and John, 1990). cAMP efflux from cells has been shown to occur via a unidirectional, energy-dependent anion efflux pump (Henderson and Strauss, 1991), although other transport mechanisms may exist. The ability of cells to extrude cAMP is especially interesting considering the resemblance between adenylyl cyclase and P-glycoprotein, an anion transporter capable of transporting cAMP (Henderson and Strauss, 1991; Gottesman and Pastan, 1988; Krupinski *et al.*, 1989). Specific receptors for cAMP have not been demonstrated, and researchers have long debated about the function of released cAMP (see Rosenberg, 1992, for an excellent summary). Extracellular conversion of cAMP to adenosine has been demonstrated in the hippocampus (Gereau and Conn, 1994; Dunwiddie and Hoffer, 1980), spinal cord synaptosomes (Nicholson *et al.*, 1991), cerebral cortex cell cultures (Rosenberg and Dichter, 1989), and the ventral tegmental area (Bonci and Williams, 1996), suggesting the presence of an extracellular phosphodiesterase (PDE) (EC 3.1.4.17) as well as ecto-5′-nucleotidase. Hence, several researchers have considered the possibility that efflux of cAMP and subsequent extracellular degradation is a physiological mechanism for elevating extracellular adenosine.

Sweeney *et al.* (1990, 1991) hypothesized that the release of cAMP may be an important source of physiologically active adenosine in the spinal cord. This idea was based on the observation that intrathecal perfusion of spinal cord with 5-hydroxytryptamine and morphine induced the release of both cAMP and adenosine (Sweeney *et al.*, 1990, 1991), and that adenosine release from spinal cord synaptosomes depended on the actions of ecto-5′-nucleotidase (Sweeney *et al.*, 1988). However, a clear demonstration that released cAMP is converted to adenosine is difficult to accomplish due to the lack of selective ecto-phosphodiesterase inhibitors. Nicholson *et al.* (1991) examined the effects of several phosphodiesterase inhibitors on the ability of spinal cord synaptosomes to degrade exogenously applied cAMP to adenosine and found that 3-isobutyl-1-methylxanthine (IBMX), but not RO 20-1724 and rolipram, was able to inhibit degradation, suggesting that only IBMX inhibits the ecto-enzyme. However, all three of these phosphodiesterase inhibitors increased the basal release of adenosine and decreased morphine-evoked release. This may reflect the ability of these inhibitors to decrease the activity of intracellular, as well as extracellular, phosphodiesterase, thereby altering cAMP levels and cAMP release as well as extracellular metabolism. Craig *et al.* (1994) found equally confusing results when they investigated the role of cAMP in mediating the NMDA-evoked release of adenosine from cortical slices. They showed that IBMX decreased and forskolin, an activator of adenylyl cyclase, increased adenosine release, but probenecid, an inhibitor of cAMP efflux, failed to inhibit adenosine release.

They then systematically tested selective inhibitors of phosphodiesterase types I, II, and IV, and found that none of these could decrease NMDA-evoked adenosine release. Although it is possible that IBMX is the only inhibitor capable of inhibiting the ecto-phosphodiesterase, the inability of probenecid to block adenosine release may suggest that IBMX is working through a mechanism other than phosphodiesterase inhibition.

Rosenberg *et al.* (1994) have also observed the release of cAMP together with adenosine from mixed astrocyte/neuronal cortical cultures and also found confusing results with phosphodiesterase inhibitors. They found that agonists of β-adrenergic receptors stimulated the efflux of cAMP from astrocytes in culture, but that a mixed population of neurons and astrocytes were necessary for the efflux of adenosine. Furthermore, probenecid decreased the efflux of both cAMP and adenosine. These data are consistent with the idea that astrocytes release cAMP, and the extracellular phosphodiesterase necessary to convert the cAMP to adenosine is associated with neurons. They also tried to inhibit adenosine formation with several different phosphodiesterase inhibitors and found that no single inhibitor decreased the efflux of adenosine. Only a combination of IBMX and RO 20-1724 decreased the release of adenosine, suggesting that there may be multiple types of phosphodiesterase in this system. However, considering that IBMX has little selectivity for the different known types of phosphodiesterase, it is unclear why adding RO 20-1724, an inhibitor of the type IV cAMP-specific phosphodiesterase (Thompson, 1991), would block adenosine formation.

Gereau and Conn (1994) demonstrated that RO 20-1724 does not inhibit the breakdown of cAMP exogenously applied to hippocampal slices, suggesting that it does not inhibit the phosphodiesterase that metabolizes extracellular cAMP. However, they also demonstrated that stimulation of adenylyl cyclase via application of agonists of β-adrenergic and metabotropic glutamate receptors induced the release of adenosine and that this release was inhibited by RO 20-1724. These data suggest that activation of adenylyl cyclase caused the release of adenosine subsequent to the *intracellular* degradation of cAMP. Bonci and Williams (1996) examined the A_1 receptor-mediated inhibition of $GABA_B$ receptor-mediated inhibitory potentials in the ventral tegmental area. They found that application of dopamine D1 receptor agonists can stimulate cAMP formation and increase extracellular adenosine in drug-withdrawn animals. They too found that RO 20-1724 could inhibit the apparent release of adenosine, but also found that probenecid prevented the release of adenosine, presumably by preventing cAMP efflux into the extracellular space. Unfortunately, they did not evaluate the ability of RO 20-1724 to block the extracellular conversion of exogenous cAMP to adenosine, and neither Bonci and Williams (1996) nor Gereau and Conn (1994) attempted to block the extracellular conversion of 5′-AMP to adenosine with α,β-methylene ADP, which would have provided further information about the form adenosine was in when it crossed the cell membrane and entered the extracellular space. In any case, the lack of selective ecto-phosphodiesterase inhibitors has made it difficult to conclusively demonstrate that cAMP release from cells is a significant source of extracellular adenosine, but it seems clear that stimulation of cAMP formation in the brain can elevate adenosine levels in the extracellular space, although the site of adenosine formation is uncertain.

B. Direct Release of Adenosine into the Extracellular Space

Another mechanism by which extracellular adenosine could become elevated is by direct release of intracellularly formed adenosine. One of the first demonstrations of adenosine release as adenosine per se, and not as a nucleotide, was by Daval and Barberis (1981), who showed that labeled adenosine could be released from cortical synaptosomes by chemical depolarization and electrical stimulation and that this release was not decreased by the ecto-5′-nucleotidase inhibitor AOPCP. Since that time, numerous investigators have used AOPCP to determine whether increases in extracellular adenosine are derived from released nucleotides. It has thus been demonstrated that adenosine released by hypoxia, electrical stimulation (Lloyd *et al.,* 1993), metabolic poisoning (Meghji *et al.,* 1989), and synaptic stimulation (Manzoni *et al.,* 1994; Mitchell *et al.,* 1993) is not prevented by inhibiting ecto-5′-nucleotidase activity, suggesting that adenosine is directly released into the extracellular space. Interestingly, Manzoni *et al.* (1994) found that adenosine released by synaptic activity in the hippocampus was dependent on the activation of NMDA receptors and could be mimicked by exogenous application of NMDA, but AOPCP did not prevent this adenosine release. This is in contrast to the NMDA-mediated release of adenosine from the cortex seen by Craig and White (1993), which was inhibited by AOPCP. It is possible that this is due to the different brain regions being studied, but it may also be due to the way in which NMDA receptors were activated and adenosine was measured. Craig and White (1993) measured the adenosine concentration in the superfusate of cortical slices with biochemical techniques and stimulated adenosine release with high (100 μM) concentrations of NMDA, whereas Manzoni *et al.* (1994) observed the effects of adenosine on synaptic activity in hippocampal slices and induced adenosine release by synaptic stimulation, which only allowed them to observe the pool of adenosine near the presynaptic terminals. It is possible that the synaptic activation of NMDA receptors can modulate further synaptic activity by the direct release of adenosine, whereas perfusion of the brain with high concentrations of NMDA induces the release of adenosine by multiple mechanisms, including the release of nucleotides. Indeed, Craig and White (1993) observed a 68% decrease in adenosine release by AOPCP, leaving open the possibility that the remaining portion was released as adenosine per se.

In order for adenosine formed in the intracellular space to interact with adenosine receptors, it must be transported across the cell membrane into the extracellular space. Adenosine transport across the cell membrane occurs via a facilitated diffusional nucleoside transport mechanism (Plagemann and Wohlhueter, 1984; Bender *et al.,* 1980). The nucleoside transporters mediating this transfer have not been cloned, and a detailed molecular characterization of these molecules is not available. However, it appears that there are at least two types of nucleoside transporters (Plagemann and Wohlhueter, 1984; Bender *et al.,* 1980), although additional subtypes have been proposed (Geiger and Fyda, 1991). These nucleoside transporters are primarily differentiated by their sensitivity or insensitivity to inhibition by nitrobenzylthioinosine (NBTI) (Lee and Jarvis, 1988; Plagemann and Wohlhueter, 1984), since other inhibitors appear to be less selective. Much of the original work in which adenosine transport was characterized focused on the role of these transporters in mediating adenosine uptake into cells, thus providing a way for cells to maintain a low extracellular adenosine concentration. However, the observation that these transporters are bidirectional (Gu *et al.,* 1995; Bender *et al.,* 1981) has led to the hypothesis that they may also be important mediators of the release of adenosine into the extracellular space. This agreed with data showing that metabolic inhibition can release adenosine and led to the hypothesis that the rapid breakdown of ATP during metabolic inhibition causes an increase in intracellular adenosine and that subsequent diffusion out of the cell via a bidirectional transporter causes an increase in extracellular adenosine. Many investigators have used inhibitors of nucleoside transport to try to confirm this hypothesis, but these experiments have resulted in conflicting results. The nonselective nucleoside transport inhibitor dipyridamole has been shown to decrease morphine-evoked adenosine release from spinal cord synaptosomes (Sweeney *et al.,* 1989), as well as adenosine release induced by electrical stimulation in hippocampal slices (Jonzon and Fredholm, 1985). The transport inhibitor dilazep was also found to decrease adenosine efflux from metabolically poisoned chick ganglia cells in culture (Meghji *et al.,* 1989). These studies seem to support the idea that adenosine efflux occurs via a nucleoside transporter. However, numerous studies have shown that the transport inhibitors dipyridamole (Mitchell *et al.,* 1993; Dunwiddie and Diao, 1994; Craig and White, 1993; Ballarin *et al.,* 1991; Phillis *et al.,* 1989; Sanderson and Scholfield, 1986), NBTI (Craig and White, 1993; Ballarin *et al.,* 1991; Sanderson and Scholfield, 1986), soluflazine (Boissard and Gribkoff, 1993), lidoflazine (Ballarin *et al.,* 1991), and dilazep (Delaney and Geiger, 1995; Sanderson and Scholfield, 1986) increased the extracellular adenosine concentration in several brain regions under a variety of conditions, consistent with the idea that adenosine is released by another mechanism (e.g., release as a nucleotide), and suggesting that the nucleoside transporters primarily mediate uptake, not efflux. Newby (1986) has provided a possible explanation for these conflicting data by using a mathematical model to demonstrate that a single transporter can mediate both adenosine release and reuptake, and that inhibition of transporter activity can potentially increase or decrease extracellular adenosine levels, depending on the relative rates of formation and inactivation. This model assumes that there are different sites within the system that mediate either influx or efflux and that both are inhibited during application of nucleoside transport inhibitors. While the model of Newby (1986) suggests that a single transporter could account for the contrasting results of previous experiments, the exact transport mechanisms involved in adenosine release from intact tissues have not been clearly defined.

VI. Localized Adenosine Release and Synaptic Modulation

As outlined in the introduction, adenosine has been suggested to serve a wide variety of functions in the nervous system. However, evidence has provided new support for a role in short-term synaptic modulation and suggests that adenosine may play a unique role as an active feedback modulator of synaptic activity. Although it has long been known that electrical and chemical stimuli can release adenosine, most of these studies involved widespread depolarization of brain tissue. Therefore, these studies cannot tell us whether adenosine plays a role in normal neuronal activity or is released only during pathological conditions such as metabolic inhibition or excitotoxicity. Evidence that adenosine may be released during normal activity has been provided by Grover and Teyler (1993), who demonstrated that heterosynaptic depression, a short-term form of synaptic plasticity in the hippocampus, was partially mediated by adenosine. In these experiments, Grover and Teyler (1993) stimulated one set of axons at 25 Hz for 15 sec and found that the responses of a second set of axons were inhibited for the next 30 sec. This synaptic inhibition could be reversed by adenosine A_1 receptor antagonists, and thus appeared to be due to released adenosine. This was significant in that it was the first demonstration of a transient increase in endogenous adenosine levels under relatively nonpathological conditions, i.e., that do not produce neuronal damage. At the same time, Mitchell *et al.* (1993) reported a similar finding using a similar type of heterosynaptic stimulation in the hippocampal slice. However, they used an extremely brief stimulation period in which four stimulating pulses were given over 40 msec. This stimulation protocol induced an extremely transient release of adenosine that occurred over a time course of about 1 sec. Mitchell *et al.* (1993) went on to show that uptake via dipyridamole-sensitive transporters and deamination by adenosine deaminase were both involved in termination of the adenosine-mediated responses and that inhibition of ecto-5′-nucleotidase did not prevent the rise in extracellular adenosine, suggesting that the adenosine was released as adenosine, not as a nucleotide. These data strongly support a role for adenosine as a transient modulator of synaptic activity during normal physiological processes, at least in the hippocampus.

Further insights into the mechanism by which adenosine is released in the hippocampus came from Manzoni *et al.* (1994), who used a heterosynaptic stimulation protocol to determine the receptor dependence of evoked adenosine release. They found that stimulation of one excitatory pathway at 100 Hz for 1 sec elicited a profound inhibition of the heterosynaptic pathway that lasted for 5 to 10 min and could be blocked by adenosine receptor antagonists. This inhibition could also be blocked with NMDA receptor antagonists, and a similar, adenosine-mediated inhibition was induced by direct application of NMDA. Thus, the stimulation of NMDA receptors by synaptically released glutamate appears to be responsible for the adenosine release in this system, in agreement with other studies showing NMDA receptor-dependent release of adenosine in the brain (Chen *et al.,* 1992; Hoehn and White, 1993). Manzoni *et al.* (1994) also demonstrated that the adenosine was released as such and did not derive from a nucleotide catabolized by ecto-5′-nucleotidase. Furthermore, they showed that enkephalin could decrease adenosine-mediated inhibition, suggesting that some of the adenosine came from interneurons, which are selectively inhibited by enkephalin. However, it is not known whether other sources of adenosine are also involved. One interesting aspect of these data is that Manzoni *et al.* (1994) stimulated adenosine release with a protocol that induced long-term potentiation in the stimulated pathway, whereas adenosine inhibited the surrounding synapses. It is possible that adenosine, by temporarily depressing the synapses surrounding the active pathways, is increasing the signal-to-noise ratio within this system, thereby contributing to other forms of synaptic plasticity.

These studies support a role for adenosine as a synaptic modulator during normal brain activity, but they leave several questions unanswered. Although two of the studies ruled out extracellular degradation of a nucleotide as the source of adenosine (Manzoni *et al.,* 1994; Mitchell *et al.,* 1993), the metabolic pathway of adenosine formation and the roles of adenosine-forming enzymes such as cytoplasmic 5′-nucleotidase and *S*-adenosylhomocysteine hydrolase are still unknown. It is also unclear how the stimulation protocols used induce the formation and release of adenosine. Manzoni *et al.* (1994) demonstrated a dependence on NMDA receptor activation, and presumably Ca^{2+} influx, but whether this releases adenosine by increasing the rate of ATP degradation, by modulating the activity of adenosine-metabolizing enzymes such as 5′-nucleotidase and adenosine kinase, or by increasing the rate of formation of cAMP is unknown. It is also unclear how adenosine is released into the extracellular space. Although transport via a bidirectional nucleoside transporter is a likely mechanism, this has yet to be demonstrated. Finally, none of these experiments conclusively show where the adenosine is coming from. Although Manzoni *et al.* (1994) showed that inhibiting interneurons with enkephalin blocked some of the adenosine release, it is not clear whether the remaining adenosine comes from pyramidal neurons or from other cell types or processes within the hippocampus.

Brundege and Dunwiddie (1996) have attempted to address some of these issues by inducing adenosine release from individual neurons in a hippocampal slice preparation. It was found that directly elevating the adenosine concentration in a single CA1 pyramidal neuron induced the release of adenosine into the extracellular space and inhibited the excitatory inputs to that cell via presynaptic adenosine receptors. Furthermore, the synaptic inhibition was relatively selective in that there was no significant effect on postsynaptic adenosine receptors or on the synaptic responses of neighboring cells. While these data do not provide information about the ability of normal physiological activity to induce the release of adenosine, they do demonstrate that CA1 pyramidal neurons can release adenosine from their postsynaptic processes in such a way as to presynaptically inhibit excitatory inputs. These results support the idea that adenosine may be a retrograde feedback messenger in the hippocampus, such that postsynaptic activity can presynaptically inhibit excitatory synapses. Although more data are needed on the mechanisms of adenosine release in this system, preliminary results (Brundege and Dunwiddie, 1996) show that inhibition of adenosine kinase in a single pyramidal neuron can also release adenosine (Fig. 3), although it is not known if modulation of the activity of this enzyme is a mechanism for elevating adenosine levels under normal conditions. Furthermore, the presence of high concentrations of uridine inside a single neuron can block the release of adenosine from that cell, suggesting that adenosine is being transported into the extracellular space by a saturable transport system for which uridine is a substrate. Although it appears likely that this is one of the nucleoside transporters, experiments with selective inhibitors will be needed to further characterize this mechanism. It is hoped that future experiments will clarify these issues and provide more insight into whether adenosine can function as a retrograde inhibitor of excitatory transmission in the hippocampus.

VII. Conclusions

The experimental evidence concerning the actions of adenosine has made it clear that adenosine does not play only one role in neuronal physiology, but rather serves multiple functions throughout the nervous system. An

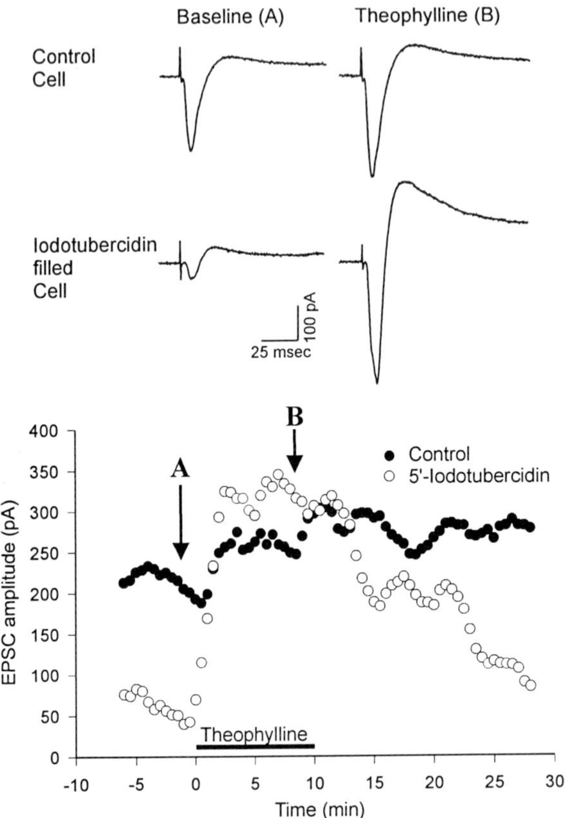

FIGURE 3 A single hippocampal pyramidal neuron can release enough endogenous adenosine to inhibit excitatory synaptic inputs. Excitatory postsynaptic current (EPSC) recordings from a control cell and a cell "loaded" with 400 μM 5′-iodotubercidin, an adenosine kinase inhibitor, by including iodotubercidin in the filling solution of the recording electrode. Cells were recorded using the whole cell voltage-clamp technique. Sample traces are shown for a control cell and a cell loaded with iodotubercidin before and during application of the adenosine receptor antagonist theophylline (200 μM). The EPSC is measured as the amplitude of the downward deflection. The graph plots the time course for the two cells. Data show that the EPSC of the cell loaded with iodotubercidin is inhibited during the baseline and that the inhibition is reversed by an adenosine receptor antagonist, suggesting that inhibition of adenosine kinase in a single cell induces the release of adenosine and the subsequent inhibition of excitatory transmission via activation of presynaptic A_1 receptors (for details see Brundege and Dunwiddie, 1996).

understanding of these functions will only come through a thorough examination of both the effects of adenosine and the manner in which adenosine levels are regulated. The lack of evidence supporting a neurotransmitter role for adenosine suggests that adenosine is a neuromodulator and is released in unconventional ways to interact with its cell surface receptors. This makes it particularly challenging to clearly define the stimuli that evoke the release of adenosine and to determine how this occurs, but it also provides the opportunity to make dramatic progress toward a more complete understanding of signaling in the brain. The list of local hormones, autocoids, retrograde messengers, and synaptic modulators has been steadily growing, and it now appears that adenosine is a unique member within these groups. As the manner in which these compounds function is elucidated, our view of how cells communicate with one another is greatly broadened.

Studies on the actions of exogenous adenosine have conclusively shown that adenosine can act as a potent and effective modulator of synaptic activity and neuronal function. Although this would seem to suggest that adenosine has a neuromodulatory function during normal physiological processes, the clear ability of pathological stimuli to release adenosine and the predominantly inhibitory actions of this compound raise the issue of whether adenosine has any function other than as a neuroprotectant, springing into action only under harmful conditions. The purpose of this review has not been to determine whether other such functions exist, but rather to summarize what is known about how cells synthesize, release, and regulate adenosine, thereby providing a base upon which we can build a more complete understanding of how adenosine acts as a neuromodulator. Data showing that adenosine is transiently released under nonpathological conditions provide the best evidence to date that adenosine functions as a modulator of synaptic activity during normal brain function. The challenge thus shifts to defining how neuronal activity triggers adenosine release and how the periodic release of endogenous adenosine affects overall neuronal activity. Further experiments should help clarify the position of adenosine among the numerous chemical signaling agents of the brain.

References

Abbracchio, M. P., Brambilla, R., Ceruti, S., Kim, H. O., von Lubitz, D. K. J. E., Jacobson, K. A., and Cattabeni, F. (1995). G protein-dependent activation of phospholipase C by adenosine A_3 receptors in rat brain. *Mol. Pharmacol.* **48**, 1038–1045.

Andy, R. J., and Kornfeld, R. (1982). The adenosine deaminase binding protein of human skin fibroblasts is located on the cell surface. *J. Biol. Chem.* **257**, 7922–7925.

Arch, J. R., and Newsholme, E. A. (1978a). Activities and some properties of 5′-nucleotidase, adenosine kinase and adenosine deaminase in tissues from vertebrates and invertebrates in relation to the control of the concentration and the physiological role of adenosine. *Biochem. J.* **174**, 965–977.

Arch, J. R., and Newsholme, E. A. (1978b). The control of the metabolism and the hormonal role of adenosine (review). *Essays Biochem.* **14**, 82–123.

Ballarin, M., Fredholm, B. B., Ambrosio, S., and Mahy, N. (1991). Extracellular levels of adenosine and its metabolites in the striatum of awake rats: Inhibition of uptake and metabolism. *Acta Physiol. Scand.* **142**, 97–103.

Bender, A. S., Wu, P. H., and Phillis, J. W. (1980). The characterization of [3H] adenosine uptake into rat cerebral cortical synaptosomes. *J. Neurochem.* **35**, 629–640.

Bender, A. S., Wu, P. H., and Phillis, J. W. (1981). The rapid uptake and release of [3H]adenosine by rat cerebral cortical synaptosomes. *J. Neurochem.* **36**, 651–660.

Bennett, M. R., and Ho, S. (1991). Probabilistic secretion of quanta from nerve terminals in avian ciliary ganglia modulated by adenosine. *J. Physiol.* (*London*) **440**, 513–527.

Bennett, M. R., and Ho, S. (1992). Adenosine modulation of potassium currents in preganglionic nerve terminals of avian ciliary ganglia. *Neurosci. Lett.* **137**, 41–44.

Berne, R. M., Rubio, R., and Curnish, R. R. (1974). Release of adenosine from ischemic brain. *Circ. Res.* **35**, 262–271.

Berne, R. M., Winn, H. R., and Rubio, R. (1981). The local regulation of cerebral blood flow (review). *Prog. Cardiovasc. Dis.* **24**, 243–260.

Birnstiel, S., Gerber, U., and Greene, R. W. (1992). Adenosine-mediated synaptic inhibition: Partial blockade by barium does not prevent anti-epileptiform activity. *Synapse* **11**, 191–196.

Boissard, C. G., and Gribkoff, V. K. (1993). The effects of the adenosine reuptake inhibitor soluflazine on synaptic potentials and population hypoxic depolarizations in area CA1 of rat hippocampus in vitro. *Neuropharmacology* **32**, 149–155.

Bonci, A., and Williams, J. T. (1996). A common mechanism mediates long-term changes in synaptic transmission after chronic cocaine and morphine. *Neuron* **16**, 631–639.

Brown, S. J., James, S., Reddington, M., and Richardson, P. J. (1990). Both A_1 and A_{2a} purine receptors regulate striatal acetylcholine release. *J. Neurochem.* **55**, 31–38.

Brundege, J. M., and Dunwiddie, T. V. (1996). Modulation of excitatory synaptic transmission by adenosine released from single hippocampal pyramidal neurons. *J. Neurosci.* **16**, 5603–5612.

Bruns, R. F., Lu, G. H., and Pugsley, T. A. (1986). Characterization of the A_2 adenosine receptor labeled by [^{3}H]-NECA in rat striatal membranes. *Mol. Pharmacol.* **29**, 331–346.

Capogna, M., Gähwiler, B. H., and Thompson, S. M. (1996). Presynaptic inhibition of calcium-dependent and -independent release elicited with ionomycin, gadolinium, and α-latrotoxin in the hippocampus. *J. Neurophysiol.* **75**, 2017–2028.

Cass, W. A., and Zahniser, N. R. (1991). Potassium channel blockers inhibit D_2 dopamine, but not A_1 adenosine, receptor-mediated inhibition of striatal dopamine release. *J. Neurochem.* **57**, 147–152.

Ceballos, G., Tuttle, J. B., and Rubio, R. (1994). Differential distribution of purine metabolizing enzymes between glia and neurons. *J. Neurochem.* **62**, 1144–1153.

Centelles, J. J., Franco, R., Canela, E. I., and Bozal, J. (1986). Kinetics of the 5′-nucleotidase and the adenosine deaminase in subcellular fraction of rat brain. *Neurochem. Res.* **11**, 471–479.

Chen, Y., Graham, D. I., and Stone, T. W. (1992). Release of endogenous adenosine and its metabolites by the activation of NMDA receptors in the rat hippocampus in vivo. *Br. J. Pharmacol.* **106**, 632–638.

Craig, C. G., and White, T. D. (1993). NMDA and Non-NMDA evoked adenosine release from rat cortical slices: Distinct purinergic sources and mechanisms of release. *J. Neurochem.* **60**, 1073–1080.

Craig, C. G., Temple, S. D., and White, T. D. (1994). Is cyclic AMP involved in excitatory amino acid-evoked adenosine release from rat cortical slices? *Eur. J. Pharmacol.* **269**, 79–85.

Cunha, R. A., Johansson, B., Constantino, M. D., Sebastiao, A. M., and Fredholm, B. B. (1996). Evidence for high affinity binding sites for the adenosine A_{2A} receptor agonist [^{3}H] CGS 21680 in the rat hippocampus and cerebral cortex that are different from striatal A_{2A} receptors. *Naunyn Schmiedeberg's Arch. Pharmacol.* **353**, 261–271.

Daly, J. W., Butts-Lamb, P., and Padgett, W. (1983). Subclasses of adenosine receptors in the central nervous system: Interaction with caffeine and related methylxanthines. *Cell. Mol. Neurobiol.* **3**, 69–80.

Da Prada, M., and Pletscher, A. (1968). Isolated 5-hydroxytryptamine organelles of rabbit blood platelets: Physiological properties and drug-induced changes. *Br. J. Pharmacol.* **34**, 591–597.

Daval, J. L., and Barberis, C. (1981). Release of radiolabelled adenosine derivatives from superfused synaptosome beds. *Biochem. Pharmacol.* **30**, 2559–2567.

Davies, L. P., and Cook, A. F. (1995). Inhibition of adenosine kinase and adenosine uptake in guinea-pig CNS tissue by halogenated tubercidin analogues. *Life Sci.* **56**, PL345–PL349.

Deckert, J., and Jorgensen, M. B. (1988). Evidence for pre- and postsynaptic localization of adenosine A_1 receptors in the CA1 region of the rat hippocampus: A quantitative autoradiographic study. *Brain Res.* **446**, 161–164.

Delaney, S. M., and Geiger, J. D. (1995). Enhancement of NMDA-induced increases in levels of endogenous adenosine by adenosine deaminase and adenosine transport inhibition in rat striatum. *Brain Res.* **702**, 72–76.

Deussen, A., Lloyd, H. G., and Schrader, J. (1989). Contribution of S-adenosylhomocysteine to cardiac adenosine formation. *J. Mol. Cell. Cardiol.* **21**, 773–782.

Dolphin, A. C., and Archer, E. R. (1983). An adenosine agonist inhibits and a cyclic AMP analogue enhances the release of glutamate but not GABA from slices of rat dentate gyrus. *Neurosci. Lett.* **43**, 49–54.

Dolphin, A. C., Forda, S. R., and Scott, R. H. (1986). Calcium-dependent currents in cultured rat dorsal root ganglion neurones are inhibited by an adenosine analogue. *J. Physiol. (London)* **373**, 47–61.

Dragunow, M. (1988). Purinergic mechanisms in epilepsy (review). *Prog. Neurobiol.* **31**, 85–108.

Dragunow, M., and Faull, R. L. (1988). Neuroprotective effects of adenosine. *Trends Pharmacol. Sci.* **9**, 193–194.

Drury, A. N., and Szent-Györgyi, A. (1929). The physiological activity of adenine compounds with especial reference to their action upon the mammalian heart. *J. Physiol. (London)* **68**, 213–237.

Duner-Engström, M., and Fredholm, B. B. (1988). Evidence that prejunctional adenosine receptors regulating acetylcholine release from rat hippocampal slices are linked to an N-ethylmaleimide-sensitive G-protein, but not to adenylate cyclase or dihydropyridine-sensitive Ca^{2+}-channels. *Acta Physiol. Scand.* **134**, 119–126.

Dunwiddie, T. V. (1980). Endogenously released adenosine regulates excitability in the in vitro hippocampus. *Epilepsia* **21**, 541–548.

Dunwiddie, T. V., and Diao, L. (1994). Extracellular adenosine concentrations in hippocampal brain slices and the tonic inhibitory modulation of evoked excitatory responses. *J. Pharmacol. Exp. Ther.* **268**, 537–545.

Dunwiddie, T.V., and Fredholm, B. B. (1989). Adenosine A_1 receptors inhibit adenylate cyclase activity and neurotransmitter release and hyperpolarize pyramidal neurons in rat hippocampus. *J. Pharmacol. Exp. Ther.* **249**, 31–37.

Dunwiddie, T. V., and Haas, H. L. (1985). Adenosine increases synaptic facilitation in the in vitro rat hippocampus: Evidence for a presynaptic site of action. *J. Physiol. (London)* **369**, 365–377.

Dunwiddie, T. V., and Hoffer, B. J. (1980). Adenine nucleotides and synaptic transmission in the in vitro rat hippocampus. *Br. J. Pharmacol.* **69**, 59–68.

Dunwiddie, T. V., and Miller, K. K. (1993). Effects of adenosine and cadmium on presynaptic fiber spikes in the CA1 region of rat hippocampus in vitro. *Neuropharmacology* **32**, 1061–1068.

Dunwiddie, T. V., Hoffer, B. J., and Fredholm, B. B. (1981). Alkylxanthines elevate hippocampal excitability: Evidence for a role of endogenous adenosine. *Naunyn-Schmiedeberg's Arch. Pharmacol.* **316**, 326–330.

Dunwiddie, T. V., Diao, L., Kim, H. O., and Jacobson, K. A. (1997). Activation of hippocampal adenosine A_3 receptors produces a heterologous desensitization of A_1 receptor mediated responses in rat hippocampus. *J. Neurosci.* **17**, 607–614.

Ebstein, R. P., and Daly, J. W. (1982). Release of norepinephrine and dopamine from brain vesicular preparations: Effects of adenosine analogs. *Cell. Mol. Neurobiol.* **2**, 193–204.

Fastbom, J., Pazos, A., and Palacios, J. M. (1987). The distribution of adenosine A1 receptors and 5′-nucleotidase in the brain of some commonly used experimental animals. *Neuroscience* **22,** 813–826.

Ferre, S., von Euler, G., Johansson, B., Fredholm, B. B., and Fuxe, K. (1991). Stimulation of high-affinity adenosine A_2 receptors decreases the affinity of dopamine D2 receptors in rat striatal membranes. *Proc. Natl. Acad. Sci. U.S.A.* **88,** 7238–7241.

Feuerstein, T. J., Hertting, G., and Jackisch, R. (1985). Modulation of hippocampal serotonin (5-HT) release by endogenous adenosine. *Eur. J. Pharmacol.* **107,** 233–242.

Fiebich, B. L., Biber, K., Gyufko, K., Berger, R., Bauer, J., and van Calker, D. (1996). Adenosine A_{2b} receptors mediate an increase in interleukin (IL)-6 mRNA and IL-6 protein synthesis in human astroglioma cells. *J. Neurochem.* **66,** 1426–1431.

Fink, J. S., Weaver, D. R., Rivkees, S. A., Peterfreund, R. A., Pollack, A. E., Adler, E. M., and Reppert, S. M. (1992). Molecular cloning of the rat A_2 adenosine receptor: Selective co-expression with D2 dopamine receptors in rat striatum. *Brain Res. Mol. Brain Res.* **14,** 186–195.

Fowler, J. C. (1989). Adenosine antagonists delay hypoxia-induced depression of neuronal activity in hippocampal brain slice. *Brain Res.* **490,** 378–384.

Fozard, J. R., Pfannkuche, H. J., and Schuurman, H. J. (1996). Mast cell degranulation following adenosine A_3 receptor activation in rats. *Eur. J. Pharmacol.* **298,** 293–297.

Franco, R., Canela, E. I., and Bozal, J. (1986). Heterogeneous localization of some purine enzymes in subcellular fraction of rat brain and cerebellum. *Neurochem. Res.* **11,** 423–435.

Fredholm, B. B. (1990). Differential sensitivity to blockade by 4-aminopyridine of presynaptic receptors regulating [3H]acetylcholine release from rat hippocampus. *J. Neurochem.* **54,** 1386–1390.

Fredholm, B. B., and Altiok, N. (1994). Adenosine A_{2B} receptor signalling is altered by stimulation of bradykinin or interleukin receptors in astroglioma cells. *Neurochem. Int.* **25,** 99–102.

Fredholm, B. B., Fried, G., and Hedqvist, P. (1982). Origin of adenosine released from rat vas deferens by nerve stimulation. *Eur. J. Pharmacol.* **79,** 233–243.

Fredholm, B. B., Jonzon, B., and Lindgren, E. (1983). Inhibition of noradrenaline release from hippocampal slices by a stable adenosine analogue. *Acta Physiol. Scand. Suppl.* **515,** 7–10.

Fredholm, B. B., Dunwiddie, T. V., Bergman, B., and Lindström, K. (1984). Levels of adenosine and adenine nucleotides in slices of rat hippocampus. *Brain Res.* **295,** 127–136.

Fredholm, B. B., Proctor, W. R., Van der Ploeg, I., and Dunwiddie, T. V. (1989). In vivo pertussis toxin treatment attenuates some, but not all, adenosine A_1 effects in slices of the rat hippocampus. *Eur. J. Pharmacol.* **172,** 249–262.

Fredholm, B. B., Abbracchio, M. P., Burnstock, G., Daly, J. W., Harden, T. K., Jacobson, K. A., Leff, P., and Williams, M. (1994). Nomenclature and classification of purinoceptors. *Pharmacol. Rev.* **46,** 143–156.

Freissmuth, M., Schutz, W., and Linder, M. E. (1991). Interactions of the bovine brain A_1-adenosine receptor with recombinant G protein alpha-subunits. Selectivity for rGi alpha-3. *J. Biol. Chem.* **266,** 17778–17783.

Geiger, J. D., and Fyda, D. (1991). Adenosine transport in the CNS. *In* "Adenoosine in the Nervous System" (T. W. Stone, ed.), pp. 1–23. Academic Press, San Diego, CA.

Geiger, J. D., and Nagy, J. I. (1986). Distribution of adenosine deaminase activity in rat brain and spinal cord. *J. Neurosci.* **6,** 2707–2714.

Gerber, U., Greene, R. W., Haas, H. L., and Stevens, D. R. (1989). Characterization of inhibition mediated by adenosine in the hippocampus of the rat in vitro. *J. Physiol (London)* **417,** 567–578.

Gereau, R. W., IV, and Conn, P. J. (1994). Potentiation of cAMP responses by metabotropic glutamate receptors depresses excitatory synaptic transmission by a kinase-independent mechanism. *Neuron* **12,** 1121–1129.

Glass, M., Faull, R. L. M., Bullock, J. Y., Jansen, K., Mee, E. W., Walker, E. B., Synek, B. J. L., and Dragunow, M. (1996). Loss of A_1 adenosine receptors in human temporal lobe epilepsy. *Brain Res.* **710,** 56–68.

Gottesman, M. M., and Pastan, I. (1988). The multidrug transporter, a double-edged sword (review). *J. Biol. Chem.* **263,** 12163–12166.

Gribkoff, V. K., Bauman, L. A., and VanderMaelen, C. P. (1990). The adenosine antagonist 8-cyclopentyltheophylline reduces the depression of hippocampal neuronal responses during hypoxia. *Brain Res.* **512,** 353–357.

Grover, L. M., and Teyler, T. J. (1993). Role of adenosine in heterosynaptic, posttetanic depression in area CA1 of hippocampus. *Neurosci. Lett.* **154,** 39–42.

Gu, J. G., Foga, I. O., Parkinson, F. E., and Geiger, J. D. (1995). Involvement of bidirectional adenosine transporters in the release of L-[3H]adenosine from rat brain synaptosomal preparations. *J. Neurochem.* **64,** 2105–2110.

Harms, H. H., Wardeh, G., and Mulder, A. H. (1978). Adenosine modulates depolarization-induced release of 3H-noradrenaline from slices of rat brain neocortex. *Eur. J. Pharmacol.* **49,** 305–308.

Harms, H. H., Wardeh, G., and Mulder, A. H. (1979). Effect of adenosine on depolarization-induced release of various radiolabelled neurotransmitters from slices of rat corpus striatum. *Neuropharmacology* **18,** 577–580.

Haulica, I., Ababei, L., Branisteanu, D., and Topoliceanu, F. (1973). Preliminary data on the possible hypnogenic role of adenosine. *J. Neurochem.* **21,** 1019–1020.

Headley, P. M., and O'Shaughnessy, C. T. (1986). The use of cyclic AMP efflux studies in attempts to determine the effects of morphine on cyclic AMP formation in striatal slices. *Neuropharmacology* **25,** 919–922.

Hellewell, P. G., and Pearson, J. D. (1983). Metabolism of circulating adenosine by the porcine isolated perfused lung. *Circ. Res.* **53,** 1–7.

Henderson, G. B., and Strauss, B. P. (1991). Evidence for cAMP and cholate extrusion in C6 rat glioma cells by a common anion efflux pump. *J. Biol. Chem.* **266,** 1641–1645.

Heurteaux, C., Lauritzen, I., Widmann, C., and Lazdunski, M. (1995). Essential role of adenosine, adenosine A_1 receptors, and ATP-sensitive K+ channels in cerebral ischemic preconditioning. *Proc. Natl. Acad. Sci. U.S.A.* **92,** 4666–4670.

Hoehn, K., and White, T. D. (1990a). Role of excitatory amino acid receptors in K+- and glutamate-evoked release of endogenous adenosine from rat cortical slices. *J. Neurochem.* **54,** 256–265.

Hoehn, K., and White, T. D. (1990b). Glutamate-evoked release of endogenous adenosine from rat cortical synaptosomes is mediated by glutamate uptake and not by receptors. *J. Neurochem.* **54,** 1716–1724.

Hoehn, K., and White, T. D. (1993). N-Methyl-D-Aspartate, Kainate and Quisqualate release endogenous adenosine from rat cortical slices. *Neuroscience* **39,** 441–450.

Hoehn, K., Craig, C. G., and White, T. D. (1990). A comparison of N-methyl-D-aspartate-evoked release of adenosine and [3H]-norepinephrine from rat cortical slices. *J. Pharmacol. Exp. Ther.* **255,** 174–181.

Holgate, S. T., Lewis, R. A., and Austen, K. F. (1980). Role of adenylate cyclase in immunologic release of mediators from rat mast cells: Agonist and antagonist effects of purine- and ribose-modified adenosine analogs. *Proc. Natl. Acad. Sci. U.S.A.* **77,** 6800–6804.

Hunt, J. M., Redman, R. S., and Silinsky, E. M. (1994). Reduction by intracellular calcium chelation of acetylcholine secretion without occluding the effects of adenosine at frog motor nerve endings. *Br. J. Pharmacol.* **111,** 753–758.

Jackisch, R., Strittmatter, H., Kasakov, L., and Hertting, G. (1984). Endogenous adenosine as a modulator of hippocampal acetylcholine release. *Naunyn Schmiedeberg's Arch. Pharmacol.* **327,** 319–325.

Jacobson, K. A., Nikodijevic, O., Shi, D., Gallo-Rodriguez, C., Olah, M. E., Stiles, G. L., and Daly, J. W. (1993). A role for central A_3-adenosine receptors. Mediation of behavioral depressant effects. *FEBS Lett.* **336,** 57–60.

James, S., and Richardson, P. J. (1993). Production of adenosine from extracellular ATP at the striatal cholinergic synapse. *J. Neurochem.* **60,** 219–227.

Jin, S., Johansson, B., and Fredholm, B. B. (1993). Effects of adenosine A_1 and A_2 receptor activation on electrically evoked dopamine and acetylcholine release from rat striatal slices. *J. Pharmacol. Exp. Ther.* **267,** 801–808.

Jockers, R., Linder, M. E., Hohenegger, M., Nanoff, C., Bertin, B., Strosberg, A. D., Marullo, S., and Freissmuth, M. (1994). Species difference in the G protein selectivity of the human and bovine A_1-adenosine receptor. *J. Biol. Chem.* **269,** 32077–32084.

Johansson, B., and Fredholm, B. B. (1995). Further characterization of the binding of the adenosine receptor agonist [3H]CGS 21680 to rat brain using autoradiography. *Neuropharmacology* **34,** 393–403.

Johansson, B., Georgiev, V., Parkinson, F. E., and Fredholm, B. B. (1993). The binding of the adenosine A_2 receptor selective agonist [3H]CGS 21680 to rat cortex differs from its binding to rat striatum. *Eur. J. Pharmacol.* **247,** 103–110.

Jonzon, B., and Fredholm, B. B. (1985). Release of purines, noradrenaline, and GABA from rat hippocampal slices by field stimulation. *J. Neurochem.* **44,** 217–224.

Katims, J. J., Annau, Z., and Snyder, S. H. (1983). Interactions in the behavioral effects of methylxanthines and adenosine derivatives. *J. Pharmacol. Exp. Ther.* **227,** 167–173.

Krupinski, J., Coussen, F., Bakalyar, H. A., Tang, W.-J., Feinstein, P. G., Orth, K., Slaughter, C., Reed, R. R., and Gilman, A. G. (1989). Adenylyl cyclase amino acid sequence: Possible channel- or transporter-like structure. *Science* **244,** 1558–1564.

Kuroda, Y. (1978). Physiological roles of adenosine derivatives which are released during neurotransmission in mammalian brain. *J. Physiol. (Paris)* **74,** 463–470.

Lambert, N. A., and Teyler, T. J. (1991). Adenosine selectively depresses excitatory synaptic transmission in area CA1 of the rat hippocampus. *Neurosci. Lett.* **122,** 50–52.

Latini, S., Corsi, C., Pedata, F., and Pepeu, G. (1995). The source of brain adenosine outflow during ischemia and electrical stimulation. *Neurochem. Int.* **27,** 239–244.

Lee, C. W., and Jarvis, S. M. (1988). Kinetic and inhibitor specificity of adenosine transport in guinea pig cerebral cortical synaptosomes: Evidence for two nucleoside transporters. *Neurochem. Int.* **12,** 483–492.

Li, Y. O., and Fredholm, B. B. (1985). Adenosine analogues stimulate cyclic AMP formation in rabbit cerebral microvessels via adenosine A_2-receptors. *Acta Physiol. Scand.* **124,** 253–259.

Lin, Y., and Phillis, J. W. (1991). Characterization of the depression of rat cerebral cortical neurons by selective adenosine agonists. *Brain Res.* **540,** 307–310.

Linden, J. (1994). Cloned adenosine A_3 receptors: Pharmacological properties, species differences and receptor functions. *Trends Pharmacol. Sci.* **15,** 298–306.

Lipton, P., and Whittingham, T. S. (1982). Reduced ATP concentration as a basis for synaptic transmission failure during hypoxia in the in vitro Guinea-pig hippocampus. *J. Physiol. (London)* **325,** 51–65.

Lloyd, H. G. E., and Fredholm, B. B. (1995). Involvement of adenosine deaminase and adenosine kinase in regulating extracellular adenosine concentration in rat hippocampal slices. *Neurochem. Int.* **26,** 387–395.

Lloyd, H. G. E., Lindstrom, K., and Fredholm, B. B. (1993). Intracellular formation and release of adenosine from rat hippocampal slices evoked by electrical stimulation or energy depletion. *Neurochem. Int.* **23,** 173–185.

Lupica, C. R., Cass, W. A., Zahniser, N. R., and Dunwiddie, T. V. (1990). Effects of the selective adenosine A_2 receptor agonist CGS 21680 on in vitro electrophysiology, cAMP formation and dopamine release in rat hippocampus and striatum. *J. Pharmacol. Exp. Ther.* **252,** 1134–1141.

Lupica, C. R., Proctor, W. R., and Dunwiddie, T. V. (1992). Presynaptic inhibition of excitatory synaptic transmission by adenosine in rat hippocampus: Analysis of unitary EPSP variance measured by whole-cell recording. *J. Neurosci.* **12,** 3753–3764.

Luthin, D.R., and Linden, J. (1995). Comparison of A_4 and A_{2a} binding sites in striatum and COS cells transfected with adenosine A_{2a} receptors. *J. Pharmacol. Exp. Ther.* **272,** 511–518.

MacDonald, R. L., Skerritt, J. H., and Werz, M. A. (1986). Adenosine agonists reduce voltage-dependent calcium conductance of mouse sensory neurones in cell culture. *J. Physiol. (London)* **370,** 75–90.

Manzoni, O. J., Manabe, T., and Nicoll, R. A. (1994). Release of adenosine by activation of NMDA receptors in the hippocampus. *Science* **265,** 2098–2101.

Mayfield, R. D., Suzuki, F., and Zahniser, N. R. (1993). Adenosine A_{2a} receptor modulation of electrically evoked endogenous GABA release from slices of rat globus pallidus. *J. Neurochem.* **60,** 2334–2337.

Mayfield, R. D., Larson, G., Orona, R. A., and Zahniser, N. R. (1996). Opposing actions of adenosine A_{2a} and dopamine D_2 receptor activation on GABA release in the basal ganglia: Evidence for an A_{2a}/D_2 receptor interaction in globus pallidus. *Synapse* **22,** 132–138.

McIlwain, H., and Poll, J. D. (1985). Interaction between adenosine generated endogenously in neocortical tissues, and homocysteine and its thiolactone. *Neurochem. Int.* **7,** 103–110.

McIlwain, H., and Poll, J. D. (1986). Adenosine in cerebral homeostatic role: Appraisal through actions of homocysteine, colchicine, and dipyridamole. *J. Neurobiol.* **17,** 39–49.

Meghji, P., Middleton, K. M., and Newby, A. C. (1988). Absolute rates of adenosine formation during ischaemia in rat and pigeon hearts. *Biochem. J.* **249,** 695–703.

Meghji, P., Tuttle, J. B., and Rubio, R. (1989). Adenosine formation and release by embryonic chick neurons and glia in cell culture. *J. Neurochem.* **53,** 1852–1860.

Meyerhof, W., Muller-Brechlin, R., and Richter, D. (1991). Molecular cloning of a novel putative G-protein coupled receptor expressed during rat spermiogenesis. *FEBS Lett.* **284,** 155–160.

Michaelis, M. L., Michaelis, E. K., and Myers, S. L. (1979). Adenosine modulation of synaptosomal dopamine release. *Life Sci.* **24,** 2083–2092.

Mitchell, J. B., Lupica, C. R., and Dunwiddie, T. V. (1993). Activity-dependent release of endogenous adenosine modulates synaptic responses in the rat hippocampus. *J. Neurosci.* **13,** 3439–3447.

Mogul, D. J., Adams, M. E., and Fox, A. P. (1993). Differential activation of adenosine receptors decreases N-type but potentiates P-type Ca^{2+} current in hippocampal CA3 neurons. *Neuron* **10,** 327–334.

Mons, N., and Cooper, D. M. F. (1995). Adenylate cyclases: Critical foci in neuronal signaling. *Trends Neurosci.* **18,** 536–542.

Montero, J. M., and Fes, J. B. (1982). Purification and characterization of bovine brain 5′-nucleotidase. *J. Neurochem.* **39,** 982–989.

Mori, A., Shindou, T., Ichimura, M., Nonaka, H., and Kase, H. (1996). The role of adenosine A_{2a} receptors in regulating GABAergic synaptic transmission in striatal medium spiny neurons. *J. Neurosci.* **16,** 605–611.

Mynlieff, M., and Beam, K. G. (1994). Adenosine acting at an A_1 receptor decreases N-type calcium current in mouse motoneurons. *J. Neurosci.* **14,** 3628–3634.

Nagy, J. I., Geiger, J. D., and Daddona, P. E. (1985). Adenosine uptake sites in rat brain: Identification using [3H]nitrobenzylthioinosine and co-localization with adenosine deaminase. *Neurosci. Lett.* **55,** 47–53.

Nagy, J. I., Geiger, J. D., and Staines, W. A. (1990). Adenosine deaminase and purinergic neuroregulation. *Neurochem. Int,* **16,** 211–221.

Newby, A. C. (1980). Role of adenosine deaminase, ecto-(5′-nucleotidase) and ecto-(non-specific phosphatase) in cyanide-induced adenosine monophosphate catabolism in rat polymorphonuclear leucocytes. *Biochem. J.* **186,** 907–918.

Newby, A. C. (1984). Adenosine and the concept of "retaliatory metabolites." *Trends Biochem. Sci.* **9,** 42–44.

Newby, A. C. (1986). How does dipyridamole elevate extracellular adenosine concentration? *Biochem. J.* **237,** 845–851.

Newby, A. C. (1988). The pigeon heart 5′-nucleotidase responsible for ischaemia-induced adenosine formation. *Biochem. J.* **253,** 123–130.

Nicholson, D., White, T. D., and Sawynok, J. (1991). Forskolin and phosphodiesterase inhibitors release adenosine but inhibit morphine-evoked release of adenosine from spinal cord synaptosomes. *Can. J. Physiol. Pharmacol.* **69**, 877–885.

Pak, M. A., Haas, H. L., Decking, U. K., and Schrader, J. (1994). Inhibition of adenosine kinase increases endogenous adenosine and depresses neuronal activity in hippocampal slices. *Neuropharmacology* **33**, 1049–1053.

Palmer, T. M., and Stiles, G. L. (1995). Adenosine receptors. *Neuropharmacology* **34**, 683–694.

Palmer, T. M., Gettys, T. W., and Stiles, G. L. (1995a). Differential interaction with and regulation of multiple G-proteins by the rat A_3 adenosine receptor. *J. Biol. Chem.* **270**, 16895–16902.

Palmer, T. M., Benovič, J. L., and Stiles, G. L. (1995b). Agonist-dependent phosphorylation and desensitization of the rat A_3 adenosine receptor—Evidence for a G-protein-coupled receptor kinase-mediated mechanism. *J. Biol. Chem.* **270**, 29607–29613.

Parkinson, F. E., and Fredholm, B. B. (1990). Autoradiographic evidence for G-protein coupled A_2-receptors in rat neostriatum using [3H]-CGS 21680 as a ligand. *Naunyn-Schmiedeberg's Arch. Pharmacol.* **342**, 85–89.

Patel, B. T., and Tudball, N. (1986). Localization of S-adenosylhomocysteine hydrolase and adenosine deaminase immunoreactivities in rat brain. *Brain Res.* **370**, 250–264.

Pearson, J. D. (1985). Ectonucleotidases: Measurement of activities and use of inhibitors. *Methods Pharmacol.* **6**, 83–108.

Pedata, F., Latini, S., Pugliese, A. M., and Pepeu, G. (1993). Investigations into the adenosine outflow from hippocampal slices evoked by ischemia-like conditions. *J. Neurochem.* **61**, 284–289.

Phillis, J. W., and Wu, P. H. (1981). The role of adenosine and its nucleotides in central synaptic transmission. *Prog. Neurobiol.* **16**, 187–239.

Phillis, J. W., Edström, J. P., Kostopoulos, G. K., and Kirkpatrick, J. R. (1979). Effects of adenosine and adenine nucleotides on synaptic transmission in the cerebral cortex. *Can. J. Physiol. Pharmacol.* **57**, 1289–1312.

Phillis, J. W., Walter, G. A., O'Regan, M. H., and Stair, R. E. (1987). Increases in cerebral cortical perfusate adenosine and inosine concentrations during hypoxia and ischemia. *J. Cereb. Blood Flow Metab.* **7**, 679–686.

Phillis, J. W., O'Regan, M. H., and Walter, G. A. (1989). Effects of two nucleoside transport inhibitors, dipyridamole and soluflazine, on purine release from the rat cerebral cortex. *Brain Res.* **481**, 309–316.

Plagemann, P. G., and Wohlhueter, R. M. (1984). Nucleoside transport in cultured mammalian cells. Multiple forms with different sensitivity to inhibition by nitrobenzylthioinosine or hypoxanthine. *Biochim. Biophys. Acta* **773**, 39–52.

Porter, J. T., and McCarthy, K. D. (1995). Adenosine receptors modulate $[Ca^{2+}]_i$ in hippocampal astrocytes in situ. *J. Neurochem.* **65**, 1515–1523.

Potter, P., and White, T. D. (1980). Release of adenosine 5′-triphosphate from synaptosomes from different regions of rat brain. *Neuroscience* **5**, 1351–1356.

Pull, I., and McIlwain, H. (1972). Adenine derivatives as neurohumoral agents in the brain. *Biochem. J.* **130**, 975–981.

Rainnie, D. G., Grunze, H. C. R., McCarley, R. W., and Greene, R. W. (1994). Adenosine inhibition of mesopontine cholinergic neurons: Implications for EEG arousal. *Science* **263**, 689–692.

Regenold, J. T., Haas, H. L., and Illes, P. (1988). Effects of purinoceptor agonists on electrophysiological properties of rat mesencephalic trigeminal neurones in vitro. *Neurosci. Lett.* **92**, 347–350.

Ribeiro, J. A., and Sebastiao, A. M. (1987). On the role, inactivation and origin of endogenous adenosine at the frog neuromuscular junction. *J. Physiol. (London)* **384**, 571–585.

Richardson, P. J., and Brown, S. J. (1987). ATP release from affinity-purified rat cholinergic nerve terminals. *J. Neurochem.* **48**, 622–630.

Richardson, P. J., Brown, S. J., Bailyes, E. M., and Luzio, J. P. (1987). Ectoenzymes control adenosine modulation of immunoisolated cholinergic synapses. *Nature* (*London*) **327,** 232–234.

Rosenberg, P. A. (1992). Functional significance of cyclic AMP secretion in cerebral cortex (review). *Brain Res. Bull.* **29,** 315–318.

Rosenberg, P. A., and Dichter, M. A. (1989). Extracellular cAMP accumulation and degradation in rat cerebral cortex in dissociated cell culture. *J. Neurosci.* **9,** 2654–2663.

Rosenberg, P. A., Knowles, R., Knowles, K. P., and Li, Y. (1994). Beta-adrenergic receptor-mediated regulation of extracellular adenosine in cerebral cortex in culture. *J. Neurosci.* **14,** 2953–2965.

Sajjadi, F. G., Takabayashi, K., Foster, A. C., Domingo, R. C., and Firestein, G. S. (1996). Inhibition of TNF-a expression by adenosine—Role of A_3 adenosine receptors. *J. Immunol.* **156,** 3435–3442.

Sanderson, G., and Scholfield, C. N. (1986). Effects of adenosine uptake blockers and adenosine on evoked potentials of guinea-pig olfactory cortex. *Pfluegers Arch.* **406,** 25–30.

Sattin, A., and Rall, T. W. (1970). The effect of adenosine and adenine nucleotides on the cyclic adenosine 3′, 5′-phosphate content of guinea pig cerebral cortex slices. *Mol. Pharmacol.* **6,** 13–23.

Scanziani, M., Capogna, M., Gahwiler, B. H., and Thompson, S. M. (1992). Presynaptic inhibition of miniature excitatory synaptic currents by baclofen and adenosine in the hippocampus. *Neuron* **9,** 919–927.

Schiffmann, S. N., Libert, F., Vassart, G., Dumont, J. E., and Vanderhaeghen, J. J. (1990). A cloned G protein-coupled protein with a distribution restricted to striatal medium-sized neurons. Possible relationship with D1 dopamine receptor. *Brain Res.* **519,** 333–337.

Scholfield, C. N., and Steel, L. (1989). Presynaptic K-channel blockade counteracts the depressant effect of adenosine in olfactory cortex. *Neuroscience* **24,** 81–91.

Scholz, K. P., and Miller, R. J. (1992). Inhibition of quantal transmitter release in the absence of calcium influx by a G protein-linked adenosine receptor at hippocampal synapses. *Neuron* **8,** 1139–1150.

Schrader, J., Wahl, M., Kuschinsky, W., and Kreutzberg, G. W. (1980). Increase of adenosine content in cerebral cortex of the cat during bicuculline-induced seizure. *Pfluegers Arch.* **387,** 245–251.

Schubert, P., Heinemann, U., and Lee, K. S. (1986). Differential effect of adenosine on pre- and postsynaptic calcium fluxes. *Brain Res.* **376,** 382–386.

Schwabe, U., and Trost, T. (1980). Characterization of adenosine receptors in rat brain by (-)[3H]N6-phenylisopropyladenosine. *Naunyn Schmiedeberg's Arch. Pharmacol.* **313,** 179–187.

Sebastiao, A. M., and Ribeiro, J. A. (1992). Evidence for the presence of excitatory A_2 adenosine receptors in the rat hippocampus. *Neurosci. Lett.* **138,** 41–44.

Segal, M. (1982). Intracellular analysis of a postsynaptic action of adenosine in the rat hippocampus. *Eur. J. Pharmacol.* **79,** 193–199.

Shimizu, H., Creveling, C. R., and Daly, J. (1970). Stimulated formation of adenosine 3′,5′-cyclic phosphate in cerebral cortex: Synergism between electrical activity and biogenic amines. Proc. Natl. Acad. Sci. U.S.A. **65,** 1033–1040.

Silinsky, E. M. (1984). On the mechanism by which adenosine receptor activation inhibits the release of acetylcholine from motor nerve endings. *J. Physiol.* (*London*) **346,** 243–256.

Silinsky, E. M., and Hubbard, J. I. (1973). Release of ATP from rat motor nerve terminals. *Nature* (*London*) **243,** 404–405.

Silinsky, E. M., and Solsona, C. S. (1992). Calcium currents at motor nerve endings: Absence of effects of adenosine receptor agonists in the frog. *J. Physiol.* (*London*) **457,** 315–328.

Skladanowski, A. C., Sala, G. B., and Newby, A. C. (1989). Inhibition of IMP-specific cytosolic 5′-nucleotidase and adenosine formation in rat polymorphonuclear leucocytes by 5′-deoxy-5′- isobutylthio derivatives of adenosine and inosine. *Biochem. J.* **262,** 203–208.

Smith, D. O. (1991). Sources of adenosine released during neuromuscular transmission in the rat. *J. Physiol. (London)* **432,** 343–354.

Snyder, S. H., Katims, J. J., Annau, Z., Bruns, R. F., and Daly, J. W. (1981). Adenosine receptors and behavioral actions of methylxanthines. *Proc. Natl. Acad. Sci. U.S.A.* **78,** 3260–3264.

Stehle, J. H., Rivkees, S. A., Lee, J. J., Weaver, D. R., Deeds, J. D., and Reppert, S. M. (1992). Molecular cloning and expression of the cDNA for a novel A_2-adenosine receptor subtype. *Mol. Endocrinol.* **6,** 384–393.

Stone, E. A., and John, S. M. (1990). In vivo measurement of extracellular cyclic AMP in the brain: Use in studies of beta-adrenoceptor function in nonanesthetized rats. *J. Neurochem.* **55,** 1942–1949.

Stoof, J. C., and Kebabian, J. W. (1981). Opposing roles for D-1 and D-2 dopamine receptors in efflux of cyclic AMP from rat neostriatum. *Nature (London)* **294,** 366–368.

Sweeney, M. I., White, T. D., and Sawynok, J. (1988). 5-Hydroxytryptamine releases adenosine from primary afferent nerve terminals in the spinal cord. *Brain Res.* **462,** 346–349.

Sweeney, M. I., White, T. D., and Sawynok, J. (1989). Morphine-evoked release of adenosine from the spinal cord occurs via a dipyridamole-sensitive carrier. *J. Neurochem.* **52,** S99B (abstr.).

Sweeney, M. I., White, T. D., and Sawynok, J. (1990). 5-Hydroxytryptamine releases adenosine and cyclic AMP from primary afferent nerve terminals in the spinal cord in vivo. *Brain Res* **528,** 55–61.

Sweeney, M. I., White, T. D., and Sawynok, J. (1991). Intracerebroventricular morphine releases adenosine and adenosine 3′,5′-cyclic monophosphate from the spinal cord via a serotonergic mechanism. *J. Pharmacol. Exp. Ther.* **259,** 1013–1018.

Terrian, D. M., Hernandez, P. G., Rea, M. A., and Peters, R. I. (1989). ATP release, adenosine formation, and modulation of dynorphin and glutamic acid release by adenosine analogues in rat hippocampal mossy fiber synaptosomes. *J. Neurochem.* **53,** 1390–1399.

Thompson, S. M., Haas, H. L., and Gahwiler, B. H. (1992). Comparison of the actions of adenosine at pre- and postsynaptic receptors in the rat hippocampus in vitro. *J. Physiol. (London)* **451,** 347–363.

Thompson, W. J. (1991). Cyclic nucleotide phosphodiesterases: Pharmacology, biochemistry and function (review). *Pharmacol. Ther.* **51,** 13–33.

Truong, V. L., Collinson, A. R., and Lowenstein, J. M. (1988). 5′-Nucleotidases in rat heart. Evidence for the occurrence of two soluble enzymes with different substrate specificities. *Biochem. J.* **253,** 117–121.

Trussell, L. O., and Jackson, M. B. (1987). Dependence of an adenosine-activated potassium current on a GTP-binding protein in mammalian central neurons. *J. Neurosci.* **7,** 3306–3316.

Ueland, P. M. (1982). Pharmacological and biochemical aspects of S-adenosylhomocysteine and S-adenosylhomocysteine hydrolase (review). *Pharmacol. Rev.* **34,** 223–253.

Ulrich, D., and Huguenard, J. R. (1995). Purinergic inhibition of GABA and glutamate release in the thalamus: implications for thalamic network activity. *Neuron* **15,** 909–918.

Umemiya, M., and Berger, A. J. (1994). Activation of adenosine A_1 and A_2 receptors differentially modulates calcium channels and glycinergic synaptic transmission in rat brainstem. *Neuron* **13,** 1439–1446.

van Calker, D., Muller, M., and Hamprecht, B. (1979). Adenosine regulates via two different types of receptors, the accumulation of cyclic AMP in cultured brain cells. *J. Neurochem.* **33,** 999–1005.

Van den Berghe, G., van Pottelsberghe, C., and Hers, H. G. (1977). A kinetic study of the soluble 5′-nucleotidase of rat liver. *Biochem. J.* **162,** 611–616.

Von Lubitz, D. K. J. E., Lin, R. C. S., Melman, N., Ji, X. D., Carter, M. F., and Jacobson, K. A. (1994a). Chronic administration of selective adenosine A_1 receptor agonist or antagonist in cerebral ischemia. *Eur. J. Pharmacol.* **256,** 161–167.

Von Lubitz, D. K. J. E., Lin, R. C. S., Popik, P., Carter, M. F., and Jacobson, K. A. (1994b). Adenosine A_3 receptor stimulation and cerebral ischemia. *Eur. J. Pharmacol.* **263,** 59–67.

Wan, W., Sutherland, G. R., and Geiger, J. D. (1990). Binding of the adenosine A_2 receptor ligand [3H]CGS 21680 to human and rat brain: Evidence for multiple affinity sites. *J. Neurochem.* **55,** 1763–1771.

Wieraszko, A., Goldsmith, G., and Seyfried, T. N. (1989). Stimulation-dependent release of adenosine triphosphate from hippocampal slices. *Brain Res.* **485,** 244–250.

Worku, Y., and Newby, A. C. (1983). The mechanism of adenosine production in rat polymorphonuclear leucocytes. *Biochem. J.* **214,** 325–330.

Wu, L. G., and Saggau, P. (1994a). Adenosine inhibits evoked synaptic transmission primarily by reducing presynaptic calcium influx in area CA1 of hippocampus. *Neuron* **12,** 1139–1148.

Wu, L. G., and Saggau, P. (1994b). Presynaptic calcium is increased during normal synaptic transmission and paired-pulse facilitation, but not in long-term potentiation in area CA1 of hippocampus. *J. Neurosci.* **14,** 645–654.

Wu, P. H., and Phillis, J. W. (1978). Distribution and release of adenosine triphosphate in rat brain. *Neurochem. Res.* **3,** 563–571.

Wu, P. H., Barraco, R. A., and Phillis, J. W. (1984). Further studies on the inhibiton of adensoine uptake into rat brain synaptosomes by adenosine derivatives and methylxanthines. *Gen. Pharmacol.* **15,** 251–254.

Wu, Y., Mercuri, N. B., and Johnson, S. W. (1995). Presynaptic inhibition of gamma-aminobutyric acidB-mediated synaptic current by adenosine recorded in vitro in midbrain dopamine neurons. *J. Pharmacol. Exp. Ther.* **273,** 576–581.

Yawo, H., and Chuhma, N. (1993). Preferential inhibition of conotoxin-sensitive presynaptic Ca^{2+} channels by adenosine autoreceptors. *Nature (London)* **365,** 256–258.

Yoneda, K., and Okada, Y. (1989). Effects of anoxia and recovery on the neurotransmission and level of high-energy phosphates in thin hippocampal slices from the guinea-pig. *Neuroscience* **28,** 401–407.

Yoon, K. W., and Rothman, S. M. (1991). Adenosine inhibits excitatory but not inhibitory synaptic transmission in the hippocampus. *J. Neurosci.* **11,** 1375–1380.

Zetterström, T., and Fillenz, M. (1990). Adenosine agonists can both inhibit and enhance in vivo striatal dopamine release. *Eur. J. Pharmacol.* **180,** 137–143.

Zetterström, T., Vernet, L., Ungerstedt, U., Tossman, U., and Jonzon, B. (1982). Purine levels in the intact rat brain. Studies with an implanted perfused hollow fibre. *Neurosci. Lett.* **29,** 111–115.

Zgombick, J. M., Beck, S. G., Mahle, C. D., Craddock-Royal, B., and Maayani, S. (1989). Pertussis toxin-sensitive guanine nucleotide-binding protein(S) couple adenosine A_1 and 5-hydroxytryptamine1A receptors to the same effector systems in rat hippocampus: biochemical and electrophysiological studies. *Mol. Pharmacol.* **35,** 484–494.

Zhang, G., Franklin, P. H., and Murray, T. F. (1993). Manipulation of endogenous adenosine in the rat prepiriform cortex modulates seizure susceptibility. *J. Pharmacol. Exp. Ther.* **264,** 1415–1424.

Zhou, Q., Li, C., Olah, M. E., Johnson, R. A., and Stiles, G. L. (1992). Molecular cloning and characterization of an adenosine receptor: the A_3 adenosine receptor. *Proc. Natl. Acad. Sci. U.S.A.* **89,** 7432–7436.

Zimmermann, H. (1992). 5′-Nucleotidase: Molecular structure and functional aspects. *Biochem. J.* **285,** 345–365.

Zimmermann, H., Dowdall, M. J., and Lane, D. A. (1979). Purine salvage at the cholinergic nerve endings of the torpedo electric organ: The central role of adenosine. *Neuroscience* **4,** 979–993.

Ronald W. Ellis*
Kenneth R. Brown†

*Vaccine Research and Development
Astra Research Center Boston
Cambridge, Massachusetts 02139

†Regulatory Liaison, Biologics/Vaccines
Merck Research Laboratories
West Point, Pennsylvania 19486

Combination Vaccines

I. Introduction

Breakthroughs in molecular biology, immunology, protein and polysaccharide biochemistry, and related fields have created the opportunity for developing new vaccines and improving current ones. Some of the newer vaccines that have become available over the past decade include those for hepatitis B, *Haemophilus influenzae* type *b*, hepatitis A, acellular pertussis ($_{ac}$P), and varicella. Other pediatric vaccines currently in large clinical trials, which may become available soon for widespread use, include those for rotavirus, *Streptococcus pneumoniae* (pneumococcal), and *Neisseria meningitidis* (meningococcal). The availability of these vaccines is providing society with the unprecedented opportunity to prevent serious infectious diseases in many age groups, especially pediatric, and to significantly reduce associated morbidity and mortality. In order to achieve these results, it will be critical

Advances in Pharmacology, Volume 39

1054-3589/97/$25.00

to assure maximal compliance of the population so that vaccines are taken at their proper times. For this reason, vaccine developers, regulatory agencies, and health practitioners seek to schedule immunizations in a way that minimizes the total number of visits by the patient. However, because almost all licensed vaccines (with the exception of oral polio) and experimental vaccines in advanced clinical trials (other than rotavirus) are injected, each new vaccine entails the need for additional needlesticks which can become so numerous as to discourage immunization. Surveys have indicated that multiple childhood immunizations are of concern to physicians and parents (Woodin *et al.*, 1995). In addition, the need to administer multiple vaccines at a single time can complicate recordkeeping, an additional factor also affecting compliance.

Given the increasing number of available vaccines, the successful development of combination vaccines is a major way for assuring better compliance with immunization programs. A combination vaccine is defined as a mixture of individual vaccines before administration *in vivo* so that the multiple vaccines are administered in an individual injection (or by another route of administration). There are two types of combination vaccines. Some vaccines for an individual disease are multivalent in that the particular pathogen has multiple types (usually serotypes). For such products, hereinafter referred to as "multitype combinations," the several types, which are of the same design, are mixed together at the time of manufacturing into a combination vaccine. Other combinations are mixtures of vaccines already licensed for different diseases. For such products, hereinafter referred to as "multitarget combinations," mixing is performed typically at three points: (1) preferably at the time of manufacturing and filling into a single vial or syringe; (2) alternatively by combining at the moment of injection vaccines filled into separate chambers of a dual-chambered syringe; or (3) by mixing vaccines immediately before administration in a vial and then injecting them. All major vaccine developers have programs for the development of combination vaccines. Regulatory agencies have begun to define tentative regulations for the development and licensure of combination vaccines. No more than one separately administered vaccine would be expected for a pathogen with multiple types; development would be for a multitype combination from the outset. However, before a multitarget combination is developed, each individual vaccine is developed separately and needs to meet the criteria for licensure before being combined into a multitarget combination vaccine.

Health-care providers and parents are both eager to have children fully protected from diseases for the prevention of which there are safe and effective vaccines. Because parents are not always able or willing to bring their children to the provider's office for all the necessary visits to meet the schedules for the many injections needed to provide full protection, the objective of putting multiple antigens together into a single injection is a laudable goal. Because such a program would require fewer visits, fewer injections, and fewer syringes (Hadler, 1994), this goal would seem to have only proponents. Thus, combination vaccines are ideal for the sake of convenience and compliance. However, we have only to look back as far as the oral polio vaccine programs to remember that there may be interactions among components that could have profound effects on one of the desired responses, in that case efficacy. In other cases there could be lower tolerability or immunogenicity than with single components or there may be physical or chemical incompatibility of the components one might intend to combine. In theory, each potential interaction should be studied in order to ensure that the results to be achieved with a combination are at least as beneficial as those with the multiple injections given separately. Exhaustive study of all the potential combinations becomes impossible in the time frame in which the combinations are needed in the field. Similarly important in considering the use of combinations is the question of the adequacy of the proposed surrogate marker that is used to "stand in" for efficacy, given that a new efficacy trial usually is impossible, impractical, or unethical.

This review describes current and potential future combinations and their rationales based on the compatibility of components and dosing schedules and discusses the numerous challenges in development, which include technical, formulation, analytical, clinical, regulatory, manufacturing, quality control, and marketing. This will include the results of clinical trials of combinations currently in development or recently licensed; key parameters include interactions among vaccines in combination affecting safety and immunological compatibility.

II. Currently Available Combination Vaccines

For the purpose of combinations, vaccines can be divided into two general categories; live-attenuated vaccines and inactivated/killed/subunit vaccines. Live-attenuated vaccines consist of strains of live viruses or bacteria that have been grown *in vitro* in a way which reduces their infectivity for humans. Such attenuated strains are able to infect humans and sometimes replicate, but not cause significant disease. Vaccines that use chemical or genetic means of inactivating infectivity are known as inactivated or killed vaccines. Other vaccines that make use of components purified from the pathogen of interest or expressed by recombinant systems are called subunit vaccines. Such subunits can include virus-like particles, protein antigens, or polysaccharides either used per se or with adjuvants or conjugated to a carrier protein for immunological reasons.

Six combination vaccines are licensed and available for routine immunization in many countries worldwide (Table I). The following, of which only

TABLE I Widely Used Combination Vaccines

Disease	*Type of vaccine*	*Date first available*	*Number of valences*
Diphtheria Tetanus Pertussis	Inactivated toxins and inactivated whole bacteria	1940s	3
Pneumococcal	Polysaccharides	1977	23
Meningococcal	Polysaccharides	1979	4
Influenza	Inactivated virion	1950	3
Polio	Inactivated virion (injected)	1955	3
Polio	Live-attenuated virus (oral)	1960	3
Measles Mumps Rubella	Live-attenuated virus	1971	3

the first is multitarget, are combinations of inactivated/killed/subunit vaccines:

1. Diphtheria (D)–tetanus (T)–pertussis (P), known as "DTP." D and T combined, known as "Td."
2. Pneumococcal (Pn).
3. Polio, which comes in two types, one of which is a killed virion vaccine.
4. Influenza, which is either a killer virion or a subunit vaccine.

There are two combinations of live-attenuated virus vaccines, the first of which is multitarget in nature:

1. Measles–mumps–rubella.
2. Oral polio vaccine.

Each of these vaccines is described in terms of its properties, historical development, and challenges regarding issues for combinations.

A. Multitarget

1. DTP

DTP vaccine is a required pediatric vaccine in virtually every country worldwide. It is produced by over 20 manufacturers in both developed and developing countries. As described later in this section, it is the "backbone" of most pediatric combination vaccines currently under development. In addition, the Td vaccine is used in adolescents and adults as a booster vaccine after DTP.

Diphtheria is a serious respiratory infection with associated cardiac toxicity caused by the D toxin of *Corynebacterium diphtheriae,* a gram-positive bacillus. This exotoxin, which could elicit long-term immunity against D, was shown to be inactivated with heat and formalin so as to lose its toxicity yet retain its immunogenicity (Holmes, 1940). This resultant D toxoid, which came into widespread use during the 1930s, is the basis for all current D vaccines. D toxin is naturally secreted from *C. diphtheriae.* A strain of this organism is selected for its ability to secrete large quantities of the toxin in large-scale liquid cultures. Filtered culture broth containing the toxin is incubated with formalin, typically at 37°C, for conversion into the toxoid, which is then purified and concentrated; alternatively, D toxin can be purified before treatment with formalin. Following verification of potency and assurance of the absence of toxin activity, the toxoid is adsorbed onto an aluminum adjuvant, aluminum phosphate or hydroxide, with the addition of a preservative, either thimerosal or 2-phenoxyethanol. This concentrated bulk is stored at 4°C for mixture with T and P vaccines to constitute DTP. The potency of D toxoid is quantified in terms of lethal flocculating units (Lf). The administration of D vaccine to adults as a booster resulted in unacceptably high rates of serious adverse events (AEs), which appeared to be delayed-type hypersensitivity (DTH) reactions (Edsall, 1952) associated with residual *C. diphtheriae* proteins cross-linked to D toxin during the formalin incubation step. Thus, the general practice has been to use lower levels of D toxoid in the adult formulation of the combination with T, which is known as "Td."

Tetanus, an often fatal systemic disease characterized by tonic spasms primarily of extensor muscles ("lockjaw"), is a noncommunicable disease caused by *Clostridium tetani,* a gram-positive bacillus. With the appreciation that the symptoms of T disease were caused by T toxin, tetanus antitoxin came into widespread use in the 1910s for the treatment of symptomatic T disease. Given the successful development of D toxoid as an active vaccine, it was shown that T toxin could be chemically inactivated and that the resultant toxoid would still be immunogenic. T toxoid as a vaccine came into widespread and very successful use during World War II (Long and Sartwell, 1947). The production process for T toxin is analogous to that of D toxin. Detoxification with formalin after the purification of the toxin offers the opportunity to remove contaminating *C. tetani* proteins from the preparation that would not be cross-linked by formalin treatment to T toxin. Following the addition of an aluminum adjuvant and preservative, the bulk T toxoid vaccine is stored at 4°C for combination with D and P vaccines. Potency is quantified in terms of Lf.

Pertussis, a serious lower respiratory infection with a characteristic severe cough that can last for a few weeks to several months, is caused by *Bordetella pertussis,* a gram-negative bacillus. Two kinds of vaccines have been developed, the whole cell P ($_{wc}$P) and the acellular P ($_{ac}$P) vaccine. The initial vaccines made in the 1930s consisted of inactivated whole *B. pertussis* organisms. The production techniques were refined in the 1940s, resulting in the current $_{wc}$P vaccines (Manclark and Cowell, 1984). The bacteria may be grown on solid or in liquid media. Following harvesting, the bacteria are inactivated by one of several different techniques. The preparation is then adsorbed to aluminum adjuvant (which can decrease reactogenicity due to bacterial lipopolysaccharide), and a preservative is added. The vaccine preparations are standardized on the basis of opacity units, which quantifies the number of organisms, and a mouse protection test which assures immunogenic potency. The $_{wc}$P vaccine is probably the least well-characterized licensed vaccine. Because immunization with the $_{wc}$P vaccine is associated with a significant level of AEs, particularly fever and injection site reactions, several groups investigated the use of purified proteins of *B. pertussis* as components of a $_{ac}$P vaccine (Sato *et al.*, 1984). These $_{ac}$P vaccines first became widely used in Japan in the 1980s as DT$_{ac}$P. More recently, six of these DT$_{ac}$P vaccines have been demonstrated to be efficacious in clinical studies of different designs (Greco *et al.*, 1996; Gustaffson *et al.*, 1996; Schmitt *et al.*, 1996). As a result, $_{ac}$P vaccines are expected to become licensed widely in developed countries in the near future (Cherry, 1993). Nevertheless, many countries, particularly developing ones, are expected to continue to use the $_{wc}$P vaccine, largely due to cost and supply issues. The major vaccine antigens in almost all $_{ac}$P vaccines are P toxoid (PT) and filamentous hemaggutinin (FHA), with pertactin present in some vaccines and fimbriae (agglutinogens) in a few. Either $_{wc}$P or $_{ac}$P vaccine is combined with D and T into DT$_{wc}$P or DT$_{ac}$P vaccine, which is the platform for further combination vaccines.

The DT$_{wc}$P vaccine first became available in the 1940s. This combination was made initially based on the convenience of combining the vaccines for the immunization of infants at the same age. The vaccine is currently indicated for immunization of infants at ages 2, 4, 6, and 15 months of age in the United States and at similar ages in other countries. Few, if any, controlled clinical studies have compared the immunogenicity and efficacy of the DT vaccine to each of the D, T, and $_{wc}$P vaccines separately. Nevertheless, the effectiveness of the DT$_{wc}$P vaccine has been substantiated through decades of use, which have been associated with a substantial reduction in disease. The incidence rates of the three diseases have been reduced by up to 99% in areas where the vaccine been widely utilized. Three developed countries, Sweden, Great Britain, and Japan, either suspended their use of $_{wc}$P vaccine or experienced significant decreases in $_{wc}$P vaccination rates for periods in the 1970s–1980s due to adverse publicity surrounding serious AEs temporally associated with immunization. In all cases, there was a resurgence in the rate of clinical pertussis disease. The introduction of the $_{ac}$P vaccine in Japan at that time then led to a major reduction in the incidence of P disease. However, it should be noted that there has been a wide variation in rates of protective efficacy in controlled trials of DT$_{wc}$P.

One of the principle challenges for all DTP vaccines as combination vaccines has been the lack of a surrogate assay for pertussis vaccine. i.e., a quality control assay on the product that correlates with clinical performance. This becomes a further issue when $DT_{wc}P$ or $DT_{ac}P$ is combined with other vaccines (see Section III,A,1). Furthermore, for neither $DT_{wc}P$ nor $DT_{ac}P$ vaccines is there a specific type of antipertussis immune response that correlates with protection from pertussis disease. Because there is no serological correlate of efficacy (see Section IV,B,3), this means that it is difficult to make any changes in the process for making the P component vaccine. Moreover, for combination vaccines including DTP and other vaccine antigens, there should be an equivalent antipertussis immune response in the DTP combination vaccine as in the DTP vaccine *per se*.

2. *Measles–Mumps–Rubella*

The measles–mumps–rubella vaccine is a routine pediatric vaccine in many developed countries worldwide. Most developing countries use the measles vaccine. Some countries use the measles–rubella vaccine. The process for developing these vaccines has been an empirical one involving the isolation of each virus from a clinical case and the passaging of its serially in one or more cell types *in vitro*. This process results in a reduction in virulence for humans while maintaining infectivity and ability to elicit a long-lasting protective immune response. In that sense, a fine line exists between overattenuation, whereby the vaccine virus does not replicate sufficiently in humans in order to elicit protective immunity, and underattenuation, whereby the vaccine virus still produces some symptom of clinical disease. There is usually no test for degree of attenuation short of testing the vaccine in humans.

The measles virus, a paramyxovirus, causes a serious systemic infection characterized by a widespread maculopapular rash, fever, and sometimes meningoencephalitis. The progenitor of virtually all measles vaccine strains in current use was isolated by passage at 35°C serially in primary human kidney cells, human amnion cells, chicken embryos, and chicken embryo cells (Enders *et al.*, 1960). The measles vaccine is produced in chicken embryo cells in large bioreactors. The conditioned culture media are harvested and filtered. The vaccine, either *per se* or after mixing with mumps and rubella vaccines, is filled and lyophilized. The vaccine, which is stored at 4°C, is reconstituted in sterile water at the time of injection. Potency of the vaccine is quantified in an *in vitro* cell culture infectivity assay, either by plaque-forming units (pfu) or by tissue culture infectious doses ($TCID_{50}$). The initial measles vaccine, which was licensed in 1963, showed a significant rate of AEs. Therefore, the initial strain was subjected to additional passages in chicken embryo cells in order to further attenuate its virulence in humans (Hilleman *et al.*, 1968). These successor strains, which were shown to be better tolerated than the original strain, were licensed later in the 1960s and have been used widely ever since. A balance exists between immunogenicity and safety of the measles vaccine. Studies had shown that a high-dose measles vaccine was highly immunogenic in children less than 1 year of age.

However, use of the vaccine was also associated with statistically significant excess mortality, especially in immunized female infants (Aaby *et al.*, 1994).

The mumps virus, a paramyxovirus, causes systemic illness, usually including parotitis but also less frequently orchitis and meningoencephalitis. The original mumps vaccine strain, Jeryl-Lynn, was isolated in the 1960s (Buynak and Hilleman, 1966). This virus strain was passed in embryonated hen eggs followed by chicken embryo cell cultures. The production process and testing of the mumps vaccine are highly similar to that of measles vaccine. Several other mumps strains have been developed, *e.g.*, Urabe (Ehrengut *et al.*, 1983). The empirical nature of the attenuation process for live-attenuated viral vaccines has been highlighted by the results of the postmarketing surveillance of these vaccines. For example, after the administration of millions of doses, it was shown that the use of the Urabe strain was accompanied by a rate of aseptic mumps meningitis on the order of 1 : 10,000 (in contrast to <1 : 1,000,000 for the Jeryl-Lynn strain), which was indicative of incomplete attenuation (Brown *et al.*, 1991). As a consequence, the use of the Urabe strain has been curtailed in some developed countries.

The rubella virus, a lipid-enveloped togavirus, causes malaise, fever, and rash. Infection of pregnant woman can cause congenital rubella syndrome in the newborn, whose symptoms may include blindness, deafness, other central nervous system symptoms, and serious cardiac malformations. The original rubella strains were isolated in the 1960s, attenuated and grown in dog or rabbit cells, and licensed in the late 1960s. At that time, the RA27/3 strain was isolated by Plotkin and passaged directly onto human WI-38 diploid fibroblasts, in which it was attenuated by growth first at 37°C then at 30°C (Plotkin *et al.*, 1965). This strain has since supplanted the use of most other strains in measles–mumps—rubella vaccines. Final production of the rubella vaccine is in WI-38 or MRC-5 human fibroblasts. Processing and testing of the rubella vaccines are similar to those of measles and mumps vaccines.

The first measles–mumps—rubella vaccine was developed in the late 1960s and licensed in 1971 (Stokes *et al.*, 1971). The vaccine consists of a mixture of three different culture media from cells infected by each of the viruses along with a vaccine stabilizer. The basis for combining these vaccines was serological studies in which it was shown that the measles–mumps–rubella vaccine elicited similar titers of antibody as each of the three vaccines separately. The effectiveness of the combined vaccine has been demonstrated by a ≥99% reduction in the incidence of each of the three diseases since the early 1970s in areas where the vaccine has been widely used. As long as a high rate of vaccination is maintained, these rates of disease reduction have persisted. The vaccine initially was indicated as a single dose early in the second year of life. However, since the early 1990s, it has been recommended in many countries that a second dose of vaccine be given upon entry to either elementary school or middle school in order to provide protection to individuals with primary vaccine failure (insufficient immunity after immunization) or secondary vaccine failure (waning immunity). Because the need for protection against rubella peaks in the reproductive age, some authorities recommend an additional dose at 11–12 years instead of at school entry.

A significant issue for measles–mumps–rubella as a combination vaccine is the issue of stability upon short-term storage at elevated temperatures and long-term storage at 2–8°C. Stabilizing three live viruses with different structures and properties is an empirical challenge. The vaccine must maintain potency levels well above the minimum immunizing dose for each virus component that would provide high levels and persistence of protection. A second issue is the potential for immunological interaction among the vaccine viruses. Because different companies use different strains of virus, especially measles and mumps, each set of strains needs to be extensively evaluated and dose ranged in clinical studies to assure robust immunogenicity.

B. Multitype

1. Pneumococcal

Pneumococci (*Streptococcus pneumoniae*) are a leading cause of significant and oftentimes fatal infection in virtually every part of the world. Perhaps more than those caused by many other organisms, such infections illustrate that to become infected there must be a breakdown of the normal immune or resistance mechanisms. There are 84 known Pn serotypes, which are displayed on the capsular polysaccharide (Ps). Defense against pneumococci depends on the presence of type-specific anti-Pn Ps antibodies. It has been shown experimentally that without the presence of an opsonizing antibody that is specific to the type of capsular Ps present, phagocytosis and subsequent killing do not occur (Johnston, 1981). The anti-Pn Ps antibody is generated in normal healthy persons in response to previous encounters with the organism, to organisms which may comprise part of the nasopharyngeal flora and have similar or identical immunogenic structures on their surface, or to immunization with a Pn Ps vaccine. Although lower respiratory infection, *i.e.,* bronchopneumonia or labor pneumonia, may be the most important infections numerically, they are not necessarily the most serious. Patients may develop bacteremia, meningitis, or other forms of invasive disease such as sinusitis and/or even soft tissue infections. In each of these types of infections, it is important to note that recovery is more rapid and complete if there is antibody directed against the Ps of the infecting/invading Pn organism. Before modern antibiotics became available, the typing of Pn Ps was important to treatment and was not just of epidemiological interest. It is much less common today to perform typing unless one needs to look specifically for serotypes that may be epidemiologically important in a specific hospital setting or population.

In the United States, about 23 Pn serotypes account for most of the disease that is seen in adults (Bolan *et al.*, 1986). The 23 valent Pn Ps vaccine has more components than any other combination. This poses a significant issue in terms of manufacturing in that the reproducible supply depends on 23 separate processes all working well. In children, the number of serotypes is more limited, *i.e.*, for children less than 2 years of age the serotypes 6B, 14, 19F, and 23F are the most common; adding type 3 to that list, we can account for about two-thirds of the bacteremic isolates in children (Grey and Dillon, 1986). Unfortunately, younger children are poor responders to almost all capsular Ps (Koskela *et al.*, 1986). The earliest vaccines were produced for adults and for children older than 2 years of age. Initially a 14 valent product was licensed in the United States (Austrian *et al.*, 1976), following which 9 additional serotypes were added. Approximately 65% of elderly immunocompetent adults respond to immunization with the pneumococcal vaccine (Roghman *et al.*, 1987). Because very few children under the age of 2 respond to Pn Ps, several laboratories have begun to study Pn conjugate vaccines in which the Pn Ps are conjugated to specific carrier proteins (Section III,B,1).

2. *Polio*

Poliomyelitis is an infection of the gray matter of the central nervous system, chiefly involving the lower motor neurons of the pons, medulla, and spinal cord. Polioviruses, of which there are three types (1, 2, 3), had been nearly ubiquitous; however, because of intensive use of the oral polio vaccines (OPV), the disease has disappeared in the western hemisphere since 1991 (de Quadros *et al.*, 1992). Polioviruses, which are transmitted by the fecal/oral route, are capable of infecting the upper respiratory tract as well as the gastrointestinal tract. Because of these loci of infection and replication in the adjacent lymph nodes (cervical and celiac, respectively), secretory IgA is an important mechanism of initial protection from infection at the local mucosal sites. If this local antibody fails to prevent infection, the viruses gain access to the submucosal lymph nodes and replicate, causing a minor viremia which is generally asymptomatic. In the absence of secretory IgA, the serum antibody can still protect against progression of infection. In most cases, poliomyelitis infection is not recognized unless there is a major viremia, which may lead to symptoms, including lower motor neuron paralysis infection. This component of the illness occurs in $<0.1\%$ of infected persons, but is the major cause for concern and constitutes the rationale for the development and use of a vaccine.

In 1952, Salk and colleagues performed studies which showed the potential utility of vaccines that were formalin inactivated and could prevent clinical disease (Salk *et al.*, 1953). Prior to the use of the vaccines, most paralytic disease was caused by type 1 poliovirus [Centers for Disease Control (CDC), 1973]. Although the rates of paralytic polio dropped substantially after the use of inactivated polio vaccines (IPV), these vaccines were not efficient at eliciting secretory IgA in the gastrointestinal and respiratory tracts, which represents the route of natural infection. Based on the work of Sabin and colleagues (Sabin and Boulger, 1973), OPV was introduced, which could induce IgA formation efficiently. As was the case for measles–mumps–rubella vaccines, a significant development issue was the need for these live-attenuated vaccine viruses to be dose ranged in order to assure that each of the three virus serotypes was sufficiently immunogenic. Such studies initially required the use of hundreds of monkeys. In the case of these vaccines, serotype 2 was able to generate such a vigorous response that in some persons the responses to types 1 and 3 were overwhelmed. Current vaccines contain 800,000, 100,000, and 500,000 infectious doses ($TCID_{50}$) of the respective types, allowing for more nearly equivalent responses to types 1, 2, and 3. Thus, doses of the trivalent oral vaccine given at 2 and 4 months yield protective titers of neutralizing antibody in >90% of vaccinated infants (McBean *et al.*, 1988).

An IPV of enhanced potency (eIPV) which engenders more effective responses to the vaccine than was previously possible with earlier vaccines has become available (Swartz *et al.*, 1986); this may allow the use of a reduced schedule of immunizations. With the eradication of the wild-type disease in the western hemisphere, all current paralytic polio is related to OPV administration; there are approximately 8–10 cases per year in the United States of vaccine-associated paralytic polio. Therefore, the recommendation has been to use eIPV instead of OPV for the first two doses of the regimen. Furthermore, with little exposure from the wild-type virus *per se,* there is less need for mucosal protection against invasion by the poliovirus (Hinman *et al.*, 1988). The eIPV will be utilized in combination with other childhood vaccines, but it will be important to show in each case that the coformulation of such products does not result in decreased immunogenicity for any combination.

3. *Influenza*

The disease referred to as influenza, or simply "the flu," is caused by one of two major strains of influenza viruses; A or B. These viruses cause annual waves of clinical influenza infection or epidemics and may be so pervasive as to develop into pandemics or infections which virtually cover the globe. In the United States alone, influenza epidemics may cause up to several tens of thousands of deaths annually. Some infected individuals may develop only upper respiratory infections, whereas others develop full-blown pneumonia, but most infected patients develop some upper respiratory infection and moderate to severe systemic disease, including muscle pain, fever, and headache. In otherwise healthy individuals, the disease is usually relatively benign and is not accompanied by any sequelae. However, in elderly patients, influenza often destroys or damages enough of the respiratory epithelium to allow easy access to bacterial pathogens such as pneumococci or staphylococci, which aggravate morbidity and mortality.

The surface of the influenza viruses consists of two protein antigens with important pathogenic contributions, known as hemagglutinin (HA) and neuraminidase (NA) (Schild *et al.*, 1980). There is a moderate degree of stability in the stucture of the surface antigens, but point mutations in the genetic structure cause minor variations from year to year (drift) (Martinez *et al.*, 1983). The influenza virus has a segmented genome. New influenza viruses can arise following coinfection with two virus types and reassortment of genomic segments. Reassortment results in major changes in the antigenic structure (shift). The neutralizing antibody parallels the specific anti-HA antibody that prevents the agglutination of red blood cells. Because neutralizing antibodies are more difficult to measure, the HA inhibition test is a reasonable surrogate of the amount of neutralizing antibody following either infection with the wild-type virus or immunization with one of the vaccines. Thus, the HA is the major surface antigen of the virus in terms of defining virus serotype.

A major development issue for this combination vaccine is the need to select virus serotypes on an annual basis and to be able to rapidly produce vaccines in a short time frame. The influenza virus is trivalent because types A and B are antigenically distinct and because there are at least two antigenic subtypes of A that are prevalent in causing disease. Each year vaccines are manufactured to contain components from three different strains, *i.e.*, two A strains and one B strain. These are formulated as an inactivated whole virus or inactivated subunit virus and have been available since the 1950s. The neutralizing antibody and other antibodies to various components of the surface are not long lived, *i.e.*, not much more than 6 months in most people. Therefore, even if the virus surface was stable from 1 year to another, revaccination is necessary. In fact, drift and shift do occur, and it is a difficult task for manufacturers as well as advisory and regulatory bodies to decide on an annual basis what components should be in the current year's vaccines. This means that a decision is made early in each calendar year regarding viral strains to be included. The manufacturer must then produce millions of doses of the vaccine by summertime in order to be ready for vaccination in the fall. In the United States, such decisions are made by the Center for Biologics Evaluation and Research (CBER) of the FDA working closely with the Centers for Disease Control and manufacturers. Decisions on what components should be included in the vaccine are made on the basis of the epidemiology of the disease to the west of the United States, i.e., in the Far East, and also on what strains have been predominant in the previous year(s).

Among the currently licensed combinations, the most effort at improving a vaccine has been directed at influenza vaccine due to (1) the short-lived antibody response, (2) shift and drift, (3) the difficulty in selecting new strains, and (4) the apparent absence of any meaningful cell-mediated immune (CMI) response that might overcome shift and drift. Live-attenuated cold-adapted vaccines have been developed because live vaccines usually offer a higher level of immunity than inactivated/subunit vaccines. Such cold-adapted strains, attenuated as gauged by their inability to grow at temperatures >37.8°C (Wright and Karzan, 1987), have been formulated into vaccines (Edwards *et al.*, 1994). The final verdict on the relative utility of live-attenuated versus killed or subunit influenza vaccines is not yet in. Some of these challenges may be overcome by newer approaches to vaccines such as the DNA vaccines, which have been shown in animal models to elicit antibody as well as broad CMI responses that can protect against drifted strains (Donnelly *et al.*, 1995). However, there is no prospect of any dramatic "quick fix" to prevent the recurrence of annual epidemics or even a pandemic of global proportions.

III. New Combinations

There are two general principles by which combination vaccines are conceived as products. The individual vaccines must be pharmaceutically stable in the combination under a defined set of storage conditions for a significant period of time, typically 2 years (Section IV,A,1). The vaccines also must be indicated for vaccination at the same time intervals so that the combination can substitute readily for the vaccines given individually. New combination vaccines (some of which are listed in Table II) include multitarget and multivalent vaccines.

TABLE II New Combination Vaccines

Disease	*Current number of valences*
Diphtheria	
Tetanus	
Pertussis (whole cell and acellular)	
+ Hib conjugate[a]	4
+ Hepatitis B[a]	4
+ Polio (injected)	6
+ Hib conjugate + polio (injected)[a]	7
+ Hib conjugate + polio (injected) + hepatitis B	8
Hib conjugate + hepatitis B	2
Hib conjugate + hepatitis B + polio (injected)	3
Pneumococcal conjugate	7–9
Rotavirus	4–5
Meningococcal conjugate	2–4

[a] Licensed in a developed country as a $DT_{wc}P$ combination.

A. Multitarget Vaccines

1. Combinations Based on DTP

Most combination vaccines either recently licensed or in advanced stages of clinical evaluation have been for pediatric immunization. Office visits for infants are at ages 2, 4, 6, and 12–18 months in the United States, with similar timings in other developed countries. Thus, DTP and polio vaccines have been given routinely at these office visits. The only oral vaccine other than polio that is not licensed but which has been extensively evaluated for pediatric use is the rotavirus vaccine. Therefore, DTP has become the "backbone" for the development of combinations of inactivated/killed/subunit-injected vaccines for pediatric use. For this reason and in order to avoid the inconvenience and expense of additional visits to the clinic, new pediatric vaccines have been developed for dosing schedules of 2, 4, and 6 months, with a booster dose early in year 2.

H. influenzae type *b* (Hib) is a gram-negative encapsulated bacterium that was the major cause of meningitis and bacteremia in young children and infants prior to the successful development of a vaccine. The Hib capsular polysaccharide PRP (polyribosylribitol phosphate) is conserved in all Hib strains and elicits protective antibodies. Because PRP is nonimmunogenic in children under the age of 18–24 months, PRP has been conjugated to (one of four different) carrier proteins: D toxoid, a natural mutant D toxoid, T toxoid, or an outer membrane protein complex from *Neisseria meningitidis* type B. The resultant Hib conjugate vaccines have been demonstrated to be immunogenic and efficacious in preventing invasive Hib diseases in young children and infants and are licensed in many developed countries (Kniskern *et al.*, 1995). These vaccines were evaluated using a dosing schedule of 2, 4, 6, and 12–15 months or a similar schedule in other countries, which has made them compatible for combination with DTP. Several DTP–Hib combination vaccines have been evaluated using both $DT_{wc}P$ and $DT_{ac}P$; a $DT_{wc}P$–Hib combination has been licensed in the United States (Avendano *et al.*, 1993; Paradiso *et al.*, 1993).

The hepatitis B virus (HBV) is responsible for acute and chronic liver infections in over 300 million people worldwide. Infection is most common from infected mother to newborn or young child. Infection also occurs among adults during sexual relations or parenteral exposure to blood. The hepatitis B (HB) vaccine was developed initially for the immunization of adults in developed countries, then for use in adolescents. Given the relatively low compliance of at-risk adults with immunization, the vaccine then became recommended for use in children and infants. The long persistence of immunity for this vaccine makes this strategy attractive for the long-term control of disease (Stevens *et al.*, 1992). The HB vaccine was evaluated as three to four doses with flexible schedules in infants; efficacy did not need to be shown again in pediatric use for the vaccine, which already had been licensed for older age groups. In addition, some countries provide an initial dose of the HB vaccine at birth. A $DT_{wc}P$–HB combination vaccine has been evaluated extensively (Papaevangelou *et al.*, 1995) and licensed in Europe.

Most countries worldwide have used OPV as its polio vaccine. However, some have preferred to use IPV (Drucker, 1991). Moreover, with the eradication of polio in the western hemisphere and other developed countries, the use of IPV is becoming more widely recommended in these areas. Because the polio vaccine has been administered at the same time as the DTP vaccine, combining these vaccines has been attractive (Swartz *et al.*, 1986); both $DT_{wc}P$ and $DT_{ac}P$ combinations with eIPV have been developed.

Additional combinations of $DT_{wc}P$ and $DT_{ac}P$ have been developed or are being evaluated clinically. These include $DT_{wc}P$–Hib–IPV, $DT_{ac}P$–Hib–HB, $DT_{ac}P$–Hib–HB–IPV, and $DT_{ac}P$–Hib–IPV (Dagan *et al.*, 1994; Guasparini and Medd, 1994). A Hib–HB combination also has been developed. The most complicated of these combinations contains D, T, five P antigens, Hib, HB, and three IPV serotype antigens, for a total of 12 antigens which must be tracked for pharmaceutical stability and immunogenicity. This is a formidable technical task.

2. *Measles–Mumps–Rubella–Varicella*

Varicella (chickenpox) has been the last major highly infectious childhood disease in most developed countries for which a vaccine was not available. A live-attenuated vaccine is now available for healthy children over 12 months of age in Japan, South Korea, the United States, and Germany and is becoming available elsewhere. The causative virus, varicella-zoster virus (VZV), is spread by aerosols and causes disease at a very high rate in nonimmune hosts. The infection is manifest as a maculopapular then vesicular rash with fever that appears 10–14 days after infection. Varicella infection is most serious in immunocompromised or older individuals, yet exacts a high rate of morbidity in younger children, which may be manifest as pneumonia, hepatitis, or meningoencephalitis.

A VZV strain was attenuated by *in vitro* passage and growth in human MRC-5 diploid fibroblasts (Takahashi *et al.*, 1974). Because VZV grows in a highly cell-associated manner in cell culture, the final vaccine consists of a lysate of MRC-5 cells which contains the live-attenuated Oka strain of VZV. Because the vaccines are indicated for immunization at the same ages, a combined measles–mumps–rubella–varicella vaccine has been considered an attractive product candidate. This vaccine has shown good immunogenicity for each of its viral components (Watson *et al.*, 1996). The major development challenges for this four-component combination live vaccine are the same as for the three-component measles–mumps–rubella vaccine, *i.e.*, stability and lack of potential immune interference. However, having four rather than three viral components, the stability challenge has become more formidable, especially since varicella vaccine as a cell lysate is added to culture media containing the other three viral components. Moreover, an additional viral vaccine presents an additional opportunity for immune interference.

3. *Hepatitis A–Hepatitis B*

The hepatitis A virus (HAV) is the major cause of enterically transmitted hepatitis. Infection is transmitted most commonly when ingesting the virus in contaminated water or food or from close personal contact with infected individuals. Following an incubation period of several weeks, acute liver infection is accompanied by fever, pain, jaundice, nausea, and vomiting. Although infection is relatively innocuous in children, symptoms are more severe with increased age; rates of hospitalization are approximately 50% in older adults. The risk of infection is enhanced by traveling to highly endemic areas. Before the availability of a vaccine, individuals who were planning to travel would receive an injection of hyperimmune globulin containing relatively high levels of anti-HA antibodies. An inactivated HA vaccine has become available (Andre *et al.,* 1990). It is prepared by growing the HAV in cell culture. HAV in the infected cell lysate is purified, inactivated by incubation in formalin, and adsorbed to an aluminum adjuvant. The inactivated HA vaccine can be administered in a two- or three-dose schedule.

Even though the two forms of viral hepatitis are transmitted in different ways, adults and adolescents are considered at-risk groups for both HA and HB diseases. Therefore, a HA–HB vaccine has been considered an attractive combination vaccine (Ambrosch *et al.,* 1994). Because both vaccines are aluminum-adsorbed inactivated/subunit vaccines, their development into a combination vaccine would have been considered relatively straightforward compared to other multidisease combinations such as those based on DTP or live-attenuated viruses. Nevertheless, there can still be stability and immunological interaction issues that need to be resolved for this combination vaccine. In addition, even though it has been developed initially as a three-dose regimen, given that HA vaccine is licensed as a two-dose regimen, there is the possibility of developing a two-dose HA–HB combination if there is suitable augmentation of the immune response to the HB vaccine.

B. Multitype Vaccines

Many of the diseases for which vaccines are available have only one vaccine antigen or attenuated virus type. However, for most vaccines currently being developed, there are multiple serotypes or genotypes. Thus, many newer combination vaccines will be multivalent.

1. *Pneumococcal Conjugate*

S. pneumoniae has 84 serotypes carried by the capsular Ps which elicit protective antibody. Although there are 23 types responsible for most adult

Pn diseases, there are 7–9 serotypes responsible for most pediatric Pn diseases, depending on the geographical area. As is the case for Hib, the Pn Ps are nonimmunogenic in children under 18–24 months of age, in which a substantial amount of pediatric Pn disease occurs. Therefore, the Pn Ps have been conjugated individually to one of the four different carrier proteins used for Hib conjugate vaccines. Plans are to incorporate from 7 to 9 or more serotypes designed to ensure coverage not only for otitis media but also for serious invasive disease in children.

The formulation of multivalent pneumococcal conjugate vaccines should be more straightforward than with multitarget combination vaccines. These Pn Ps vaccines have been combined in powder form in the unconjugated state and generally are stable. The issue of interference by one serotype on the response to another, as well as the possibility of combining several subtypes of one conjugation with those of another, is an intriguing consideration, especially if there is evidence that the protein carrier might have some undesirable immunologic effects, *e.g.*, inducing tolerance.

The pneumococcal conjugate vaccines are well into Phase III studies, in which they are being examined for their ability to prevent Pn otitis media as well as invasive disease, especially meningitis and bacteremia in children (Klein, 1995). The results have great potential to dramtically influence the health of children throughout the world as serious respiratory disease is a major cause of infant mortality, especially in the developing world. Furthermore, the impact such a multitype vaccine could have on both otitis media and invasive disease in the more medically sophisticated countries is of similar great importance.

2. Meningococcal Conjugate

With the near eradication of Hib meningitis in countries where the Hib conjugate vaccine is widely used, meningococcal meningitis has bcome more visible as a pediatric disease. In addition, meningitis caused by *N. meningitidis* has higher rates of case–fatality and sequelae than those caused by pneumococci or Hib. A quadrivalent meningococcal Ps vaccine (types A, C, W, Y) is licensed and is immunogenic in adults and children >2 years of age. However, as in the case of Hib and Pn, these Ps are nonimmunogenic in <2-year-old children. Three serotypes of meningococci (A, B, C) cause almost all pediatric meningococcal meningitis, with group B predominant; serotype is carried by the capsular Ps. The group B Ps has the structure of polysialic acid, a self-antigen, and therefore is nonimmunogenic in humans. Using the same carrier proteins as the previously mentioned Ps, group A and C Ps have been developed into a bivalent meningococcal conjugate vaccine in clinical trials (Twumasi *et al.*, 1995). Because the prevalence of meningococcal meningitis may not be high enough to justify a separate immunization, this vaccine may be combined with other pediatric vaccines given in the routine pediatric immunization schedule.

3. *Rotavirus*

Rotavirus is the major cause of severe diarrhea worldwide, being responsible for close to 1 million deaths annually. The case–fatality rate is much lower in developed countries. Nevertheless, rotavirus infections cause up to 100,000 hospitalizations and 100 deaths annually in the United States (Smith *et al.,* 1995). Live-attenuated rotavirus vaccines are being developed based on rotaviruses of bovine and simian origin. The serotype of rotavirus is carried by the virion glycoprotein; four serotypes are responsible for almost all disease. The vaccine virus consits of an animal rotavirus into which the gene encoding the human rotavirus glycoprotein has been introduced by reassortment. Thus, the vaccine candidate consists of a mixture of four reassortant rotaviruses, each of which carries a human glycoprotein serotype (Bernstein *et al.,* 1995). Such vaccines have been in Phase III efficacy studies.

IV. Issues in Making New Combination Vaccines

A. Technical Development

1. *Formulation Development and Stability*

In creating new combination vaccines, the final product must be pharmaceutically acceptable and stable in terms of physical interactions among component vaccines and excipients, including adjuvants and preservatives. For multitype combinations, the different antigens usually have similar physiochemical properties such that interactions among components are usually not significant. However, multitarget combinations usually have antigens of different properties, sometimes associated with different types of aluminum salts or other adjuvants or preservatives. Multitarget combinations of live-attenuated viral vaccines have viruses of different types, which may be challenging to formulate in a way whereby all viruses are equally stable. Thus, development issues are the most challenging for multitarget combinations.

Different types of excipients, *i.e.,* additives including buffers, stabilizers, and adjuvants, may be brought into the final combination vaccine along with individual component vaccines. Such excipients do not necessarily contribute to the stability of the final formulation. In cases where they are deleterious in the final combination, the processes for making the individual component vaccines may need to be altered. Appropriate buffers may ensure long-term stability and may control physical interactions such as aggregation. Preservatives may be needed for processes that cannot assure sterility of the final vaccine, *e.g.,* where there is no final sterilization step. Preservatives are also used in multidose vials to assure against the inadvertent introduction of a microorganism through multiple needle punctures of the stopper. As an example of preservative interaction, in a combined $DT_{wc}P$/IPV combination, the thimerosal used to preserve the $DT_{wc}P$ vaccine is deleterious to the potency of the IPV vaccine (Sawyer *et al.*, 1994). A very important excipient in most inactivated/subunit vaccines is the adjuvant, which is a nonantigenic component that increases the immunogenicity of the vaccine antigens. Although there are many new adjuvants under development (Allison and Byars, 1992), only aluminum salts such as phosphate and hydroxide are currently licensed, having been used in billions of doses of vaccines over decades. Antigens bind noncovalently to aluminum salts or other adjuvants; as a result, there may be physical interactions among different antigens on their own aluminum salts in combination. If an antigen that is not adsorbed as a monovalent vaccine is mixed with other antigens in a combination that is aluminum adsorbed, that antigen itself may become adsorbed, which may increase or decrease its immunogenicity. In addition, any extraneous protein carried along with an unadsorbed antigen may itself become adsorbed to an adjuvant in the combination.

Physical interactions among all component antigens and excipients can affect the consistency, appearance, and stability of the final combination. Noncovalent binding or aggregation can make the final vaccine appear clumpy, discolored, or nonuniform in appearance. This may require vigorous mixing to ensure uptake into a syringe for delivery. It can also lead to the medical practitioner questioning the quality of the product and to regulatory agencies becoming concerned about the consistency of production and stability of the product. This means that the formulation must be systematically optimized for all component antigens and excipients, which can become a tremendous challenge as the number of vaccine components increases. As a result, there is a yet to be determined limit so to the number of antigens that can be accommodated in any given combination while maintaining stability and acceptable appearance and properties.

A vaccine should be stable for at least 18 to 24 months following manufacture in order to assure ease of use in the field and adequate time for distribution channels. The vaccine developer defines the expiration date, which is printed on each vial of vaccine as the end of the dating period of the final filled product. The dating period is established by stability studies of each of the component vaccines in combination by means of analytical tests which should measure stability of the product, especially tests that correlate with immunogenicity. The dating period is established for each presentation, *i.e.*, syringe, single-dose vial, or mutidose vial, at the intended temperature of storage in the field.

2. *Manufacturing and Quality Control*

Numerous quality control assays are performed on each component vaccine before mixing and on both the final filled vials and bulk combination vaccine. Every assay on all components and on the combination must give a satisfactory result before the vaccine is released for clinical evaluation or to the market. During development, three to five consecutive manufacturing lots must be produced as consistency lots for proving that the combination can be produced consistently as judged by quality control assays as well as the results of clinical evaluation. Stability studies on the consistency lots are used to validate the dating period for the vaccine. Because there are many more quality control assays on a combination than for a single-component vaccine, combination vaccines are inherently much more complex from a manufacturing and regulatory perspective.

Given all these technical and analytical complexities, as well as immunological interactions (Section IV,B,4), there will be practical limitations as to how many individual vaccines can be combined successfully.

B. Clinical and Regulatory Development

1. Introduction

The overall development of vaccines that has led to the currently utilized schedules has not been a systematic prospective approach because the availability of the various vaccines was not simultaneous; rather vaccines have been brought into use as they became available. Interestingly and fortunately, the eradication or near-eradication of any of the diseases for which vaccines have been developed has not resulted in another similar disease coming in to replace the first. Rather, following the eradication of smallpox, there is now the potential for the eradication of poliomyelitis, first in the western hemisphere and hopefully later in the remainder of the world. In addition, for Hib disease including meningitis, as the PRP vaccine became available followed by the conjugated vaccines, there was a dramatic drop in cases of disease in children as those vaccines were appropriately used. Although most pediatric bacterial meningitis is now caused by pneumococci and meningococci, the total number of cases of meningitis in small children has decreased and, hopefully, will decrease further when the pneumococcal conjugate vaccines and meningococcal vaccines become available and are widely used. The scientific bases for vaccines, the resultant use of the vaccines in the clinic, and the regulatory guidance provided for the development and uses of these vaccines are all closely intertwined. Usually, the regulatory issues and practices are guided by or driven by science (Brown and Douglas, 1994). The development of vaccines is carefully controlled by appropriate regulations prior to the broader use of vaccines after licensure.

2. Age of Vaccination and Schedules

The age at which active immunization is provided to infants should depend on two factors: (1) the age at which the child will be exposed to a given pathogen, and (2) the age after which the child may expect no further protection from maternal antibody provided either by exposure *in utero* and passage of antibodies across the placenta or through antibodies provided in colostrum and breast milk. The appropriate schedule for a given vaccine is that which will generate the optimal response in a minimum amount of time and require the fewest injections needed to provide the desired protection. A scientifically secondary consideration in the choice of a schedule is the timing that will best coincide with visits to the health-care provider engendered either by other immunization schedules or by routine checkups designed to ensure optimal developmental health. As noted earlier, the issue of compliance with proposed vaccine schedules may actually alter those schedules because it is obviously preferred to have a child receive an appropriate vaccine somewhat off the immunologically optimal schedule rather than not receive the vaccine at all.

The schedules that have developed for multitarget combination vaccines (as for monovalent vaccines) involve a wide variety of interested parties, including the manufacturers who have sponsored extensive studies to develop a profile of safety, tolerance, immunogenicity, and efficacy for each vaccine; CBER as the regulatory body in the United States; and the policy bodies which recommend the usage of vaccines such as the Red Book Committee of the American Academy of Pediatrics (AAP) and the ACIP (Advisory Committee for Immunization Practices) of the Centers for Disease Control and Prevention. These parties work together during the latter phases of development of any given vaccine to harmonize the recommendations of all the groups. This is not always fully successful because of the FDA has the ultimate responsiblity for the wording of the label and initial advertising that will be proposed by the manufacturer; however, the AAP has a responsibility to its practitioners to come up with recommendations that are functional in terms of maximizing compliance as well as approaching the best possible schedules fro the point of view of protection.

Most immunization schedules do not begin earlier than 2 months of age, although some newborns are immunized with their first dose of hepatitis B vaccine shortly after birth. In the United States (see Table III), the general immunization schedule as suggested by the AAP follows a 2-, 4-, and 6-month schedule for the first three office visits. Although some countries use a 1-month interval (Table IV), there is evidence for a variety of antigens that a 2-month interval between doses is preferred (Jilg, 1989) for eliciting higher antibody responses. Thus while there may be latitude in the time schedules for some vaccines, clearly the degree of protective efficacy may vary with the schedule, the antigen(s), the adjuvant, and the concomitant vaccines given. It is unfortunate that so many factors can come into play that ultimately determine the level of immunologic response and indirectly the efficacy of a given combination vaccine.

3. *Immune Responses and Markers of Efficacy*

As soon as any given monovalent vaccine is shown to be efficacious, an ethical question arises as to whether it is ever appropriate and fair to do

TABLE III Recommended Childhood Immunization Schedule (United States, January–June 1996)[a,b]

Age ▶ / Vaccine ▼	Birth	1 mo	2 mos	4 mos	6 mos	12 mos	15 mos	18 mos	4-6 yrs	11-12 yrs	14-16 yrs
Hepatitis B[1,2]	Hep B-1										
		Hep B-2			Hep B-3					Hep B[2]	
Diphtheria, Tetanus, Pertussis[3]			DTP	DTP	DTP	DTP[3] (DTaP at 15+ m)			DTP or DTaP	Td	
H. influenzae type b[4]			Hib	Hib	Hib[4]	Hib[4]					
Polio[5]			OPV[5]	OPV	OPV				OPV		
Measles, Mumps, Rubella[6]						MMR			MMR[6] or	MMR[6]	
Varicella Zoster Virus Vaccine[7]						Var				Var[7]	

[a] Approved by the Advisory Committee on Immunization Practices (ACIP), the American Academy of Pediatrics (AAP), and the American Academy of Family Physicians (AAFP).

[b] Vaccines are listed under the routinely recommended ages. Bars indicate range of acceptable ages for vaccination. Shaded bars indicate catch-up vaccination: at 11–12 years of age, the hepatitis B vaccine should be administered to children not previously vaccinated, and the varicella-zoster virus vaccine should be administered to children not previously vaccinated who lack a reliable history of chickenpox.

[1] Infants born to HBsAg-negative mothers should receive 2.5 μg of Merck vaccine (Recombivax HB) or 10 μg of SmithKline Beecham (SB) vaccine (Engerix-B). The second dose should be administered ≥1 month after the first dose. Infants born to HBsAg-positive mothers should receive 0.5 ml of hepatitis B immune globulin (HBIG) within 12 hr of birth and either 5 μg of Merck vaccine (Recombivax HB) or 10 μg of SB vaccine (Engerix-B) at a separate site. The second dose is recommended at 1–2 months of age and the third dose at 6 months of age. Infants born to mothers whose HBsAg status is unknown should receive either 5 μg of Merck vaccine (Recombivax HB) or 10 μg of SB vaccine (Engerix-B) within 12 hr of birth. The second dose of vaccine is recommended at 1 month of age and the third dose at 6 months of age.

[2] Adolescents who have not previously received three doses of the hepatitis B vaccine should initiate or complete the series at the 11- to 12-year-old visit. The second dose should be administered at least 1 month after the first dose, and the third dose should be administered at least 4 months after the first dose and at least 2 months after the second dose.

[3] DTP4 may be administered at 12 months of age, if at least 6 months have elapsed since DTP3. DTaP (diphtheria and tetanus toxoids and acellular pertussis vaccine) is licensed for the fourth and/or fifth vaccine dose(s) for children aged ≥15 months and may be preferred for these doses in this age group. Td (tetanus and diphtheria toxoids, adsorbed, for adult use) is recommended at 11–12 years of age if at least 5 years have elapsed since the last dose of DTP, DTap, or DT.

[4] Three *H. influenzae* type *b* (Hib) conjugate vaccines are licensed for infant use. If PRP-OMP [PedvaxHIB (Merck)] is administered at 2 and 4 months of age, a dose at 6 months is not required. After completing the primary series, any Hib conjugate vaccine may be used as a booster.

(Continues)

TABLE III (*Continued*)

[5] Oral poliovirus vaccine (OPV) is recommended for routine infant vaccination. Inactivated poliovirus vaccine (IPV) is recommended for persons with a congenital or acquired immune deficiency disease or an altered immune status as a result of disease or immunosuppressive therapy, as well as their household contacts, and is an acceptable alternative for other persons. The primary three-dose series for IPV should be given with a minimum interval of 4 weeks between the first and second doses and 6 months between the second and third doses.

[6] The second dose of MMR is routinely recommended at 4–6 years of age or at 11–12 years of age, but may be administered at any visit, provided at least 1 month has elapsed since receipt of the first dose.

[7] The varicella-zoster virus vaccine (Var) can be administered to susceptible children any time after 12 months of age. Unvaccinated children who lack a reliable history of chickenpox should be vaccinated at the 11- to 12-year-old visit.

further efficacy studies with that vaccine. Randomized, placebo-controlled, double-blinded protective efficacy studies have been completed for monovalent versions of hepatitis A, hepatitis B, Hib conjugate vaccine, measles, mumps, rubella, IPV, and OPV vaccines. Controlled studies have demonstrated the efficacy and improved safety profile of $_{ac}$P vaccines, and long-term use of diphtheria and tetanus antigens has demonstrated their value. From the perspective of defined efficacy studies, more variable results have been noted for the influenza vaccines and the whole cell pertussis-containing vaccines. Because efficacy has been shown to be afforded by these vaccines, it will be very difficult to find sites where it would be possible or even ethical to perform efficacy trials when these antigens are put into multitarget combinations.

With the inability to conduct efficacy trials in the future for most antigens we desire to put in multitarget vaccines, we should be able to use adequate measures that will be surrogates for protective efficacy. The use of surrogacy in medicine is commonplace. For example, the diagnosis of HBV infection of the liver is not made by liver biopsy, histopathology, and detection of HBV in that specimen. Rather, it is from the history (exposure to an infected

TABLE IV Vaccine Schedules Commonly Used in Europe[a]

	Age for administering vaccines (months)					
Country	*2*	*3*	*4*	*5*	*6*	*12–15*
Finland		X		X		X
France	X	X	X			X
Germany		X	X	X		X
Greece	X		X		X	X
United Kingdom	X	X	X			

[a] Adapted from Plotkin (1994).

contact), the development of typical signs and symptoms of disease (jaundice, malaise, fever, *etc.*), and laboratory confirmation (elevated serum bilirubin, elevated liver-derived transaminases, HBV antigens); these are all surrogates of the actual hepatitis B disease. Similarly, in attempting to diagnose chickenpox caused by VZV, we do not ordinarily attempt to isolate the virus; we rely on the clinical syndrome. Because most viral and bacterial infections result in antibody responses, we are able to use parallel sets of pre- and postexposure immune responses to provide information regarding the immune status of the subject, regardless of whether the response we measure has been generated by natural disease or by an immunization.

Understanding the mechanism of protection from a given infectious disease is uniquely helpful in defining what an optimal surrogate marker for efficacy might be. For example, pneumococcal infection stimulates anti-Pn Ps antibodies; we could provide passive immunity by giving people specific anti-Ps antibodies for any given Pn serotype or we could stimulate antibody by immunizing the person with purified Ps. Although the system of assuring immunity to some diseases is not exquisitely accurate, for some others we have a high level of assurance that when a given antibody level is reached, a high degree of protection will be assured. This is certainly true for hepatitis B vaccines in which case we infer protection after we see a level of anti-HBs $\geq$10 (mIU)/ml; similarly for Hib disease in infants, we infer a high degree of protection from an antibody level of 1.0 mcg anti-PRP/ml. Examples of antibody assays for individual vaccines and their use in surrogate assays for protection are shown in Table V. Note that in the case of all $_{ac}$P vaccines in which efficacy has been shown, no surrogate marker of protection has been identified. Thus in the setting of clinical development for multitarget combination vaccines, several questions come to mind, not all of which are easily answerable.

1. Are all the component antigens and adjuvants physically/chemically compatible without changes in responses (efficacy, immunogenicity, safety, tolerance)?
2. Is there a legitimate, thoughtful way to produce representative lots for consistency of manufacture, or will their purpose be simply to meet a regulatory requirement?
3. Is it possible to do a complete matrix of studies to answer the appropriate clinical questions to which we need responses (Clemens *et al.*, 1995)?
4. Might it be ethical to perform protective efficacy studies in populations that have no access at present to the vaccine(s) under study?

The issue of surrogacy, then, is critical to our ability to develop and release new multitarget combination vaccines because in almost all cases efficacy studies will not be possible; such surrogate markers must be shown to be relevant and, preferably, to have been developed from data derived in a clinical efficacy trial. Absent the ability to know what a protective level of

TABLE V Antibody Assays for Individual Vaccines in Combination

Vaccine	*Type of assay*[a]	*Specificity*	*Surrogate*
Diphtheria	RIA, ELISA, Nt	Toxoid	+
Tetanus	RIA, ELISA, Nt	Toxoid	+
Pertussis	Agglutination	Whole bacteria	–
	Nt	PT	
	ELISA	FHA	–
	ELISA	Pertactin	–
	Agglutination	Agglutinogens	–
Measles	HI, ELISA	Whole virion	+
Mumps	HI, ELISA	Whole virion	+
Rubella	HI, ELISA	Whole virion	+
Influenza	HI	Whole virion	+
Polio	Nt	Whole virion	+
Pneumococcal	RIA	Capsular Ps	+
Meningococcal	Bactericidal	Capsular Ps	+
Hepatitis B	RIA, ELISA	HBsAg	+
Haemophilus influenzae b	RIA	Capsular Ps	+
Varicella	ELISA	Viral glycoproteins	?
Pneumococcal conjugate	ELISA	Capsular Ps	?

[a] RIA, radioimmunoassay; ELISA, enzyme-linked immunosorbent assay; Nt, neutralization; HI, hemagglutination inhibition.

antibody is in a specific immunization program, it will be essential to develop some form of an early warning system to detect any breakthrough disease that might occur should the combination vaccine be less than optimal in its ability to prevent the disease for which its use is intended.

4. Controlled Clinical Studies and Vaccine Interactions

For multitype combination vaccines, early clinical studies typically evaluate monovalent vaccines followed by multivalent vaccines, leading up to large-scale trials on the final multitype combination to be licensed. The final combination is expected to have a good safety profile. However, there usually is not a controlled comparison of the tolerability of the multitype vaccine with one of its monovalent components. One or more of the monovalent components may be tested for immunogenicity, and further trials may enable comparison of the multitype vaccine with one or more of its components in terms of immunogenicity. The immunogenicity comparison is interesting but does not bear directly on licensure of the product, as only the multitype vaccine has broad enough coverage for the given disease.

In contrast, controlled clinical studies comparing multitarget combination vaccines with its component vaccines are pivotal to the evaluation of the vaccine. If the safety profile or immunogenicity of the combination is inferior to that of its component vaccines, then the combination vaccine may be an unacceptable alternative not worthy of sparing the patient the extra injection. The AE profile of the combination is expected to not be significantly worse than that of its least well-tolerated component vaccine. The AE profile is established on a certain minimum number of subjects (*e.g.*, >1000). Postmarketing surveillance and national reporting through routine vaccine usage (the vaccine adverse experience reporting system in the United States) may enable the detection of AEs so rare (*e.g.*, 1 : 50,000) as to not be detectable in thousands of subjects in prelicensure trials.

The immunogenicity of a particular vaccine generally should not be significantly lower when part of a combination than when administered separately, as revealed through comparative clinical trials. If lower, the difference may be calculated to be statistically significant. In that case, the issue would be whether the difference is clinically significant. As an example, 10 mIU anti-HBs/ml is considered to be the protective level of antibodies elicited in response to an HB vaccine. There may be a statistically significant difference in geometric mean titers (GMTs) between the monovalent HB vaccine (10,000 mIU/ml with 99% of subjects >10 mIU/ml) and HB in combination (4000 mIU/ml with 98% of subjects >10 mIU/ml), but this difference in GMTs is not clinically significant because there is no significant difference in rates of protection elicited by the different vaccines.

The greatest number of studies comparing multitarget combination vaccines with its component vaccines has been for DTP combinations. For example, separate study arms would compare a DTP/Hib combination with the concomitant administration of DTP and Hib injected simultaneously in separate anatomical sites (not each of D, T, P, and Hib as DTP *per se* is the licensed vaccine) in prospective, randomized, and multicentered studies. In these cases, both enhancement (higher antibody titers) and interference (lower antibody titers) have been observed in combinations relative to their components. For enhancement, a $DT_{wc}P$/Hib combination was statistically (not clinically) more immunogenic for all four of its component vaccines than $DT_{wc}P$ and Hib administered separately at the same time (Paradiso *et al.*, 1993). Using two other $DT_{wc}P$/Hib combinations with two different Hib components, each combination elicited higher levels of anti-T antibodies than $DT_{wc}P$ and Hib administered simultaneously at separate sites (Begg *et al.*, 1995), yet another $DT_{wc}P$/Hib study showed enhancement of anti-D antibody titers in the combined vaccine (Avendano *et al.*, 1993). However, a $DT_{wc}P$/IPV combination elicited lower levels of antibodies to four different pertussis antigens than $DT_{wc}P$ and IPV administered separately at the same time (Halperin *et al.*, 1996). A $DT_{wc}P$/IPV/Hib combination elicited lower anti-P and anti-T titers than the vaccines administered simultaneously at different sites (Gold *et al.*, 1994). Likewise, a $DT_{wc}P$/IPV/Hib combination elicited lower anti-T titers than a $DT_{wc}P$/IPV control vaccine (Dagan *et al.*, 1994). Other reports show no statistically significant difference in the immunogenicity of the combination relative to its component vaccines. Because most of these clinical immunological interactions could not have been predicted from preclinical studies in experimental animals, these results highlight the somewhat empirical nature of clinical trials of combinations.

5. Regulatory Expectations/Requirements

There is no argument that combining antigens should necessarily provide an adjuvant effect of one on the other; however, some components of older vaccines such as free endotoxin do have some adjuvant activity. From a regulatory standpoint, however, one would be expected to show the absence of interference of any two antigens that are proposed to be given together. This is exactly the case in the United States in that CBER expects that in order to be placed into a combination vaccine, each of the components must be shown to be useful and efficacious in its own right or, in the case of a component that has never been used alone or never will be used alone, that its contribution to the utility of the new combination must be licensable. If the immunogenicity of a single component in combination is less than that when the component is used by itself, it is necessary to show that the actual level of protection anticipated is not less than the monovalent component would afford. In this case, this presumes that the surrogate marker is fully adequate and predictive and that under ordinary circumstances its monovalent use provides levels of antibody that are well above those that are minimally protective.

In the United States, CBER prepares documents for the guidance of sponsors who develop biological products. These are issued as Points-to-Consider which offer guidance and do not have the force of regulations. However, they frequently represent the most matured and recent thought by the agency on a given topic and thus may be the basis for the next approvals to be granted. Therefore, it is prudent to heed such guidance when it is available because the alternative sources of guidance may be only the code of federal regulations (in this case 12 CFR610) or licensing precedent from the recent or remote past. The practice of applying regulations relating to a licensed product considerably different from the one currently under consideration is not an impossibility. Draft guidelines are available upon request from CBER at HFM 635, 1401 Rockville Pike, Rockville, MD 20852.

In the EC, the quality and efficacy requirements for new combination vaccines of licensed components will generally comply with European Pharmacopoeia monographs for each particular vaccine component. However, a European expert group for vaccines recognizes that such requirements may be modified if compliance is affected by the presence of other components. The modifications, as decided and approved by a competent authority, ensure compliance for efficacy in humans subject to the vaccination schedule recommended in a country.

C. Marketing

Multitype combination vaccines offer coverage for a particular disease and may be used in the same way as other vaccines such as influenza and HB vaccines. Medical practitioners will need to understand that such vaccines may cover most but not all serotypes of a particular pathogen, in contrast to vaccines such as HA and HB which have only one major serotype.

Multitarget combination vaccines offer the opportunity to decrease the number of injection per immunization visit. However, especially for DTP-based combinations, there are many related products licensed or being developed (DTP/Hib, DTP/IPV, DTP/HB, Hib/HB, Hib/HB/IPV, DTP/HB/Hib, DTP/HB/Hib/IPV with $_{ac}$P and $_{wc}$P for several of these) that could confuse medical practitioners in both private and public sectors. Thus, companies will need to simplify and clarify the presentation of their products, assuring clear labeling, with respect to identity of component vaccines, compatibility for simultaneous immunization with other vaccines, and flexibility of dosing schedule. The needs of different groups of practitioners for different presentations of syringes or vials will need to be met to assure compliance in the field. In other cases, *e.g.*, HA–HB, there will be the need to educate the medical community as to the availability and benefits of such products. The most widely used combination products may be those which meet the needs of practitioners and of the patients in each country.

References

Aaby, P., Samb, B., Simondon, F., Knudsen, K., Seck, A. M. C., Bennet, J., Markowitz, L., Rhodes, P., and Whittle, H. (1994). Sex-specific differences in mortality after high-titre measles immunization in rural Senegal. *Bull. W.H.O.* **72,** 761–770.

Allison, A. C., and Byars, N. E. (1992). Immunological adjuvants and their mode of action. *In* "Vaccines: New Approaches to Immunological Problems" (R. W. Ellis, ed.), pp. 431–449. Butterworth, Stoneham.

Ambrosch, F., Wiedermann, G., André, F. E., Delem, A., Gregor, H., Hofmann, H., D'Hondt, E., Kundi, M., Wynen, J., and Kunz, C. (1994). Clinical and immunological investigation of a new combined hepatitis A and hepatitis B vaccine. *J. Med. Virol.* **44,** 452–456.

Andre, F. E., Hepburn, A., and D'Hondt, E. (1990). Inactivated candidate vaccine for hepatitis A. *In* "Progress in Medical Virology" (J. Melnick, ed.) pp. 72–95. Karger, Basel.

Austrian, R., Douglas, R. M., Schiffman, G., Coetzee, A. M., Koornhof, H. J., Hayden-Smith, S., and Reid, R. D. (1976). Prevention of pneumococcal pneumonia by vaccination. *Trans. Assoc. Am. Physicians* **89,** 184–194.

Avendano, A., Ferreccio, C., Lagos, R., Horwitz, I., Cayazzo, M., Fritzell, B., Meschievitz, C., and Levine, M. (1993). *Haemophilus influenzae* type *b* polysaccharide-tetanus protein conjugate vaccine does not depress serologic responses to diphtheria, tetanus or pertussis antigens when coadministered in the same syringe with diphtheria-tetanus-pertussis vaccine at two, four and six months of age. *Pediatr. Infect. Dis. J.* **12,** 638–643.

Begg, N. T., Miller, E., Fairley, C. K., Chapel, H. M., Griffiths, H., Waight, P. A., and Ashworth, L. A. E. (1995). Antibody responses and symptoms after DTP and either tetanus or

diphtheria *Haemophilus influenzae* type *b* conjugate vaccines given for primary immunization by separate or mixed injection. *Vaccine* **13,** 1547–1550.
Bernstein, D. I., Glass, R. I., Rodgers, G., Davidson, B. L., and Sack, D. A. (1995). Evaluation of rhesus rotavirus monovalent and tetravalent reassortant vaccines in US children. *J. Am. Med. Assoc.* **273,** 1191–1196.
Bolan, G., Broome, C., and Facklam, R. R. (1986). Pneumococcal vaccine efficacy in selected populations in the United States. *Ann. Intern. Med.* **104,** 1–6.
Brown, E. G., Furesz, J., Dimock, K., Yarosh, W., and Contreras, G. (1991). Nucleotide sequence analysis of Urabe mumps vaccine strain that caused meningitis in vaccine recipients. *Vaccine* **9,** 840–842.
Brown, K. R., and Douglas, R. G. (1994). New challenges in quality control and licensure: Regulation. *Int. J. Tech. Assess. Health Care* **10**(1), 55–64.
Buynak, E. B., and Hilleman, M. R. (1966). Live attenuated mumps virus vaccine. I. Vaccine development. *Proc. Soc. Exp. Biol. Med.* **123,** 768–775.
Centers for Disease Control (CDC) (1973). "Neurotropic Diseases Surveillance. Annual Poliomyelitis Summary." CDC, Atlanta, GA.
Cherry, J. D. (1993). Acellular pertussis vaccines—a solution to the problem. *J. Infect. Dis.* **168,** 21–24.
Clemens, J., Brenner, R., and Rao, M. (1995). Interactions between PRP-T vaccine against *Haemophilus influenzae* type *b* and conventional infant vaccines: Lessons for future studies of simultaneous immunization and combined vaccines. *Ann. N. Y. Acad. Sci.* **754,** 255–266.
Dagan, R., Botujansky, C., Watemberg, N., Arbelli, Y., Belmaker, I., Ethevenaux, C., and Fritzell, B. (1994). Safety and immunogenicity in young infants of *Haemophilus* b-tetanus protein conjugate vaccine, mixed in the same syringe with diphtheria-tetanus-pertussis-enhanced inactivated poliovirus vaccine. *Pediatr. Infect. Dis. J.* **13,** 356–361.
deQuadros, C. A., Andrus, J. K., Olive, J. M., and deMacedo, C. G. (1992). Polio eradication from the Western Hemisphere. *Annu. Rev. Public Health* **13,** 239–252.
Donnelly, J. J., Friedman, A., Martinez, D., Montgomery, D. L., Shiver, J. W., Motzel, S. L., Ulmer, J. B., and Liu, M. L. (1995). Preclinical efficacy of a prototype DNA vaccine: Enhanced protection against antigenic drift in influenza virus. *Nat. Med.* **1,** 583–587.
Drucker, J. (1991). Poliomyelitis in France. Epidemiology and vaccination status. *Pediatr. Infect. Dis. J.* **20,** 967–969.
Edsall, G. (1952). Immunization of adults against diphtheria and tetanus. *Am. J. Hyg.* **42,** 393–400.
Edwards, K. M., Dupont, W. D., Westrich, M. K., Plummer, W. D., Palmer, P. S., and Wright, P. F. (1994). A randomized controlled trial of cold-adapted and inactivated vaccines for the prevention of influenza A disease. *J. Infect Dis.* **169,** 68–76.
Ehrengut, W., Georges, A. M., and Andre, F. E. (1983). The reactogenicity and immunogenicity of the Urabe Am 9 live mumps vaccine and persistence of vaccine-induced antibodies in healthy young children. *J. Biol. Stand.* **11,** 105–113.
Enders, J. F., Katz, S. L., Milovanocič, M. V., and Holloway, A. (1960). Studies on an attenuated measles-virus vaccine. I. Development and preparation of the vaccine: Technics for assay of effects of vaccination. *N. Engl. J. Med.* **263,** 153–159.
Gold, R., Scheifele, D., Barreto, L., Wiltsey, S., Bjornson, G., Meekison, W., Guasparini, R., and Medd, L. (1994). Safety and immunogenicity or *Haemophilus influenzae* vaccine (tetanus toxoid conjugate) administered concurrently or combined with diphtheria and tetanus toxoids, pertussis vaccine and inactivated poliomyelitis vaccine to healthy infants at two, four and six months of age. *Pediatr. Infect. Dis. J.* **13,** 348–355.
Greco, D., Salmaso, S., Mastrantonio, P., Giuliano, M., Tozzi, A. E., Anemona, A., Ciofi, M. L., Giammanco, A., Panei, P., Blackwelder, W. C., Klein, D. L., Wassilak, S. G. F., and the Progetto Pertosse Working Group (1996). A controlled trial of two acellular vaccines and one whole-cell vaccine against pertussis. *N. Engl. J. Med.* **334,** 341–348.

Grey, B. M., and Dillon, H. C. (1986). Clinical and epidemiologic studies of pneumococcal infection in children. *Pediatr. Infect. Dis.* **5**, 201–207.

Guasparini, R., and Medd, L. (1994). Safety and immunogenicity of *Haemophilus influenzae* vaccine (tetanus toxoid conjugate) administered concurrently or combined with diphtheria and tetanus toxoids, pertussis vaccine and inactivated poliomyelitis vaccine to healthy infants at two, four and six months of age. *Pediatr. Infect. Dis. J.* **13**, 348–355.

Gustafsson, L., Hallander, H. O., Olin, P., Reizenstein, E., and Storsaeter, J. (1996). A controlled trial of a two-component acellular, a five-component accelular, and a whole-cell pertussis vaccine. *N. Engl. J. Med.* **334**, 349–355.

Hadler, S. C. (1994). Cost-benefit of combining antigens. *Biologicals* **22**, 415–418.

Halperin, S. A., Langley, J. M., and Eastwood, B. J. (1996). Effect of inactivated poliovirus vaccine on the antibody response to *Bordetella pertussis* antigens when combined with diphtheria-pertussis-tetanus vaccine. *Clin. Infect. Dis.* **22**, 59–62.

Hilleman, M. R., Buynak, E. G., Weibel, R. E., Stokes, J., Whitman, J. E., and Leagus, M. B. (1968). Development and evaluation of the Moraten measles virus vaccine. *JAMA, J. Am. Med. Assoc.* **206**, 587–590.

Hinman, A. R., Koplan, J. P., Orenstein, W. A., Brink, E. W., and Nkowane, B. M. (1988). Live or inactivated poliovirus vaccine: An analysis of the benefits and risks. *Am. J. Public Health* **78**, 291–295.

Holmes, W. H. (1940). "Diphtheria: History, Bacillary and Rickettseal Infections." Macmillan, New York.

Jilg, W. (1989). Vaccination against hepatitis B: Comparison of three different vaccination schedules. *J. Infect. Dis.* **160**, 766–769.

Johnston, R. B., Jr. (1981). The host response to invasion by *Streptococcus pneumoniae:* Protection and the pathogenesis of tissue damage. *Rev. Infect. Dis.* **3**, 282–288.

Klein, D. L. (1995). Pneumococcal conjugate vaccines: Review and update. *Microb. Drug Resistance* **1**, 49–58.

Kniskern, P. J., Marburg, S., and Ellis, R. W. (1995). *Haemophilus influenzae* type b conjugate vaccines. *In* "Vaccine Design: The Subunit and Adjuvant Approach" (M. F. Powell and M. J. Newman, eds.), pp. 673–694. Plenum, New York.

Koskela, M., Leinonen, M., Haiva, V., Timonen, M., and Makela, P. H. (1986). First and second dose antibody responses to pneumococcal polysaccharide vaccine in infants. *Pediatr. Infect. Dis. J.* **5**, 45–50.

Long, A. P., and Sartwell, P. E. (1947). Tetanus in the U.S. Army in World War II. *Bull. U.S. Army Med. Dep.* **7**, 371–385.

Manclark, C. R., and Cowell, J. (1984). Pertussis. *In* "Bacterial Vaccines" (R. Germanier, ed.), pp. 69–106. Academic Press, New York.

Martinez, C., DelRio, L., Portela, A., Domingo, E., and Ortin, J. (1983). Evolution of influenza virus neuraminidase gene during drift of the N2 subtype. *Virology* **130**, 539–545.

McBean, A. M., Thoms, M. L., Albrecht, P., Cuthie, J. C., and Bernier, R. (1988). The serologic response to oral polio vaccine and enhanced potency inactivated polio vaccines. *Am. J. Epidemiol.* **128**, 615–628.

Papaevangelou, G., Karvelis, E., Alexiou, D., Kiossoglou, K., Roumeliotou, A., Safary, A., Collard, F., and Vandepapeliere, P. (1995). Evaluation of a combined tetravalent diphtheria, tetanus, whole-cell pertussis and hepatitis B candidate vaccine administered to healthy infants according to a three-dose vaccination schedule. *Vaccine* **13**, 175–178.

Paradiso, P. R., Hogerman, D. A., Madore, D. V., Keyserling, H., King, J., Reisinger, K. S., Blatter, M. M., Rothstein, E., Bernstein, H. H., Pennridge Pediatric Associates, and Hackell, J. (1993). Safety and immunogenicity of a combined diphtheria, tetanus, pertussis and *Haemophilus influenzae* type b vaccine in young infants. *Pediatrics* **92**, 827–832.

Plotkin, S. A. (1994). Problems in the choice of combined vaccines for Europe. *Biologicals* **22**, 411–414.

Plotkin, S. A., Cornfeld, D., and Ingalls, T. H. (1965). Studies of immunization with living rubella virus: Trials in children with a strain cultured from an aborted fetus. *Am. J. Dis. Child.* **110,** 381–389.

Roghman, K. J., Tabloski, P. A., Bentley, D. W., and Schiffman, G. (1987). Immune response of elderly adults to pneumococcus: 2. Variation by age, sex and functional impairment. *J. Gerontol.* **42,** 265–70.

Sabin, A. B., and Boulger, L. R. (1973). History of Sabin attenuated poliovirus oral live vaccine strains. *Biol. Stand.* **1,** 115–125.

Salk, J. E., Bennett, B. L., Lewis, L. J., Ward, E. M., and Youngner, J. S. (1953). Studies in human subjects in active immunization against poliomyelitis: I. A preliminary report of experiments in progress. *JAMA, J. Am. Med. Assoc.* **151,** 1081–1098.

Sato, Y., Kimura, M., and Fukumi, H. (1984). Development of a pertussis component vaccine in Japan. *Lancet* **1,** 122–126.

Sawyer, L. A., McInnis, J., Patel, A., Horne, A. D., and Albrecht, P. (1994). Deleterious effect of thimerosal on the potency of inactivated poliovirus vaccine. *Vaccine* **12,** 851–855.

Schild, G. C., Newman, R. W., Webster, R. G., Major, D., and Hinshaw, V. S. (1980). Antigenic analysis of influenza A virus surface antigens: Consideration for the nomenclature of influenza virus. *Arch. Virol.* **63,** 171–184.

Schmitt, H.-J., Wirsing von König, C. H., Neiss, A., Bogaerts, H., Bock, H. L., Schulte-Wissermann, H., Gahr, M., Schult, R., Folkens, J. U., Rauh, W., and Clemens, R. (1996). Efficacy of acellular pertussis vaccine in early childhood after household exposure. *JAMA, J. Am. Med. Assoc.* **275,** 37–41.

Smith, J. C., Haddix, A. C., Teutsch, S. M., and Glass, R. I. (1995). Cost-effectiveness analysis of a rotavirus immunization program for the United States. *Pediatrics* **96,** 609–615.

Stevens, C. E., Toy, P. T., Taylor, P. E., Lee, T., and Yip, H.-Y. (1992). Prospects for control of hepatitis B virus infection: Implications of childhood vaccination and long-term protection. *Pediatrics* **90,** 170–173.

Stokes, J., Weibel, R. E., Villarejos, V. M., Arguedes, G., Buynak, E. B., and Hilleman, M. R. (1971). Trivalent combined measles-mumps-rubella vaccine. Findings in clinical-laboratory studies. *JAMA, J. Am. Med. Assoc.* **218,** 57–61.

Swartz, T. A., Roumiantzeff, M., Peyron, L., Stopler, T., Drucker, J., Epstein, I., Leitner, L., and Goldblum, M. (1986). Use of a combined DTP-polio vaccine in a reduced schedule. *Dev. Biol. Stand.* **65,** 159–166.

Takahashi, M., Otsuka, T., Okuno, Y., Asano, Y., Yazaki, T., and Isomura, S. (1974). Live vaccine used to prevent the spread of varicella in children in hospital. *Lancet* **2,** 1288–1290.

Twumasi, P. A., Jr., Kumah, S., Leach, A., O'Dempsey, T. J. D., Ceesay, S. J., Todd, J., Broome, C. V., Carlone, G. M., Pais, L. B., Holder, P. K., Plikaytis, B. D., and Greenwood, B. M. (1995). A trial of a group A plus group C meningococcal polysaccharide-protein conjugate vaccine in African infants. *J. Infect. Dis.* **171,** 632–638.

Watson, B. M., Laufer, D. S., Kuter, B. J., Staehle, B., and White, C. J. (1996). Safety and immunogenicity of a combined measles, mumps, rubella, and Varicella vaccine (MMRIIV) in healthy children. *J. Infect. Dis.* **173,** 731–734.

Woodin, K. A., Rodewald, L. E., Humiston, S. G., Carges, M. S., Schaffer, S. J., and Szilagyi, P. G. (1995). Physician and parent opinions. Are children becoming pincushions from immunizations? *Arch. Pediar. Adolesc. Med.* **149,** 845–849.

Wright, P. F., and Krazan, D. T. (1987). Live attenuated influenza vaccine. *Prog. Med. Virol.* **34,** 70–88.

Maria L. Garcia*
Markus Hanner*
Hans-Günther Knaus†
Robert Koch†
William Schmalhofer*
Robert S. Slaughter*
Gregory J. Kaczorowski*

*Department of Membrane Biochemistry and Biophysics
Merck Research Laboratories
Rahway, New Jersey 07065

†Institute for Biochemical Pharmacology
A-6020 Innsbruck, Austria

Pharmacology of Potassium Channels

I. Introduction

Potassium channels represent the largest and most diverse family of ion channels. As a first approximation, K^+ channels can be divided into two major groups, voltage-gated and ligand-gated channels, depending on the stimulus that triggers the conformational changes leading to channel opening. K^+ channels share in common the feature of having high selectivity for K^+ as the permeating ion. Because of this property, and given the wide tissue distribution of these proteins, K^+ channels have been postulated to be involved in a variety of physiologic processes, such as control of cell excitability, release of neurotransmitters, secretion of hormones, regulation of fluid secretion, and clonal expansion of cells of the immune system. In order to delineate the role of K^+ channels in the physiology of a given target tissue, it is necessary to have a thorough understanding of the nature and

Advances in Pharmacology, Volume 39

1054-3589/97/$25.00

properties of the specific channels that are present. Second, selective and high-affinity modulators for the different types of channels must be identified and characterized in order to provide probes for assessing the functional role of a specific K^+ channel in cell function.

Molecular biology has been pivotal in the progress of K^+ channel research. A large number of proteins belonging to different K channel subfamilies have been cloned and functionally expressed. At the present time, it is believed that most K^+ channels have been identified and, by the time that this review reaches the reader, it is most likely that the primary structure of those remaining proteins will have also be determined.

A large number of voltage-dependent K^+ channels are known to exist (Chandy and Gutman, 1995; Pongs, 1995). The best characterized ones represent the mammalian counterparts of the *Drosophila* channels *Shaker* (K_v1), *Shab* (K_v2), *Shaw* (K_v3), and *Shal* (K_v4). Each of these families contains several members. In addition, two other families, K_v5 and K_v6, are known to exist; few functional data have been reported for these later proteins to date. The predicted secondary structure for the K_v1–6 families is similar (Fig. 1). Thus, they are presumed to contain six α-helical transmembrane domains (S1–S6) with a segment between S5 and S6, termed the P region, that contributes to the formation of the channel's pore. The P region is the most conserved domain among all different types of K^+ channels and, because it is not large enough to cross the membrane in an α-helical conformation, it has been proposed to form a β-hairpin-like structure. Another common feature of these proteins resides in the S4 segment where positively charged residues are located every fourth residue and, therefore, are expected to face the same side of the helix. These cationic residues are believed to be involved in the initial conformational changes that the protein undergoes, which eventually leads to channel opening when the membrane potential becomes depolarized. In this respect, it is worth noting that the inward rectifier family of K^+ channels is predicted to have a much simpler organization with only two transmembrane domains connected by the pore region (Fig. 1). Although their pore region is highly conserved, inward rectifiers do not possess the typical S4 segment of the K_v1–6 family, consistent with the fact that channel gating of these proteins is not dependent on voltage.

Within the ligand-gated family of K^+ channels, the best characterized members represent the mammalian counterparts of the *Drosophila slowpoke* gene product, *Slo* (Kaczorowski *et al.*, 1996). *Slo* channels are Ca^{2+}- and voltage-dependent and display the highest single channel conductance for K^+ of all K^+ channels. The secondary structure of these proteins is predicted to be similar to that of K_v1–6 channels (Fig. 1). However, *Slo* possess a very large C terminus; although the topology of this segment is unknown, the potential for four additional transmembrane domains exists. Other intermediate- and small-conductance Ca^{2+}-activated K^+ channels have also been identified. However, efforts directed toward cloning these proteins have not been successful until very recently.

ATP-dependent K^+ channels represent another class of ligand-gated proteins (Fig. 1). Perhaps the best studied of these channels is the one present in pancreatic β cells because it represents the target of sulfonylureas, a class of antidiabetic drugs. The receptor for sulfonylurea drugs has been cloned, but it does not express functional channels, suggesting that it is an auxiliary protein associated with the K^+ channel pore-forming subunit. This idea has been confirmed in coexpression experiments employing a new member of the inward rectifier family of K^+ channels and the sulfonylurea receptor. The resulting channel is modulated by ATP and displays all pharmacological properties expected for the pancreatic β-cell ATP-dependent K^+ channel.

The large number of K^+ channels that have been identified is indicative of the high diversity of this family of ion channels. However, molecular differences are not the only contributors to this functional diversity. It is known that K^+ channels are tetrameric structures made up by association of identical or related subunits. In addition, K^+ channels can exist *in vivo* in complexes with auxiliary proteins that modify the functional and pharmacological properties of the pore-forming subunit. Therefore, as a result of these phenomena, the diversity of K^+ channels is theoretically enormous and a large amount of time is currently devoted to understanding which K^+ channel subunits contribute *in vivo* to the biophysical and pharmacological properties of currents found in given cell types. To aid in such studies, pharmacological reagents represent a very important tool. Unfortunately, the pharmacology of K^+ channels, unlike that of Na^+ and Ca^{2+} channels, has only emerged fairly recently. Most of the progress in this area has been possible due to the discovery of high-affinity peptidyl K^+ channel inhibitors in venoms from bee, scorpions, snakes, and spiders. The use of these peptides has facilitated the purification of channels from native tissues and determination of their subunit composition, study of the functional role that K^+ channels play in given target tissues, and, in some cases, discovery of small organic molecules that modulate channel activity. Some of these peptidyl blockers have also provided unique tools with which to study K^+ channel structure and function at the molecular level.

Although there is not a facile way of organizing a review describing the pharmacology of K^+ channels, given the fact that some peptidyl blockers display a broad spectrum of interaction with different family members, this review is divided into three major areas; voltage-gated K^+ channels, Ca^{2+}-activated K^+ channels, and ATP-dependent K^+ channels.

II. Voltage-Gated K^+ Channels

For reasons that are not entirely clear, the richest pharmacology that exists for voltage-gated K^+ channels is associated with the K_v1 family. The

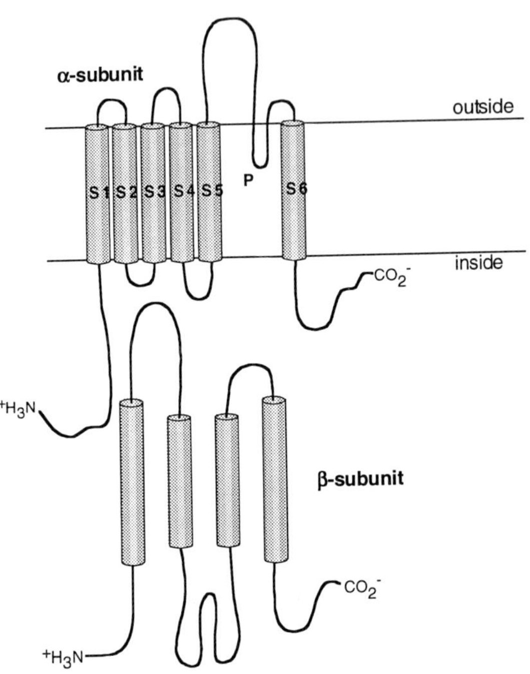

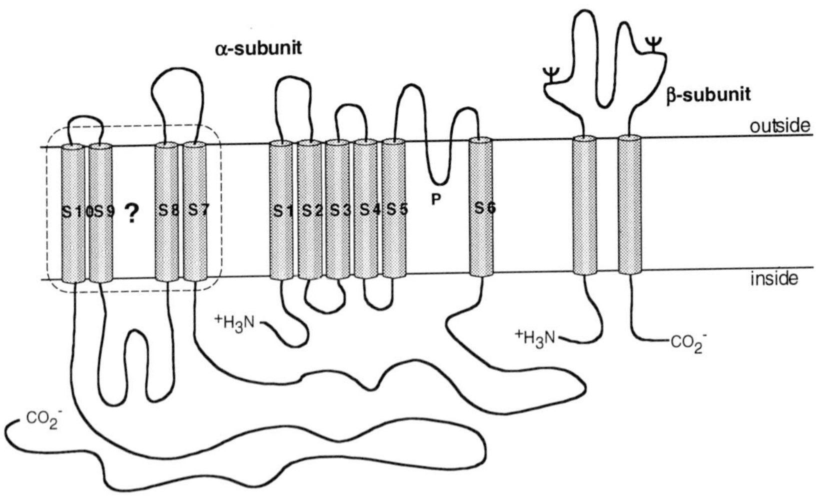

FIGURE 1 Schematic representation of the putative secondary structure of the different families of K^+ channels.

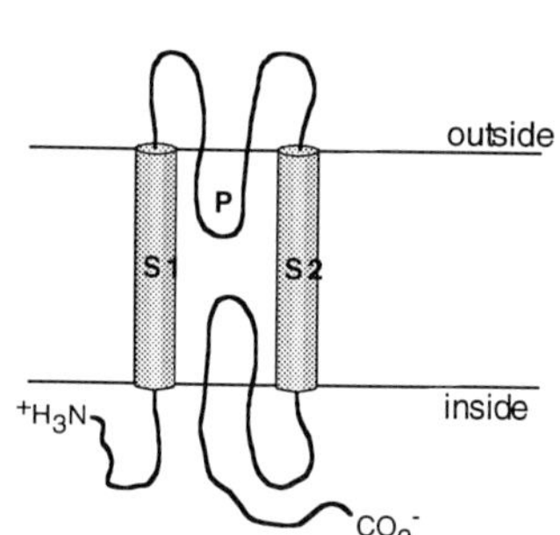

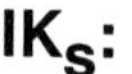

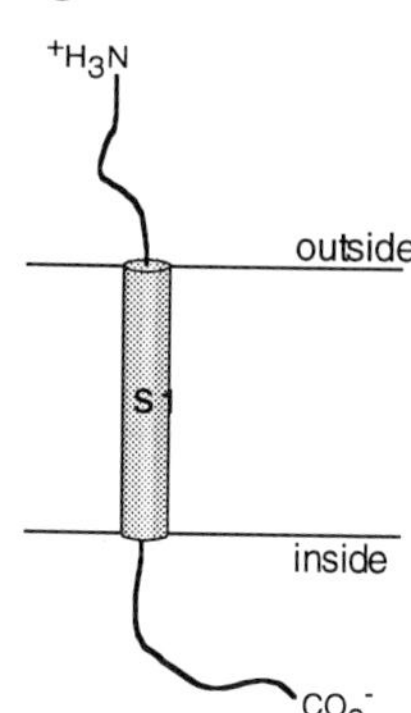

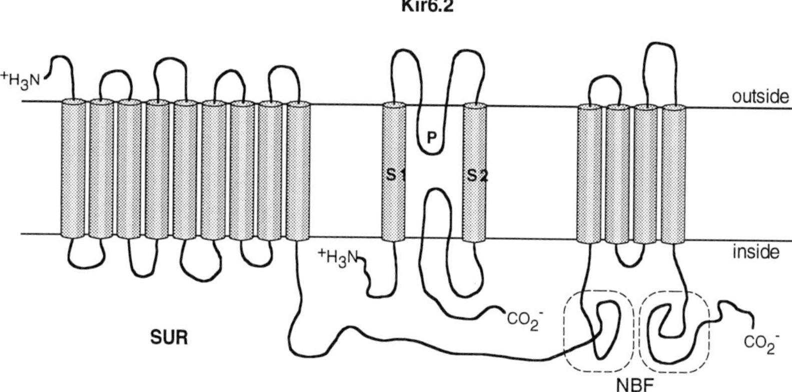

FIGURE 1 *Continued*

major contributor to this phenomenon is nature, which has provided us with a large number of peptidyl K^+ channel blockers that are present in venoms from a variety of invertebrate species. The only other type of channel from the K_v1–6 family known to be sensitive to peptide inhibitors is K_v2, whose activity has been shown to be blocked by a novel peptide isolated from spider venom. The entire K_v1–6 family of channels is sensitive to blockade by the nonselective inhibitors, tetraethylammonium ion (TEA) and 4-aminopyridine, although sensitivity to these agents varies dramatically between members of these families. Another class of proteins known as IK_r are the target for a series of compounds that are under development as Class III anti-arrhythmic agents (Colatsky and Argentieri, 1994), and the molecular components of this channel have been identified. A protein (minK) that was believed to underlie the cardiac delayed rectifier current, IK_s, has been cloned from several tissues, and it has a much different structure than that of other K^+ channels (Fig. 1). However, it has just been reported that minK coassembles with a newly identified K^+ channel, K_vLQT_1, to form functional channels that possess all the characteristics of the native cardiac myocyte current, and that minK, by itself, does not form channels (Sanguinetti *et al.*, 1996a). The pharmacology of IK_s is still under development (Colatsky and Argentieri, 1994).

A. Peptidyl Blockers Derived from Scorpion Venoms

A large amount of work has been devoted to the identification of agents that interact at high affinity with voltage-gated K^+ channels (Fig. 2). Scorpion venoms have provided a rich source of peptides that block these channels. At the present time, a large number of these peptides have been characterized. They can be classified into four different families based on sequence homology and specificity. All are 37–39 amino acids in length and have six cysteine residues which bridge their backbone structures with three disulfide linkages.

1. Charybdotoxin

Although chronologically this was not the first peptidyl K^+ channel blocker identified, charybdotoxin (ChTX; Fig. 2) is perhaps the most extensively studied of the scorpion venom-derived peptides. ChTX was identified in venom of the scorpion *Leiurus quinquestriatus* var. *hebraeus* (Miller *et al.*, 1985). Soon after its discovery, ChTX was purified to homogeneity by a combination of ion-exchange and reversed-phase chromatographies, and its complete amino acid sequence was determined (Gimenez-Gallego *et al.*, 1988). ChTX is a 37 amino acid peptide with its six cysteines forming three disulfide bridges. It has a high content of positively charged residues which confers a net charge of +5 onto the peptide. Some of these residues have been shown to be very important in the mechanism of K^+ channel blockade. ChTX has been produced by solid-phase synthesis using fluorenylmethyloxy carbonyl (FMOC) pentafluorophenyl ester methodologies (Sugg *et al.*, 1990). The reduced synthetic peptide can be oxidized to yield biologically active material that is indistinguishable from native material. Analysis of peptide fragments obtained after enzymatic digestion of either native or synthetic oxidized ChTX allowed the assignment of the disulfide bonds as: Cys_7–Cys_{28}, Cys_{13}–Cys_{33}, and Cys_{17}–Cys_{35}.

Biologically active ChTX can also be produced in large quantities by recombinant techniques (Park *et al.*, 1991). In this approach, not only can large amounts of material be made (i.e., ~3 mg per liter of *Escherichia coli* culture), but also through the use of site-directed mutagenesis, specific residues in the molecule can be altered for structure–function investigation.

```
Position   1 2 3 4 5 6 7 8 9 10 11 ... 61 (one character per aligned position)

I
ChTX       " ZFTNVSCTTSKECWSVCQRLHNTSRG KCMNKKCRCYS"
Lq2        " ZFTQESCTASNQCWSICKRLHNTNRG KCMNKKCRCYS"

MgTX       " TIINVKCTSPKQCLPPCKAQFGQSAGAKCMNGKCKCYPH"
NxTX       " TIINVKCTSPKQCSKPCKELYGSSAGAKCMNGKCKCYNN"
C.I.I. I   " ITINVKCTSPQQCLRPCKDRFGQHAGGKCINGKCKCYP"

AgTX1      "GVPINVKCTGSPQCLKPCKDA GMRFG KCINGKCHCTPK"
AgTX2      "GVPINVSCTGSPQCIKPCKDA GMRFG KCMNRKCHCTPK"
AgTX3      "GVPINVPCTGSPQCIKPCKDA GMRFG KCMNRKCHCTPK"
KTX        "GVEINVKCSGSPQCLKPCKDA GMRFG KCMNRKCHCTPK"
KTX2       " VRIPVSCKHSGQCLKPCKDA GMRFG KCMNGKCDCTPK"

TyKα       " VFINAKCRGSPECLPKCKEAIGKAAG KCMNGKCKCYP"

II
α-DaTX     "ZPRRKLCILHRNPGRCYDKIPAFYYNQKKKQCERFDWSGCGGNSNRFKTIEECRRTCIG"
β-DaTX     "   GXGCPLTLPFGR  TXEENSXYK     CLPFLFSGCGGNANRFQTIGECR"
γ-DaTX     "        LPAEXGR    QFXSFY      CLPFLFSGCGG A  FQTIGECR"
δ-DaTX     "  AAKYCKLPVRYGPCKKKIPSFYYKWKAKQCLPFDYSGCGGNANRFKTIEECRRTCVG"
AsKC1      "  INKDCLLPMDVGRCRASHPRYYYNSSSKRCEKFIYGGCRGNANNFHTLEECEKVCGVR"
AsKC2      "  INKDCLLPMDVGRCRARHPRYYYNSSSRRCEKFIYGGCRGNANNFITKKECEKVCGVR"
AsKC3      "  INGDCELPKVVGRCRARFPRYYYNLSSRRCEKFIYGGCGGNANNFHTLEECEKVCGVRS"

III
BgK        " VCRDWFKETACRHAKSLGNCRTSQKYRAN CAKTLQC C"
ShK        "RSCIDTIPKSRCTAFQ    CKHSMKYRLSFCRKTCGT C"
AsKS       " ACKDNFAAATCKHVKENKNC GSQKYATN CAKTCGK C"

IV
HaTX1      "ECRYLFGGCKTTSDCCKHLGCKFRDKYCAWDFTFS"
HaTX2      "ECRYLFGGCKTTADCCKHLGCKFRDKYCAWDFTFS"

Position   1 2 3 4 5 6 7 8 9 10 11 ... 61
```

For these studies, knowledge of the three-dimensional solution structure of ChTX as determined by nuclear magnetic resonance (NMR) techniques has been of great importance (Bontems *et al.*, 1991a,b; Lambert *et al.*, 1990). ChTX is a globular structure with dimensions of 20 × 20 × 25 Å; the polypeptide backbone consists of a three turn α-helix linked by disulfide bridges to a three strand antiparallel β-sheet. The rigidity of the structure is maintained by the three disulfide bonds which comprise the entire internal volume of the peptide. All other residue side chains lie on the surface and project into aqueous solution.

ChTX inhibits the $K_v1.3$ channel that is present in human T lymphocytes and neuronal tissue with high affinity (Sands *et al.*, 1989; Swanson *et al.*, 1990). In addition, $K_v1.2$ channels are also highly sensitive to the peptide (Grissmer *et al.*, 1994; Werkman *et al.*, 1992) and, as will be described later, ChTX interacts potently with high-conductance Ca^{2+}-activated K^+ channels. Initially, ChTX was also reported to be a high-affinity inhibitor of native *Shaker* K^+ channels (MacKinnon *et al.*, 1988). Although it was later discovered that the blocking activity was due to a contaminating homologous peptide present in that ChTX preparation, *Shaker* K^+ channels have become a useful substrate by which to study the ChTX receptor site. This is due to the fact that a single amino acid substitution at position 425 (Gly for Phe) in the wild-type *Shaker* K^+ channel confers high ChTX sensitivity (Goldstein and Miller, 1993). The mechanism by which ChTX blocks *Shaker* channels has been extensively studied. ChTX binds to a receptor site in the external vestibule of the K^+ channel in a bimolecular fashion and prevents ion conduction by a simple plugging mechanism (Goldstein and Miller, 1993). All residues in the peptide exposed to the solvent have been mutated in order to identify which part of the toxin makes direct contact with the channel. Five residues, Lys_{27}, Met_{29}, Asn_{30}, Arg_{34}, and Tyr_{36}, were found to be critical for the toxin–channel interaction (Goldstein *et al.*, 1994). These residues are well separated from unimportant ones and lie together in an area of 530 Å^2, which represents 17% of the toxin's molecular surface. Lys_{27} is a particularly interesting residue because its neutralization abolishes the voltage dependence of the toxin blockade. These data indicate that once ChTX is bound to the channel, Lys_{27} enters the pore and interacts with K^+ in the conduction pathway of the ion channel.

Because the ChTX interaction surface must mirror a complementary surface on the *Shaker* channel, it may be possible to deduce the shape of the external opening of the channel (Goldstein *et al.*, 1994). Two considerations should be taken into account, however: (1) the channel is a fourfold symmetric structure with its center of symmetry lying along the pore axis, and (2) there are four equivalent configurations for ChTX to bind, but only one can be occupied at any given time. By placing the fourfold axis on Lys_{27} of ChTX, the channel surface can be resolved by rotating the ChTX interaction surface in fourfold symmetry around this residue. The shape of this surface suggests that the narrow K^+ conduction pore widens at its external face to a 25×35-Å plateau. Complementary mutagenesis of both ChTX and *Shaker* indicates that Phe_{425} in the channel makes contact with an area in ChTX close to Thr_8 and Thr_9. This interaction reduces toxin-binding affinity, but toxin binding can be enhanced by mutating these two Thr residues to smaller ones. When the residue at Phe_{425} is made smaller, the destabilizing contact is lost, toxin binds more strongly, and binding is no longer sensitive to the size of the two residues on the toxin. Given these data, Phe_{425} in *Shaker* must be located at a 20-Å radial distance from the pore axis and 10–15 Å above the receptor floor. Complementary mutagenesis has also identified a pair of residues, *Shaker* Lys_{427} and ChTX Lys_{11}, that sense each other via through-space electrostatic forces (Stocker and Miller, 1994). These studies suggest that Lys_{427} in *Shaker* is at the same elevation as Phe_{425}. These two *Shaker* residues appear to form a low wall enveloping the floor of the receptor.

Because ChTX contains a single Tyr residue, the molecule can be iodinated to high specific activity with ^{125}I and the resulting monoiodotyrosine ChTX (I-ChTX) can be separated from nonlabeled material by reversed-phase chromatography (Vazquez *et al.*, 1989). In rat brain membranes, ^{125}I-ChTX binds to a single class of receptor sites with pharmacological properties predicted for an interaction of toxin with $K_v1.3/K_v1.2$ channels (Vazquez *et al.*, 1990). In both human T lymphocytes and membranes derived from Jurkat cells (a human T-cell leukemic line), ^{125}I-ChTX binds to receptor sites associated with the $K_v1.3$ channel (Deutsch *et al.*, 1991; Slaughter *et al.*, 1991). In human T cells, toxin binding is upregulated after stimulation of the T-cell receptor with anti-CD3 (Deutsch *et al.*, 1991). A ChTX mutant containing a Cys residue at position 19 has been produced and shown to have the same biological activity as native toxin (Shimony *et al.*, 1994). This ChTX mutant can be derivatized with thiol-alkylating reagents such as [^3H]*N*-ethylmaleimide (NEM) or fluorescence derivatives of maleimide to yield novel ChTX adducts. [^3H]NEM–ChTX has been used to study the expression of *Shaker* K^+ channels after transient transfection of COS cells with a plasmid carrying a cDNA for that channel (Sun *et al.*, 1994).

2. *Noxiustoxin*

Noxiustoxin (NxTX; Fig. 2) is a 39 amino acid peptide isolated from venom of the scorpion *Centruroides noxius* (Possani *et al.*, 1982). NxTX was the first peptidyl blocker of K^+ channels to be identified. However, it has not been as extensively studied as ChTX. For some time, the high-affinity K^+ channel target of NxTX was a matter of controversy. Initially, it was reported that NxTX inhibited the delayed rectifier K^+ channel in squid axon, although high concentrations (μM) were needed to produce this effect (Carbone *et al.*, 1982). NxTX was also shown to increase [^3H]GABA release and block $^{86}Rb^+$ efflux from superfused mouse brain synaptosomes, consistent with the finding that the peptide affects K^+ permeability of neurons (Sitges *et al.*, 1986). During the last period of time, the identity of the high-affinity receptor for NxTX has been discerned. $K_v1.3$ K^+ channels present in Jurkat cells (Sands *et al.*, 1989) or obtained by heterologous expression in *Xenopus* oocytes (Swanson *et al.*, 1990) are inhibited with high affinity by NxTX. Consistent with this finding, ^{125}I-ChTX binding to purified rat brain synaptic plasma membranes, human T lymphocytes, or Jurkat cells is inhibited by low concentrations of NxTX (Deutsch *et al.*, 1991; Slaughter *et al.*, 1991; Vazquez *et al.*, 1990). It has been shown that NxTX also inhibits $K_v1.2$ channels stably transfected into mammalian cells with similar affinity to that observed for inhibition of $K_v1.3$ (Grissmer *et al.*, 1994).

The solid-phase synthesis of NxTX has been accomplished using FMOC chemistry (Drakopoulou *et al.*, 1995). Two synthetic forms, containing either an amidated C terminus or the C-terminal free acid, have been produced. Comparison of the two synthetic forms with native toxin indicates that native NxTX possesses an amidated C terminus. Although few mechanistic studies have been performed with NxTX, this peptide is also predicted to function as a channel pore blocker. The three-dimensional structure of the peptide has been elucidated by NMR and molecular modeling, and has been shown to be similar to that of ChTX, although the β-sheet is longer in NxTX (Dauplais *et al.*, 1995). NxTX has been a useful probe for defining the physiologic role that $K_v1.3$ channels play in human T lymphocytes (Lin *et al.*, 1993).

3. *Margatoxin*

In the search for selective toxins directed against the $K_v1.3$ channel, the ^{125}I-ChTX-binding assay was used to screen different scorpion venoms for inhibitory activity against the rat brain membrane receptor. From crude venom of the scorpion *Centruroides margaritatus,* a novel peptide termed margatoxin (MgTX; Fig. 2) was purified and characterized (Garcia-Calvo *et al.*, 1993). MgTX is a 39 amino acid peptide that displays 79% identity in its primary amino acid sequence with NxTX. The amino acid sequence of MgTX was confirmed by producing the peptide in *E. coli* using recombinant techniques, as well as by solid-phase synthesis. The three-dimensional structure of MgTX in solution has been resolved through ^2H, ^{13}C, ^{15}N triple-resonance NMR spectroscopy (Johnson *et al.*, 1994). The global structure is very similar to that of ChTX. A helix is present from residues 11 through 20 and includes two prolines at positions 15 and 16. There is a two strand antiparallel sheet from residues 25 to 38, with a turn occurring at residues 30–33. The additional two amino acids in MgTX extend the β-sheet by one residue relative to ChTX.

MgTX is a high-affinity blocker of $K_v1.3$ channels and displays a K_d of 50 p*M* in electrophysiological experiments employing either human T cells or channels heterologously expressed in *Xenopus* oocytes (Garcia-Calvo *et al.,* 1993; Leonard *et al.,* 1992). Importantly, MgTX has no effect on other ChTX-sensitive K^+ channels, such as maxi-K channels or the small-conductance Ca^{2+}-activated K^+ channels present in human T lymphocytes. Among the K_v1 family of K^+ channels, only $K_v1.2$ is highly sensitive to MgTX (K_d similar to that of Kv1.3; R. Leonard, personal communication), whereas $K_v1.6$ displays 100-fold less sensitivity for inhibition.

MgTX has been radiolabeled in a biologically active form and its interaction with rat brain synaptic plasma membrane vesicles has been characterized (Knaus *et al.,* 1995). Toxin binding occurs through a simple bimolecular reaction to a class of receptor sites that display a K_d of 0.1 p*M* under the experimental conditions of the assay. MgTX, therefore, represents the highest affinity ligand for any membrane receptor or ion channel identified to date. Binding of ^{125}I-MgTX is inhibited with high affinity by native MgTX, NxTX, α-dendrotoxin, kaliotoxin, or the agitoxins 1 and 2. The pharmacology of the binding site suggests that the brain MgTX receptor must be a heteromultimer of at least $K_v1.2/K_v1.3$ channels because none of the individual K_v1 channels display these overall pharmacological features. This idea has been tested further by immunoprecipitation studies of solubilized rat brain MgTX receptors employing site-directed antibodies raised against unique sequences of either $K_v1.2$ or $K_v1.3$ channel proteins. Each antibody was able to immunoprecipitate, in a dose-dependent manner, ^{125}I-MgTX bound to its receptor. Importantly, the addition of saturating concentrations of one antibody did not cause any additional effect over that produced by the other. These data are consistent with the notion that the rat brain MgTX receptor is a heteromultimeric structure, made up of at least $K_v1.2$ and $K_v1.3$ subunits. High-affinity binding of ^{125}I-MgTX has also been observed in human peripheral T lymphocytes and Jurkat plasma membranes (Felix *et al.,* 1995). In these cases, the channel complex has been shown to be a homomultimer of $K_v1.3$ subunits.

MgTX and NxTX have been very valuable in evaluating the role that $K_v1.3$ channels play in human T lymphocyte function as $K_v1.3$ is the only high-affinity target of these peptides in T cells. When the membrane potential of nonactivated peripheral human T lymphocytes is monitored with the lipophilic cation [^{3}H]tetraphenylphosphonium ion, the cells display a resting potential of approximately -50 mV. In the presence of increasing concentrations of MgTX, NxTX, or ChTX, the cells depolarize to new value of -30 mV, and the concentrations of the peptides required to produce this effect correlate well with their ability to block the $K_v1.3$ channel (Leonard *et al.,* 1992). These data indicate that the $K_v1.3$ channel controls the resting potential in nonactivated human T cells. Interestingly, the membrane potential of Chinese hamster ovary cells stably transfected with $K_v1.3$ also appears to be determined by the activity of this channel as MgTX also elicits depolarization in those cells (DeFarias *et al.,* 1995).

Mitogen-induced T-cell activation involves a number of different processes which ultimately lead to the production of lymphokines such as IL-2. This lymphokine serves as an autocrine factor for clonal expansion and proliferation of T cells. The initial step in T-cell activation is a rise in cytoplasmic Ca^{2+} levels due to the release of this ion from thapsigargin-sensitive intracellular stores, coupled with the influx of extracellular Ca^{2+} through plasmalemmal Ca^{2+} channels activated by the depletion of intracellular Ca^{2+} stores. T-cell proliferation appears to require the sustained entry of extracellular Ca^{2+}. MgTX, NxTX, and ChTX inhibit the rise in intracellular Ca^{2+} and, as expected, these peptides also inhibit lymphokine production and T-cell proliferation (Lin *et al.*, 1993). These data suggest that membrane depolarization caused by inhibition of $K_v1.3$ is sufficient to prevent the rise in Ca^{2+} required for human T-cell activation. The precise mechanism by which membrane depolarization alters Ca^{2+} homeostasis in T cells is not well understood at present. It is speculated that the internal negative membrane potential of T lymphocytes contributes to the driving force for Ca^{2+} influx and that, after depolarization, the entry of Ca^{2+} into the cell is blunted. Regardless of the mechanism, these data suggest that selective blockers of $K_v1.3$ may represent novel immunosuppresive agents. This has been verified by demonstrating that MgTX has immunosuppressant properties *in vivo* (Koo *et al.*, 1996).

4. *Kaliotoxin*

Kaliotoxin (KTX; Fig. 2) is a 38 amino acid peptide isolated from venom of the scorpion *Androctonus mauretanicus*. Although only 37 residues were identified in the first attempt to determine the sequence of the peptide (Crest *et al.*, 1992), in a later report the last residue of the peptide was characterized and the sequence corrected (Romi *et al.*, 1993). KTX has been produced by solid-phase synthesis and by recombinant techniques using an *E. coli* expression system. It is surprising, therefore, that several commercial sources only have KTX_{1-37} available, but not the correct native peptide. The three-dimensional structure of KTX has been determined by NMR techniques independently in two laboratories. In one study, where KTX_{1-37} was used, it was found that the helical region of the toxin is shorter, as well as distorted, when compared with ChTX. In addition, the N-terminal strand and α-helix interact with opposite sides of the β-sheet, whereas in ChTX they interact with the same face of the β-sheet structure (Fernandez *et al.*, 1994). In a study employing full-length KTX, it was shown that the tertiary folding of KTX has the same features as those found in ChTX (Aiyar *et al.*, 1995). It is possible, therefore, that the differences found between the two toxin structures in these studies may be related to the use of a truncated form in one case, which could have led to altered peptide folding.

Although initial reports on the pharmacological target of KTX were confusing, it is now clear that KTX blocks $K_v1.3$ with very high affinity

(Aiyar *et al.*, 1995; Grissmer *et al.*, 1994). Consistent with this, KTX is a potent inhibitor of ^{125}I-MgTX binding to rat brain membranes (unpublished observations). The affinity of KTX against other K_v1 channels is much reduced. Complementary mutagenesis between $K_v1.3$ and KTX has been employed to determine the shape and dimensions of the outer vestibule of this channel (Aiyar *et al.*, 1995). Asp_{386} in $K_v1.3$ was found to interact electrostatically with Arg_{24} in KTX, and from electrostatic compliance, the distance between the two residues was estimated to be 3–4 Å. In addition, Gly_{380} of $K_v1.3$, which appears to lie in the outer margin of the external vestibule, is close to Leu_{15} and Arg_{31} in KTX, whereas His_{404} in $K_v1.3$ is close to Phe_{25} in KTX. Based on these data, the vestibule is estimated to be 28–32 Å wide at its outer margin, 28–34 Å at its base, and ~4–8 Å deep. The pore is 9–14 Å wide at its external entrance and the ion conduction pathway narrows to 4–5 Å at a distance of about 5–7 Å from the base of the vestibule.

Another related toxin, KTX_2 (Fig. 2), has been isolated from venom of the scorpion *Androctonus australis*, based on its ability to inhibit ^{125}I-KTX_{1-37} binding to rat brain synaptosomes (Laraba-Djebari *et al.*, 1994). KTX_2 contains 37 amino acids and displays 76% identity with KTX; it is five-fold weaker than KTX as either an inhibitor of binding or in toxicity studies in mice, where the LD_{50} doses are 25 and 110 ng for KTX and KTX_2, respectively.

5. Agitoxins

$Agitoxin_{1-3}$ ($AgTX_{1-3}$; Fig. 2) are three closely related 38 amino acid peptides isolated from *L. quinquestriatus* venom. They also display high homology in their amino acid sequence with KTX (Garcia *et al.*, 1994). The identity of $AgTX_1$ and $AgTX_2$ has been confirmed by producing recombinant peptides in *E. coli.* The three-dimensional structure of $AgTX_2$ has been determined by NMR techniques and has similar backbone folding as ChTX (Krezel *et al.*, 1995). The AgTX's are a very interesting class of peptides because they possess the blocking activity reported against *Shaker* that was previously attributed to ChTX. In addition, they display a distinct pharmacological profile against other K_v1 channels. $AgTX_2$ is the most potent peptidyl inhibitor of $K_v1.3$ discovered so far. This peptide blocks the $K_v1.3$ channel expressed in *Xenopus* oocytes with a K_i of 4 p*M;* it also inhibits $K_v1.1$ and $K_v1.6$ channels, although with 10-fold reduced potency. As cited earlier, both $AgTX_1$ and $AgTX_2$ are very potent inhibitors of ^{125}I-MgTX binding to rat brain membranes. A single point mutant of $AgTX_2$, $Asp_{20}Cys$, has been constructed and the resulting peptide has been covalently modified with [^{3}H]*N*-ethylmaleimide to yield a radiolabeled derivative of the toxin that is biologically active. [^{3}H]NEM–$AgTX_2$ has been used to determine expression levels of *Shaker* channels in *Xenopus* oocytes. By using this peptide along with a *Shaker* mutant that does not display ion conduction, but in which gating is unaffected, it has been possible to correlate the number of gating charges present per channel molecule (Aggarwal and MacKinnon, 1994).

Complementary mutagenesis between the *Shaker* channel and $AgTX_2$, using a thermodynamic cycle analysis, has allowed the identification of pair residues that make close contact. This technique has been used to deduce the dimensions of the channel's outer vestibule (Hidalgo and MacKinnon, 1995). Asp_{431} in *Shaker* was found to interact electrostatically with Arg_{31} in $AgTX_2$. Moreover, Arg_{24} in the toxin interacts with Asp_{431} of the channel through short-range molecular forces, most likely via formation of a salt bridge. These data imply that the distance separating residues Arg_{24} and Arg_{31} (about 25 Å) is a measure of the spacing between Asp_{431} residues on diagonally opposed channel subunits. Thus, Asp_{431} is 12–15 Å from the central axis of the K^+ channel pore.

$AgTX_2$ has also been used as a probe of the transfer of toxin sensitivity from $K_v1.3$ to the toxin-insensitive K^+ channel, $K_v2.1$ (Gross *et al.*, 1994). This was accomplished by transferring the stretch of amino acids between transmembrane domains S_5 and S_6 (the P region) from one channel to the other. Such studies indicate that this region represents the only part of the ion channel that makes direct contact with the bound toxin. The presence of two residues in $K_v2.1$, Lys_{356} and Lys_{386}, appears to be the reason for the native channel's insensitivity to $AgTX_2$ blockade.

6. Other Peptidyl Blockers

Several additional peptidyl blockers of K^+ channels have also been identified in scorpion venoms (Fig. 2). Although these peptides have not been as thoroughly characterized as the toxins described earlier, they have still contributed to the pharmacology of these channels. Lq_2 toxin has been purified and characterized from venom of the scorpion *L. quinquestriatus* (Lucchesi *et al.*, 1989). This peptide consists of 37 amino acids and displays high sequence identity with ChTX. Lq_2 blocks the *Shaker* H_4 channel expressed in *Xenopus* oocytes, but with reduced potency when compared with the AgTX's. Its selectivity against K_v1 channels has not been determined. Lq_2 toxin has also been shown to block the inward rectifier K^+ channel, ROMK1, with a K_i of 0.4 μM (Lu *et al.*, 1996). In addition, this peptide blocks the maxi-K channel (see later); in this respect Lq_2 is 10-fold weaker than ChTX due to a combination of faster dissociation and slower association rates.

Two novel peptides have been purified from venom of the Mexican scorpion *Centruroides limpidus limpidus,* using an immunoassay based on antibodies raised against NxTX (Martin *et al.*, 1994). *C. limpidus limpidus* toxin I contains 38 amino acid residues and has 74, 64, 51, 37, and 37% sequence identity with MgTX, NxTX, KTX, ChTX, and Lq_2 toxin, respectively. The complete amino acid sequence of *C. limpidus limpidus* toxin 2 has not been fully described. Both toxins potently inhibit the binding of ^{125}I-

NxTX to rat brain synaptosomes. They also block a transient voltage-dependent K^+ current present in cultured rat cerebellar granule cells, but with much reduced potency. The specificity of these toxins against other types of K^+ channels has not been determined. It has been reported that β scorpion toxin 2 from *C. noxius*, which is known to affect Na^+ channel activation kinetics, inhibits currents through $K_v1.3$ channels in human peripheral T lymphocytes by accelerating channel inactivation (Gaspar *et al.*, 1994). This effect, however, occurred at much higher toxin concentrations than needed for the Na^+ channel interaction, with a half-blocking concentration of about 5 μM.

Two nonhomologous peptides, tityustoxin Kα (TsTX-Kα) and tityustoxin Kβ (TsTX-Kβ), have been purified from venom of the Brazilian scorpion *Tityus serrulatus* (Rogowski *et al.*, 1994). These peptides block voltage-gated noninactivating K^+ channels in rat brain synaptosomes with IC_{50}'s of 8 and 30 nM, respectively. TsTX-Kα inhibits the binding of ^{125}I-α-dendrotoxin to synaptic membranes, whereas TsTX-Kβ has no effect here. In experiments monitoring $^{86}Rb^+$ efflux from synaptosomes, it was shown that TsTX-Kα causes unblocking of rapidly inactivating voltage-gated K^+ channels when they are blocked by α-dendrotoxin, but not when they are blocked by ChTX. TsTX-Kα appears to bind to a site on the inactivating K^+ channel that does not occlude the pore, and its binding must prevent α-dendrotoxin, but not ChTX, from interacting with the pore.

B. Peptidyl Inhibitors Isolated from Snake Venoms

Neurotransmitter release is stimulated at peripheral (Harvey and Karlsson, 1982) and central (Docherty *et al.*, 1983; Dolly *et al.*, 1984) neurons by a group of homologous peptides derived from snake venoms that selectively modify voltage-gated K^+ channels (dendrotoxins; Fig. 2). These toxins have been identified in venom from several related species of snakes, two types of green mamba, *Dendroaspis angusticeps* and *Dendroaspis viridus*, and a species of black mamba, *Dendroaspis polylepsis*.

Four peptides have been purified and characterized from *D. angusticeps* venom. The most studied is α-dendrotoxin (α-DaTX), a basic 7-kDa polypeptide that contains 59 amino acids with six Cys residues which exist in three disulfide bridges (Harvey and Anderson, 1985). δ-DaTX contains 57 amino acids and has marked sequence homology with α-DaTX in the C-terminal region, where 25 out of 30 amino acids in the primary structure are identical. The amino acid sequences of β- and γ-DaTX have been partially resolved, and their primary structures are very similar to that of α- and δ-DaTX in the C-terminal region, where 20 out of 23 amino acids are conserved in all four dendrotoxins. The crystal structure of α-DaTX has been determined (Skarzynski, 1992). In addition to a short α-helical configuration made up of residues 50 to 58, there is a region composed of a double-stranded, antiparallel β-sheet comprising residues 19 to 27 and 31 to 38. In this structure, the β-sheet is twisted about 180°. Three Lys residues are located between the β-sheets which may be important for peptide–channel interactions. α-DaTX has been synthesized by solid-phase techniques and folded to yield a biologically active species (Byrnes *et al.*, 1995). Synthetic α-DaTX was shown to coelute with native toxin upon reverse-phase, high-performance liquid chromatography and to have identical biological activity to the native peptide. α-DaTX has also been expressed in *E. coli* as a fusion protein that is secreted into the culture medium, and recombinant toxin was subsequently generated by chemical treatment (Danse *et al.*, 1994). Using this approach, an α-DaTX mutant was constructed in which the Lys triplet (residues 28–30) was changed into Ala–Ala–Gly. The mutated peptide exhibits only a small decrease in biological activity, suggesting that the positively charged Lys triplet 28–30 of α-DaTX does not constitute part of the toxin interaction site.

α-DaTX reduces a transient, voltage-dependent K^+ current in intracellular recordings of CA1 neurons from hippocampal slices (Halliwell *et al.*, 1986). However, α-DaTX has also been shown to inhibit a slowly inactivating K^+ current present in various neurons (Penner *et al.*, 1986; Stansfeld *et al.*, 1986). Thus, electrophysiological data obtained from a variety of neuronal sources indicate that α-DaTX inhibits a family of K^+ channels that differ greatly in their inactivation kinetics. The pharmacological target of α-DaTX has been elucidated after expression of individual K_v channel subunits in *Xenopus* oocytes or mammalian cell lines, followed by determination of their sensitivity to the peptide. Only members of the K_v1 family of voltage-gated K^+ channels were found to be blocked by α-DaTX (Chandy and Gutman, 1995). From this family, $K_v1.1$, $K_v1.2$, and $K_v1.6$, all of which display noninactivating K^+ currents, were found to be more sensitive to α-DaTX inhibition than the inactivating channels, $K_v1.3$ and $K_v1.4$, or another noninactivating channel, $K_v1.5$. In a different set of experiments where the activity of K^+ channels was monitored measuring $^{86}Rb^+$ efflux from rat brain synaptosomes, α-DaTX preferentially blocked a component of flux mediated by rapidly inactivating K^+ channels (Benishin *et al.*, 1988). It appears that the α-DaTX sensitivity of inactivating K^+ channels that has been observed in biological preparations could be due to either heteromultimeric channel formation or the presence of an auxiliary subunit that alters the inactivation kinetics of the pore-forming subunit (see later).

The expression of chimeras formed between α-DTX-sensitive and -insensitive channels supports the idea that the putative extracellular loop between transmembrane domains S_5 and S_6 is a major determinant of α-DTX sensitivity. Furthermore, the toxin association rate depends on the number of wild-type subunits making up the functional channel (Hurst *et al.*, 1991; Tytgat *et al.*, 1995). Moreover, there is a linear relationship between the number of wild-type subunits in the channel complex and the free energy for α-DTX binding, suggesting that all four subunits must interact with α-DTX to produce a high-affinity binding site.

α-DaTX has been radiolabeled with ^{125}INa, and ^{125}I-α-DaTX has been used to identify receptor sites for this toxin in various membrane preparations. High-affinity binding sites have been identified in synaptosomal membranes and these have been localized in the mammalian central nervous system (Bidard *et al.*, 1987; Breeze and Dolly, 1989; Halliwell *et al.*, 1986; Rehm *et al.*, 1988; Rehm and Lazdunski, 1988a; Sorensen and Blaustein, 1989). Binding of α-DaTX is modulated by other dendrotoxins, and also by mast cell degranulating peptide (MCD), isolated from venom of the bee *Apis mellifera,* as well as by β-bungarotoxin (β-BTX), a protein from the Formosan krait. Such studies have identified two subtypes of α-DaTX-binding proteins. In one subtype, binding of either ^{125}I-α-DaTX or ^{125}I-MCD is inhibited by β-BTX with low affinity, whereas in the second subtype, β-BTX inhibits these interactions with high affinity.

The receptor for α-DaTX has been purified from bovine and rat brain and is composed of two noncovalently linked subunits with apparent M_r of 78,000 and 39,000 (Parcej and Dolly, 1989; Rehm and Lazdunski, 1988b). The larger subunit binds both α-DaTX and β-BTX. Reconstitution of the purified rat brain receptor into artificial bilayers results in the appearance of a K^+ conductance displaying up to seven levels of unitary current (Rehm *et al.*, 1989). This heterogeneity in unitary current expression suggests that the purified α-DaTX receptor may be a mixture of closely related K^+ channel structures. The N-terminal amino acid sequence from the larger subunit of the purified bovine α-DaTX receptor has been obtained (Scott *et al.*, 1990). The 27 identified residues indicate that this receptor is highly homologous to K_v1.2. Another minor sequence was also observed that is homologous with the N terminus of K_v1.1. Specific antibodies raised against K_v1 family members have been employed to identify which subunits are present in the purified α-DaTX receptor preparation (Muniz *et al.*, 1992; Scott *et al.*, 1994a). K_v1.1, K_v1.2, K_v1.4, and K_v1.6 were shown to copurify with α-DaTX-binding sites from bovine cerebral cortex. When α-DaTX receptors were purified from other brain regions, the distribution of K_v1.2 and K_v1.6 subunits was found to be constant, whereas K_v1.1 reactivity was highest in brain stem and lowest in cerebellum; K_v1.4 was most prevalent in hippocampus. These data indicate that K_v1 subunits associate to form heteromultimeric complexes; this phenomena could account for the α-DaTX sensitivity found for different types of K^+ channels present in various biological preparations.

The smaller (β) subunit of the α-DaTX receptor was initially cloned from bovine brain (Scott *et al.*, 1994b). The cDNA predicts a protein of 367 amino acids that possesses no transmembrane domains based on hydropathy analysis, suggesting that it must be firmly associated with the pore-forming subunit on the inside of the membrane (Figure 1). Other β subunits from rat brain, ferret, and human heart have been isolated (England *et al.*, 1995a,b;

Majumder *et al.*, 1995; Morales *et al.*, 1995; Rettig *et al.*, 1994). The β subunits have been shown to alter the inactivation properties of members of the *Shaker* family of K^+ channels (Castellino *et al.*, 1995; England *et al.*, 1995a,b; Majumder *et al.*, 1995; McCormack *et al.*, 1995; Morales *et al.*, 1995; Pongs, 1995; Rettig *et al.*, 1994; Sasaki *et al.*, 1995; Stephens *et al.*, 1996; Uebele *et al.*, 1996).

Twenty-eight different peptides have been purified from venom of the snake *D. polylepis* (Schweitz *et al.*, 1990). The 14 most cationic peptides form a group of closely related analogs. DaTX I, a toxin that is structurally similar to α-DaTX, is the most well-characterized peptide of this group (Hollecker *et al.*, 1993). These peptides recognize antibodies raised against DaTX I, as well as ^{125}I-α-DaTX-binding sites in brain that are sensitive to modulation by DaTX I and MCD. The structure of two members of this group, DaTX I and DaTX K, has been determined in solution by NMR techniques and is very similar to that of α-DaTX (Berndt *et al.*, 1993; Foray *et al.*, 1993). Like DaTX I, these peptides produce convulsions after intracerebroventricular injections into mice and induce GABA release from synaptosomes. mRNA isolated from glands of *D. polylepis* was used to construct a cDNA library. cDNA's encoding 14 different venom proteins were isolated, and genes coding for DaTX I, DaTX K, and DaTX E were expressed in *E. coli* (Smith *et al.*, 1995). Recombinant DaTX K has been purified in a biologically active form. This approach provides an important means for the preparation of toxin mutants that could be used for structure–activity relationship studies employing the three-dimensional structure of α-DaTX and the toxin-binding site identified on cloned K^+ channels.

C. Peptidyl Blockers from Sea Anemone

Three peptide toxins that block voltage-dependent K^+ channels, BgK, ShK, and AsKS, have been isolated from the sea anemones *Bunodosoma granulifera* (Aneiros *et al.*, 1993), *Stichodactyla helianthus* (Castañeda *et al.*, 1995), and *Anemonia sulcata* (Schweitz *et al.*, 1995), respectively (Fig. 2). These peptides consist of 35–37 amino acids and contain six Cys residues. There is sequence homology among these peptides, but there is no structural similarity to other groups of peptidyl blockers of K^+ channels. The disulfide bonding pattern in ShK has been determined.

ShK suppresses a K^+ current in cultured rat dorsal root ganglion neurons and inhibits binding of ^{125}I-DaTX I and ^{125}I-α-DaTX to rat brain synaptosomal membranes (Castañeda *et al.*, 1995). ShK also inhibits the $K_v1.3$ channel in Jurkat cells with a K_i of 133 p*M* (Pennington *et al.*, 1995). ShK, as well as a number of synthetic analogs, has been produced by solid-phase synthesis and tested for biological activity against ^{125}I-α-DaTX binding to rat brain membranes or against ^{125}I-ChTX binding to Jurkat cells (Pennington *et al.*, 1996). The ShK pharmacophore requirements for binding at these two

K^+ channel receptors appears to be different; binding to Jurkat cells is more influenced by substitutions at Lys_9, Arg_{11}, and Phe_{15}, whereas Lys_{22} appears to be essential for binding to brain.

AsKS inhibits binding of ^{125}I-α-DTX to rat brain with a K_i of 10 nM through an apparently competitive mechanism (Schweitz *et al.*, 1995). Electrophysiological experiments indicate that AsKS inhibits the $K_v1.2$ channel expressed in *Xenopus* oocytes with a K_i of 140 nM.

Three 57–60 amino acid peptides homologous to serine protease inhibitors of the Kunitz type, as well as to the dendrotoxins, have been purified from the sea anemone *A. sulcata:* kalicludines 1, 2, and 3 (AsKC1, 2, and 3) (Schweitz *et al.*, 1995). These peptides inhibit binding of ^{125}I-α-DTX to rat brain with IC_{50} values of 60 nM for AsKC2, 375 nM for AsKC1, and 500 nM for AsKC3. They are, however, weak inhibitors of $K_v1.2$ expressed in *Xenopus* oocytes, displaying K_i values of 1.1 μM for AsKC2, 1.3 μM for AsKC3, and 2.8 μM for AsKC1. Kalicludines also inhibit trypsin in a stoichiometric manner with K_d values below 30 nM.

D. Peptidyl Blockers Isolated from Spider Venom

Two peptides have been isolated from venom of the Chilean tarantula *Granulosa spatulata* that inhibit the Kv2.1 channel (Swartz and MacKinnon, 1995). The two peptides, hanatoxin 1 (HaTX1) and hanatoxin 2 (HaTX2), which are not related in their primary amino acid sequence to other K^+ channel inhibitors, define a new class of toxins (Fig. 2). They are, however, related to grammotoxin (43% identity), an inhibitor of voltage-gated Ca^{2+} channels isolated from the same spider. HaTX1 and HaTX2 consist of 35 residues and differ only at position 13. The sequence of HaTX1 has been confirmed by producing the peptide in *E. coli* using recombinant methods. HaTX blocks the $K_v2.1$ channel with a K_d of 42 nM, displaying bimolecular kinetics of inhibition. The association rate constant for HaTX is about 1000-fold slower than that of ChTX or $AgTX_2$ for the K_v1 channels. All members of the *Shaker* family of K^+ channels tested are quite insensitive to HaTX. Thus, $K_v1.1$, 1.3, and 1.6 are not blocked by 500 nM HaTX, with only weak inhibition of the *Shaker* K^+ channel, at this toxin concentration. $K_v3.1$ is also insensitive to 500 nM HaTX, but, surprisingly, $K_v4.2$ is sensitive to the peptide. Unlike peptidyl blockers derived from scorpion venoms, HaTX appears to interact with a region of K^+ channels distinct from the S_5–S_6 linker. This was inferred from studies with a chimeric channel in which the S_5–S_6 linker from $K_v2.1$ was transferred to the *Shaker* K^+ channel; as expected, $AgTX_2$ sensitivity is lost, but HaTX sensitivity is not acquired.

E. Nonpeptidyl Blockers

Certain K^+ channels such as $K_v1.1$ and $K_v3.1$–3.4 are extremely sensitive to inhibition by externally applied TEA (K_i of 0.1–1 mM). This sensitivity appears to be due to the presence of a Tyr residue at the C-terminal portion of the P region of these channels (Kavanaugh *et al.*, 1992; MacKinnon and Yellen, 1990). A direct correlation exists between the number of subunits containing Tyr and the degree of TEA block, suggesting that four channel subunits interact simultaneously with TEA to form a high-affinity binding site.

Internally applied TEA blocks K_v channels by interacting at a distinct site on the inner surface of the pore. $K_v1.1$, $K_v1.3$, $K_v1.6$, $K_v2.1$, and the *Shaker* K^+ channel are half-blocked by ~0.3 m*M* TEA (Taglialatela *et al.*, 1991). Block by internal TEA is voltage dependent, being less pronounced at depolarized potentials. The TEA-binding site is located approximately 20% within the electric field of the membrane (Kirsch *et al.*, 1991; Taglialatela *et al.*, 1991) and has been characterized by mutagenesis studies. Two residues in the P region of *Shaker* (TM$\underline{T}$T$\underline{V}$GYG) appear to participate in the binding of internal TEA (Aiyar *et al.*, 1993; Kirsch *et al.*, 1992a,b; Yellen *et al.*, 1991). In addition, some residues from S_6 are also involved in the interaction with TEA (Choi *et al.*, 1993).

4-Aminopyridine blocks all K_v channels with moderate potency (K_i from 0.2–9 m*M*), with $K_v3.1$ being the most sensitive to inhibition. The 4-aminopyridine-binding site appears to be formed from the association of the N-terminal region of S_5 and the C-terminal end of S_6, both of which are thought to lie in the inner vestibule of the channel's pore (Kirsch *et al.*, 1993).

A series of 4-alkylimino-1,4-dihydroquinolines (Fig. 3) have been shown to be inhibitors of the $K_v1.3$ channel present in human T lymphocytes, displaying IC_{50} values between 10^{-7} and 10^{-5} *M* (Michne *et al.*, 1995). These compounds also inhibit ^{125}I-ChTX binding to $K_v1.3$ with IC_{50} values ranging from 10^{-8} to 10^{-6} *M*. The activity of these compounds is very sensitive to changes at the 4-imino position. Lengthening the alkyl chain results in an increase in potency against ^{125}I-ChTX binding, whereas bulky alkyl derivatives are much less potent. Incorporation of an acidic group, or a permanently charged cation, into the alkyl chain abolishes activity. Moreover, the direct attachment of a phenyl group to the position of the imino nitrogen causes a large drop in activity compared to a similarly substituted benzyl analog. The *in vitro* biological activity of one of these compounds, WIN 17317-3 (1-benzyl-7-chloro-4-*n*-propylimino-1,4-dihydroquinoline hydrochloride), has been more extensively evaluated (Hill *et al.*, 1995). In human T lymphocytes, WIN 17317-3 inhibits ^{125}I-ChTX binding to the $K_v1.3$ channel with an IC_{50} value of 83 n*M*, and inhibition of toxin binding occurs by an apparently competitive mechanism. WIN 17317-3 appears to act as an open channel blocker and inhibits the $K_v1.3$ current with an IC_{50} value of 335 n*M*. This compound appears to display much reduced potency against ChTX-sensitive, Ca^{2+}-activated K^+ channels from smooth muscle. It also displays selectivity as a $K_v1.3$ inhibitor among members of the K_v1 channel family (Nguyen *et al.*, 1996). IL-2 production from activated $CD4^-$ lymphocytes

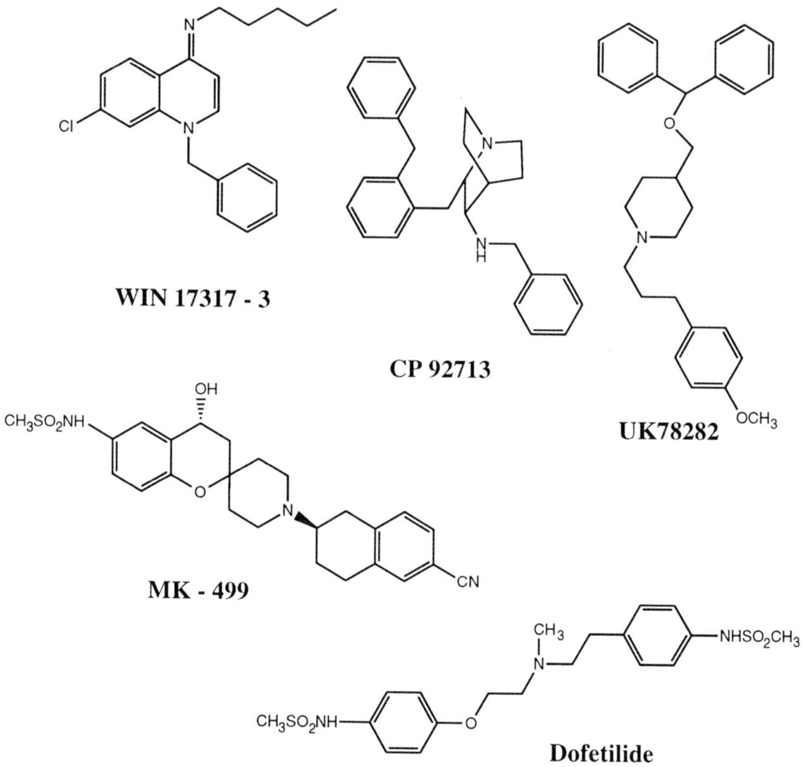

WIN 17317 - 3

CP 92713

UK78282

MK - 499

Dofetilide

FIGURE 3 Nonpeptidyl blockers of voltage-gated K^+ channels.

was inhibited by WIN 17317-3 in a concentration-dependent manner with an EC_{50} of about 1 μM. Furthermore, WIN 17317-3 appears to have no effect on $CD4^-$ lymphocyte viability at concentrations up to 10 μM. This structural series represents the first small molecule $K_v1.3$ inhibitor to be publically disclosed.

Scientists from Pfizer have also revealed two other structural classes of small molecule $K_v1.3$ inhibitors (Keystone Symposium, "Ion Channels as Therapeutic Targets," February 1996). Using a functional assay in which $^{86}Rb^+$ flux through $K_v1.3$ channels in human T cells was monitored, screening of the Pfizer sample collection yielded two molecules, CP 92713 and UK 78282 (Fig. 3), with micromolar activity against $K_v1.3$ (IC_{50} of 1.0 and 0.4 μM, respectively). The UK compound was subjected to further medicinal chemistry efforts because of its better profile in ion channel selectivity assays; this compound has >10-fold selectivity against $K_v1.1$, 1.2, 1.5, and 3.1 channels. UK 78282 was active in inhibiting both phytohemagglutinin-induced human T-cell proliferation and a human mixed lymphocyte reaction *in vitro,* and showed efficacy in blocking a murine delayed-type hypersensitivity reaction *in vivo*. In cell biology experiments, UK 78282 inhibited IL-2 production, but had no effect on either IL-2 receptor synthesis or protein synthesis in general. In functional studies to address the mechanism of action of this compound (electrophysiology, ^{125}I-ChTX binding, channel mutagenesis) UK 78282 was shown to act as a pore blocker and to bind to H_{404} in the P region of $K_v1.3$. This apparently occurs through an interaction between the imidazole of H_{404} and the benzhydryl group of UK 78282. To test this hypothesis, the mono-benzyl derivative of UK 78282 was synthesized; it is predicted to bind less well to H_{404} and, indeed, the compound was 10-fold weaker as an inhibitor of $K_v1.3$. It appears that this lead structure is no longer under active investigation because of difficulties in increasing potency and defining the SAR for biological activity of this class.

Class III antiarrhythmic drugs (Fig. 3) such as E-4031, dofetilide, and MK-499 are potent and specific blockers of IK_r, a rapidly activating current that exhibits strong inward rectification in cardiac myocytes. Interestingly, mutations in the gene coding for the K^+ channel, HERG, produce long QT syndrome, an inherited disorder that causes sudden death from ventricular tachyarrhythmia, *torsade de pointes* (Curran *et al.*, 1995). Heterologous expression of HERG in *Xenopus* oocytes reveals that this channel has biophysical properties identical to Ik_r (Sanguinetti *et al.*, 1996). In addition, MK-499 blocks HERG currents in oocytes by preferentially affecting the open channel conformation, supporting the idea that HERG subunits form IK_r channels in cardiac myocytes (Spector *et al.*, 1996). The target of E-4031, dofetilide, and MK-499 appears to be identical. Although dofetilide has no significant blocking effect on human $K_v1.2$, $K_v1.4$, $K_v1.5$, or $K_v2.1$ channels, it blocks an inward rectifier K^+ channel cloned from human heart at submicromolar concentrations (Kiehn *et al.*, 1995).

III. Ca^{2+}-Activated K^+ Channels

The family of Ca^{2+}-activated K^+ channel proteins which share in common a dependence on intracellular Ca^{2+} for channel activation can be divided into distinct categories according to their biophysical properties (McManus, 1991). Because the pharmacology of these subfamilies can be well distinguished, they will be discussed in two separate sections corresponding to (a) high-conductance and (b) small-conductance Ca^{2+}-activated K^+ channels.

A. High-Conductance Ca^{2+}-Activated K^+ Channels

High-conductance Ca^{2+}-activated K^+ (maxi-K) channels are activated by both cytoplasmic Ca^{2+} and depolarizing voltage. In the absence of other divalent cations, binding of at least 2–4 Ca^{2+} is required for channel opening. Increasing the concentration of internal Ca^{2+} causes a shift in the voltage dependence of activation of maxi-K channels along the voltage axis toward more negative potentials. A unique property of these channels is their large conductance, as well as high cation selectivity. Maxi-K channels from bovine tracheal and aortic smooth muscle have been purified to homogeneity and are composed of two subunits, α and β (see later; Garcia-Calvo *et al.*, 1994; Giangiacomo *et al.*, 1995). The α pore-forming subunit is a member of the *Slo* family of maxi-K channels (Knaus *et al.*, 1994a), whereas the β subunit is a novel protein that modulates the biophysical and pharmacological properties of α (Knaus *et al.*, 1994b; McManus *et al.*, 1995). Several *Slo* cDNA's have been cloned from different tissues and species (Butler *et al.*, 1993; Dworetzky *et al.*, 1994; Pallanck and Ganetzky, 1994; Tseng-Crank *et al.*, 1994; Wallner *et al.*, 1995). The first mammalian cDNA was obtained based on expected homologies between *Slo* and the *Drosophila slow poke* Ca^{2+}-activated K^+ channel gene (Adelman *et al.*, 1992). It appears that *Slo* is coded for by a single gene, but that alternative splicing gives rise to a number of different molecular entities. These individual proteins produce maxi-K channels that differ in their Ca^{2+} sensitivity when expressed in *Xenopus* oocytes (Tseng-Crank *et al.*, 1994; Wei *et al.*, 1994), and this phenomena could explain, at least in part, the large diversity of maxi-K channels described in different tissues. Two types of agents have been described that define the pharmacology of maxi-K channels: peptidyl inhibitors derived from scorpion venoms and small molecule channel modulators.

1. Peptidyl Inhibitors Derived from Scorpion Venoms

The initial discovery of ChTX as a minor component of *L. quinquestriatus* var. *hebraeus* venom was related to its ability to block maxi-K channels (Miller *et al.*, 1985). The general properties of ChTX have been described earlier; this section will be restricted to the interaction of the peptide with maxi-K channels. In single channel recordings of skeletal muscle t-tubular maxi-K channels reconstituted into planar lipid bilayers, ChTX added at the external face of the channel causes the appearance of long silent periods, interspersed between bursts of normal channel activity. These silent periods represent the times at which a single toxin molecule is bound in the mouth of the channel to block ion conduction. Because toxin binding is a freely reversible process, toxin dissociation leads to normal channel behavior because channel gating kinetics are faster than those of toxin binding, until another toxin molecule binds to the channel. Consistent with the hypothesis that toxin binding occurs through a simple bimolecular reaction, the average blocked time is independent of toxin concentration, whereas the duration of the burst periods is inversely related to toxin concentration (Smith *et al.*, 1986). Binding of ChTX is also driven by electrostatic interactions between positively charged residues on the toxin molecule and negatively charged residues located in the external vestibule of the channel (MacKinnon and Miller, 1988, 1989).

Mutations at all residues of ChTX exposed to solvent have been produced and analyzed for maxi-K channel-blocking properties (Stampe *et al.*, 1994). Eight residues were found to be critical in that their modification leads to an increase in toxin dissociation of eight-fold or greater. These residues are Ser_{10}, Trp_{14}, Arg_{25}, Lys_{27}, Met_{29}, Asn_{30}, Arg_{34}, and Tyr_{36}. They cover approximately 25% of the molecular surface of ChTX, and these amino acids are spatially separated from unimportant residues. Lys_{27} is a particularly interesting residue because it is responsible for the interaction between the peptide and K^+ entering the ion conduction pathway from the inside (MacKinnon and Miller, 1988). If position 27 of ChTX carries a positively charged residue, internal K^+ accelerates the dissociation rate of toxin in a voltage-dependent manner (Park and Miller, 1992). However, if a neutral Asn or Gln is substituted at this position, the dissociation rate is completely insensitive to either internal K^+ or applied voltage. These studies suggest that when ChTX is bound to the channel, Lys_{27} lies in close physical proximity to a K^+-specific binding site located externally along the ion conduction pathway. Occupancy of this site by K^+ destabilizes ChTX via direct electrostatic repulsion of the ε-amino group of Lys_{27}. The interaction surface of ChTX predicts that a triangular area on the flat surface formed by the three antiparallel β strands of ChTX will bind to a complementary surface on the maxi-K channel. The peptide makes close contact with an area which may span several channel subunits of the tetrameric complex (Stampe *et al.*, 1994). This interaction prevents ion conduction by physical occlusion of the pore.

^{125}I-ChTX has been useful in identifying receptors associated with maxi-K channels, as well as aiding in their purification (see later). Furthermore, toxin binding to maxi-K channels has been used as a means of identifying and characterizing other specific high-affinity blockers of this channel. A peptide termed iberiotoxin (IbTX; Fig. 4) was purified to homogeneity and characterized from venom of the scorpion *Buthus tamulus* (Galvez *et al.*, 1990). IbTX is a 37 amino acid peptide that displays 68% homology with ChTX, but it is less positively charged. IbTX has been produced by chemical synthesis and biosynthesis. The three-dimensional structure of IbTX in solution reveals that its backbone configuration is identical to that of ChTX, as is the position of those residues critical for the interaction of ChTX with the maxi-K channel (Johnson and Sugg, 1992). A series of three single looped analogs of IbTX, in which four of the six cysteine residues were replaced by alanine, has been synthesized (Flinn *et al.*, 1995). None of the analogs were biologically active, indicating that no individual loop is the mediator of channel-blocking activity. IbTX inhibits maxi-K channels by a reversible bimolecular reaction identical to ChTX, although the silent periods caused by IbTX are of much longer duration than those produced by ChTX (Candia *et al.*, 1992; Giangiacomo *et al.*, 1992). This is due to a slower off-rate of IbTX, suggesting that IbTX must overcome a much higher energy barrier

ChTX	Z	F	T	N	V	S	**C**	T	T	S	K	E	**C**	W	S	V	**C**	Q	R	L	H	N	T	S	R	G	K	**C**	M	N	K	K	**C**	R	**C**	Y	S
IbTX	Z	F	T	D	V	D	**C**	S	V	S	K	E	**C**	W	S	V	**C**	K	D	L	F	G	V	D	R	G	K	**C**	M	G	K	K	**C**	R	**C**	Y	Q
Lq$_2$	Z	F	T	Q	E	S	**C**	T	A	S	N	Q	**C**	W	S	I	**C**	K	R	L	H	N	T	N	R	G	K	**C**	M	N	K	K	**C**	R	**C**	Y	S
LbTX	V	F	I	D	V	S	**C**	S	V	S	K	E	**C**	W	A	P	**C**	K	A	A	V	G	T	D	R	G	K	**C**	M	G	K	K	**C**	K	**C**	Y	...
	1	2	3	4	5	6	7	8	9	10	11	12	13	14	15	16	17	18	19	20	21	22	23	24	25	26	27	28	29	30	31	32	33	34	35	36	37

to dissociate from the channel. Perhaps the most interesting feature of IbTX is its high selectivity for maxi-K channels, as it does not affect other ChTX-sensitive K^+ channels, such as $K_v1.3$, and other small conductance Ca^{2+}-activated K^+ channels (Giangiacomo *et al.*, 1993; Leonard *et al.*, 1992). IbTX is the most potent and selective peptidyl blocker of the maxi-K channels described to date and represents a useful probe with which to explore the physiological role of maxi-K channels in different tissues.

A biologically active radiolabeled derivative of IbTX has been prepared by substituting Cys at position 19 and reacting this residue with [^{3}H]*N*-ethylmaleimide (Knaus *et al.*, 1996). [^{3}H]NEM–IbTX has been useful in identifying maxi-K channel receptor sites in rat brain membranes, a tissue where use of ^{125}I-ChTX to study maxi-K channels was hampered by the presence of relatively high densities of ChTX-sensitive, voltage-gated K^+ channels.

A novel peptide termed limbatustoxin (LbTX; Fig. 4) has been purified and characterized from venom of the scorpion *Centruroides limbatus* (Novick *et al.*, 1991). LbTX has high sequence homology with both IbTX and ChTX. LbTX blocks maxi-K channels by a reversible bimolecular reaction in which the duration of the silent periods is similar to those produced by IbTX. Furthermore, LbTX does not block other ChTX-sensitive K^+ channels. The specificity of IbTX and LbTX for maxi-K channels appears, therefore, to be identical.

2. *Nonpeptidyl Maxi-K Channel Modulators*

In addition to peptidyl channel inhibitors, both small molecule channel agonists and antagonists have been identified employing the ^{125}I-ChTX-binding assay in smooth muscle as a screen for such channel modulators. Extracts of the African herb *Desmodium adscendens,* which is used in Ghanan folk medicine as a treatment for asthma, dysmenorrhea, and other conditions associated with smooth muscle dysfunction, were found to inhibit ^{125}I-ChTX binding to smooth muscle sarcolemmal membranes. Three active components of the plant were purified and their structures were shown to be known glycosylated triterpenes: dehydrosoyasaponin I (DHS-1; Fig. 5), soyasaponin I, and soyasaponin III (McManus *et al.*, 1993). The most potent of these compounds in the binding assay is DHS-1 (K_i of 120 n*M*). These agents modulate ^{125}I-ChTX binding through an allosteric mechanism and display a defined structure–activity relationship for inhibition of the toxin–channel interaction. In single channel recordings, DHS-1 (10 n*M*) increases the open probability of maxi-K channels in a reversible fashion, but only when added to the intracellular face of the channel. Because ChTX binds in the external vestibule of the channel, and the glycosylated triterpenes are only effective when added at the intracellular channel surface, this is a further indication of allosteric coupling between toxin and drug receptors. This phenomena can also be observed in electrophysiological experiments

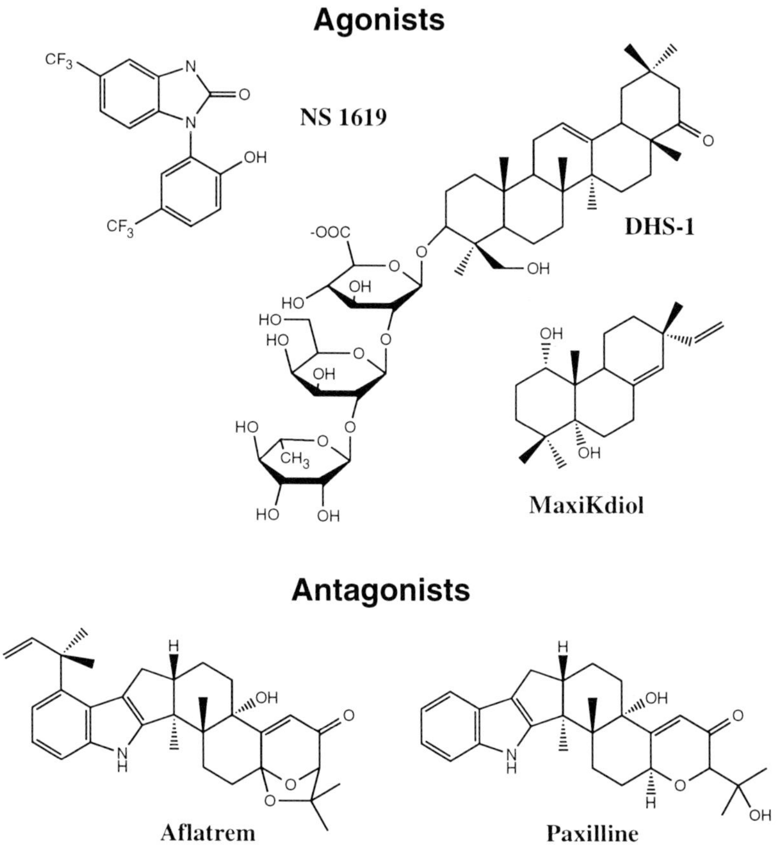

FIGURE 5 Nonpeptidyl modulators of maxi-K channels.

where DHS-1 was shown to enhance dissociation of ChTX bound to the channel. Because DHS-1 does not affect other types of ion channels, it represents the most potent and selective K^+ channel opener discovered to date.

A compound termed maxiKdiol (Fig. 5) was purified from the fermentation broth of a coelomycete based on its ability to inhibit ^{125}I-ChTX binding to smooth muscle (Singh *et al.*, 1994). MaxiKdiol is a novel 1,5-dihydroxyisoprimane diterpenoid that reversibly increases the activity of smooth muscle maxi-K channels, but with low potency (1–10 μM). Although maxiKdiol inhibits binding of ^{125}I-ChTX to aortic smooth muscle sarcolemmal membranes, it has no significant effect on ^{125}I-ChTX binding to voltage-dependent K^+ channels in rat brain synaptic plasma membranes, indicating specificity in the interaction of this compound with maxi-K channels.

The first series of potent nonpeptidyl maxi-K channel blockers was also discovered using the ^{125}I-ChTX binding assay with smooth muscle membranes (Fig. 5). These agents were identified as a series of indole diterpene members of the tremorgenic mycotoxin family (Knaus *et al.*, 1994d). Various indole diterpenes such as paspalitrem A and C, aflatrem, penitrem A, and paspalinine inhibit toxin binding, whereas three structurally related compounds, paxilline, verruculogen, and paspalicine, stimulate ^{125}I-ChTX binding in a concentration-dependent fashion. All of these compounds function as allosteric modulators of toxin binding as indicated by their effects on equilibrium and kinetic parameters of the binding reaction. In electrophysiological experiments, all of these agents are potent maxi-K channel blockers ($K_i < 10$ nM), and they are also very selective because they do not affect other types of voltage-gated ion channels at these low concentrations. Interestingly, paspalicine, a des-hydroxy analog of paspalinine which lacks tremorgenic activity, is also a potent maxi-K channel blocker, suggesting that tremorgenic activity can be dissociated from inhibition of the channel. The indole diterpenes therefore represent the most potent and selective nonpeptidyl inhibitors of the maxi-K channel identified to date.

Other small molecule maxi-K channel modulators have also been identified. A series of novel benzimidazolones typified by NS004 and NS1619 (Fig. 5) have been shown to reversibly enhance maxi-K channel activity at micromolar concentrations (Olesen, 1994; Olesen *et al.*, 1994). However, these compounds display Ca^{2+}-entry blocker activity and they also inhibit other types of voltage-gated K^+ channels. A substituted diphenylurea, NS 1608, has also been shown to enhance the activity of *hSlo* channels expressed in HEK 293 cells by shifting the voltage dependency of activation to more hyperpolarized potentials (Olesen *et al.*, 1996). Addition of NS 1608 causes a hyperpolarization of HEK 293 cells expressing *hSlo* from their resting potential to up to 50 mV. Although members of the cromakalim series are not agonists of maxi-K channels, one analog, BRL 55834, has been reported to promote opening of both ATP-dependent and maxi-K channels in bovine airway smooth muscle (Ward *et al.*, 1992). Consistent with its ability to activate maxi-K channels, BRL 55834 has been shown in *in vivo* experiments to display some selectivity as a bronchodilator when compared to its ability to reduce blood pressure (Bowring *et al.*, 1993).

Through the use of purified bovine smooth muscle sarcolemmal membranes derived from either aortic or tracheal tissue, it has been shown that ^{125}I-ChTX binds to a single class of receptor sites that display the pharmacological properties expected for an interaction with maxi-K channels (Vazquez *et al.*, 1990). Thus, toxin binding is a freely reversible reaction, sensitive to the ionic strength of the incubation medium, and blocked by a number of metal ions that are known to bind with high affinity to sites located along the ion conduction pathway of the channel. In addition, IbTX and TEA block toxin binding with K_i values similar to those found for their inhibition of maxi-K channels in functional studies.

^{125}I-ChTX has also been used as a marker for the purification of the maxi-K channel from bovine tracheal and aortic smooth muscle. The purified receptor (Fig. 1) consists of two subunits, α and β, and possesses maxi-K channel activity upon reconstitution into planar lipid bilayers (Garcia-Calvo *et al.*, 1994; Giangiacomo *et al.*, 1995). Partial amino acid sequence obtained from proteolytic fragments of the tracheal α subunit indicate that it is a member of the *Slo* family of K^+ channels (Knaus *et al.*, 1994a). A unique 28 amino acid sequence obtained from the β subunit led to the isolation of a full-length cDNA from bovine tracheal and aortic smooth muscle (Knaus *et al.*, 1994b). The deduced amino acid sequence predicts a novel protein of approximately 22,000 that contains two α-helical transmembrane domains connected by a large extracellular loop, with two putative sites for N-linked glycosylation. Both the amino- and carboxy-terminals are postulated to be cytoplasmic. This subunit is the protein to which ^{125}I-ChTX becomes covalently attached in the presence of a bifunctional cross-linking reagent, despite the fact that ChTX binds to its receptor site in the external vestibule of the α subunit. Proteolytic digestion of the ^{125}I-ChTX–cross-linked β subunit has identified the residue to which ChTX is covalently attached (Lys_{69}) and has confirmed the postulated topology of this protein (Knaus *et al.*, 1994c). Evidence for functional association of the α and β subunits has been obtained from immunoprecipitation studies and from coexpression experiments. Site-directed antibodies against sequences of either the α or the β subunit are able to immunoprecipitate, under nondenaturing conditions, the α–β complex (Knaus *et al.*, 1994a,b). Coexpression of the β subunit with the α pore-forming subunit of the maxi-K channel shifts the voltage dependence of channel activation by 80 to 100 mV in the hyperpolarized direction (McManus *et al.*, 1995; Wallner *et al.*, 1995). This shift is equivalent to that produced by approximately a 10-fold increase in Ca^{2+} concentration. Importantly, the effects of the maxi-K channel activator DHS-1 require the presence of the β subunit, as maxi-K channel activation is not observed when the α subunit is expressed alone (McManus *et al.*, 1995). These data indicate that the β subunit functionally associates with the pore-forming subunit and has pronounced effects on the biophysical and pharmacological properties of the maxi-K channel complex. Four α–β complexes are thought to comprise a functional channel.

A site-directed antibody against *Slo* that is able to immunoprecipitate [^{3}H]NEM–IbTX receptor sites from rat brain membranes has been used to study the distribution of maxi-K channels in rat brain (Knaus *et al.*, 1996). *Slo* immunoreactivity appears highly concentrated in terminal areas of prominent fiber tracts such as the substantia nigra pars reticulata, globus pallidus, olfactory system, interpeduncular nucleus, hippocampal formation, and pyramidal tract, as well as in cerebellar Purkinje cells. The high immunoreactivity within terminal areas and the fact that *Slo* mRNA is expressed in the same neurons suggest a functional role for the maxi-K channel at the presynaptic nerve ending.

B. Small-Conductance Ca^{2+}-Activated K^+ Channels

Small-conductance Ca^{2+}-activated K^+ (SK) channels are in general very sensitive to internal Ca^{2+} and can be divided into two different categories: voltage-dependent SK channels, such as those present in *Aplysia* and *Helix* neurons, and voltage-independent channels that are found in muscle, olfactory neurons, erythrocytes, liver, and human T cells (Latorre *et al.*, 1989). Some of these SK channels, such as the 35 pS SK channel present in *Aplysia* neurons, the red cell Gardos channel, and the SK channels of human T cells, are sensitive to inhibition by ChTX. Out of these channels, the best characterized pharmacologically is the Gardos channel. Ca^{2+}-activated K^+ channel fluxes in human red cells when carried out under low ionic strength conditions are inhibited with high affinity by ChTX, ShK, MgTX, and KTX, but they are insensitive to IbTX, α-DTX, apamin, and scyllatoxin (Brugnara *et al.*, 1995). Interestingly, under physiological ionic strength conditions, only ChTX and ShK display high-affinity inhibition, with KTX and MgTX producing no significant effects. In addition to peptidyl blockers, various small molecule inhibitors of the red cell Gardos channel have been described: quinine (IC_{50} = 100 μM), carbocyanine (IC_{50} = 20–50 nM), nifedipine (IC_{50} = 4 μM), nitrendipine (IC_{50} = 130 nM), and clotrimazole (IC_{50} = 50 nM).

The SK channel in rat skeletal muscle displays a conductance of 10–14 pS and is linked to after-hyperpolarization responses in myotubes (Blatz and Magleby, 1986). This channel is blocked by low concentrations of three peptidyl toxins (Fig. 6): apamin isolated from bee venom, scyllatoxin isolated from scorpion venom, and PO5, another scorpion venom peptide. Apamin is an 18 amino acid peptide containing two disulfide bridges. Structure–activity studies indicate that Arg_{13} and Arg_{14} are critical residues for toxin action (Romey *et al.*, 1984). The solid-phase synthesis of apamin and related analogs has been achieved (Granier *et al.*, 1978), and the structure of apamin has been determined using NMR techniques (Pease and Wemmer, 1988). These studies indicate that the toxin is a highly ordered structure with an α-helical core consisting of residues 9–17 and a region consisting of β-type turns. Radiolabeled apamin can be prepared by incorporation of iodine into the imidazole ring of His_{18}, the C-terminal residue of the toxin. ^{125}I-apamin has been employed to identify high-affinity receptors for this toxin in several tissues, including rat brain synaptosomes (Hugues *et al.*, 1982a), cultured rat embryonic neurons (Seagar *et al.*, 1984), neuroblastoma cells (Hugues *et al.*, 1982c), membranes prepared from cultured rat muscle cells (Hugues *et al.*, 1982d), smooth muscle tissue (Hugues *et al.*, 1982b), and hepatocytes

	1	2	3	4	5	6	7	8	9	10	11	12	13	14	15	16	17	18	19	20	21	22	23	24	25	26	27	28	29	30	31	
Apamin	**C**	N	**C**	K	A	P	E	T	A	L	**C**	A	R	R	**C**	Q	Q	H	NH_2													
LeTX	A	F	**C**	N	L	R	M	**C**	Q	L	S	**C**	R	S	L	G	L	L	G	K	**C**	I	G	D	K	C	E	C	V	K	H	NH_2
PO5	T	V	**C**	N	L	R	R	**C**	Q	L	S	**C**	R	S	L	G	L	L	G	K	**C**	I	G	V	K	C	E	C	V	K	H	

(Cook *et al.*, 1983). Interaction of ^{125}I-apamin with its receptor is of high affinity, with K_d's in the range of 10–400 p*M*. However, the maximum density of binding sites is very low, with B_{max} values between 1 and 30 fmol/mg protein. Fifty-fold higher levels of apamin receptors have been found in undifferentiated pheochromocytoma cells (Schmid-Antomarchi *et al.*, 1986). Interestingly, the apamin receptor in rat muscle is only expressed in noninnervated cells. In normal adult rat muscle, binding of apamin is not detectable and the action potential in this preparation is insensitive to apamin (Schmid-Antomarchi *et al.*, 1985). After denervation, binding sites for apamin and an apamin-sensitive after-hyperpolarization current both appear in a synchronized fashion.

Attempts to identify the molecular components of the apamin receptor have yielded conflicting data. Photoreactive apamin derivatives were prepared with aryl azide groups located at two different positions within the molecule (Leveque *et al.*, 1990; Seagar *et al.*, 1986). The Lys_4 derivative labeled polypeptides of 33 and 22 kDa in both cultured neurons and synaptic plasma membranes, whereas the Cys_1 derivative labeled only an 86-kDa polypeptide, or 86- and 59-kDa components, in these two preparations, respectively. In a different study, photoreactive derivatives of apamin, together with the cross-linking reagent disuccinimidyl suberate, were used to identify the components of the apamin receptor in rat brain membranes and pheochromocytoma cell membranes (Auguste *et al.*, 1989). A variety of polypeptides are labeled using these techniques. One major component has a molecular mass of about 30 kDa, but other polypeptides of 45, 58, and 86 kDa were also identified. cDNA's encoding apamin-sensitive and -insensitive SK channels have recently been identified (Köhler *et al.*, 1996).

Two other toxins that block SK channels, but which are structurally unrelated to apamin, have been purified and characterized from scorpion venoms. A 31 amino acid peptide, leiurotoxin I (Fig. 6), was purified from *L. quinquestriatus* var. *hebraeus* venom, based on its ability to inhibit apamin binding (Chicchi *et al.*, 1988). Leiurotoxin I completely inhibits ^{125}I-apamin binding to rat brain synaptic plasma membranes by an apparently noncompetitive mechanism. Like apamin, leiurotoxin I blocks epinephrine-induced relaxation of guinea pig taenia coli, but has no effect on the rate, or force of contraction, of guinea pig atria or rabbit portal vein. In addition, leiurotoxin I blocks the apamin-sensitive, Ca^{2+}-dependent, after-hyperpolarization K^+ current in bullfrog ganglion B cells (Goh *et al.*, 1992). The independent purification of leiurotoxin I was later reported by another laboratory, and they assigned the name scyllatoxin (ScyTX) to this peptide (Auguste *et al.*, 1990). ScyTX and two analogs have been synthesized by solid-phase methodologies. One of these analogs, in which a Tyr residue is introduced at position 2 as a replacement for Phe, displays identical activity to the native toxin and has been used to obtain a radiolabeled derivative for binding studies. As found for the interaction of apamin, ^{125}I-ScyTX binding is activated by low K^+ levels and is blocked by Ca^{2+}, Na^+, and guanidinium ions. In addition, in cross-linking experiments with ScyTX, two polypeptides of 27 and 57 kDa were identified (Auguste *et al.*, 1990). Chemical modifications of ScyTX have shown that Arg_6 and Arg_{13} are essential both for binding and for the functional effects of the toxin (Auguste *et al.*, 1992).

The three-dimensional structure of ScyTX has been determined using NMR techniques (Martins *et al.*, 1995). The assignment of the disulfide bridges was achieved from a statistical analysis of characteristic intercystinyl distances in a set of preliminary structures. There is an α-helix spanning residues Leu_5 to Ser_{14} and an antiparallel β-sheet from Leu_{18} to Val_{29}, with a β turn centered around residues Gly_{23} and Asp_{24}. The global fold of these structural elements in ScyTX is dictated by the disulfide bridges Cys_8–Cys_{26} and Cys_{12}–Cys_{28}, which connect one face of the α-helix with the C-terminal strand of the β-sheet. The disulfide bridge between Cys_3 and Cys_{21} further constrains the N-terminal residues to the first β-sheet strand. The general folding pattern adopted by the backbone of ScyTX is the same as found in ChTX and related toxins. The structures only differ in the number of additional strands in the sheet and in the location and extent of loops and turns.

A novel leiurotoxin I-like toxin, called PO5 (Fig. 6), has been characterized from venom of the scorpion *Androctonus mauretanicus mauretanicus* (Sabatier *et al.*, 1993). This toxin possesses binding and functional properties similar to those of apamin and leiurotoxin I. Its three-dimensional structure is practically identical to that of leiurotoxin I as well. Structure–activity studies with PO_5 indicate that the residues Arg_6, Arg_7, and the carboxyl C-terminal His_{31} are involved in interaction with its receptor (Sabatier *et al.*, 1994). These three residues are located on the same side of the molecule.

IV. ATP-Dependent K^+ Channels

ATP-sensitive K^+ (K_{ATP}) channels (Fig. 1) are found in a variety of tissues such as cardiac muscle, pancreatic β cells, skeletal muscle, and vascular/nonvascular smooth muscle. In pancreatic β cells, K_{ATP} channels regulate glucose-induced insulin secretion by controlling membrane potential and are the target for sulfonylureas (e.g., glibenclamide; Fig. 7), oral hypoglycemic agents used in the treatment of noninsulin-dependent diabetes mellitus, as well as for the potassium channel opener, diazoxide. The sulfonylurea receptor (SUR) has been cloned and shown to be a member of the ATP-binding cassette superfamily with multiple transmembrane-spanning domains and two potential nucleotide-binding folds (Aguilar-Bryan *et al.*, 1995). The SUR, by itself, does not express functional channels. However, coexpression of SUR with a new member of the inward rectifying potassium channel family, $K_{ir}6.2$, reconstitutes the pharmacological properties expected for a K_{ATP} channel (Inagaki *et al.*, 1995; Sakura *et al.*, 1995). Although neither

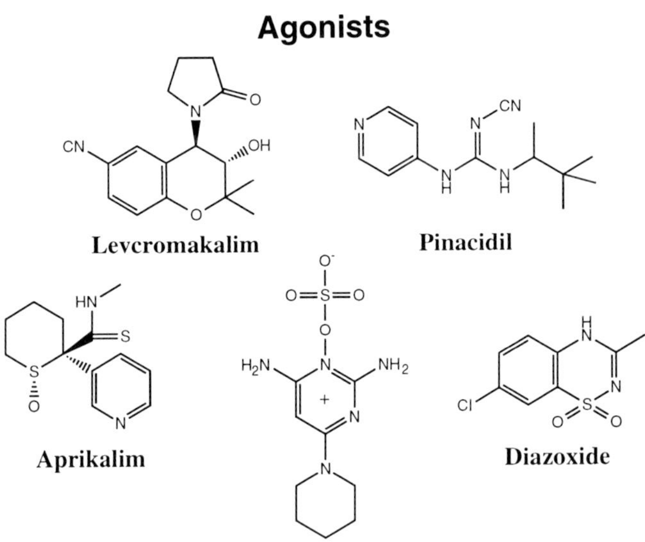

FIGURE 7 Modulators of ATP-dependent K^+ channels.

protein alone can function as a channel, coexpression of both subunits leads to the appearance of an inwardly rectifying potassium channel of 76 pS that is sensitive to ATP, inhibited by sulfonylureas, and activated by diazoxide. These results suggest that native K_{ATP} channels are a complex composed of at least two subunits; the stoichiometry of the members in this complex is currently unknown.

SUR appears to couple promiscuously with different inward rectifier K^+ channels, such as the endogenous K_{ir} channel of HEK 293 cells, $K_{ir}1.1a$, and $K_{ir}6.1$ (Ämmälä *et al.*, 1996). In all cases, sensitivity to inhibition by tolbutamide is determined primarily by SUR and does not appear to be influenced by the K_{ir} channel with which it interacts. In the case of the endogenous K_{ir} channel of HEK 293 cells, SUR does not confer ATP sensitivity.

Openers of K_{ATP} channels (Fig. 7) constitute the largest number and most structurally diverse class of small molecule K^+ channel modulators described to date. Pharmacologically they can be distinguished because their effects are antagonized by the sulfonylurea glibenclamide, but are unaffected by ChTX (Edwards and Weston, 1995). Because of differences in their chemical structures, they can be subdivided into groups: benzopyrans are typified by cromakalim and levcromakalim, the more active enatiomer of cromakalim (Edwards and Weston, 1990); cyanoguanidines are represented by pinacidil and closely related derivatives such as P1060 and P1075; aprikalim is the prototype of the thioformamides; within the pyrimidines, the prototype member of this group is minoxidil sulfate; and the most investigated member of the benzothiadiazines is diazoxide. The hyperglycemic actions of diazoxide are due to its ability to open K_{ATP} channels in pancreatic β cells (Zünkler *et al.*, 1988), and its vasodilator effects are also associated with the opening of K_{ATP} channels in smooth muscle (Quast and Cook, 1989). All of these K_{ATP} openers increase the membrane conductance to potassium, causing membrane hyperpolarization, which can result in the reduction of Ca^{2+} influx through voltage-gated Ca^{2+} channels. In vascular smooth muscle cells, these agents promote vasodilation. In cardiac muscle, K_{ATP} openers cause a concentration-dependent shortening of the action potential, and this property could manifest itself by effects on cardiac rhythmicity.

Benzoic acid derivatives of glibenclamide, such as meglitinide and AZ-DF265, both of which lack the sulfonylurea moiety, are also capable of inhibiting pancreatic β-cell $K_{ATP,}$ thereby stimulating insulin secretion (Edwards and Weston, 1993). Two inhibitors of K_{ATP} that exhibit tissue selectivity are 5-hydroxydecanoate and ZM 181,037. The former agent appears to inhibit only cardiac K_{ATP}, and in cardiac muscle it has a preference for ischemic tissue (McCullough *et al.*, 1991). In contrast, ZM 181,037 antagonizes the stimulatory effects of cromakalim on ^{86}Rb fluxes in rat detrusor muscle and portal vein, without increasing plasma insulin levels *in vivo* (Kau *et al.*, 1994).

V. Conclusions

Although work on the structure and function of K^+ channels has progressed rapidly, the molecular pharmacology of these proteins is relatively undeveloped. This is in marked contrast to the well-known pharmacology of other classes of ion channels (e.g., Na^{2+} Ca^{2+} and ligand-gated channels). The situation with K^+ channels is improving, however. With the discovery of specific, high-affinity peptidyl probes for various K^+ channels, it has been possible to characterize channel function in target tissues of interest, to validate new ion channel targets, and to advance the pharmacology of specific ion channels by designing high capacity screens to detect small molecule channel modulators. Because ion channels are multidrug receptors, it is possible to screen for allosterically acting agents by monitoring peptide binding in the pore region of a given channel. This approach has succeeded in identifying both agonists and antagonists of the maxi-K channel, as well as inhibitors of $K_v1.3$. Furthermore, with the cloning of various K^+ channels and their β subunits, as well as the construction of cell lines stably expressing these proteins, a high capacity functional screen can also be developed as a means of searching for novel channel agonists and antagonists. These screening approaches, together with the assay of large libraries of synthetic or natural product molecules, provide a strategy for the very rapid development of new pharmacologies for specific K^+ channels. The expected progress in this area will ultimately lead to the identification and development of novel therapeutic agents targeting K^+ channels.

References

Adelman, J. P., Shen, K.-Z., Kavanaugh, M. P., Warren, R. A., Wu, Y.-N., Lagrutta, A., Bond, C. T., and North, R. A. (1992) Calcium-activated potassium channels expressed from cloned complementary DNAs. *Neuron* **9**, 209–216.

Aggarwal, S. K., and MacKinnon, R. (1994). Determination of *Shaker* K^+ channel number and gating charge in individual *Xenopus* oocytes. *Biophys. J.* **66**, A136.

Aguilar-Bryan, L., Nichols, C. G., Wechsler, S. W., Clement, J. P., Boyd, A. E., Gonzalez, G., Herrera-Sosa, H., Nguy, K., Bryan, J., and Nelson, D. A. (1995). Cloning of the β cell high-affinity sulfonylurea receptor: A regulator of insulin secretion. *Science* **268**, 423–425.

Aiyar, J., Grissmer, S., and Chandy, K. G. (1993). The L401V mutation in Kv3.1 does not alter single channel conductance or K^+/Rb^+ selectivity. *Biophys. J.* **64**, 197a.

Aiyar, J., Withka, J. M., Rizzi, J. P., Singleton, D. H., Andrews, G. C., Lin, W., Boyd, J., Hanson, D. C., Simon, M., Dethlefs, B., Lee, C.-L., Hall, J. E., Gutman, G. A., and Chandy, K. G. (1995). Topology of the pore-region of a K^+ channel revealed by the NMR-derived structures of scorpion toxins. *Neuron* **15**, 1169–1181.

Ämmälä, C., Moorhouse, A., Gribble, F., Ashfield, R., Proks, P., Smith, P. A., Sakura, H., Coles, B., Ashcroft, S. J. H., and Ashcroft, F. M. (1996). Promiscuous coupling between the sulphonylurea receptor and inwardly rectifying potassium channels. *Nature* (*London*) **379**, 545–548.

Aneiros, A., García, I., Martínez, J. R., Harvey, A. L., Anderson, A. J., Marshall, D. L., Engström, A., Hellman, U., and Karlsson, E. (1993). A potassium channel toxin from the secretion of the sea anemone *Bunodosoma granulifera.* Isolation, amino acid sequence and biological activity. *Biochim. Biophys. Acta* **1157**, 86–92.

Auguste, P., Hughes, M., and Lazdunski, M. (1989). Polypeptide constitution of receptors for apamin, a neurotoxin which blocks a class of Ca^{2+}-activated K^+ channels. *FEBS Lett.* **248**, 150–154.

Auguste, P., Hugues, M., Gravé, B., Gesquiere, J.-C., Maes, P., Tartar, A., Romey, G., Schweitz, H., and Lazdunski, M. (1990). Leiurotoxin I (Scyllatoxin), a peptide ligand for Ca^{2+}-activated K^+ channels. *J. Biol. Chem.* **265**, 4753–4759.

Auguste, P., Hugues, M., Mourre, C., Moinier, D., Tartar, A., and Lazdunski, M. (1992). Scyllatoxin, a blocker of Ca^{2+}-activated K^+ channels: Structure-function relationships and brain localization of the binding sites. *Biochemistry* **31**, 648–654.

Benishin, C. G., Sorensen, R. G., Brown, W. E., Krueger, B. K., and Blaustein, M. P. (1988). Four polypeptide components of green mamba venom selectively block certain potassium channels in rat brain synaptosomes. *Mol. Pharmacol.* **34**, 152–159.

Berndt, K. D., Güntert, P., and Wüthrich, K. (1993). Nuclear magnetic resonance solution structure of dendrotoxin K from venom of *Dendroaspis polylepis polylepis*. *J. Mol. Biol.* **234,** 735–750.

Bidard, J.-N., Mourre, C., and Lazdunski, M. (1987). Two potent central convulsant peptides, a bee venom toxin, the MCD peptide, and a snake venom toxin, dendrotoxin I, known to block K^+ channels, have interacting receptors sites. *Biochem. Biophys. Res. Commun.* **143,** 383–389.

Blatz, A. L., and Magleby, K. L. (1986). Single apamin blocked Ca-activated K^+ channels of small conductance in cultured rat skeletal muscle. *Nature* (*London*) **323,** 718–720.

Bontems, F., Roumestand, C., Boyot, P., Gilquin, B., Doljansky, Y., Menez, A., and Toma, F. (1991a). Three-dimensional structure of natural charybdotoxin in aquous solution by ^{1}H-NMR. Charybdotoxin possesses a structural motif found in other scorpion toxins. *Eur. J. Biochem.* **196,** 19–28.

Bontems, F., Roumestand, C., Gilquin, B., Menez, A., and Toma, F. (1991b). Refined structure of charybdotoxin: Common motifs in scorpion toxins and insect defensins. *Science* **254,** 1521–1523.

Bowring, N. E., Arch, J. R. S., Buckle, D. R., and Taylor, J. F. (1993). Comparison of the airways relaxant and hypotensive potencies of the potassium channel activators BRL 55834 and levcromakalim (BRL 38227) *in vivo* in guinea-pigs and rats. *Br. J. Pharmacol.* **109,** 1133–1139.

Breeze, A. L., and Dolly, J. O. (1989). Interactions between discrete neuronal membrane binding sites for the putative K^+-channel ligands β-bungarotoxin, dendrotoxin and mast-cell-degranulating peptide. *Eur. J. Biochem.* **178,** 771–778.

Brugnara, C., Armsby, C. C., Franceschi, L. D., Crest, M., Euclaire, M.-F. M., and Alper, S. L. (1995). Ca^{2+}-activated K^+ channels of human and rabbit erythrocytes display distinctive patterns of inhibition by venom peptide toxins. *J. Membr. Biol.* **147,** 71–82.

Butler, A., Tsunoda, S., McCobb, D. P., Wei, A., and Salkoff, L. (1993). mSlo, a complex mouse gene encoding "maxi" calcium-activated potassium channels. *Science* **261,** 221–224.

Byrnes, M. E., Mahnir, V. M., Kem, W. R., and Pennington, M. W. (1995). Synthesis and characterization of dendrotoxin: A potent potassium channel inhibitor. *Protein Pept. Lett.* **1,** 239–245.

Candia, S., Garcia, M. L., and Latorre, R. (1992). Mode of action of iberiotoxin, a potent blocker of the large conductance Ca^{2+}-activated K^+ channel. *Biophys. J.* **63,** 583–590.

Carbone, E., Wanke, E., Prestipino, G., Possani, L. D., and Maelicke, A. (1982). Selective blockage of voltage-dependent K^+ channels by a novel scorpion toxin. *Nature* (*London*) **296,** 90–91.

Castañeda, O., Sotolongo, V., Amor, A. M., Stöcklin, R., Anderson, A. J., Harvey, A. L., Engström, A., Wernstedt, C., and Karlsson, E. (1995). Characterization of a potassium channel toxin from the Caribbean sea anemone *Stichodactyla helianthus*. *Toxicon* **33,** 603–613.

Castellino, R., Morales, M. J., Strauss, H. C., and Rasmusson, R. L. (1995). Time- and voltage-dependent modulation of a Kv1.4 channel by a β-subunit (Kvβ3) cloned from ferret ventricle. *Am. J. Physiol.* **269,** H385–H391.

Chandy, K. G., and Gutman, G. A. (1995). Voltage-gated potassium channel genes. *In* "Ligand- and Voltage-gated Ion Channels" (R. A. North, ed.), 1–71. CRC Press, Boca Raton, FL.

Chicchi, G. G., Gimenez-Gallego, G., Ber, E., Garcia, M. L., Winquist, R., and Cascieri, M. A. (1988). Purification and characterization of a unique, potent inhibitor of apamin binding from *Leiurus quinquestriatus habraeus* venom. *J. Biol. Chem.* **263,** 10192–10197.

Choi, K. L., Mossman, C., Aube, J., and Yellen, G. (1993). The internal quaternary ammonium receptor site of *Shaker* potassium channels. *Neuron* **10,** 533–541.

Colatsky, T. J., and Argentieri, T. M. (1994). Potassium channel blockers as antiarrhythmic drugs. *Drug Dev. Res.* **33,** 235–249.

Cook, N. S., Haylett, D. N., and Strong, P. (1983). High affinity binding of ^{125}I-monoiodo apamin to isolated guinea-pig hepatocytes. *Febs Lett.* **152,** 265–269.

Crest, M., Jacquet, G., Gola, M., Zerrouk, H., Benslimane, A., Rochat, H., Mansuelle, P., and Martin-Eauclaire, M.-F. (1992). Kaliotoxin, a novel peptidyl inhibitor of neuronal BK-type Ca^{2+}-activated K^+ channels characterized from *Androctonus mauretanicus mauretanicus* venom. *J. Biol. Chem.* **267,** 1640–1647.

Curran, M. E., Splawski, I., Timothy, K. W., Vincent, G. M., Green, E. D., and Keating, M. T. (1995). A molecular basis for cardiac arrhythmia: HERG mutations cause long QT syndrome. *Cell (Cambridge, Mass.)* **80,** 795–803.

Danse, J. M., Rowan, E. G., Gasparini, S., Ducancel, F., Vatanpour, H., Young, L. C., Poorheidari, G., Lajeunesse, E., Drevet, P., Ménez, R., Pinkasfeld, S., Boulain, J.-C., Harvey, A. L., and Ménez, A. (1994). On the site by which α-dendrotoxin binds to voltage-dependent potassium channels: Site-directed mutagenesis reveals that the lysine triplet 28–30 is not essential for binding. *FEBS Lett.* **356,** 153–158.

Dauplais, M., Gilquin, B., Possani, L. D., Gurrola-Briones, G., Roumestand, C., and Menez, A. (1995). Determination of the three-dimensional solution structure of noxiustoxin: Analysis of structural differences with related short-chain scorpion toxins. *Biochemistry* **34,** 16563–16573.

DeFarias, F. P., Stevens, S. P., and Leonard, R. J. (1995). Stable expression of human Kv1.3 potassium channels resets the resting membrane potential of cultured mammalian cells. *Recept. Channels* **3,** 273–281.

Deutsch, C., Price, M., Lee, S., King, V. F., and Garcia, M. L. (1991). Characterization of high affinity binding sites for charybdotoxin in human T lymphocytes: Evidence for association with the voltage-gated K^+ channel. *J. Biol. Chem.* **266,** 3668–3674.

Docherty, R. J., Dolly, J. O., Halliwell, J. V., and Othman, I. (1983). Excitatory effects of dendrotoxin on the hippocampus in vitro. *J. Physiol. (London)* **336,** 58–59.

Dolly, J. O., Halliwell, J. V., Black, J. D., Williams, R. S., Pelchen-Matthews, A., Breeze, A., Mehraban, F., Othman, I. B., and Black, A. R. (1984). Botulinum neurotoxin and dendrotoxin as probes for studies of neurotransmitter release. *J. Physiol. (Paris)* **79,** 280–303.

Drakopoulou, E., Cotton, J., Virelizier, H., Bernardi, E., Schoofs, A. R., Partiseti, M., Choquet, D., Gurrola, G., Possani, L. D., and Vita, C. (1995). Chemical synthesis, structural and functional characterization of noxiustoxin, a powerful blocker of lymphocyte voltage-dependent K^+ channels. *Biochem. Biophys. Res. Commun.* **213,** 901–907.

Dworetzky, S. I., Trojnacki, J. T., and Gribkoff, V. K. (1994). Cloning and expression of a human large-conductance calcium-activated potassium channel. *Mol. Brain Res.* **27,** 189–193.

Edwards, G., and Weston, A. H. (1990). Structure-activity relationship of K^+ channel openers. *Trends Pharmacol. Sci.* **11,** 417–422.

Edwards, G., and Weston, A. H. (1993). The pharmacology of ATP-sensitive potassium channels. *Annu. Rev. Pharmacol. Toxicol.* **33,** 597–637.

Edwards, G., and Weston, A. H. (1995). Pharmacology of the potassium channel openers. *Cardiovasc. Drugs Thera.* **9,** 185–193.

England, S. K., Uebele, V. N., Kodali, J., Bennett, P. B., and Tamkun, M. M. (1995a). A novel K^+ channel β-subunit (hKvβ1.3) is produced via alternative mRNA splicing. *J. Biol. Chem.* **270,** 28531–28534.

England, S. K., Uebele, V. N., Shear, H., Kodali, J., Bennett, P. B., and Tamkun, M. M. (1995b). Characterization of a voltage-gated K^+ channel β subunit expressed in human heart. *Proc. Natl. Acad. Sci. U.S.A.* **92,** 6309–6313.

Felix, J. P., Bugianesi, R. M., Abramsom, A. A., and Slaughter, R. S. (1995). Binding of mono- and di-iodinated margatoxin to human peripheral T lymphocytes and to Jurkat plasma membranes. *Biophys. J.* **68,** 267a.

Fernandez, I., Romi, R., Szendeffy, S., Martin-Eauclaire, M. F., Rochat, H., Rietschoten, J. B., Pons, M., and Giralt, E. (1994). Kaliotoxin (1–37) shows structural differences with related potassium channel blockers. *Biochemistry* **33,** 14256–14263.

Flinn, J. P., Murphy, R., Johns, R. B., Kunze, W. A. A., and Angus, J. A. (1995). Synthesis and biological characterisation of a series of iberiotoxin analogues. *Int. J. Pep. Protein Res.* **45,** 320–325.

Foray, M.-F., Lancelin, J.-M., Hollecker, M., and Marion, D. (1993). Sequence-specific ^{1}H-NMR assignment and secondary structure of black mamba dendrotoxin I, a highly selective blocker of voltage-gated potassium channels. *Eur. J. Biochem.* **211,** 813–820.

Galvez, A., Gimenez-Gallego, G., Reuben, J. P., Roy-Contancin, L., Feigenbaum, P., Kaczorowski, G. J., and Garcia, M. L. (1990). Purification and characterization of a unique, potent, peptidyl probe for the high conductance calcium-activated potassium channel from venom of the scorpion Buthus tamulus. *J. Biol. Chem.* **265,** 11083–11090.

Garcia, M. L., Garcia-Calvo, M., Hidalgo, P., Lee, A., and MacKinnon, R. (1994). Purification and characterization of three inhibitors of voltage-dependent K^+ channels from *Leiurus quinquestriatus* var. *hebraeus* venom. *Biochemistry* **33,** 6834–6839.

Garcia-Calvo, M., Leonard, R. J., Novick, J., Stevens, S. P., Schmalhofer, W., Kaczorowski, G. J., and Garcia, M. L. (1993). Purification, characterization, and biosynthesis of margatoxin, a component of *Centruroides margaritatus* venom that selectively inhibits voltage-dependent potassium channels. *J. Biol. Chem.* **268,** 18866–18874.

Garcia-Calvo, M., Knaus, H.-G., McManus, O. B., Giangiacomo, K. M., Kaczorowski, G. J., and Garcia, M. L. (1994). Purification and reconstitution of the high-conductance calcium-activated potassium channel from tracheal smooth muscle. *J. Biol. Chem.* **269,** 676–682.

Gaspar, R., Bene, L., Damjanovich, S., Munoz-Garay, C., Calderon-Aranda, E. S., and Possani, L. D. (1995). β-Scorpion toxin 2 from Centruroides noxius blocks voltage-gated K^+ channels in human lymphocytes. *Biochem. Biophys. Res. Commun.* **213,** 419–423.

Giangiacomo, K. M., Garcia, M. L., and McManus, O. B. (1992). Mechanism of iberiotoxin block of the large-conductance calcium-activated potassium channel from bovine aortic smooth muscle. *Biochemistry* **31,** 6719–6727.

Giangiacomo, K. M., Sugg, E. E., Garcia-Calvo, M., Leonard, R. J., McManus, O. B., Kaczorowski, G. J., and Garcia, M. L. (1993). Synthetic charybdotoxin-iberiotoxin chimeric peptides define toxin binding sites on calcium-activated and voltage-dependent potassium channels. *Biochemistry* **32,** 2363–2370.

Giangiacomo, K. M., Garcia-Calvo, M., Knaus, H.-G., Mullmann, T. J., Garcia, M. L., and McManus, O. (1995). Functional reconstitution of the large-conductance, calcium-activated potassium channel purified from bovine aortic smooth muscle. *Biochemistry* **34,** 15849–15862.

Gimenez-Gallego, G., Navia, M. A., Reuben, J. P., Katz, G. M., Kaczorowski, G. J., and Garcia, M. L. (1988). Purification, sequence, and model structure of charybdotoxin, a potent selective inhibitor of calcium-activated potassium channels. *Proc. Natl. Acad. Sci. U.S.A.* **85,** 3329–3333.

Goh, J. W., Kelley, M. E. M., Pennefather, P. S., Chicchi, G. G., Cascieri, M. A., Garcia, M. L., and Kaczorowski, G. J. (1992). Effect of charybdotoxin and leiurotoxin I on potassium currents in bullfrog sympathetic ganglion and hippocampal neurons. *Brain Res.* **591,** 165–170.

Goldstein, S. A. N., and Miller, C. (1993). Mechanism of charybdotoxin block of a voltage-gated K^+ channel. *Biophys. J.* **65,** 1613–1619.

Goldstein, S. A. N., Pheasant, D. J., and Miller, C. (1994). The charybdotoxin receptor of a *Shaker* K^+ channel: Peptide and channel residues mediating molecular recognition. *Neuron* **12,** 1377–1388.

Granier, C., Pedroso-Müller, E., and Rietschoten, J. V. (1978). Use of synthetic analogs for a study on the structure-activity relationship of apamin. *Eur. J. Biochem.* **82,** 293–299.

Grissmer, S., Nguyen, A. N., Aiyar, J., Hanson, D. C., Mather, R. J., Gutman, G. A., Karmilowicz, M. J., Auperin, D. D., and Chandy, K. G. (1994). Pharmacological characterization of five cloned voltage-gated K^+ channels, types $K_v1.1$, 1.2, 1.3, 1.5, and 3.1, stably expressed in mammalian cell lines. *Mol. Pharmacol.* **45,** 1227–1234.

Gross, A., Abramson, T., and MacKinnon, R. (1994). Transfer of the scorpion toxin receptor to an insensitive potassium channel. *Neuron* **13,** 961–966.

Halliwell, J. V., Othman, I. B., Pelchen-Matthews, A., and Dolly, J. O. (1986). Central action of dendrotoxin: Selective reduction of a transient K conductance in hippocampus and binding to localized acceptors. *Proc. Natl. Acad. Sci. U.S.A.* **83,** 493–497.

Harvey, A. L., and Anderson, A. (1985). Dendrotoxins: Snake toxins that block potassium channels and facilitate neurotransmitter release. *Pharmacol. Ther.* **31,** 33–55.

Harvey, A. L., and Karlsson, E. (1982). Protein inhibitor homologues from Mamba venoms: Facilitation of acetylcholine release and interactions with prejunctional blocking toxins. *Br. J. Pharmacol.* **77,** 153–161.

Hidalgo, P., and MacKinnon, R. (1995). Revealing the architecture of a K^+ channel pore through mutant cycles with a peptide inhibitor. *Science* **268,** 307–310.

Hill, R. J., Grant, A. M., Volberg, W., Rapp, L., Faltynek, C., Miller, D., Pagani, K., Baizman, E., Wang, S., Guiles, J. W., and Krafte, D. S. (1995). WIN 17317-3: Novel nonpeptide antagonist of voltage-activated K^+ channels in human T lymphocytes. *Mol. Pharmacol.* **48,** 98–104.

Hollecker, M., Marshall, D. L., and Harvey, A. L. (1993). Structural features important for the biological activity of the potassium channel blocking dendrotoxins. *Br. J. Pharmacol.* **110,** 790–794.

Hugues, M., Duval, D., Kitabi, P., Lazdunski, M., and Vincent, J. P. (1982a). Preparation of a pure monoiodo derivative of the bee venom neurotoxin apamin and its binding properties to rat brain synaptosomes. *J. Biol. Chem.* **257,** 2762–2769.

Hugues, M., Duval, D., Schmid, H., Kitabgi, P., and Lazdunski, M. (1982b). Specific binding and pharmacological interactions of apamin, the neurotoxin from bee venom, with guinea-pig colon. *Life Sci.* **31,** 437–443.

Hugues, M., Schmid, H., Romey, G., Duval, D., Frelin, C., and Lazdunski, M. (1982c). Apamin as a selective blocker of the calcium dependent potassium channel in neuroblastoma cells: Voltage clamp and biochemical characterization of the toxin receptor. *Proc. Natl. Acad. Sci. U.S.A.* **79,** 1308–1312.

Hugues, M., Schmid, H., Romey, G., Duval, D., Frelin, C., and Lazdunski, M. (1982d). The Ca^{2+}-dependent slow K^+ conductance in cultured rat muscle cells: Characterization with apamin. *EMBO J.* **1,** 1039–1042.

Hurst, R. S., Busch, A. E., Kavanaugh, M. P., Osborne, P. B., North, R. A., and Adelman, J. P. (1991). Identification of amino acid residues involved in dendrotoxin block of rat voltage-dependent potassium channels. *Mol. Pharmacol.* **40,** 572–576.

Inagaki, N., Gonoi, T., IV, J. P. C., Namba, N., Inazawa, J., Gonzalez, G., Aguilar-Bryan, L., Seino, S., and Bryan, J. (1995). Reconstitution of I_{KATP}: An inward rectifier subunit plus the sulfonylurea receptor. *Science* **270,** 1166–1170.

Johnson, B. A., and Sugg, E. E. (1992). Determination of the three-dimensional structure of iberiotoxin in solution by ^1H nuclear magnetic resonance spectroscopy. *Biochemistry* **31,** 8151–8159.

Johnson, B. A., Stevens, S. P., and Williamson, J. M. (1994). Determination of the three-dimensional structure of margatoxin by ^1H, ^{13}C, ^{15}N triple-resonance nuclear magnetic resonance spectroscopy. *Biochemistry* **33,** 15061–15070.

Kaczorowski, G. J., Knaus, H.-G., Leonard, R. J., McManus, O. B., and Garcia, M. L. (1996). High conductance calcium-activated potassium channels; structure, pharmacology and function. *J. Biomembr. Bioenerg.* **28,** 253–265.

Kau, S. T., Zografos, P., Do, M. L., Halterman, T. J., McConville, M. W., Yochim, C. L., Trivedi, S., Howe, B. B., and Li, J. H. Y. (1994). Characterization of ATP-sensitive potassium channel-blocking activity of Zeneca ZM181,037, a eukalemic diuretic. *Pharmacology* **49**, 238–248.

Kavanaugh, M. P., Hurst, R. S., Yakel, J., Varnum, M. D., Adelman, J. P., and North, R. A. (1992). Multiple subunits of a voltage-dependent potassium channel contribute to the binding site for tetraethylammonium. *Neuron* **8**, 493–497.

Kiehn, J., Wible, B., Ficker, E., Taglialatela, M., and Brown, A. M. (1995). Cloned human inward rectifier K^+ channel as a target for class III methanesulfonanilides. *Circ. Res.* **77**, 1151–1155.

Kirsch, G. E., Taglialatela, M., and Brown, A. M. (1991). Internal and external TEA block in single cloned K^+ channels. *Am. J. Physiol.* **261**, C583–C590.

Kirsch, G. E., Drewe, J. A., Hartmann, H. A., Taglialatela, M., DeBiasi, M., Brown, A. M., and Joho, R. H. (1992a). Differences between the deep pores of K^+ channels determined by an interacting pair of nonpolar amino acids. *Neuron* **8**, 499–505.

Kirsch, G. E., Drewe, J. A., Taglialatela, M., Joho, R. H., DeBiasi, M., Hartman, H. A., and Brown, A. M. (1992b). A single nonpolar residue in the deep pore of related K^+ channels acts as $K^+:Rb^+$ conductance switch. *Biophys. J.* **62**, 136–143.

Kirsch, G. E., Shieh, C. C., Drewe, J. A., Vener, D. F., and Brown, A. M. (1993). Segmental exchanges define 4-aminopyridine binding and the inner mouth of K^+ pores. *Neuron* **11**, 1–20.

Knaus, H.-G., Garcia-Calvo, M., Kaczorowski, G. J. and Garcia, M. L. (1994a). Subunit composition of the high conductance calcium-activated potassium channel from smooth muscle, a representative of the *mSlo* and *slowpoke* family of potassium channels. *J. Biol. Chem.* **269**, 3921–3924.

Knaus, H.-G., Folander, K., Garcia-Calvo, M., Garcia, M. L., Kaczorowski, G. J., Smith, M., and Swanson, R. (1994b). Primary sequence and immunological characterization of the β-subunit of the high-conductance Ca^{2+}-activated K^+ channel from smooth muscle. *J. Biol. Chem.* **269**, 17274–17278.

Knaus, H.-G., Eberhart, A., Kaczorowski, G. J., and Garcia, M. L. (1994c). Covalent attachment of charybdotoxin to the β-subunit of the high-conductance Ca^{2+}-activated K^+ channel. *J. Biol. Chem.* **269**, 23336–23341.

Knaus, H.-G., McManus, O. B., Lee, S. H., Schmalhofer, W. A., Garcia-Calvo, M., Helms, L. M. H., Sanchez, M., Giangiacomo, K., Reuben, J. P., Smith, A. B., III, Kaczorowski, G. J., and Garcia, M. L. (1994d). Tremorgenic indole alkaloids potently inhibit smooth muscle high-conductance Ca^{2+}-activated K^+ channels. *Biochemistry* **33**, 5819–5828.

Knaus, H.-G., Koch, R. O. A., Eberhart, A., Kaczorowski, G. J., Garcia, M. L. and Slaughter, R. S. (1995). $[^{125}I]$Margatoxin, an extraordinarily high affinity ligand for voltage-gated potassium channels in mammalian brain. *Biochemistry* **34**, 13627–13634.

Knaus, H.-G., Schwarzer, C., Koch, R. O. A., Eberhart, A., Kaczorowski, G. J., Glossmann, H., Wunder, F., Pongs, O., Garcia, M. L., and Sperk, G. (1996). Distribution of high-conductance Ca^{2+}-activated K^+ channels in rat brain: Targeting to axons and nerve terminals. *J. Neurosci.* **16**, 955–963.

Köhler, M., Hirschberg, B., Bond, C. T., Kinzie, J. M., Marrion, N. V., Maylie, J. and Adelman, J. P. (1996). Small-conductance, calcium-activated potassium channels from mammalian brain. *Science* **273**, 1709–1714.

Koo, G. C., Blake, J. T., Talento, A., Nguyen, M., Lin, S., Sirotina, A., Shah, K., Mulvany, K., Hora, D., Jr., Cunningham, P., Slaughter, R., Bugianesi, R., Felix, J., Garcia, M., Williamson, J., Kaczorowski, G., Sigal, N., Springer, M., and Feeney, W. (1996). Margatoxin, a blocker of Kv1.3 channels, inhibits immune responses in vivo. *Fed. Proc., Fed. Am. Soc. Exp. Biol.* **10**, A 1447.

Krezel, A. M., Kasibhatla, C., Hidalgo, P., MacKinnon, R., and Wagner, G. (1995). Solution structure of the potassium channel inhibitor agitoxin 2: Caliper for probing channel geometry. *Protein Sci.* **4**, 1478–1489.

Lambert, P., Kuroda, H., Chino, N., Watanabe, T. X., Kimura, T., and Sakakibara, S. (1990). Solution synthesis of charybdotoxin (ChTX), a K^+ channel blocker. *Biochem. Biophys. Res. Commun.* **170,** 684–690.

Laraba-Djebari, F., Legros, C., Crest, M., Ceard, B., Romi, R., Mansuelle, P., Jacquet, G., von Rietschoten, J., Gola, M., Rochat, H., Bougis, P. E., and Martin-Eauclaire, M.-F. (1994). The kaliotoxin family enlarged. *J. Biol. Chem.* **269,** 32835–32843.

Latorre, R., Oberhauser, A., Labarca, P., and Alvarez, O. (1989). Varieties of calcium-activated potassium channels. *Annu. Rev. Physiol.* **51,** 385–399.

Leonard, R. J., Garcia, M. L., Slaughter, R. S., and Reuben, J. P. (1992). Selective blockers of voltage-gated K^+ channels depolarize human T lymphocytes: Mechanism of the antiproliferative effect of charybdotoxin. *Proc. Natl. Acad. Sci. U.S.A.* **89,** 10094–10098.

Leveque, C., Marqueze, B., Couraud, F., and Seagar, M. (1990). Polypeptide components of the apamin receptor associated with a calcium activated potassium channel. *FEBS Lett.* **275,** 185–189.

Lin, C. S., Boltz, R. C., Blake, J. T., Nguyen, M., Talento, A., Fischer, P. A., Springer, M. S., Sigal, N. H., Slaughter, R. S., Garcia, M. L., Kaczorowski, G. J., and Koo, G. C. (1993). Voltage-gated potassium channels regulate calcium-dependent pathways involved in human T lymphocyte activation. *J. Exp. Med.* **177,** 637–645.

Lu, Z., Lewis, J. H., and MacKinnon, R. (1996). Probing the pore of an inward-rectifier K^+ channel with a scorpion toxin. *Biophys. J.* **70,** 145a.

Lucchesi, K., Ravindran, A., Young, H., and Moczydlowski, E. (1989). Analysis of the blocking activity of charybdotoxin homologs and iodinated derivatives against Ca^{2+}-activated K^+ channels. *J. Membr. Biol.* **109,** 269–281.

MacKinnon, R., and Miller, C. (1988). Mechanism of charybdotoxin block of the high-conductance, Ca^{2+}-activated K^+ channel. *J. Gen. Physiol.* **91,** 335–349.

MacKinnon, R., and Miller, C. (1989). Functional modification of a Ca^{2+}-activated K^+ channel by trimethyloxonium. *Biochemistry* **28,** 8087–8092.

MacKinnon, R., and Yellen, G. (1990). Mutations affecting TEA blockade and ion permeation in voltage-activated K^+ channels. *Science* **250,** 276–279.

MacKinnon, R., Reinhart, P. H., and White, M. M. (1988). Charybdotoxin block of *Shaker* K^+ channels suggests that different types of K^+ channels share common structural features. *Neuron* **1,** 997–1001.

Majumder, K., Biasi, M. D., Wang, Z., and Wible, B. A. (1995). Molecular cloning and functional expression of a novel potassium channel β-subunit from human atrium. *FEBS Lett.* **361,** 13–16.

Martin, B. M., Ramirez, A. N., Gurrola, G. B., Nobile, M., Prestipino, G., and Possani, L. D. (1994). Novel K^+-channel-blocking toxins from the venom of the scorpion *Centruroides limpidus limpidus* Karsch. *Biochem. J.* **304,** 51–56.

Martins, J. C., Van de Ven, F. J. M., and Borremans, F. A. M. (1995). Determination of the three-dimensional solution structure of scyllatoxin by ^1H nuclear magnetic resonance. *J. Mol. Biol.* **253,** 590–603.

McCormack, K., McCormack, T., Tanouye, M., Rudy, B., and Stühmer, W. (1995). Alternative splicing of the human *Shaker* K^+ channel $\beta 1$ gene and functional expression of the $\beta 2$ gene product. *FEBS Lett.* **370,** 32–36.

McCullough, J. R., Normandin, D. E., Conder, M. L., Sleph, P. G., Dzwonczyk, S., and Grover, G. J. (1991). Specific block of the anti-ischemic actions of cromakalim by sodium 5-hydroxydecanoate. *Circ. Res.* **69,** 949–958.

McManus, O. B. (1991). Calcium-activated potassium channels: Regulation by calcium. *J. Bioenerg. Biomembr.* **23,** 537–560.

McManus, O. B., Harris, G. H., Giangiacomo, K. M., Feigenbaum, P., Reuben, J. P., Addy, M. E., Burka, J. F., Kaczorowski, G. J., and Garcia, M. L. (1993). An activator of calcium-dependent potassium channels isolated from a medicinal herb. *Biochemistry* **32,** 6128–6133.

McManus, O. B., Helms, L. M. H., Pallanck, L., Ganetzky, B., Swanson, R., and Leonard, R. J. (1995). Functional role of the β subunit of high-conductance calcium-activated potassium channels. *Neuron* **14**, 1–20.

Michne, W. F., Miles, J. W., Treasurywala, A. M., Castonguay, L. A., Weigelt, C., Oconnor, B., Volberg, W. A., Grant, A. M., Chadwick, C. C., Kraft, D. S., and Hill, R. J. (1995). Novel inhibitors of potassium ion channels on human T lymphocytes. *J. Med. Chem.* **38**, 1877–1883.

Miller, C., Moczydlowski, E., Latorre, R., and Phillips, M. (1985). Charybdotoxin, a protein inhibitor of single Ca^{2+}-activated K^+ channels from mammalian skeletal muscle. *Nature (London)* **313**, 316–318.

Morales, M. J., Castellino, R. C., Crews, A. L., Rasmusson, R. L., and Strauss, H. C. (1995). A novel β subunit increases rate of inactivation of specific voltage-gated potassium channel α subunits. *J. Biol. Chem.* **270**, 6272–6277.

Muniz, Z. M., Parcej, D. N., and Dolly, J. O. (1992). Characterization of monoclonal antibodies against voltage-dependent K^+ channels raised using α-dendrotoxin acceptors purified from bovine brain. *Biochemistry* **31**, 12297–12303.

Nguyen, A., Kath, J., Hanson, D., Dethlefs, B., Gutman, G., Cahalan, M. D., and Chandy, K. G. (1996). A novel class of potent organic blockers of the T-cell K channel, Kv1.3, that are selective for histidine 404. *Biophys. J.* **70**, A446.

Novick, J., Leonard, R. J., King, V. F., Schmalhofer, W., Kaczorowski, G. J., and Garcia, M. L. (1991). Purification and characterization of two novel peptidyl toxins directed against K^+ channels from venom of new world scorpions. *Biophys. J.* **59**, 78a.

Olesen, S.-P. (1994). Activators of large-conductance Ca^{2+}-dependent K^+ channels. *Exp. Opin. Invest. Drugs* **3**, 1181–1188.

Olesen, S.-P., Munch, E., Moldt, P., and Drejer, J. (1994). Selective activation of Ca^{2+}-dependent K^+ channels by novel benzimidazolone. *Eur. J. Pharmacol.* **251**, 53–59.

Olesen, S.-P., Mathiasen, D., Christophersen, P., Ahring, P. K., and Johansen, T. E. (1996). The substituted diphenylurea NS 1608 activates the α-subunit of the human BK channel (hSlo). *Biophys. J.* **70**, 129a.

Pallanck, L. and Ganetzky, B. (1994). Cloning and characterization of human and mouse homologs of the *Drosophila* calcium-activated potassium channel gene, *slowpoke*. *Hum. Mol. Genet.* **3**, 1239–1243.

Parcej, D. N., and Dolly, J. O. (1989). Dendrotoxin acceptor from bovine synaptic plasma membranes: Binding properties, purification and subunit composition of a putative constituent of certain voltage-activated K^+ channels. *Biochem. J.* **257**, 899–903.

Park, C.-S., and Miller, C. (1992). Interaction of charybdotoxin with permeant ions inside the pore of a K^+ channel. *Neuron* **9**, 307–313.

Park, C.-S., Hausdorff, S. F., and Miller, C. (1991). Design, synthesis, and functional expression of a gene for charybdotoxin, a peptide blocker of K^+ channels. *Proc. Natl. Acad. Sci. U.S.A.* **88**, 2046–2050.

Pease, J. H. B., and Wemmer, D. E. (1988). Solution structure of apamin determined by nuclear magnetic resonance and distance geometry. *Biochemistry* **27**, 8491–8498.

Penner, R., Petersen, M., Pierau, F.-K., and Dreyer, F. (1986). Dendrotoxin: a selective blocker of a non-inactivating potassium current in guinea pig dorsal root ganglion neurons. *Pflüeger's Arch.* **407**, 365–369.

Pennington, M. W., Byrnes, M. E., Zaydenberg, I., Khaytin, I., Chastonay, J. D., Krafte, D. S., Hill, R., Mahnir, V. M., Volberg, W. A., Gorczyca, W., and Kem, W. R. (1995). Chemical synthesis and characterization of ShK toxin: A potent potassium channel inhibitor from a sea anemone. *Int. J. Pept. Protein Res.* **46**, 354–358.

Pennington, M. W., Mahnir, V. M., Krafte, D. S., Zaydenberg, I., Byrnes, M. E., Khaytin, I., Crowley, K., and Kem, W. R. (1996). Identification of three separate binding sites on SHK toxin, a potent inhibitor of voltage-dependent potassium channels in human T-lymphocyte and rat brain. *Biochem. Biophys. Res. Commun.* **219**, 696–701.

Pongs, O. (1995). Regulation of the activity of voltage-gated potassium channels by β subunits. *Semin. Neurosci.* **7**, 137–146.

Possani, L. D., Martin, B. M., and Svendsen, I. B. (1982). The primary structure of Noxiustoxin: A K^+ channel blocking peptide, purified from the venom of the scorpion *Centruroides noxius* Hoffmann. *Carlsberg Res. Commun.* **47**, 285–289.

Quast, U., and Cook, N. S. (1989). In vitro and in vivo comparison of two K^+ channel openers diazoxide and cromakalim and their inhibition by glibenclamide. *J. Pharmacol. Exp. Ther.* **250**, 261–271.

Rehm, H., and Lazdunski, M. (1988a). Existence of different populations of the dendrotoxin I binding protein associated with neuronal K^+ channels. *Biochem. Biophys. Res. Commun.* **153**, 231–240.

Rehm, H., and Lazdunski, M. (1988b). Purification and subunit structure of a putative K^+-channel protein identified by its binding properties for dendrotoxin I. *Proc. Natl. Acad. Sci. U.S.A.* **85**, 4919–4923.

Rehm, H., Bidard, J.-N., Schweitz, H., and Lazdunski, M. (1988). The receptor site for bee venom mast cell degranulating peptide. Affinity labeling and evidence for a common target for mast cell degranulating peptide and dendrotoxin I, a snake toxin active on K^+ channels. *Biochemistry* **27**, 1827–1832.

Rehm, H., Pelzer, S., Cochet, C., Chambaz, E., Temple, B. L., Trautwein, W., Pelzer, D., and Lazdunski, M. (1989). Dendrotoxin-binding brain membrane protein displays a K^+ channel activity that is stimulated by both cAMP-dependent and endogenous phosphorylations. *Biochemistry* **28**, 6455–6460.

Rettig, J., Heinemann, S. H., Wunder, F., Lorra, C., Parcej, D. N., Dolly, J. O., and Pongs, O. (1994). Inactivation properties of voltage-gated K^+ channels altered by presence of β-subunit. *Nature (London)* **369**, 289–294.

Rogowski, R. S., Krueger, B. K., Collins, J. H., and Blaustein, M. P. (1994). Tityustoxin Kα blocks voltage-gated noninactivating K^+ channels and unblocks inactivating K^+ channels blocked by α-dendrotoxin in synaptosomes. *Proc. Natl. Acad. Aci. U.S.A.* **91**, 1475–1479.

Romey, G., Hugues, M., Schmid-Antomarchi, H., and Lazdunski, M. (1984). Apamin: a specific toxin to study a class of Ca^{2+}-dependent K^+ channels. *J. Physiol. (Paris)* **79**, 259–264.

Romi, R., Crest, M., Gola, M., Sampieri, F., Jacquet, G., Zerrouk, H., Mansuelle, P., Sorokine, O., Dorsselaer, A. V., Rochat, H., Martin-Eauclaire, M.-F., and Rietschoten, J. V. (1993). Synthesis and characterization of kaliotoxin. *J. Biol. Chem.* **268**, 26302–26309.

Sabatier, J.-M., Zerrouk, H., Darbon, H., Mabrouk, K., Benslimane, A., Rochat, H., Martin-Eauclaire, M.-F., and Rietschoten, J. V. (1993). P05, a new leiurotoxin I-like scorpion toxin: Synthesis and structure-activity relationships of the α-amidated analog, a ligand of Ca^{2+}-activated K^+ channels with increased affinity. *Biochemistry* **32**, 2763–2770.

Sabatier, J.-M., Fremont, V., Mabrouk, K., Crest, M., Darbon, H., Rochat, H., Rietschoten, J. V., and Martin-Eauclaire, M.-F. (1994). Leiurotoxin I, a scorpion toxin specific for Ca^{2+}-activated K^+ channels: Structure-activity analysis using synthetic analogs. *Int. J. Pept. Protein Res.* **43**, 486–495.

Sakura, H., Ämmälä, C., Smith, P. A., Gribble, F. M., and Ashcroft, F. M. (1995). Cloning and functional expression of the cDNA encoding a novel ATP-sensitive potassium channel subunit expressed in pancreatic β-cells, brain, heart and skeletal muscle. *FEBS Lett.* **377**, 338–344.

Sands, S. B., Lewis, R. S., and Cahalan, M. D. (1989). Charybdotoxin blocks, voltage-gated K^+ channels in human and murine T lymphocytes. *J. Gen. Physiol.* **93**, 1061–1074.

Sanguinetti, M. C., Curran, M. E., Spector, P. S., and Keating, M. T. (1996). Spectrum of HERG K^+-channel dysfunction in an inherited cardiac arrhythmia. *Proc. Natl. Acad. Sci. U.S.A.* **93**, 2208–2212.

Sanguinetti, M. C., Curran, M. E., Zou, A., Shen, J., Spector, P. S., Atkinson, D. L. and Keating, M. T. (1996a). Coassembly of K_vLQT1 and minK (IsK) proteins to form cardiac I_{Ks} potassium channel. *Nature* **384**, 80–83.

Sasaki, Y., Ishii, K., Nunoki, K., Yamagishi, T., and Taira, N. (1995). The voltage-dependent K^+ channel (Kv1.5) cloned from rabbit heart and facilitation of inactivation of the delayed rectifier current by the rat β subunit. *FEBS Lett.* **372,** 20–24.

Schmid-Antomarchi, H., Renaud, J. F., Romey, G., Hugues, M., Schmid, A., and Lazdunski, M. (1985). The all-or-none role of innervation in expression of apamin-sensitive calcium-activated potassium channel in mammalian skeletal muscle. *Proc. Natl. Acad. Sci. U.S.A.* **82,** 2188–2191.

Schmid-Antomarchi, H., Hugues, M., and Lazdunski, M. (1986). Properties of the apamin-sensitive Ca^{2+}-activated K^+ channel in PC12 pheochromocytoma cells which hyper-produce the apamin receptor. *J. Biol. Chem.* **261,** 8633–8637.

Schweitz, H., Bidard, J.-N., and Lazdunski, M. (1990). Purification and pharmacological characterization of peptide toxins from the black mamba (*Dendroaspis polylepis*) venom. *Toxicon* **28,** 847–856.

Schweitz, H., Bruhn, T., Guillemare, E., Moinier, D., Lancelin, J.-M., Béress, L., and Lazdunski, M. (1995). Kalicludines and kaliseptine. Two different classes of sea anemone toxins for voltage-sensitive K^+ channels. *J. Biol. Chem.* **270,** 25121–25126.

Scott, V. E. S., Parcej, D. N., Keen, J. N., Keen, J. B. C., and Dolly, J. O. (1990). α-Dendrotoxin acceptor from bovine brain is a K^+ channel protein. *J. Biol. Chem.* **265,** 20094–20097.

Scott, V. E. S., Muniz, Z. M., Sewing, S., Lichtinghagen, R., Parcej, D. N., Pongs, O., and Dolly, J. O. (1994a). Antibodies specific for distinct Kv subunits unveil a heterooligomeric basis for subtypes of α-dendrotoxin-sensitive K^+ channels in bovine brain. *Biochemistry* **33,** 1617–1623.

Scott, V. E. S., Rettig, J., Parcej, D. N., Keen, J. N., Findlay, J. B. C., Pongs, O., and Dolly, J. O. (1994b). Primary structure of a β subunit of α-dendrotoxin-sensitive K^+ channels from bovine brain. *Proc. Natl. Acad. Sci. U.S.A.* **91,** 1637–1641.

Seagar, M. J., Granier, C., and Couraud, F. (1984). Interactions of the neurotoxin apamin with a Ca^{++} activated K^+ channel in primary cultured neurons. *J. Biol. Chem.* **259,** 1491–1495.

Seagar, M. J., Labbe-Jullie, C., Granier, C., Goll, A., Glossmann, H., Rietschoten, J. V., and Couraud, F. (1986). Molecular structure of rat brain apamin receptor: differential photoaffinity labelling of putative K^+ channel subunits and target size analysis. *Biochemistry* **25,** 4051–4057.

Shimony, E., Sun, T., Kolmakova-Partensky, L., and Miller, C. (1994). Engineering a uniquely reactive thiol into a cysteine-rich peptide. *Protein Eng.* **7,** 503–507.

Singh, S. B., Goetz, M. A., Zink, D. L., Dombrowski, A. W., Polishook, J. D., Garcia, M. L., Schmalhofer, W., McManus, O. B., and Kaczorowski, G. J. (1994). MaxiKdiol: A novel dihydroxyisoprimane as an agonist of maxi-K channels. *J. Chem. Soc., Perkin Trans.* **1,** pp. 3349–3352.

Sitges, M., Possani, L. D., and Bayón, A. (1986). Noxiustoxin, a short-chain toxin from the Mexican scorpion *Centruroides noxius,* induces transmitter release by blocking K^+ permeability. *J. Neurosci.* **6,** 1570–1574.

Skarzynski, T. (1992). Crystal structure of α-dendrotoxin from the green mamba venom and its comparison with the structure of bovine pancreatic trypsin inhibitor. *J. Mol. Biol.* **224,** 671–683.

Slaughter, R. S., Shevell, J. L., Felix, J. P., Lin, C. S., Sigal, N. H., and Kaczorowski, G. J. (1991). Inhibition by toxins of charybdotoxin binding to the voltage-gated potassium channel of lymphocytes: Correlation with block of activation of human peripheral T-lymphocytes. *Biophys. J.* **59,** 213a.

Smith, C., Phillips, M., and Miller, C. (1986). Charybdotoxin, a specific inhibitor of the high conductance Ca^{2+}-activated K^+ channel. *J. Biol. Chem.* **261,** 14607–14613.

Smith, L. A., Olson, M. A., Lafaye, P. J., and Dolly, J. O. (1995). Cloning and expression of mamba toxins. *Toxicon* **33,** 459–474.

Sorensen, R. G., and Blaustein, M. P. (1989). Rat brain dendrotoxin receptors associated with voltage-gated potassium channels: Dendrotoxin binding and receptor solubilization. *Mol. Pharmacol.* **36,** 689–698.

Spector, P. S., Curran, M. E., Keating, M. T., and Sanguinetti, M. C. (1996). Class III antiarrhythmic drugs block HERG, a human cardiac delayed rectifier K^+ channel. *Circ. Res.* **78,** 499–503.

Stampe, P., Kolmakova-Partensky, L., and Miller, C. (1994). Intimations of K^+ channel structure from a complete functional map of the molecular surface of charybdotoxin. *Biochemistry* **33,** 443–450.

Stansfeld, C. E., Marsh, S. J., Halliwell, J. V., and Brown, D. A. (1986). 4-Aminopyridine and dendrotoxin induce repetitive firing in rat visceral sensory neurones by blocking a slowly inactivating outward current. *Neurosci. Lett.* **64,** 299–304.

Stephens, G. J., Cockett, M. I., Nawoschik, S. P., Schecter, L. E., and Owen, D. G. (1996). The modulation of the rate of inactivation of the mKv1.1 K^+ channel by the β subunit, Kvβ1 and lack of effect of a Kvβ1 N-terminal peptide. *FEBS Lett.* **378,** 250–252.

Stocker, M., and Miller, C. (1994). Electrostatic distance geometry in a K^+ channel vestibule. *Proc. Natl. Acad. Sci. U.S.A.* **91,** 9509–9513.

Sugg, E. E., Garcia, M. L., Reuben, J. P., Patchett, A. A., and Kaczorowski, G. J. (1990). Synthesis and structural characterization of charybdotoxin, a potent peptidyl inhibitor of the high conductance Ca^{2+}-activated K^+ channel. *J. Biol. Chem.* **265,** 18745–18748.

Sun, T., Naini, A. A., and Miller, C. (1994). High-level expression and functional reconstitution of *Shaker* K^+ channels. *Biochemistry* **33,** 9992–9999.

Swanson, R., Marshall, J., Smith, J. S., Williams, J. B., Boyle, M. B., Folander, K., Luneau, C. J., Antanavage, J., Oliva, C., Buhrow, S. A., Bennett, C., Stein, R. B., and Kaczmarek, L. K. (1990). Cloning and expression of cDNA and genomic clones encoding three delayed rectifier potassium channels in rat brian. *Neuron* **4,** 929–939.

Swartz, K. J., and MacKinnon, R. (1995). An inhibitor of the Kv2.1 potassium channel isolated from the venom of a Chilean tarantula. *Neuron* **15,** 941–949.

Taglialatela, M., VanDongen, A. M. J., Drewe, J. A., Joho, R. H., Brown, A. M., and Kirsch, G. E. (1991). Patterns of internal and external tetraethylammonium block in four homologous K^+ channels. *Mol. Pharmacol.* **40,** 299–307.

Tseng-Crank, J., Foster, C. D., Krause, J. D., Mertz, R., Godinot, N., DiChiara, T. J., and Reinhart, P. H. (1994). Cloning, expression, and distribution of functionally distinct Ca^{2+}-activated K^+ channel isoforms from human brain. *Neuron* **13,** 1315–1330.

Tytgat, J., Debont, T., Carmeliet, E., and Daenens, P. (1995). The α-dendrotoxin footprint on a mammalian potassium channel. *J. Biol. Chem.* **270,** 24776–24781.

Uebele, V. N., England, S. K., Chaudhary, A., Tamkun, M. M., and Snyders, D. J. (1996). Functional differences in Kv1.5 currents expressed in mammalian cell lines are due to the presence of endogenous Kvβ2.1 subunits. *J. Biol. Chem.* **271,** 2406–2412.

Vazquez, J., Feigenbaum, P., Katz, G., King, V. F., Reuben, J. P., Roy-Contancin, L., Slaughter, R. S., Kaczorowski, G. J., and Garcia, M. L. (1989). Characterization of high affinity binding sites for charybdotoxin in sarcolemmal membranes from bovine aortic smooth muscle: Evidence for a direct association with the high conductance calcium-activated potassium channel. *J. Biol. Chem.* **264,** 20902–20909.

Vazquez, J., Feigenbaum, P., King, V. F., Kaczorowski, G. J., and Garcia, M. L. (1990). Characterization of high affinity binding sites for charybdotoxin in synaptic plasma membranes from rat brain: Evidence for a direct association with an inactivating, voltage-dependent, potassium channel. *J. Biol. Chem.* **256,** 15564–15571.

Wallner, M., Meera, P., Ottolia, M., Kaczorowski, G. J., Latorre, R., Garcia, M. L., Stefani, E., and Toro, L. (1995). Characterization of and modulation by a β-subunit of a human maxi K_{Ca} channel cloned from myometrium. *Recept. Channels* **3,** 185–199.

Ward, J. P. T., Taylor, S. G., and Collier, M. L. (1992). The novel benzopyranol potassium channel activator BRL55834 activates two potassium channels in bovine airway smooth muscle. *Br. J. Pharmacol.* **107,** 49P.

Wei, A., Solaro, C., Lingle, C., and Salkoff, L. (1994). Calcum sensitivity of BK-type KCa channels determined by a separable domain. *Neuron* **13,** 671–681.

Werkman, T. R., Kawamura, T., Yokoyama, S., Higashida, H., and Rogawski, M. A. (1992). Charybdotoxin, dendrotoxin and mast cell degranulating peptide block the voltage-activated K^+ current of fibroblast cells stably transfected with NGK1 ($K_v1.2$) K^+ channel complementary DNA. *Neuroscience* **4**, 935–946.

Yellen, G., Jurman, M. E., Abramson, T., and MacKinnon, R. (1991). Mutations affecting internal TEA blockade identify the probable pore-forming region of a K^+ channel. *Science* **251**, 939–942.

Zünkler, B. J., Lenzen, S., Mauer, K., Panten, U., and Trube, G. (1988). Concentration-dependent effects of tolbutamide, meglitinide, glipizide, glibenclamide and diazoxide on ATP-regulated K^+ currents in pancreatic β-cells. *Naunyn-Schmiedeberg's Arch. Pharmacol.* **337**, 225–230.

Index

Contents of Previous Volumes

Volume 29A

Volume 29B

Volume 30

Volume 31

Volume 32

Volume 33

Volume 34

Volume 35

Volume 36

Volume 37

Volume 38